EMERGENCY MEDICINE SECRETS

Third Edition

EMERGENCY MEDICINE SECRETS

Third Edition

Vincent J. Markovchick, MD, FACEP
Professor of Surgery
Division of Emergency Medicine, Department of Surgery
University of Colorado Health Sciences Center
Director, Emergency Medical Services
Associate Program Director, Emergency Medicine Residency
Denver Health Medical Center
Denver, Colorado

Peter T. Pons, MD, FACEP
Attending Emergency Physician
Denver Health Medical Center
Professor, Division of Emergency Medicine
Department of Surgery
University of Colorado Health Sciences Center
Denver, Colorado

HANLEY & BELFUS, INC. / Philadelphia

Publisher: HANLEY & BELFUS, INC.
                   Medical Publishers
                   210 South 13th Street
                   Philadelphia, PA 19107
                   (215) 546-7293; 800-962-1892
                   FAX (215) 790-9330
                   Web site: http://www.hanleyandbelfus.com

Note to the reader: Although the information in this book has been carefully reviewed for correctness of dosage and indications, neither the authors nor the editors nor the publisher can accept any legal responsibility for any errors or omissions that may be made. Neither the publisher nor the editors make any warranty, expressed or implied, with respect to the material contained herein. Before prescribing any drug, the reader must review the manufacturer's current product information (package inserts) for accepted indications, absolute dosage recommendations, and other information pertinent to the safe and effective use of the product described.

Library of Congress Control Number: 2002112407

EMERGENCY MEDICINE SECRETS, 3rd edition   ISBN 1-56053-503-2

Last digit is the print number: 9   8   7   6   5   4   3   2   1

CONTENTS

CONTRIBUTORS

Jean T. Abbott, M.D., FACEP
Associate Professor, Division of Emergency Medicine, Department of Surgery, University of Colorado Health Sciences Center; Attending Physician, University of Colorado Hospital, Denver, Colorado

Paul-André C. Abboud, M.D.
Department of Emergency Medicine, Denver Health Medical Center, Denver, Colorado

Stephen L. Adams, M.D., FACP, FACEP
Professor of Medicine; Chief, Division of Sports Medicine; Chief Emeritus, Division of Emergency Medicine, Department of Medicine, Northwestern University Medical School; Attending Physician, Northwestern Memorial Hospital, Chicago, Illinois

Stephen C. Altmin, M.D., M.P.H.
Department of Emergency Medicine, Denver Health Medical Center, Denver, Colorado

Mark E. Anderson, M.D.
Assistant Professor, Department of Community Health Services–Pediatrics, University of Colorado Health Sciences Center; Kid's Care Clinic, Denver Health Medical Center, Denver, Colorado

Jonathan D. Apfelbaum, M.D.
Emergency Care and Rescue Program, Weber State University, Salt Lake City, Utah

Katherine M. Bakes, M.D.
Assistant Professor, Department of Emergency Medicine, Denver Health Medical Center, Denver, Colorado

Stacey Bangh, Pharm.D.
Clinical Coordinator, Hennepin Regional Poison Center, Minneapolis, Minnesota

Roger M. Barkin, M.D., M.P.H., FAAP, FACEP
Professor of Surgery, Division of Emergency Medicine, Department of Surgery, University of Colorado Health Sciences Center; Vice President for Pediatric and Newborn Programs, HealthONE, Denver, Colorado

F. Keith Battan, M.D., FAAP
Associate Professor, Department of Pediatrics, University of Colorado Health Sciences Center; Associate Director, Emergency and Trauma Services, Children's Hospital, Denver, Colorado

Vikhyat Bebarta, M.D.
Rocky Mountain Poison and Drug Center, Denver Health Medical Center, Denver, Colorado

Jeff S. Beckman, M.D.
Department of Emergency Medicine, Denver Health Medical Center, Denver, Colorado

Holly U. Biffl, M.D.
Arapahoe Park Pediatrics, Littleton, Colorado

Walter L. Biffl, M.D.
Associate Professor of Surgery, Brown Medical School; Chief, Division of Trauma and Surgical Critical Care, Rhode Island Hospital, Providence, Rhode Island

Diane Birnbaumer, M.D.
Professor of Medicine, University of California, Los Angeles, David Geffen School of Medicine, Westwood, California; Associate Program Director, Department of Emergency Medicine, Harbor-UCLA Medical Center, Torrance, California

Joan Bothner, M.D.
Associate Professor, Department of Pediatrics, University of Colorado Health Sciences Center; Director, Emergency and Ambulatory Services, Children's Hospital, Denver, Colorado

Patricia A. Braun, M.D.
Assistant Professor, Department of Pediatrics, University of Colorado Health Sciences Center; Denver Health Medical Center, Denver, Colorado

Russ Braun, M.D., M.P.H., M.B.A., FACEP
Assistant Clinical Professor, Department of Emergency Medicine, University of California, San Francisco, School of Medicine, San Francisco; Medical Director, Department of Emergency Medicine, Highland General Hospital, Oakland, California

Kerry B. Broderick, M.D.
Assistant Professor, Division of Emergency Medicine, Department of Surgery, University of Colorado Health Sciences Center; Denver Health Medical Center, Denver, Colorado

Alexander Brough, M.D.
Department of Emergency Medicine, University of Massachusetts Medical School; University of Massachusetts Medical Center, Worcester, Massachusetts

James E. Brown, M.D.
Assistant Professor and Program Director, Department of Emergency Medicine, Wright State University School of Medicine; Good Samaritan Hospital, Dayton, Ohio

Michael W. Brunko, M.D., FACEP
Medical Director, Flight for Life, Emergency Medical Services, St. Anthony Hospital, Denver, Colorado

Joanna M. Burch, M.D.
Instructor, Department of Dermatology, University of Colorado Health Sciences Center; University of Colorado Hospital, Denver, Colorado

Gregory W. Burcham, M.D.
Attending Physician, Department of Emergency Medicine, Swedish Medical Center, Englewood, Colorado

Charles B. Cairns, M.D.
Associate Professor, Division of Emergency Medicine, Department of Surgery, University of Colorado Health Sciences Center; Attending Staff, University of Colorado Hospital, Denver, Colorado

Stephen V. Cantrill, M.D., FACEP
Assistant Professor, Division of Emergency Medicine, Department of Surgery, University of Colorado Health Sciences Center; Associate Director, Department of Emergency Medicine, Denver Health Medical Center, Denver, Colorado

Justin C. Chang, M.D.
Department of Emergency Medicine, Denver Health Medical Center, Denver, Colorado

Robert G. Chin, M.D.
Assistant Professor, Department of Emergency Medicine, Albert Einstein College of Medicine of Yeshiva University; Montefiore Hospital, Bronx, New York

Christopher B. Colwell, M.D., FACEP
Assistant Professor, Division of Emergency Medicine, Department of Surgery, University of Colorado Health Sciences Center; Denver Health Medical Center, Denver, Colorado

Elizabeth A. Criss, R.N., C.E.N., M.A.Ed.
Senior Research Associate, Department of Emergency Medicine, University of Arizona College of Medicine; Clinical Educator, Emergency Services, University Medical Center, Tucson, Arizona

Patrick G. Croskerry, M.D., Ph.D.
Associate Professor, Department of Emergency Medicine, Dalhousie University Faculty of Medicine, Halifax, Nova Scotia; Dartmouth General Hospital, Dartmouth, Nova Scotia, Canada

Catherine B. Custalow, M.D., Ph.D.
Department of Emergency Medicine, University of Virginia Health System, Charlottesville, Virginia

Daniel F. Danzl, M.D.
Professor and Chair, Department of Emergency Medicine, University of Louisville School of Medicine, Louisville, Kentucky

Wyatt W. Decker, M.D.
Chair and Program Director, Department of Emergency Medicine, Mayo Medical School; Mayo Clinic, Rochester, Minnesota

Christopher Dewitt, M.D.
Medical Toxicology Fellow, Rocky Mountain Poison and Drug Center, Denver, Colorado

Steven E. Doerr, M.D.
Attending Physician, Emergency Department, Lutheran Medical Center, Wheat Ridge, Colorado

Thomas R. Drake, M.D.
Medical Director, Emergency Department, Porter Hospital, Denver, Colorado

Michael P. Earnest, M.D.
Professor, Department of Neurology, University of Colorado Health Sciences Center; Medical Director of Performance Improvement, Denver Health Medical Center, Denver, Colorado

Joanne M. Edney, M.D., FACEP
Associate Medical Director, Department of Emergency Services, Lutheran Medical Center, Wheat Ridge, Colorado

Javier I. Escobar II, M.D.
Clinical Faculty, Department of Emergency Medicine, University of Florida College of Medicine; Jacksonville, Florida; Assistant Medical Director, Department of Emergency Medicine, Tallahassee Memorial Hospital, Tallahassee, Florida

Bruce Evans, M.D.
Senior Instructor, Department of Surgery, University of Colorado Health Sciences Center; Attending Physician, Department of Emergency Medicine, University of Colorado Hospital, Denver, Colorado

Neide Fehrenbacher, M.D.
Department of Emergency Medicine, Denver Health Medical Center, Denver, Colorado

Kim M. Feldhaus, M.D., FACEP
Associate Professor, Department of Surgery, University of Colorado Health Sciences Center; Attending Emergency Physician, Department of Emergency Medicine, Denver Health Medical Center, Denver, Colorado

Toby J. Feldman, D.D.S.
Department of Oral and Maxillofacial Surgery, Denver Health Medical Center, Denver, Colorado

Christopher M. B. Fernandes, M.D.
Associate Professor, Department of Medicine, McMaster University Faculty of Health Sciences; Chief, Department of Emergency Medicine, Hamilton Health Sciences Center, Hamilton, Ontario, Canada

Reginald J. Franciose, M.D.
Assistant Professor, Department of Surgery, University of Colorado Health Sciences Center; Attending, Trauma Surgery, Denver Health Medical Center, Denver, Colorado; Trauma Director, Vail Valley Medical Center, Vail, Colorado

Gayle Galleta, M.D.
Clinical Instructor, Department of Emergency Medicine, University of Massachusetts Medical School; University of Massachusetts Medical Center, Worcester, Massachusetts

Shamai A. Grossman, M.D., M.S.
Instructor of Medicine, Department of Emergency Medicine, Harvard Medical School; Director, The Cardiac Emergency Center, Beth Israel Deaconess Medical Center, Boston, Massachusetts

Kent N. Hall, M.D.
Assistant Professor, Department of Emergency Medicine, University of Cincinnati Medical Center, Cincinnati, Ohio

Glenn C. Hamilton, M.D., M.S.M.
Professor and Chair, Department of Emergency Medicine, Wright State University School of Medicine, Dayton, Ohio

Linda L. Hanson, M.D.
Attending Physician, Department of Emergency Medicine, St. Joseph Hospital, Denver, Colorado

Christina E. Hantsch, M.D., FACEP
Assistant Professor, Division of Emergency Medicine, Loyola University at Chicago Stritch School of Medicine; Medical Director, Illinois Poison Center, Chicago, Illinois; Attending Physician, Loyola University Medical Center, Maywood, Illinois

Alden H. Harken, M.D.
Professor, Department of Surgery, University of Colorado Health Sciences Center; University of Colorado Hospital; Rose Medical Center; Veterans Affairs Hospital; Denver Health Medical Center; The Children's Hospital, Denver, Colorado

Luis H. Haro, M.D.
Instructor of Emergency Medicine, Mayo Medical School; Senior Associate Consultant, Department of Emergency Medicine, Mayo Clinic, Rochester, Minnesota

Ann L. Harwood-Nuss, M.D., FACEP
Professor and Assistant Dean, Department of Emergency Medicine, University of Florida Health Science Center, Jacksonville, Florida

Edward P. Havranek, M.D.
Associate Professor, Division of Cardiology, Department of Medicine, University of Colorado Health Sciences Center; Staff Cardiologist, Denver Health Medical Center, Denver, Colorado

Kennon Heard, M.D.
Assistant Professor, Division of Emergency Medicine, Department of Surgery, University of Colorado Health Sciences Center, Denver, Colorado

Philip L. Henneman, M.D., FACEP
Professor and Chair, Department of Emergency Medicine, Tufts University School of Medicine, Boston, Massachusetts; Department of Emergency Medicine, Baystate Medical Center, Springfield, Massachusetts

Gwendolyn J. Hewitt, M.D.
Department of Emergency Medicine, Denver Health Medical Center, Denver, Colorado

Jeffrey S. Hill, M.D., FACEP
Director of Emergency Services, Suburban Emergency Associates, St. Francis Regional Medical Center, Shakopee, Minnesota

Robert S. Hockberger, M.D.
Professor of Medicine, University of California, Los Angeles, David Geffen School of Medicine, Westwood, California; Harbor-UCLA Medical Center, Torrance, California

Benjamin Honigman, M.D., FACEP
Professor, Division of Emergency Medicine, Department of Surgery, University of Colorado Health Sciences Center; University of Colorado Hospital, Denver, Colorado

Debra Houry, M.D., M.P.H.
Assistant Professor, Department of Emergency Medicine; Associate Director, Center for Injury Control, Emory University School of Medicine, Atlanta, Georgia

John M. Howell, M.D., FACEP
Clinical Professor, Department of Emergency Medicine, Georgetown University School of Medicine, Washington, DC; Director of Academic Affairs, Inova Fairfax Hospital, Falls Church, Virginia

Richard L. Hughes, M.D.
Chief, Department of Neurology, Denver Health Medical Center, Denver, Colorado

Katherine M. Hurlbut, M.D.
Clinical Assistant Professor, Department of Surgery, University of Colorado Health Sciences Center; Attending Physician, Denver Health Medical Center, Denver, Colorado

Grant D. Innes, M.D., FRCPC
Associate Professor, Department of Emergency Medicine, University of British Columbia Faculty of Medicine; St. Paul's Hospital, Vancouver, British Columbia, Canada

Eric D. Isaacs, M.D., FACEP, FAAEM
Associate Clinical Professor, Department of Emergency Medicine, University of California, San Francisco, School of Medicine; San Francisco General Hospital, San Francisco, California

Kenneth C. Jackimczyk, M.D.
Associate Chairman, Department of Emergency Medicine, Maricopa Medical Center, Phoenix, Arizona

Timothy G. Janz, M.D.
Associate Professor, Department of Emergency Medicine and Division of Pulmonary and Critical Care, Department of Medicine, Wright State University School of Medicine; Veterans Affairs Medical Center; Greene Memorial Hospital, Dayton, Ohio

Christina Johnson, M.D.
Attending Physician, Department of Emergency Medicine, Exempla Lutheran Medical Center, Wheat Ridge, Colorado

Richard O. Jones, M.D.
Assistant Professor, Department of Obstetrics and Gynecology, University of Colorado Health Sciences Center; Denver Health Medical Center, Denver, Colorado

Robert C. Jorden, M.D., FACEP
Chairman, Department of Emergency Medicine, Maricopa Medical Center, Phoenix, Arizona

Nicholas J. Jouriles, M.D., FACEP
Associate Professor and Residency Director, Department of Emergency Medicine, Case Western Reserve University School of Medicine; MetroHealth Medical Center; Cleveland Clinic Foundation, Cleveland, Ohio

Juliana Karp, M.D.
Attending Physician, Department of Emergency Medicine, Lakeland Regional Medical Center, Lakeland, Florida

John L. Kendall, M.D., FACEP
Associate Professor, Division of Emergency Medicine, Department of Surgery, University of Colorado Health Sciences Center; Denver Health Medical Center, Denver, Colorado

Eugene E. Kercher, M.D., FACEP
Associate Clinical Professor, Department of Internal Medicine, University of California, Los Angeles, David Geffen School of Medicine, Westwood, California; Chair, Department of Emergency Medicine, Kern Medical Center, Bakersfield, California

Samuel J. Killian, M.D., FACEP
Attending Physician, Department of Emergency Medicine, Swedish Medical Center, Englewood, Colorado

Michael J. Klevens, M.D.
Department of Emergency Medicine, Temple University Hospital, Philadelphia, Pennsylvania

Andrew L. Knaut, M.D., Ph.D.
Assistant Professor, Division of Emergency Medicine, Department of Surgery, University of Colorado Health Sciences Center; Attending Physician, Department of Emergency Medicine, Denver Health Medical Center, Denver, Colorado

Carolyn Sprinthall Knaut, J.D.
Attorney, Golden, Colorado

Michael A. Kohn, M.D., M.P.P.
Assistant Professor, Department of Epidemiology and Biostatistics, University of California, San Francisco, School of Medicine, San Francisco, California; Attending Emergency Physician, Mills-Peninsula Medical Center, Burlingame, California

Ken Kulig, M.D., FACEP, FAACT
Associate Clinical Professor, Division of Emergency Medicine, Department of Surgery, University of Colorado Health Sciences Center; Chair, Department of Medicine, Porter Adventist Hospital, Denver, Colorado

Shirley H. Kung, M.D.
Department of Emergency Medicine, Denver Health Medical Center, Denver, Colorado

Ryan P. Lamb, M.D.
Department of Emergency Medicine, Kaiser Permanente Medical Center, Santa Clara, California

Mark I. Langdorf, M.D., MHPE, FACEP, FAAEM
Associate Professor of Clinical Emergency Medicine, Residency Director, and Interim Chair, Department of Emergency Medicine, University of California, Irvine, College of Medicine; Medical Director, Emergency Department, UCI Medical Center, Orange, California

Lela A. Lee, M.D.
Professor, Departments of Dermatology and Medicine, University of Colorado Health Sciences Center; Chief of Dermatology, Denver Health Medical Center, Denver, Colorado

Louis J. Ling, M.D., FACEP, FACMT
Professor, Department of Emergency Medicine, University of Minnesota Medical School; Medical Director, Hennepin Regional Poison Center; Associate Medical Director, Hennepin County Medical Center, Minneapolis, Minnesota

Gayle E. Long, M.D.
Assistant Professor, Division of Emergency Medicine, Department of Surgery, University of Colorado Health Sciences Center; University of Colorado Hospital, Denver, Colorado

K. Alexander Malone, M.D.
Department of Emergency Medicine, University of Arizona College of Medicine; University Medical Center, Tucson, Arizona

Catherine A. Marco, M.D.
Associate Professor, Department of Surgery, Medical College of Ohio; St. Vincent Mercy Medical Center, Toledo, Ohio

Vincent J. Markovchick, M.D., FACEP
Professor of Surgery, Division of Emergency Medicine, Department of Surgery, University of Colorado Health Sciences Center; Director, Emergency Medical Services; Associate Program Director, Emergency Medicine Residency, Denver Health Medical Center, Denver, Colorado

Ann B. Marshall, M.D.
Assistant Clinical Professor, Department of Emergency Medicine, University of California, San Francisco, School of Medicine; Attending Physician, San Francisco General Hospital, San Francisco, California

John P. Marshall, M.D.
Department of Emergency Medicine, Denver Health Medical Center, Denver, Colorado

John A. Marx, M.D.
Clinical Professor of Emergency Medicine, University of North Carolina at Chapel Hill School of Medicine, Chapel Hill; Chair and Chief, Department of Emergency Medicine, Carolinas Medical Center, Charlotte, North Carolina

James Mathews, M.D.
Professor, Department of Medicine, Northwestern University Medical School; Northwestern Memorial Hospital, Chicago, Illinois

Tracy R. McCubbin, M.D.
Department of Emergency Medicine, Exempla St. Joseph Hospital, Denver, Colorado

John McGoldrick, M.D.
Emergency Department, Central Maine Medical Center, Lewiston, Maine

Richard L. McLain, D.D.S.
Department of Oral and Maxillofacial Surgery, Denver Health Medical Center, Denver, Colorado

Robert M. McNamara, M.D., FAAEM
Professor, Department of Emergency Medicine, Temple University School of Medicine; Temple University Hospital, Philadelphia, Pennsylvania

Harvey W. Meislin, M.D., FACEP
Professor and Chief, Division of Emergency Medicine, Department of Surgery, University of Arizona College of Medicine, Tucson, Arizona

Cheryl Melick-Casanova, M.D.
Attending Physician, Department of Emergency Medicine, Swedish Medical Center, Englewood, Colorado

James R. Miner, M.D.
Assistant Professor, Department of Emergency Medicine, University of Minnesota Medical School; Department of Emergency Medicine, Hennepin County Medical Center, Minneapolis, Minnesota

Scott Miner, M.D.
Department of Emergency Medicine, Denver Health Medical Center, Denver, Colorado

James C. Mitchiner, M.D., M.P.H.
Clinical Assistant Professor, Department of Emergency Medicine, University of Michigan Medical School; Staff Physician, Emergency Department, St. Joseph Mercy Hospital, Ann Arbor, Michigan

Ernest E. Moore, M.D.
Vice Chairman and Professor, Department of Surgery, University of Colorado Health Sciences Center; Chief of Surgery and Trauma, Denver Health Medical Center, Denver, Colorado

John C. Moorhead, M.D., M.S.
Professor, Department of Emergency Medicine, Oregon Health and Science University; Oregon Health and Science University Hospitals, Portland, Oregon

Steven J. Morgan, M.D.
Assistant Professor, Department of Orthopaedics, University of Colorado Health Sciences Center; Denver Health Medical Center, Denver, Colorado

Larry A. Nathanson, M.D.
Instructor, Department of Emergency Medicine, Harvard Medical School; Attending Physician, Department of Emergency Medicine, Beth Israel Deaconess Medical Center, Boston, Massachusetts

Christopher R. H. Newton, M.D.
Department of Emergency Medicine, University of Michigan Medical Center, Ann Arbor, Michigan

Edward Newton, M.D., FACEP
Associate Professor and Chairman, Department of Emergency Medicine, University of Southern California Keck School of Medicine; Los Angeles County–University of Southern California Medical Center, Los Angeles, California

Richard A. Nockowitz, M.D.
Neuropsychiatry Consultants, Inc., Lima, Ohio

Owen P. O'Meara, M.D.
Associate Professor, Department of Pediatrics, University of Colorado Health Sciences Center; Director of Neonatology, Denver Health Medical Center, Denver, Colorado

Christopher J. Ott, M.D.
Attending Staff, Department of Emergency Medicine, St. Anthony Central Level I Trauma Center, Denver, Colorado

Polly E. Parsons, M.D.
Professor, Department of Medicine; Director, Pulmonary and Critical Care Medicine Unit, University of Vermont College of Medicine, Fletcher Allen Health Care, Burlington, Vermont

Shawna J. Perry, M.D., FACEP
Director of Clinical Operations, Assistant Chair, and Assistant Professor, Department of Emergency Medicine, University of Florida Health Sciences Center; Shands Jacksonville, Jacksonville, Florida

Peter T. Pons, M.D., FACEP
Professor, Division of Emergency Medicine, Department of Surgery, University of Colorado Health Sciences Center; Attending Emergency Physician, Denver Health Medical Center, Denver, Colorado

Thomas B. Purcell, M.D.
Adjunct Assistant Professor, Department of Medicine, University of California, Los Angeles, David Geffen School of Medicine, Westwood, California; Kern Medical Center, Bakersfield, California

Jedd Roe, M.D., M.B.A., FACEP
Medical Director, Emergency Services, Legacy Emanuel Hospital, Portland, Oregon

Carlo L. Rosen, M.D.
Assistant Professor, Department of Medicine, Harvard Medical School; Program Director, Beth Israel Deaconess Medical Center Harvard Affiliated Emergency Medicine Residency, Boston, Massachusetts

Peter Rosen, M.D., FACS, FACEP
Department of Medicine, Harvard Medical School; Attending Physician, Emergency Department, Beth Israel Deaconess Medical Center, Boston, Massachusetts; St. John's Hospital, Jackson, Wyoming

Scott E. Rudkin, M.D.
Director of Medical Informatics and Assistant Clinical Professor, Department of Emergency Medicine, University of California, Irvine, College of Medicine, Irvine, California; UCI Medical Center, Orange, California

Douglas A. Rund, M.D., FACEP
Professor and Chairman, Department of Emergency Medicine; Associate Dean, The Ohio State University College of Medicine and Public Health; The Ohio State University Medical Center, Columbus, Ohio

Jeffrey J. Schaider, M.D.
Associate Chairman, Department of Emergency Medicine, Cook County Hospital, Chicago, Illinois

Nicola E. E. Schiebel, M.D., FRCPC
Assistant Professor, Department of Emergency Medicine, Mayo Clinic; Consultant, Mayo Medical Center, Rochester, Minnesota

Robert D. Schmidt, M.D.
Assistant Director, St. Anthony Hospital, Denver, Colorado

Robert E. Schneider, M.D.
Academic Faculty, Department of Emergency Medicine, Carolinas Medical Center, Charlotte, North Carolina

Elaine Norman Scholes, M.D.
Clinical Professor, Department of Pediatrics, University of Colorado Health Sciences Center; Medical Director, Denver Health Medical Plan Clinic, Denver Health Medical Center, Denver, Colorado

W. Jared Scott, M.D.
Emergency Medical Services, Denver Health Medical Center, Denver, Colorado

Julie Seaman, M.D.
Department of Emergency Medicine, Lutheran Medical Center, Wheat Ridge, Colorado

Donna L. Seger, M.D., FACEP, ABMT
Assistant Professor of Medicine, Center for Clinical Toxicology, Vanderbilt University School of Medicine; Chief, Medical Toxicology, Vanderbilt University Medical Center; Medical Director, Tennessee Poison Center, Nashville, Tennessee

Fred A. Severyn, M.D., FACEP
Assistant Professor, Division of Emergency Medicine, Department of Surgery, University of Colorado Health Sciences Center; Denver Health Medical Center, Denver, Colorado

Kaushal H. Shah, M.D.
Department of Emergency Medicine, Harvard Medical School, Beth Israel Deaconess Medical Center, Boston, Massachusetts

Lee W. Shockley, M.D., FACEP
Residency Program Director and Associate Professor, Division of Emergency Medicine, Department of Surgery, University of Colorado Health Sciences Center; Denver Health Medical Center, Denver, Colorado

Barry C. Simon, M.D.
Associate Clinical Professor of Medicine, Department of Internal Medicine, University of California, San Francisco, School of Medicine, San Francisco, California; Highland General Hospital, Oakland, California

Corey M. Slovis, M.D., FACP, FACEP
Professor of Emergency Medicine and Medicine; Chairman, Department of Emergency Medicine, Vanderbilt University School of Medicine; Vanderbilt University Medical Center; Medical Director, Nashville Fire and Emergency Medical Services, Nashville, Tennessee

Rodney W. Smith, M.D.
Department of Emergency Medicine, St. Joseph Mercy Hospital, Ann Arbor, Michigan

Wade R. Smith, M.D.
Assistant Professor, Department of Orthopaedic Surgery, University of Colorado Health Sciences Center; Director of Orthopaedic Surgery, Denver Health Medical Center; Veterans Affairs Medical Center, Denver, Colorado

Shannon Sovndal, M.D.
Department of Emergency Medicine, Stanford University Medical Center, Palo Alto, California

Daniel W. Spaite, M.D., FACEP
Professor, Department of Emergency Medicine, University of Arizona College of Medicine; Director, Emergency Services, University Medical Center, Tucson, Arizona

Harold Thomas, M.D.
Professor, Department of Emergency Medicine, Oregon Health and Science University School of Medicine, Portland, Oregon

Bryce R. Tiller, M.D.
Department of Emergency Medicine, University of Florida Health Science Center, Jacksonville, Florida

G. Winston Tripp, M.D.
Department of Emergency Medicine, Maricopa Medical Center, Phoenix, Arizona

Alexander T. Trott, M.D.
Professor, Department of Emergency Medicine, University of Cincinnati College of Medicine; Associate Chief of Staff, University of Cincinnati Hospital, Cincinnati, Ohio

Robert S. Van Hare, M.D., FACEP
Department of Emergency Medicine, Overlake Hospital Medical Center, Bellevue, Washington

W. Peter Vellman, M.D., FACEP
Director, Emergency Services, St. Anthony Hospitals, Denver, Colorado

Salvator J. Vicario, M.D.
Associate Professor, Department of Emergency Medicine, University of Louisville School of Medicine; University of Louisville Hospital, Louisville, Kentucky

David J. Vukich, M.D., FACEP

Professor and Chairman, Department of Emergency Medicine, University of Florida College of Medicine; Shands Jacksonville, Jacksonville, Florida

Robert L. Wears, M.D., M.S.

Professor, Department of Emergency Medicine, University of Florida College of Medicine, Jacksonville, Florida

Richard E. Wolfe, M.D.

Assistant Professor of Medicine, Division of Emergency Medicine, Harvard Medical School; Chief of Emergency Medicine, Beth Israel Deaconess Medical Center, Boston, Massachusetts

Allan B. Wolfson, M.D.

Professor, Department of Emergency Medicine, University of Pittsburgh School of Medicine; Program Director, University of Pittsburgh Affiliated Residency in Emergency Medicine; University of Pittsburgh Medical Center; Mercy Hospital of Pittsburgh; West Penn Hospital, Pittsburgh, Pennsylvania

Michael Yaron, M.D.

Associate Professor of Surgery, Division of Emergency Medicine, Department of Surgery, University of Colorado Health Sciences Center; University of Colorado Hospital, Denver, Colorado

William F. Young, Jr., M.D.

Assistant Clinical Professor, Department of Emergency Medicine, University of Kentucky College of Medicine, Lexington, Kentucky

Richard D. Zallen, D.D.S., M.D.

Director of Dentistry and Oral Maxillofacial Surgery, Denver Health Medical Center, Denver, Colorado

Andrew B. Ziller, M.D.

Assistant Clinical Professor, Department of Family Medicine, University of Colorado Health Sciences Center; Attending, Emergency Department, Rose Medical Center, Denver, Colorado

DEDICATION

To my wife, Leslie, and daughters, Nicole, Tasha, and Nadia—the four greatest ladies in my world. I wish to thank them for their lifelong support of all my endeavors and, in particular, for their understanding in the time the editing of this manuscript has taken away from my time with them. I would also like to acknowledge all the medical students and residents with whom I have had the pleasure of working at the Denver Health Emergency Department over the past 25 years. Their enthusiasm and intellectual curiosity have stimulated many of the questions in this book.

VJM

To my wife, Kathy, whose love, support and remarkable patience make every day worthwhile.

PTP

The editors would like to express their heartfelt thanks to Carol Lucas for her tenacity, good humor, hard work, and incredible dedication to the preparation of the third edition. We could not have accomplished this without her help.

PREFACE TO THE THIRD EDITION

This book is designed to be read by all students of emergency medicine, both novice and experienced. As emergency medicine continues to evolve as a specialty, we have added several new chapters to our third edition. We hope it continues to be a valuable and enjoyable method of providing information and knowledge. Knowing the important questions about a particular presentation or problem is the first step to obtaining the answers needed at the patient's bedside. It is with this concept in mind that we prepared this text.

Vincent J. Markovchick, M.D., FACEP
Peter T. Pons, M.D., FACEP

PREFACE TO THE FIRST EDITION

The art of emergency medicine is the ability to evaluate, diagnose, and treat—often with minimal data and time. Knowing the questions and answers that routinely confront the physician on the front line of medicine is the first step in surviving the chaotic atmosphere of the emergency medicine department. The use of the Socratic method is well recognized by most bedside teachers as a way to actively involve the student in the learning process. Through the questions and answers contained here, we have attempted to emphasize the information needed for the decisive and safe practice of emergency medicine. We hope that this book will stimulate the student to seek further knowledge from the comprehensive textbooks and the scientific literature of our field.

PREFACE TO THE SECOND EDITION

In this second edition, we have updated all the chapters featured in the first edition and added several new chapters based on the expanded body of knowledge in emergency medicine. The question-and-answer format provides a unique approach to offering information in emergency medicine. The stimuli for new questions and chapters were provided by the numerous emergency medicine technicians, nurses, medical students, and residents we and the chapter authors encounter every day in our emergency departments. We hope that the readers will assist us with future editions by providing suggestions for new questions and new topics.

Vincent J. Markovchick, M.D., FACEP
Peter T. Pons, M.D., FACEP

I. Decision Making in Emergency Medicine

1. DECISION MAKING IN EMERGENCY MEDICINE

Vincent J. Markovchick, M.D.

1. Is there anything unique about emergency medicine?

Although there is significant crossover between emergency medicine and all other clinical specialties, emergency medicine has unique aspects, such as the approach to patient care and the decision-making process.

2. Describe the conventional method of evaluating a patient.

A comprehensive history, physical examination, "routine" laboratory diagnostic studies, special diagnostic procedures, and the formulation of a problem-oriented medical record and rational course of therapy constitute the "ideal" approach to patient care because it is so comprehensive.

3. Why is the conventional methodology not ideal for use in the emergency department (ED)?

Even though in retrospect only 10–20% of patients presenting to an ED truly have emergent problems, it must be presumed that every patient who comes to an ED has an emergent condition. Therefore, the first and most important question that must be answered is, *What is the life threat?* The conventional approach does not ensure an expeditious answer to this question. Time constraints also impede the use of conventional methodology in the ED.

4. How do I identify the life-threatened patient?

Three components are necessary to quickly identify the life-threatened patient:
1. A chief complaint and a brief, focused history relevant to the chief complaint
2. A complete and accurate set of vital signs in the field and in the ED
3. An opportunity to visualize, auscultate, and touch the patient

5. What is so important about the chief complaint?

The chief complaint, which sometimes cannot be obtained directly from the patient but must be obtained from family members, observers, emergency medical technicians (EMTs), or others at the scene, will immediately help categorize the general type of problem (e.g., cardiac, traumatic, respiratory, etc.).

6. Why are vital signs important?

Vital signs are the most reliable, objective data that are immediately available to ED personnel. Vital signs and the chief complaint, when used as triage tools, will identify the majority of life-threatened patients. Familiarity with normal vital signs for all age groups is essential.

7. What are the determinants of (normal) vital signs?

Age, underlying physical condition, medical problems (e.g., hypertension), and current medications (e.g., beta blockers) are important considerations in determining normal vital signs for a given patient. For example, a well-conditioned, young athlete who has just sustained major trauma and arrives with a resting, supine pulse of 80 bpm must be presumed to have significant blood loss because his normal pulse is probably in the 40–50 bpm range.

8. Why do I need to compare field vital signs with ED vital signs?

Most prehospital care systems with a level of care beyond basic transport also provide therapy to patients. Because this therapy usually makes positive changes in the patient's condition, the patient may look deceptively well upon arrival in the ED. For example, a 20-year-old female with acute onset of left lower quadrant abdominal pain, who is found to be cool, clammy, and diaphoretic, with a pulse of 116 and a blood pressure of 78 palpable, and who receives 1500 cc of IV fluid en route to the ED, may arrive with normal vital signs and no skin changes. If one does not read and pay attention to the EMT's description of the patient and the initial vital signs, the presumption may be made that this is a stable patient.

9. When are "normal" vital signs abnormal?

This is where the chief complaint comes in. For example, a 20-year-old male who states he has asthma and has been wheezing for hours arrives in the ED with a respiratory rate of 14. An asthmatic who is dyspneic and wheezing should have a respiratory rate of at least 20–30/min. Thus a "normal" respiratory rate of 14 in this setting indicates the patient is fatiguing and is in respiratory failure. This is a classic example of when "normal" is extremely abnormal.

10. Why do I need to visualize, auscultate, and touch the patient?

In many instances, these measures help to identify the life threat (e.g., is it the upper airway, lower airway, or circulation?). Touching the skin is important in order to determine whether shock is associated with vasoconstriction (hypovolemic or cardiogenic) or with vasodilatation (septic, neurogenic, or anaphylactic). Auscultation will identify life threats associated with the lower airway (e.g., bronchoconstriction, tension pneumothorax).

11. Once I have identified the life threat, what do I do?

Do not go on. Stop immediately and intervene to reverse the life threat. For example, if the initial encounter with the patient identifies upper airway obstruction, take whatever measures are necessary to alleviate upper airway obstruction such as suctioning, positioning, or intubating the patient. If the problem is hemorrhage, volume restoration and hemorrhage control (when possible) are indicated.

12. Okay, I have identified and stabilized or ruled out an immediate life threat in the patient. What else is unique about the approach?

The differential diagnosis formulated in the ED must begin with the most serious condition possible to explain the patient's presentation, and proceed from there. An example is a 60-year-old male who presents with nausea, vomiting, and epigastric pain. Instead of assuming the condition is caused by a gastrointestinal disorder, one must consider that the presentation could represent an acute myocardial infarction (MI) and take the appropriate steps to stabilize (i.e., start an IV and place the patient on O_2 and a cardiac monitor) the patient and rule out an MI (an adequate history, physical exam, and electrocardiogram [ECG]).

13. Why does formulating a differential diagnosis sometimes lead to problems?

The natural tendency in formulating a differential diagnosis is to think of the most common or statistically most probable condition to explain the patient's initial presentation to the ED. If one does this, one will be right most of the time but may overlook the most serious, albeit sometimes a very uncommon, problem. Therefore, the practice of emergency medicine involves some degree of healthy paranoia in that one must consider the most serious condition possible, and, through a logical process of elimination, rule it out and thereby arrive at the correct and generally more common diagnosis.

14. Is a diagnosis always possible or necessary with information I can obtain in the ED?

Of course not. Sometimes it takes days, weeks, or months for the final diagnosis to be made. It is unreasonable to expect that every patient evaluated in the ED should or must have a diagnosis made in the ED. If you have an obsessive-compulsive personality with a need to be absolutely certain before you can act to stabilize or treat a patient, then the ED is an unhealthy work environment for you.

15. Suppose I can't make the diagnosis. What do I do?

It is advisable to be intellectually honest and admit to the patient and document in the medical record the inability to make a diagnosis. As stated earlier, it is the role of the ED physician to rule out serious or life-threatening causes of a patient's presentation, not to arrive at the definitive diagnosis. For example, a patient who presents with acute abdominal pain, who has had an appropriate history taken, who has had a physical exam and diagnostic studies performed, and who in your best judgment does not have a life-threatening or acute surgical problem should be so informed. The discharge diagnosis would be abdominal pain of unknown etiology. This avoids the trap so often encountered of labeling the patient with a benign diagnosis such as gastroenteritis or gastritis that is not supported by the medical record. More importantly, it avoids giving the patient the impression that there is a totally benign process occurring and will help to avoid the medical (and legal) problem of the patient presenting 2 days later with a ruptured appendix (see Chapter 126, Cost Containment and Risk Management in Emergency Medicine).

16. What is the most important question to ask a patient who presents with a chronic persistent, or recurrent condition?

What's different now? This question should be asked of all patients who have a chronic condition that has resulted in their visit to the ED. The classic example is migraine headache. The patient with a chronic, recurrent migraine headache who is not asked this question may, on this presentation, have had an acute subarachnoid bleed. Such a patient may not volunteer that this headache is different from the pattern of chronic migraines unless asked.

17. How do I decide if the patient needs hospitalization?

Obviously the medical condition is the first factor to consider. The question that must be answered is, "Is there a medical need that can be fulfilled only by hospitalization?" For example, does the patient need oxygen therapy or cardiac monitoring? Another factor to weigh in the decision regarding hospitalization is whether the patient can be safely observed in the outpatient setting. For example, a patient who has sustained head trauma and needs to follow head trauma precautions at home, and who is either homeless or lives alone, cannot be safely discharged. Unfortunately, the patient's ability to pay for services is also sometimes inappropriately used in ED disposition decisions.

18. If the patient does not need admission, how do I arrange a satisfactory disposition?

Every patient seen in the ED must be referred to a physician or referred back to the ED for follow-up care. Failure to do so constitutes patient abandonment. Appropriate and specific follow-up instructions should be given to all patients.

19. What is meant by specific follow-up instructions?

All follow-up instructions must include specific mention of the most serious potential complication of the patient's condition. For example, a patient who is being discharged home with the diagnosis of a probable herniated L4, 5 intervertebral disc should be instructed to return immediately if any bowel or bladder dysfunction develops. This takes into account the most serious complication of a herniated lumbar disc, which is a central mid-line herniation (cauda equina syndrome) with bowel or bladder dysfunction, and constitutes an acute neurosurgical emergency.

20. What two questions should always be asked (and answered) before a patient is discharged from the ED?

1. Why did the patient come to the ED?
2. Have I made the patient feel better?

Generally, most patients present to the ED because of pain, somatic or psychologic, and a reasonable expectation is that this pain will be acknowledged and appropriately treated. If such pain cannot be alleviated, a thorough explanation should be given to the patient regarding the reasons why. An example of this is a patient with abdominal pain of unknown etiology, which may evolve into appendicitis. Narcotics may mask the recognition of worsening symptoms and localized abdominal pain. Reassurance is sometimes all that is needed to relieve anxiety about serious medical conditions such as cancer or heart attack. Other agents such as antiemetics or antianxiety medications should be administered in the ED to alleviate presenting symptoms.

21. Why is the previous question and answer one of the most important in this chapter?
Attention to treating and alleviating a patient's pain will dramatically reduce subsequent complaints concerning care in the ED and remove one of the significant risk factors for initiation of a malpractice suit. It is also how you would want to be treated.

22. What about the chart?
The chart must reflect the answers to the preceding questions in this chapter. It need not list the entire differential diagnosis but one should be able to ascertain from reading the chart that the more serious diagnoses were indeed considered. It also must contain appropriate follow-up instructions.

---

2. MANAGEMENT OF CARDIAC ARREST AND RESUSCITATION

Charles B. Cairns, M.D.

---

1. What are the ABCs of resuscitation?
Airway, breathing, and circulation.

2. How should cardiopulmonary resuscitation (CPR) be performed?
The ABCs should guide and steady the resuscitation of all critically ill patients, including all cardiac arrest victims.
   1. Activate the EMS 911 system if out of the hospital or the cardiac arrest response team if in the hospital.
   2. Open the airway by performing a head tilt–chin lift or a head tilt–jaw thrust maneuver. These maneuvers cause anterior displacement of the mandible and lift the tongue and epiglottis away from the glottic opening. To improve airway patency, suction the mouth and oropharynx, and insert an oropharyngeal or nasopharyngeal airway.
   3. Assist breathing by performing mouth-to-mouth, mouth-to-mask, or bag-valve-mask breathing. The recommended technique depends on the clinical setting, the equipment available, and the rescuer's skill and training. Although these techniques can sustain ventilation and oxygenation indefinitely in ideal situations (e.g., in the operating room), in the emergency setting they can be suboptimal. Air leaks at the facemask result in inadequate lung ventilation. Insufflation of the stomach, followed by emesis and aspiration, is an ever-present threat. To reduce these risks, deliver slow, even breaths, pausing for full deflation between breaths and avoiding excessive peak inspiratory pressures. Use the Sellick maneuver (continuous application of digital pressure to the cricoid cartilage) to compress the esophagus and reduce the risk of vomiting and aspiration.
   4. After opening the airway and initiating rescue breathing, check for spontaneous circulation by palpating for a carotid or femoral pulse. If the patient is pulseless, begin chest compressions.

Compress the chest smoothly and forcefully 80 to 100 times per minute. If there are two rescuers, interpose one artificial breath after every five chest compressions. If only one rescuer is available, the recommended sequence is 15 compressions, followed by two breaths.

3. What are the exceptions to the rule of the ABCs?

1. **Monitored cardiac arrest.** When a patient in a monitored setting experiences sudden ventricular tachycardia or ventricular fibrillation, immediate electrical defibrillation is the priority.

2. **Traumatic arrest.** In traumatic cardiac arrest, closed-chest CPR is usually ineffective. In trauma, the cause of the arrest may be a tension pneumothorax, cardiac tamponade, or an exsanguinating hemorrhage from the thorax or abdomen. An immediate thoracotomy, not CPR, is indicated. In the setting of significant craniofacial trauma or forceful deceleration, there may be a fracture or dislocation of the cervical spine. When neck injury is suspected, a jaw thrust (*never a head tilt*) should be used to open the airway.

4. Explain the mechanism of blood flow during CPR.

Two basic models explain the mechanism of blood flow during CPR. In the **cardiac pump model**, the heart is squeezed between the sternum and the spine. Chest compression results in systole, and the atrioventricular valves close normally, ensuring unidirectional, antegrade flow. During the relaxation phase (diastole), intracardiac pressures fall, the valves open, and blood is drawn into the heart from the lungs and vena cavae.

In the **thoracic pump model**, the heart is considered a passive conduit. Chest compression results in uniformly increased pressures throughout the heart and thorax. Forward blood flow is achieved selectively in the arterial system because the stiff-walled arteries resist collapse and because retrograde flow is prevented in the great veins by one-way valves. Aspects of both models have been substantiated in animal models, and both pumps probably contribute to blood flow during CPR.

5. Is blood flow to the brain and heart adequate during CPR?

In the cardiac pump model and the thoracic pump model, blood flow to the brain is a function of the aortic-to-jugular venous pressure difference during systole (the compression phase of CPR). The cerebral flow measured experimentally is approximately 30% of normal. Blood flow to the heart occurs during the relaxation phase of CPR and is a function of the aortic-to-right atrial pressure difference in diastole. Net myocardial flow via the coronary arteries is essentially nil during closed-chest CPR, and retrograde coronary artery flow also has been shown.

6. Discuss the role of pharmacologic therapy during CPR.

The immediate goal of pharmacologic therapy is to improve myocardial blood flow, the key physiologic parameter conducive to the return of spontaneous circulation. α-Adrenergic agonists, such as epinephrine, augment the aortic-to-right atrial diastolic gradient by increasing arterial vascular tone. Reports suggest that nonadrenergic receptor agonists, including vasopressin, may be more efficacious than epinephrine in improving myocardial blood flow. Additional clinical studies suggested that amiodarone can improve rates of defibrillation. This antifibrillatory effect of amiodarone may be independent of its effects on myocardial blood flow.

7. What are the most common causes of cardiopulmonary arrest?

Most cardiopulmonary arrests in prehospital and hospital settings are caused by ventricular fibrillation, which usually occurs in patients with ischemic heart disease. Drug toxicity, electrolyte disturbances (hyperkalemia), and prolonged hypoxemia also are important inciting factors.

A significant proportion (30% to 50%) of cardiac arrests are bradyasystolic at the outset. Common causes of this rhythm are hypoxia and acidemia. Another important cause of bradyasystole is heightened vagal tone, which may be precipitated by drugs, anesthetic agents, inferoposterior myocardial infarction (Bezold-Jarisch reflex), or invasive procedures.

Pulseless electrical activity (PEA) is the third most common arrest rhythm. PEA most commonly is caused by prolonged arrest itself; typically, after 8 minutes or more of ventricular fibrillation, electrical defibrillation is futile and induces a slow, wide-complex PEA, which is usually irreversible and known as pulseless idioventricular rhythm. PEA also may present as an inciting, rather than terminal, rhythm. Tension pneumothorax, cardiac tamponade, exsanguination, anaphylaxis, and pulmonary embolus (discussed later) are examples.

8. **What are the reversible causes and immediate treatments of cardiopulmonary arrest?**
   - **Hyperkalemia**. Treatment includes calcium chloride, sodium bicarbonate, and an insulin-glucose infusion.
   - **Anaphylaxis**. Rapid tracheal intubation and administration of crystalloid and epinephrine are the cornerstones of resuscitation.
   - **Cardiac tamponade**. A pericardiocentesis or subxyphoid pericardiorrhaphy is lifesaving.
   - **Tension pneumothorax**. Immediate chest decompression is mandatory.
   - **Hypovolemia**. Treatment includes immediate IV administration of crystalloid solutions. In traumatic arrest, blood products (whole blood or packed cells) should be given concomitantly with crystalloid.
   - **Torsades de pointes**. Treatment includes cardioversion, followed by magnesium, isoproterenol, and rapid ventricular pacing.
   - **Toxic cardiopulmonary arrest**. Carbon monoxide poisoning occurs after prolonged exposure to smoke or inhalation of exhaust from an incomplete combustion. High-flow and hyperbaric oxygen and management of acidosis are the cornerstones of treatment. Cyanide poisoning occurs often, especially during fires involving synthetic materials. The antidote for this is IV sodium nitrite and sodium thiosulfate. Tricyclic antidepressants act as type Ia antiarrhythmic agents and cause cardiac conduction slowing, ventricular arrhythmias, hypotension, and seizures. Vigorous alkalinization and seizure control are required.
   - **Primary asphyxia**. In addition to anaphylaxis, obstructive asphyxia may occur after foreign body aspiration, inflammatory conditions of the hypopharynx (epiglottis or retropharyngeal abscess), or cervicofacial trauma. The last-mentioned results in edema or hematoma formation, subcutaneous emphysema, or laryngeal or tracheal disruption. Treatment includes establishment of a patent airway via endotracheal intubation or by cricothyrotomy and assisted ventilation with 100% oxygen.

9. **How should ventricular fibrillation be treated?**
   Rapid treatment is essential; the prognosis worsens with each minute of delay. An initial defibrillation dose of 200 J is recommended to minimize myocardial damage and to prevent the development of postcountershock pulseless bradyarrhythmias. Animal studies and clinical reports suggested that in prolonged cardiac arrest, augmentation of myocardial blood flow with either epinephrine or vasopressin before countershock may improve defibrillation success. A randomized, controlled clinical trial suggested that amiodarone enhances the rate of out-of-hospital defibrillation success and survival to the ED; however, amiodarone use was not associated with an improvement in mortality (see question 19).

10. **What about persistent ventricular fibrillation?**
    1. Perform endotracheal intubation and ensure adequate ventilation.
    2. Administer amiodarone (300 mg IV),which may be an effective antifibrillatory agent.
    3. Administer epinephrine (dosage is controversial; see question 16) or vasopressin (40 U IV) to augment aortic diastolic blood pressure and to improve myocardial perfusion.
    4. Administer procainamide (20 to 30 mg/min to a maximum of 17 mg/kg) or lidocaine (1.0 to 1.5 mg/kg). Neither lidocaine nor procainamide has been proved efficacious in improving defibrillation success rates or in restoring a perfusing rhythm in patients with ventricular fibrillation.

11. Is pulseless idioventricular rhythm treatable?

Delayed electrical countershock frequently results in asystole or a pulseless idioventricular rhythm, which most often is untreatable and results in death. In animal experiments, high-dose epinephrine (0.1 to 0.2 mg/kg) has helped to restore cardiac contractility and pacemaker activity, so it may improve the outcome in postcountershock bradyasystole. In the prehospital setting, pulseless idioventricular rhythm may be a transient rhythm after defibrillation. A review of such cases revealed a hospital discharge rate of 8%.

12. How should asystole be treated?

1. Confirm the absence of cardiac activity (a flat-line ECG may be recorded because of technical mistakes). Verify the absence of pulses at the carotid or femoral arteries. Check for loose or disconnected battery cables and monitor leads. Finally, rotate the monitoring leads 90°, and increase the amplitude to detect occult, fine ventricular fibrillation.

2. Atropine (1 mg IV) is given to counteract low vagal tone, which may accompany infero-posterior myocardial infarction, acidosis, drug administration, or hypoxia.

3. Administer epinephrine (dosage is controversial; see question 16) or vasopressin (40 U IV).

4. For refractory asystole, consider nonreceptor inotropic agents, such as aminophylline, 250 mg IV. At this point, many would consider this and any further pharmacologic interventions to be merely embalming fluid.

13. Is electrical defibrillation or pacemaker therapy used for asystole?

Electrical defibrillation is reserved for cases in which differentiation between asystole and fine ventricular fibrillation is difficult; in these ambiguous situations, defibrillation should be employed after administration of epinephrine. Pacemaker therapy often is attempted for asystole but is seldom effective in restoring a pulsatile rhythm.

14. What are the appropriate routes of drug administration?

IV administration is the preferred route of drug therapy during cardiopulmonary arrest. If a central venous catheter is in place, the most distal port should be used. Otherwise, use of a peripheral venous catheter results in a slightly delayed onset of action, although the peak drug effect is similar to that for the central route. Intracardiac administration should be reserved for cases of open cardiac massage. Many drugs (epinephrine, atropine, lidocaine) are absorbed systemically after endotracheal administration, yet the effectiveness of this route during CPR is suspect. Pulmonary blood flow and systemic absorption are minimal during CPR. Studies in animals suggest that comparable hemodynamic responses occur only with endotracheal doses of epinephrine 10 times that of IV doses. Virtually every drug used for resuscitation can be given in conventional doses by the intraosseous route. This method is useful in pediatric patients when an IV line cannot be established.

15. When may prehospital resuscitation efforts be terminated?

According to the most recent American Heart Association Advanced Cardiac Life Support (ACLS) guidelines, prehospital resuscitation can be discontinued by EMS authorities when a valid no-CPR order is presented to the rescuers or when a patient is deemed nonresuscitable after an adequate trial of ACLS including:
- Successful endotracheal intubation
- Achievement of IV access and administration of rhythm-appropriate medications and countershocks
- Determination that persistent asystole or agonal ECG patterns are present

Resuscitation can be discontinued when no reversible causes can be identified.

CONTROVERSIES

16. Which vasopressor should I administer for cardiac arrest, epinephrine or vasopressin?

For epinephrine: The conventional dose of epinephrine (1 mg IV every 3 to 5 minutes) was derived empirically from animal studies, then applied arbitrarily to humans. No dose-response studies were done, and the α-adrenergic receptors that epinephrine acts on have been found to be down-regulated during arrest states. The *standard* 1-mg dose of epinephrine reduces myocardial blood flow in experimental studies and has never been proved to be efficacious in human cardiac arrest. Many animal experiments and human trials indicate that *high-dose* epinephrine (0.1 to 0.2 mg/kg) improves coronary flow (coronary perfusion pressure) during CPR and results in higher rates of return of spontaneous circulation compared with standard doses. These preliminary and limited clinical trials have not shown any evidence of detrimental side effects.

Critics point out that although human trials may have shown a higher rate of return of spontaneous circulation with high-dose epinephrine, no trial has shown improved neurologic recovery. Until a well-designed study is done showing improved survival and neurologic recovery, current therapy should remain standard. This is especially true because the result of high-dose treatment may be an increased number of neurologically impaired survivors.

For vasopressin: Vasopressin acts directly on V_1-receptors, which may not be down-regulated during arrest states. In laboratory animal models of ventricular fibrillation, vasopressin improved vital organ blood flow, resuscitation rates, and neurologic recovery better than did epinephrine.

Critics note that a randomized, controlled clinical trial failed to detect any survival advantage for vasopressin (40 U IV) over epinephrine (1 mg IV). Because no evidence for a beneficial effect of vasopressin was found, the investigators "strongly" disagreed with American Heart Association ACLS guidelines, which recommend vasopressin as alternative therapy for cardiac arrest.

17. Should I routinely administer sodium bicarbonate to a cardiac arrest victim?

For: When cardiopulmonary arrest occurs, acidemia follows. Even if CPR is performed correctly, tissue perfusion is suboptimal and metabolic acidosis ensues. In addition, and more importantly, alveolar hypoventilation (respiratory acidosis) occurs. Buffering is necessary to counter the pernicious effects of acidemia. A severe drop in pH interferes with the vascular and myocardial responses to adrenergic drugs and endogenous catecholamines and reduces cardiac chronotropy and inotropy. Acidosis leads to ventricular irritability and a lower threshold for ventricular fibrillation. Below a pH of 7.2, myocardial contractile function may decline, resulting in refractory PEA.

Although the primary treatment of the acidemia of cardiac arrest is adequate ventilation, metabolic acidosis often progresses inexorably. Sodium bicarbonate is the only buffer commonly available, and its use traditionally has been recommended when the pH falls to a life-threatening range, usually below 7.2. Sodium bicarbonate may be particularly useful in attenuating postresuscitation myocardial dysfunction.

Against: The primary treatment of the acidemia of cardiac arrest is adequate ventilation, which in clinical and animal studies correlates with survival. The metabolic acidosis is usually unimportant in the first 15 to 18 minutes of resuscitation. If ventilation is maintained, arterial pH usually remains above 7.2. Moderate acidosis in this range does not interfere with defibrillation, shifts the oxyhemoglobin dissociation curve to the right, may augment cardiac contractility, and protects against, rather than precipitates, PEA.

Sodium bicarbonate is a poor buffering agent for cardiac resuscitation. Sodium bicarbonate causes volume overload, hyperosmolarity, hypernatremia, and hyperkalemia, even when used as recommended. Iatrogenic alkalosis may cause arrhythmias, cerebral vasoconstriction, lactic acid production, and a left shift of the oxyhemoglobin dissociation curve, further limiting tissue oxygen delivery. Most important, the bicarbonate ions, after combining with hydrogen ions, generate new carbon dioxide. Biologic membranes are highly permeable to carbon dioxide (but are much more slowly permeable to sodium bicarbonate). Administration of sodium bicarbonate causes a paradoxical intracellular acidosis. Studies indicate that intramyocardial hypercarbia causes a profound decline in cardiac contractile function and leads to failure of resuscitation. Myocardial PCO_2 in human resuscitation may reach levels greater than 250 mmHg, further highlighting the risks of administering carbon dioxide–generating agents such as sodium bicarbonate. Within the myocardial cell, hypercapnia impairs contractility and results in refractory PEA.

18. So, do I administer sodium bicarbonate or not?

Sodium bicarbonate is **not** recommended because no buffer therapy is needed in the first 15 minutes of arrest (if adequate lung ventilation is maintained) and because the optimal acid-base status for resuscitation has not been established. Only restoration of the spontaneous circulation—not a buffering agent—can reverse the development of intramyocardial hypercarbia.

19. What about the use of amiodarone in cardiac arrest?

Amiodarone is an antiarrhythmic agent that has been used to prevent sudden death from ventricular arrhythmias. A randomized, controlled clinical trial in patients with out-of-hospital cardiac arrest comparing amiodarone with its diluent showed that amiodarone (300 mg IV) when combined with other therapies improved defibrillation rates and resulted in a 10% increase in survivors transported to the ED.

Critics note there was no difference between the amiodarone (an expensive drug) and placebo groups in terms of neurologic status or survival to discharge. This lack of an outcome difference, similar to the data of many studies involving cardiac arrest interventions, did not deter the American Heart Association from putting amiodarone in the most recent ACLS guidelines. Some have argued that clinicians should be cautious in considering the use of agents such as amiodarone or vasopressin in a field setting for cardiac arrest until studies clearly show an outcome benefit over drugs currently in use.

BIBLIOGRAPHY

1. American Heart Association: Guidelines for cardiopulmonary resuscitation and emergency cardiac care. Circulation 102(suppl I): I-1–I-166, 2000.
2. Cairns CB, Niemann JT: Hemodynamic responses to repeated doses of epinephrine during prolonged cardiac arrest and resuscitation. Resuscitation 36:181–185, 1998.
3. Cairns CB, Paradis NA: Empiric lidocaine: Deja vu (all over again?) Ann Emerg Med 36:626–627, 2000.
4. Cobb LA, Fahrenbruch CE, Walsh TR, et al: Influence of cardiopulmonary resuscitation prior to defibrillation in patients with out-of-hospital ventricular fibrillation. JAMA 281:1182–1188, 1999.
5. Dorian P, Cass D, Schwartz B, et al: Amiodarone as compared with lidocaine for shock resistant ventricular fibrillation. N Engl J Med 346:884–890, 2002.
6. Hein HA: The use of sodium bicarbonate in neonatal resuscitation: Help or harm? Pediatrics 91:496, 1993.
7. Kudenchuk PJ, Cobb LA, Copass MK, et al: Amiodarone for resuscitation after out-of-hospital cardiac arrest due to ventricular fibrillation. N Engl J Med 341:871–878, 1999.
8. Marx JA, Hockberger RS, Walls RM (eds): Rosen's Emergency Medicine: Concepts and Clinical Practice, 5th ed. St. Louis, Mosby, 2002.
9. Niemann JT, Cairns CB, Sharma J, Lewis RJ: Treatment of prolonged ventricular fibrillation: Immediate countershock versus high-dose epinephrine and CPR prior to countershock. Circulation 95:281–287, 1992.
10. Stewart CE: Amiodarone for ACLS: A critical evaluation. Emerg Med Serv 30:61–67, 2001.
11. Stiell IG, Hebert PC, Wells GA, et al: Vasopressin versus epinephrine for inhospital cardiac arrest: A randomised controlled trial. Lancet 358:105–109, 2001.
12. Wenzel V, Lindner KH: Employing vasopressin during cardiopulmonary resuscitation and vasodilatory shock as a lifesaving vasopressor. Cardiovasc Res 51:529–541, 2001.

3. AIRWAY MANAGEMENT

Barry C. Simon, M.D.

1. Do I really need to know about airway management?

Yes. Expeditious airway management saves lives.

2. How is the adequacy of ventilation assessed?

First, look at the patient. Cyanosis suggests profound hypoxia. Diaphoresis and somnolence indicate hypercapnia and respiratory acidosis. Measure the respiratory rate, and assess the tidal volume by placing your hand over the endotracheal tube or the patient's mouth and nose. If you are still concerned, use a pulse oximeter. Mild-to-moderate hypoxia can be monitored with pulse oximetry, which measures arterial oxygen saturation. If there is a question of inadequate ventilation, an arterial blood gas or measurement of end-tidal carbon dioxide should be considered.

3. Why do patients need airway management?

Assisted ventilation can help to decrease intracranial pressure or correct hypercarbia and acidosis. **Oxygenation** may be needed in patients with severe lung disease or injury who are unable to maintain an acceptable PaO_2. **Overcoming or preventing airway obstruction** is imperative in patients with neck trauma, epiglottitis, or airway burns from smoke inhalation or ingestion of caustic substances. **Prevention of aspiration** in patients with altered mentation is best accomplished with endotracheal intubation. **Administration of intratracheal drugs (epinephrine, atropine, lidocaine)** through the endotracheal tube is indicated in resuscitation until an IV line can be established.

4. What is the most common cause of airway obstruction?

The tongue obstructs the airway far more commonly than do foreign bodies or edema. With decreasing levels of consciousness, the supporting muscles in the floor of the mouth lose tone, and the tongue falls posteriorly, obstructing the oropharynx. The fastest, least invasive treatment modality is repositioning via the head tilt–chin lift maneuver. A nasopharyngeal or oral airway should be inserted in a patient with ongoing upper airway obstruction unrelieved by repositioning. Care must be taken in patients with potential or suspected cervical spine injury.

5. What is an EOA?

The **esophageal obturator airway (EOA)** is a 34-cm-long plastic tube with a mask at the proximal end and a balloon at the distal end. This device is placed blindly in the esophagus, and the balloon is inflated to prevent air from entering the stomach and vomitus from entering the airway.

6. What are the indications for the EOA?

The EOA is acceptable only in a prehospital setting when assisted ventilation is needed and the providers are not trained or authorized to perform endotracheal intubation.

7. Is the EOA safe?

Not really. The greatest danger is the risk of inadvertent intubation of the trachea. A more common complication is aspiration because the EOA does not protect the trachea from secretions, bleeding, and emesis. Esophageal rupture has been reported in patients who have attempted to vomit with an EOA in place.

8. What are the relative contraindications to blind nasotracheal intubation (BNTI)?

Apnea is the most important contraindication because the chance of esophageal intubation is unacceptably high. Because epistaxis complicates BNTI in one third of cases, the procedure is contraindicated in patients with coagulopathies. Other routes of intubation are advisable in patients with maxillary facial or severe nasal fractures because a false passage, severe epistaxis, or, rarely, cranial placement may occur. Hematomas, epiglottitis, and infections of the upper neck are relative contraindications because of the risk of sudden airway obstruction or laryngospasm.

9. Name some complications of BNTI.

Hypoxia may occur during the intubation process. In addition to epistaxis and esophageal intubation, there are acute complications, such as avulsion of the turbinates, avulsion of the vocal cords, and pharyngeal perforations with retropharyngeal dissection. Significant elevation in intracranial pressure with coughing may precipitate uncal herniation in head-injured patients. Sinusitis may occur several days later from obstruction of the paranasal ostia.

10. What is rapid-sequence intubation (RSI)?
A method of safely paralyzing and intubating a patient with a full stomach. Because all emergency patients are at risk for aspiration, the airway must be secured as quickly as possible. Paralysis with succinylcholine facilitates visualization and tube placement and reduces complications that occur with attempts to intubate an awake, struggling patient.

11. Don't you need to be an anesthesiologist to perform RSI? How is it done?
No. The basics can be remembered as the **five** *Ps*: preparation, preoxygenation, priming, pressure, and paralysis.
1. **Prepare** equipment (e.g., suction, endotracheal tube, bag, mask, laryngoscope).
2. **Preoxygenate** with 100% oxygen (no positive-pressure) ideally for 5 minutes.
3. Pretreat with a defasciculating dose of vecuronium or pancuronium (0.01 mg/kg).
4. **Prime** with thiopental, 3 to 4 mg/kg rapid IV push.
5. Apply **pressure** with Sellick's maneuver (cricoid pressure) as consciousness is lost to prevent regurgitation and aspiration.
6. Follow thiopental immediately with 1 to 2 mg/kg of succinylcholine to **paralyze**.
7. Intubate the trachea, and verify accurate placement with an end-tidal carbon dioxide detector.
8. Release cricoid pressure.

Alternative RSI

1. Prepare equipment (e.g., suction, endotracheal tube, bag, mask, laryngoscope).
2. Preoxygenate with 100% oxygen (no positive-pressure ventilation) ideally for 5 minutes.
3. Prime with thiopental, 3 to 4 mg/kg rapid IV push.
4. Paralyze with rocuronium, 1.0 mg/kg IV push.
5. Apply Sellick's maneuver (cricoid pressure) as consciousness is lost.
6. Intubate the trachea, and verify accurate placement with an end-tidal carbon dioxide detector.
7. Release cricoid pressure.

12. How do I preoxygenate a patient before intubation?
Bag-valve-mask ventilation is the only option in the apneic patient, even though this increases the risk of aspiration by raising gastric pressure. If a patient is making effective respiratory efforts, he or she should receive passive oxygenation via a nonrebreather mask on 100% oxygen for a full 5 minutes. In the apneic patient, eight vital capacity breaths using high-flow oxygen should be administered.

13. What is Sellick's maneuver?
Sellick described a method of applying pressure over the cricoid cartilage to help prevent aspiration. Pressure should equal the amount of force it takes to cause discomfort when pressing over the bridge of one's nose. Pressure is applied after loss of consciousness and is maintained until the endotracheal tube balloon is inflated and tube placement is confirmed.

14. How do I remember the size of the endotracheal tube for children?
The easiest way is to carry a card in your wallet. The following formula works for persons 2 to 20 years old:

$$\text{Tube size} = \frac{(\text{age in years} + 16)}{4}$$

15. Describe some of the induction drugs available for RSI.

Thiopental is a short-acting barbiturate that has been used by anesthesiologists for decades. It is safe and effective with few serious complications but is a little longer acting than many of the newer agents (10 to 15 minutes). **Methohexital** is an ultra-short–acting barbiturate with a similar safety profile. The benzodiazepine **midazolam** has the added benefit of being reversible. **Propofol** is a diisopropylphenol induction agent that has become popular among anesthesiologists for outpatient procedures. Its major disadvantage is a significant decrease in blood pressure. **Etomidate** is gaining popularity in emergency settings for its rapid action, short duration, and absence of any effects on the cardiovascular system.

16. Why is succinylcholine the most common paralyzing agent in RSI?

No other neuromuscular blocking agent has as rapid an onset of action (45 to 60 seconds) or as brief a duration of activity (4 to 7 minutes). This provides added safety, with the return of spontaneous respiration within 7 minutes.

17. What are the theoretical risks of succinylcholine?

Despite its significant benefits, succinylcholine has many undesirable characteristics, some of which may be dangerous. It increases intragastric, intraocular, and intracranial pressure. Life-threatening hyperkalemia may occur in patients with neuromuscular disease or 3 to 4 days after major burns and trauma. Severe muscle contractions cause delayed pain and occasionally rhabdomyolysis. Rarely, it can precipitate malignant hyperthermia.

18. Are there any alternative paralytics?

Rocuronium has been suggested as an alternative to succinylcholine. It has few complications and has an onset of action nearly as fast as succinylcholine. Its only significant drawback is a duration of action of 20 to 40 minutes. **Vecuronium** is another alternative, but its duration is even longer at 60 to 90 minutes. Pancuronium is a poor choice for RSI because of its slow onset of action. Newer nondepolarizing drugs with properties similar to succinylcholine should be available in the near future. One of the new agents, rapacuronium, has been recalled by the manufacturer because of deaths related to bronchospasm.

19. Are there any contraindications to RSI?

Yes. Paralyze a patient only when you are sure he or she can be bag/mask ventilated if intubation is unsuccessful. Anticipation of a difficult airway based on anatomic features or traumatic anatomic distortion (e.g., patients with massive facial trauma or severe facial burns) is a relative contraindication. Inability to preoxygenate patients (e.g., patients with severe chronic obstructive pulmonary disease or asthma) is a relative contraindication to RSI. Patients with airway obstruction (foreign body, allergic reaction, airway infections, malignancies) who continue to make some respiratory effort should not be paralyzed.

20. How do I manage patients who have contraindications to RSI?

Nasotracheal intubation is a good alternative in patients with pulmonary disease. If unsuccessful, or if there is a contraindication to nasotracheal intubation, awake oral intubation with an induction agent, such as ketamine, allows the patient to maintain a certain degree of ventilation and airway protection during the procedure. Ketamine should not be used in head-injured patients because it dramatically increases intracranial pressure. Benzodiazepines, such as midazolam, may be useful for induction because they can be reversed easily with flumazenil if the need arises.

21. Summarize the alternatives available if these standard techniques fail.

1. **Laryngeal mask airway** is an irregular ovoid silicone mask with an inflatable rim connected to a tube that allows ventilation. The device can be passed blindly with a high degree of success. The nose of the mask is seated in the esophagus. When the rim is inflated, it prevents air from going into the esophagus and forces air into the trachea. This is a good temporizing device until a definitive airway can be established.

2. **Cricothyrotomy**, a surgical airway through the cricothyroid membrane, can be done rapidly, although it often is complicated by hemorrhage and is contraindicated in children younger than 8 years old.

3. **Tracheotomy** is more time-consuming but is the surgical airway of choice in children and patients with tracheal injury.

4. **Fiberoptic intubation** allows visualization of the cords and trachea but is technically difficult and time-consuming.

5. In **tactile intubation**, the practitioner uses his or her index and middle fingers to palpate the epiglottis and guide the tube through the cords. The patient needs to be comatose or heavily sedated, and the success rate is lower than that of RSI.

6. **Retrograde intubation** involves placing a wire through the cricoid membrane and securing it through the mouth. The wire is used as a guide to pass the endotracheal tube.

7. **Percutaneous transtracheal ventilation** involves inserting a catheter into the trachea and ventilating the patient with high-pressure oxygen.

The two last techniques are used rarely and require prior training or special equipment.

22. When the patient is intubated, how do I determine if the endotracheal tube is placed correctly?

The best method of confirming placement is to see the tube pass through the cords. Monitoring of oxygen saturation and the use of capnography or colorimetric end-tidal carbon dioxide devices are standard-of-care adjuncts. Other findings are helpful but are not definitive: The tube fogs and clears with ventilation; breath sounds are heard in both axillae but not over the stomach; and chest expansion is noted and symmetric.

23. Doesn't the chest radiograph confirm placement in the trachea?

No. Although the chest radiograph is helpful in ruling out bronchial intubation, the tube easily can be placed in the esophagus and appear to be in the trachea proximal to the carina.

BIBLIOGRAPHY

1. Bergen JM, Smith DC: A review of etomidate for rapid sequence intubation in the emergency department. J Emerg Med 15:221–230, 1997.
2. Dailey RH, Simon B: Pharmacologic aids in airway management. In Dailey RH, Simon B, Young GP, Stewart RD (eds): The Airway: Emergency Management. St. Louis, Mosby, 1992, pp 145–170.
3. Dufour DG, et al: Rapid sequence intubation in the emergency department. J Emerg Med 13:705–710, 1995.
4. Hamilton PY, Kang JJ: Emergency airway management. Mt Sinai J Med 64:292–301, 1997.
5. Marx JA, et al: Airway. In Marx JA, Hockberger RS, Walls RM (eds): Rosen's Emergency Medicine: Clinical Concepts. St. Louis, Mosby, 2002, pp 2–21.
6. Nordt SP, Clark RF: Midazolam: A review of therapeutic uses and toxicity. J Emerg Med 15:357–365, 1997.
7. Tryba M, et al: Rapid sequence orotracheal intubation with rocuronium: A randomized double-blind comparison with suxamethonium—preliminary communication. Eur J Anaesthesiol 9(suppl):44–48, 1994.

4. SHOCK

Robert D. Schmidt, M.D.

1. What is shock?

A clinical syndrome defined by inadequate blood flow and inadequate transport of oxygen to organs and tissues. It also has been defined as a reduction of blood flow by diminished cardiac output or maldistributed output such that potential irreversible cellular damage occurs.

2. Summarize the primary concerns when addressing a patient who presents with clinical shock.

Assessment of the **ABCs** (airway, breathing, and circulation) and **vital signs** should be included in the primary survey of all seriously ill or injured patients. All patients should receive supplemental high-flow oxygen, have large-bore intravenous access, and be placed on a cardiac monitor. Any obvious hemorrhage in trauma patients should be controlled. The initial goals are to improve oxygen delivery to the tissues and control excessive oxygen consumption. One way to control excessive oxygen consumption is by mechanical ventilation in a patient who is tachypneic and using accessory respiratory muscles.

3. Name the three pathophysiologic classifications of shock and give some examples of each class.

Hypovolemic

Examples: Gastrointestinal bleeds, ruptured aortic aneurysm, and severe diabetic ketoacidosis.

Vasogenic

Examples: Septic shock, anaphylactic shock, neurogenic shock, and shock from pharmacologic causes.

Cardiogenic

Examples: Acute myocardial infarction, cardiomyopathies, valvular abnormalities (especially severe aortic stenosis and regurgitation), arrhythmias, and pulmonary embolism (PE).

PE can be included as a separate classification—obstructive—but presents similarly to cardiogenic causes.

4. How is a patient's class of shock clinically determined?

History of blood loss, trauma, and gastrointestinal fluid losses is often evident in hypovolemic causes. One of the most helpful bedside tests is feeling the skin of the patient's extremities. Cool, moist skin suggests a hypovolemic or cardiogenic cause. Warm skin is helpful in distinguishing vasogenic causes (i.e., septic or neurogenic). The cardiovascular findings that suggest a cardiogenic cause are distention of neck veins, S3 gallop, and signs of pulmonary edema.

5. What are the body's compensatory mechanisms for loss of blood volume?

Cardiac output is decreased with loss of blood volume. A reflex tachycardia occurs to maintain adequate blood pressure. This tachycardia causes a release of epinephrine and norepinephrine, mediated by baroreceptors, by a reflex known as the **sympathoadrenal reaction**. These catecholamines increase cardiac output through improved contractility, an elevated pulse rate, and increased venous tone. Vasoconstriction is greatest in the splanchnic bed and musculoskeletal system, shunting more available blood to the heart and brain.

6. How sensitive are supine vital signs when determining volume loss?

Not very. The body can compensate for a 15% intravascular volume loss before developing a tachycardia. It may take a 30% volume loss to have a significant decrease in blood pressure.

7. Are orthostatic vital signs a sensitive indicator of hypovolemia? What determines a positive orthostatic test?

To know what is considered abnormal, you first must know what is normal. Studies on healthy *euvolemic* people showed an average increase in pulse of 12.6 to 17.9 beats/min with a large standard deviation. A pulse increase of 20 beats/min as a determinant for hypovolemia would be nonspecific because many normal individuals are within this range. A 30 beats/min increase in heart rate is a specific indicator of hypovolemia. A 20% volume loss is required to produce this change in heart rate, making this an insensitive test at best. The development of symptoms (e.g., dizziness on standing) does not occur in healthy euvolemic individuals on standing and should be considered abnormal. Patients with shock should be kept supine and not standing up, subjecting them to the effects of gravity.

8. What is a normal central venous pressure (CVP), and what are the four determinants of CVP?

Normal CVP is 5 to 12 cm H_2O. (1) Intravascular volume, (2) intrathoracic pressure, (3) right ventricular function, and (4) venous tone all affect the CVP. To reduce the variability caused by intrathoracic pressure, CVP should be measured at end expiration either in positive or negative pressure ventilation.

9. Do you need a pulmonary artery catheter to determine cardiac output?

No. Bioimpedance cardiography is becoming more available and may become a standard in some EDs in the future. By measuring change in the conduction of current across the thorax, these monitors can measure stroke volume, cardiac output, systemic vascular resistance (SVR), and diastolic cardiac function.

10. Define sepsis.

Sepsis is a condition associated with the presence of pathogenic microorganisms or their toxins in the blood. Shock from sepsis occurs from gram-negative bacteria in most cases but also can occur from gram-positive bacteria, viruses, protozoa, and fungi.

11. Name the causes of shock from sepsis.

Exotoxins and endotoxins are strong antigenic stimuli that cause the release of vasoactive substances, such as prostaglandins, cytokines, and nitric oxide, resulting in peripheral venous and arteriolar dilation. Production of myocardial depressant factors, including nitric oxide, reduce cardiac contractility. These mediators increase endothelial permeability, causing intravascular volume loss of fluid in the periphery.

12. What are the changes in SVR and cardiac output in septic shock?

Vascular tone and SVR are reduced in response to vasoactive mediators. With reduced SVR, cardiac output significantly increases initially. With progression of shock, cardiac output and ejection fraction decrease secondary to myocardial depressant factors. The heart no longer can compensate for reduced SVR, resulting in hypotension.

13. List the primary goals in the treatment of septic shock in the ED.

Maximize tissue oxygenation
Improve hemodynamic dysfunction
Correct underlying metabolic abnormalities
Treat the infection

14. What specific treatments are important when treating septic shock?

Supplemental oxygen should be given to any septic patient. All patients in septic shock have intravascular volume loss and require aggressive volume resuscitation. If blood pressure and tissue perfusion, measured by mental status and urine output, do not improve with volume, dopamine can be started as an initial pressor agent in septic shock. Studies suggest avoiding dopamine alone in high doses. Norepinephrine (Levophed) alone or with dobutamine may be used in refractory shock. Septic shock is an indication for starting antibiotics in the ED. Antibiotic choice depends on the suspected source of the infection. If the source is unknown, broad-spectrum coverage of gram-positive and gram-negative organisms is appropriate.

15. What are newer therapies on the horizen for treating septic shock?

The focus in more recent years has been to control the host's inflammatory response because the mediators produced cause many of the circulatory deficiencies in septic shock. Clinical trials using steroids, nonsteroidal antiinflammatory drugs, antiendotoxin antibodies, and anticytokine therapies have been uniformly disappointing; however, early studies using activated protein C have been encouraging. Protein C interacts with protein S to reduce thrombin formation. The inflammatory responses of sepsis cause downregulation of this process, and thrombin is formed more readily. The Food and Drug Administration has given preliminary approval of the use of human activated protein C (drotrecogin alfa) in septic shock based on a single study of 1600 people that resulted in an absolute reduction in mortality of 6.1%.

16. Describe the Killip classifications of pump dysfunction in acute myocardial infarction.

The Killip classification is based on clinical criteria that correlate the degree of pump dysfunction with acute mortality in a patient with myocardial infarction. **Class I** exhibits no evidence of left ventricular failure and has a 5% mortality. **Class II** exhibits bibasilar rales, an S3 gallop, and a 15% to 20% mortality. **Class III** patients have pulmonary edema. These patients have a 40% mortality. **Class IV** patients are in cardiogenic shock defined by (1) systolic blood pressure less than 90 mm Hg, (2) peripheral vasoconstriction, (3) oliguria, and (4) pulmonary vascular congestion. Patients in Killip class IV have an 80% mortality. Autopsy studies on patients who died of pump failure with acute myocardial infarction typically have 35% to 70% left ventricular necrosis.

17. What is the significance of a loud holosystolic murmur in acute myocardial infarction?

Loud holosystolic murmurs indicate either papillary muscle rupture or acute ventricular septal defect. These may be indistinguishable, but acute ventricular septal defect usually occurs with an anteroseptal myocardial infarction and has an associated palpable thrill. Thrill does not occur often with papillary rupture, which usually is seen in inferior myocardial infarctions. These structural abnormalities cause shock because of reduced forward blood flow and can be differentiated by echocardiogram or by a Swan-Ganz catheter. Both require emergent cardiothoracic surgery consultation for early repair.

18. Describe a treatment algorithm for cardiogenic shock in patients with myocardial infarction.

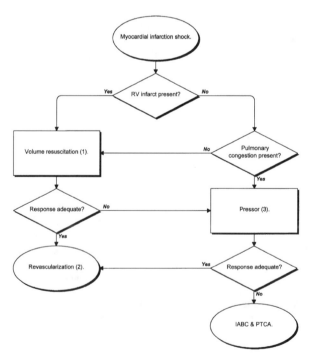

Cardiogenic shock in myocardial infarction. (1) Aliquots of 200–300 cc normal saline. (2) Thrombolytic therapy or direct PTCA. (3) See question 20. RV = right ventricular; IABC = intra-aortic balloon counterpulsation; PTCA = percutaneous transluminal coronary angioplasty.

19. Which pressors should be used in the treatment of cardiogenic shock?

In patients with systolic blood pressure of 90 to 100 mm Hg with pulmonary edema, dobutamine may be an excellent single pressor agent. Its primary β effect increases cardiac output, reduces left ventricular end-diastolic pressure (LVEDP), and reduces SVR. Studies suggest avoiding dopamine in high doses as a single pressor agent; norepinephrine and dobutamine may have significant hemodynamic advantages in the treatment of shock.

20. What determines the coronary artery filling pressure? What is its significance in cardiogenic shock?

LVEDP = coronary artery filling pressure. In cardiogenic shock, coronary artery filling pressure can be quite low and may cause further myocardial tissue necrosis in myocardial infarction. Steps must be taken to improve coronary artery filling pressure because diastolic pressure is low and LVEDP is high. Diastolic pressure in the aorta is increased by dopamine, norepinephrine, epinephrine, and intraaortic balloon counterpulsation. LVEDP is reduced by dobutamine, diuretics, and intraaortic balloon counterpulsation.

21. How does PE cause shock?

Massive PE causes shock by reducing the cross-sectional area of the pulmonary outflow tract. Shock occurs at a reduction of 50% or more of the cross-sectional area in normal individuals. With this acute reduction in area, the pulmonary artery systolic pressure maximum of 40 mm Hg is reached, blood flow is reduced, and shock ensues. Pulmonary vasoconstriction by mediators such as thromboxane A_2 and serotonin also may play a role in increasing the obstruction.

22. What is the treatment for shock from a massive PE?

Massive PE should be treated similarly to cardiogenic shock from myocardial infarction, using oxygen (intubation if necessary), volume, and pressors. Thrombolytic use has shown improved hemodynamics with reduced tricuspid regurgitation, reduced right ventricular dilation, and improved cardiac output in patients with massive PE. If right ventricular dysfunction is visable on echocardiogram, there are data showing improved mortality with thrombolytic treatment. If a patient arrests in the ED with a known PE, open thoracotomy and pulmonary artery massage may break up a saddle embolus and allow blood flow. The success rate is low, but then again so is the alternative.

23. How should I approach the patient with hemorrhagic shock?

Search for the cause of blood loss. A chest radiograph is key to look for a widened mediastinum or a hemothorax. A pelvis radiograph for fractures is important because pelvic fractures can cause rapidly progressive shock and death from hemorrhage. Obtain appropriate diagnostic studies to rule out peritoneal hemorrhage (see Chapter 111, Abdominal Trauma). Control external hemorrhage with pressure and hemorrhage from pelvic fractures with MAST pants or a sheet tied around the pelvis. A baseline hematocrit and a blood sample for type and crossmatching blood are crucial initial laboratory tests. Lactate levels and base deficit are helpful in determining need for volume resuscitation and mortality. Lactate levels greater than 4.0 mmol/L have significantly higher requirements for fluid and blood administration. A base deficit greater than 15 mmol/L correlates with significantly higher mortality.

24. How should volume resuscitation be done in the ED in patients with hypovolemic shock from trauma?

Please see Figure, top of next page.

25. What is neurogenic shock, and how should it be managed?

In acute cervical and upper thoracic spinal cord injuries, sympathetic tone is lost to regions distal to the lesion, causing arteriolar and venous dilation. Bradycardia can be seen with cervical lesions resulting from reduced sympathetic stimulation to the sinus node. Any degree of hypovolemia from other injuries can cause extremely low blood pressures.

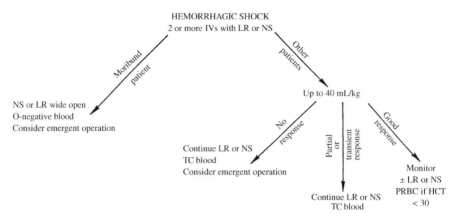

Fluid resuscitation of hemorrhagic shock. NS, normal saline; LR, lactated Ringer's solution; TC, typed and crossmatched blood; PRBC, packed red blood cells; HCT, hematocrit. (Adapted from Mannix FL: Hemorrhagic shock. In Rosen P, et al (eds): Emergency Medicine: Concepts and Clinical Practice, 2nd ed. St. Louis, Mosby, 1988, p 179.)

Neurogenic shock should be managed with volume (40 mL/kg of crystalloid), atropine if brady-cardia is present, and an α-agonist (dopamine or ephedrine) for refractory hypotension. Anaphylaxis causing cardiovascular compromise and vasodilation is another form of neurogenic shock, which although rare requires specific therapy with epinephrine (see Chapter 18, Anaphylaxis).

26. Name four causes of cardiogenic shock in trauma.
Pericardial tamponade, myocardial contusion, tension pneumothorax, and air gas embolism from bronchial tears.

27. When should pericardial tamponade be suspected?
Acute pericardial tamponade occurs in about 2% of penetrating chest wounds and is more common with stab wounds than gunshot wounds. Tamponade is rare after blunt trauma. Beck's classic triad of distended neck veins, decreased arterial pressure, and muffled heart sounds occurs in only one third of patients. A high CVP in the face of tachycardia and hypotension in penetrating trauma is a reliable indicator of tamponade. ED ultrasound should be done when this diagnosis is suspected. Physical examination and chest radiographs exclude tension pneumothorax.

CONTROVERSIES

28. Should dopamine be used as the initial pressor in cardiogenic and septic shock?
Pro: Dopamine has a long history of use in treating cardiogenic and septic shock. Its combined α and β effects make it the ideal single medication in both of these senarios.
Con: In mild cardiogenic shock in patients with systolic blood pressure of 90 to 100 mm Hg and pulmonary edema, dobutamine is an excellent single pressor agent. Its primary β effect increases cardiac output, reduces LVEDP, and reduces SVR. Studies recommend avoiding dopamine in high doses as a single pressor agent and suggest that norepinephrine and dobutamine may have significant hemodynamic advantages in the treatment of shock. In patients with septic shock, the combination of dobutamine and norepinephrine improved cardiac index and acid-base status. The combination therapy is often successful in cases of hypotension resistant to dopamine alone.

29. Should hemorrhagic shock be treated with large volumes of crystalloid before blood administration?
Pro: For years, emergency phycisians and surgeons treated hemorrhagic shock with rapid crystalloid infusion up to 60 mL/kg before infusing blood. Hemodynamics and tissue perfusion

are improved. If crystalloid is given early instead of blood, there may be less need for transfusion.

Con: More recent data suggest that rapid infusion of crystalloid may be harmful in patients with moderate hypotension, and blood should be given immediately as the initial volume expansion agent. Increasing the blood pressure in a hypotensive patient with injuries may increase blood loss because of higher pressure and thrombolysis of clot. Animal studies suggest that mortality is reduced when blood is used for initial resuscitation versus crystalloid.

30. Should drotrecogin a be used routinely in the treatment of severe sepsis?

Pro: In a randomized, controlled prospective multicenter trial, there was 6% increased survival at 28 days.

Con: The medication is expensive, it requires a 96-hour continuous infusion in the ICU, and it increases the risk of serious bleeding. It should be used only in patients with a high risk of mortality.

BIBLIOGRAPHY

1. Bernard GR, Vincent JL, et al: Efficacy and safety of recombinant human activated protein C for severe sepsis. N Engl J Med 344:699–709, 2001.
2. Bickell WH, Wall MJ, Pepe PE, et al: Immediate versus delayed fluid resuscitation for hypotensive patients with penetrating torso injuries, N Engl J Med 331:1105–1109, 1994.
3. Freeman BD, Natanson C: Anti-inflammatory therapies in sepsis and septic shock. Expert Opin Invest Drugs 9:1651–1653, 2000.
4. Hanneman L, Reinhart K, Grenzer O, et al: Comparison of dopamine to dobutamine and norepinephrine for oxygen delivery and uptake in septic shock. Crit Care Med 23:1962–1970, 1995.
5. Kline JA: Shock. In Rosen P, Barkin RM (eds): Emergency Medicine: Concepts and Clinical Practice, 4th ed. St. Louis, Mosby, 1998, pp 86–106.
6. Konstantinides S, Giebel A, Kasper W: Submassive and massive pulmonary emolism: A target for thrombolytic therapy? Thromb Haemost 82(suppl 1):104–108, 1999.
7. Kox WJ, Volk T, Kox SN, et al: Immunomodulatory therapies in sepsis. Intensive Care Med 26(suppl 1):S124–128, 2000.
8. Rosenberg P, Yancy CW: Noninvasive assessment of hemodynamics: An emphasis on bioimpedance cardiography. Curr Opin Cardiol 153:151–155, 2000.
9. Rutherford EJ, Morris JA, Reed GW, et al: Base deficit stratifies mortality and determines therapy. J Trauma 33:417–423, 1992.
10. Schoonover LL, Stewart AS, Clifton GD: Hemodynamic and cardiovascular effects of nitric oxide modulation in the therapy of septic shock. Pharmacotherapy 20:1184–1197, 2000.

5. EMERGENCY ULTRASOUND

John L. Kendall, M.D., and Katherine Bakes, M.D.

1. What is ED ultrasound all about?

An ultrasound probe in the hands of the clinician is the stethoscope of the 21st century. It is noninvasive; it is safe; and when used appropriately, it can be another tool with which to perform certain focused aspects of the physical examination.

2. Why should ultrasound be performed in the ED?

Limited ultrasound examinations performed by ED physicians allow for more timely, less invasive, and safer evaluations of patients. Ectopic pregnancy and biliary colic may be evaluated rapidly, intraabdominal traumatic hemorrhage may be diagnosed without the invasiveness of diagnostic peritoneal lavage or the delay of a CT scan, and patients with major trauma or suspected abdominal aortic aneurysm (AAA) may be evaluated quickly in the safety of the ED.

3. How does emergency ultrasound differ from ultrasound performed by the radiology department?

Emergency ultrasound is meant to be a limited, goal-directed examination. Specific findings, such as the presence of intraperitoneal fluid in blunt abdominal trauma; intrauterine pregnancy (IUP) in suspected ectopic pregnancy; gallstones, wall thickness, or sonographic Murphy's sign in right upper quadrant pain; aortic dilation in suspected AAA; and pericardial fluid in patients with possible pericardial tamponade, are used to guide patient care. In contrast, a radiologist-performed ultrasound is more comprehensive. All of the structures in the requested type of ultrasound are evaluated and commented on.

Another significant difference is that an emergency ultrasound is used primarily to *rule in* pathology. Positive findings are acted on, whereas negative or equivocal studies should be confirmed by a formal imaging study. In comparison, the radiologist uses ultrasound to rule in and rule out pathology.

4. How about some basic ultrasonography physics?

Ultrasound images are generated as sound waves at various frequencies (MHz) that reflect off tissue interfaces. The higher the ultrasound frequency, the greater the resolution, but at the cost of reduced tissue penetration. Dense tissues, such as bone or gallstones, appear bright because most of the ultrasound energy is absorbed or reflected. Solid organs, such as the liver or spleen, show a gray scale of tissue architecture. All of the ultrasound energy passes through fluid or blood, leaving a black, or anechoic, area on the screen. Ultrasound energy does not propagate through air well so that lung and hollow viscous structures are difficult to visualize. In general, abdominal and cardiac examinations are done using 3.5- to 5-MHz probes, transvaginal ultrasound examinations use 7.5- to 10-MHz probes, and vascular studies use 10- to 12-MHz specialized probes.

5. Describe the basics of the trauma ultrasound examination.

The trauma ultrasound examination is done rapidly at the patient's bedside during the secondary survey. The primary goal is to detect free intraperitoneal fluid, which appears as anechoic areas within the peritoneal cavity. Sites in the abdomen that are evaluated are the potential spaces that occur at dependent sites within the peritoneal cavity. These include the hepatorenal recess or Morison's pouch (see Figure), splenorenal recess, retrovesicular recess (pouch of Douglas), and both pericolic gutters.

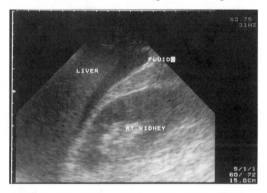

View of Morison's pouch shows intraperitoneal fluid.

Oblique views of the right and left chest are obtained to search for hemothorax, and a subxyphoid or left parasternal cardiac image is obtained to locate pericardial effusion (see Figure, top of next page).

6. Where is the best place to look for intraperitoneal fluid?

The sonographic examination should include all of the sites mentioned previously. The sensitivity increases from approximately 60% if one site is viewed to almost 90% if all sites are used. At least one study has shown the most sensitive site to be the pouch of Douglas (58% sensitive).

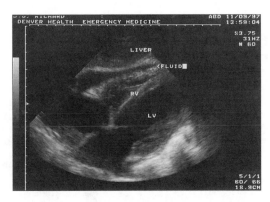

Subxyphoid cardiac view shows a pericardial effusion.

7. How does ultrasound compare with traditional means of evaluating the traumatic abdomen?

Physical examination is only 50% to 60% sensitive for detecting abdominal injuries after blunt trauma. Diagnostic peritoneal lavage is 95% sensitive but is not specific, resulting in unnecessary laparotomies. CT is sensitive for detecting abdominal injuries (> 95%) but is costly, is time-consuming, and requires the patient to leave the ED. Prospective studies of ultrasound showed an 85% to 90% sensitivity for the detection of hemoperitoneum, with sensitivity approaching 100% in patients who were hypotensive from an abdominal source. The accuracy of ultrasound to detect the underlying parenchymal lesion varies widely.

8. How should I use ultrasound in my evaluation of blunt trauma patients?

A good start would be to consider it for patient scenarios based on vital signs and ultrasound findings: (1) stable vital signs, negative ultrasound; (2) stable vital signs, positive ultrasound; (3) unstable vital signs, negative ultrasound; and (4) unstable vital signs, positive ultrasound. Patients with stable vital signs and a negative ultrasound who have no other significant injuries, have normal mental status, and are not intoxicated can be managed with observation, serial physical examinations, and serial ultrasound studies. Patients with stable vital signs and a positive ultrasound warrant an abdominal CT scan. If the vital signs are unstable and ultrasound is negative or indeterminate, a bedside diagnostic peritoneal lavage should be done. If the vital signs are unstable and the ultrasound is positive for free fluid, the patient should go directly to laparotomy.

9. Can I tell how much intraperitoneal fluid is present based on the ultrasound image?

No. Conflicting data exist, but no study has yet shown any accurate means of quantifying the amount of intraperitoneal fluid that is present based on its sonographic appearance.

10. What are some of the pitfalls I may encounter during a trauma ultrasound examination of the abdomen?

Although relatively rare, one of the more concerning aspects of emergency ultrasound is the false-negative study. In terms of abdominal trauma, clotted blood is the finding that mimics a negative study the closest. An example of clotted blood found in Morison's pouch is shown in the Figure, top of next page. It initially was interpreted to be liver parenchyma because of a similar echogenic pattern. False-positive findings simulate hemoperitoneum. Examples are ascites, urine from a ruptured bladder, bowel contents from bowel perforation, perinephric fat, and fluid-filled bowel.

11. What is the sonographic appearance of the gallbladder and related structures?

The gallbladder is cystic, so the sonographic appearance is a pearlike structure that is anechoic. Surrounding this anechoic area is a ring of midechogenicity that corresponds to the gallbladder wall. Normally, it is less than 4 mm wide but can be thicker immediately after eating or if in edematous states, such as liver disease, ascites, congestive heart failure, renal disease, or

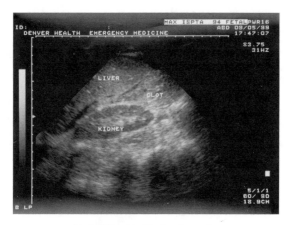

Clotted blood in Morison's pouch.

AIDS. Stones are typically circular in nature; can be of any size; and are bright, or hyperechoic, on their proximal side. Ultrasound does not penetrate stones well, so distal to the stone there is a shadow (see Figure). This also is called the *headlight sign*, signifying the presence of a calcified gallstone. Sludge is a collection of the precipitants of bile that layers within the gallbladder and appears sonographically as mildly echogenic material without any shadowing.

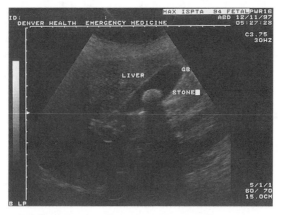

Long-axis view of the gallbladder shows a gallstone. The gallstone is represented by an echogenic proximal surface and distal attenuation shadow.

12. What findings are suggestive of acute cholecystitis?

The primary findings of the emergency gallbladder ultrasound are the presence of stones, sonographic Murphy's sign (defined as maximal tenderness over an ultrasound-detected gallbladder), and wall thickening (> 4 mm). The presence of all three primary findings has a 99% positive predictive value for the presence of gallbladder disease. Other findings, such as ductal dilation, pericholecystic fluid, sludge, and an emphysematous gallbladder, are considered to be secondary findings and are less reliably seen by emergency sonographers. Ultrasound is insensitive at detecting choledocholithiasis.

13. What are the indications for pelvic ultrasonography in the ED?

Ultrasonography is the imaging study of choice for evaluating abdominal pain or bleeding in pregnant patients in the first or second trimester. The goal of ED ultrasound is to establish the presence of an intrauterine pregnancy (IUP), so as to rule out effectively an ectopic pregnancy.

Ectopic pregnancy is the second leading cause overall of maternal mortality and the number one cause of maternal mortality during the first trimester.

14. How early can an IUP be detected using ultrasound? What value of β-human chorionic gonadotropin (HCG) does this correspond to?

An IUP may be detectable at 5 weeks by transvaginal ultrasound at a β-HCG level of 1800 mIU/mL and at 6 weeks or greater with a β-HCG of 5000 mIU/mL using transabdominal ultrasound. The **discriminatory zone**, or level of β-HCG at which one would expect to see evidence of an IUP, depends on the institution.

15. How sensitive is ultrasound for the evaluation of ectopic pregnancy?

Several studies have shown that 75% to 80% of patients have a diagnostic ultrasound (i.e., either an IUP or a demonstrable ectopic pregnancy). The problem is that in the remaining 20% of patients with nondiagnostic ultrasounds, nearly one fourth have ectopic pregnancies. This increase in ectopic pregnancy among patients with nondiagnostic ultrasound suggests that this group should have an aggressive workup, including an obstetric-gynecologic consultation in the ED.

16. Describe the pitfalls in pelvic ultrasonography.

For emergency physicians, the goal of pelvic ultrasonography is to determine whether an IUP is present. It is not clear how well emergency physicians evaluate the adnexa, pelvic free fluid, or ovaries. Cornual pregnancies may be mistaken for an IUP, with an attendant risk of rupture and hemorrhage. The question of heterotopic pregnancies (i.e., simultaneous IUP and ectopic pregnancy) must be considered. In populations without risk factors for ectopic pregnancy, the risk of a heterotopic gestation is approximately 1 in 30,000 pregnancies. The incidence increases markedly, however, in patients with preexisting pelvic inflammatory disease or scarring and is greatest for patients receiving medical fertility assistance, in whom the incidence is estimated to be 1 in 100 to 1 in 400 pregnancies. A pseudosac can be seen in 20% of ectopic pregnancies. It is formed in response to the β-HCG produced by the abdnormal pregnancy. It consists of a single-ringed structure in the endometrial cavity, and it can be mistaken for a true gestational sac, which consists of **two** concentric rings.

17. What abdominal structure can be evaluated by emergency ultrasound?

Evaluation of the abdominal aorta can be useful in elderly patients who present with a pulsatile abdominal mass, nontraumatic abdominal pain or flank pain, hypotension of unknown cause, or unexplained pulseless electrical activity. AAA is manifested by aortic diameter greater than 3 cm with most symptomatic aneurysms being greater than 5 cm (see Figure). Studies by radiologists and emergency physicians showed sensitivity and specificity of 100% for the detection of AAA. Studies showed a 90% correlation of ultrasound-determined aortic diameter to pathologic specimens.

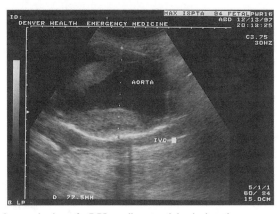

Long-axis view of a 7.75-cm diameter abdominal aortic aneurysm.

18. What is the significance of increased aortic diameter?

Longitudinal studies have shown that patients with AAA have an increase in aortic diameter of approximately 0.5 cm per year. Patients with an aortic diameter of greater than 5 cm have a 25% chance of rupture within 5 years, with larger aneurysms having a greater chance of rupture. Aneurysms that rupture have a mortality of greater than 80%, so ultrasound is an important tool in the detection of AAA.

19. Describe the uses of cardiac ultrasonography in the ED.

There are two primary indications for cardiac ultrasonography in the ED. It may be used during the trauma examination to detect pericardial effusions in patients thought to have mechanisms of injury or clinical presentations consistent with pericardial tamponade or cardiac rupture. Detection of nontraumatic pericardial effusions is also possible (i.e., malignancy, uremic, rheumatologic). The other major indication is for the evaluation of patients presenting in cardiac arrest. Contractility can be assessed in patients presenting in cardiac arrest when there is a question of pulseless electrical activity. When patients have no evidence of cardiac contractility and other reversible causes of pulseless electrical activity have been ruled out, strong consideration should be given to terminating the resuscitation.

20. How can ultrasound be used to evaluate flank pain?

Ultrasound has been used to identify hydronephrosis and urinary calculi. Hydronephrosis is dilation of the renal pelvis and ureter caused by distal obstruction of the collecting system. Urinary calculi can be seen at any point from the renal pelvis to the ureteral-vesicular junction and appear as hyperechoic, round structures with distal attenuation shadows.

21. What is the role of ultrasound in the evaluation of patients with flank pain?

The results of studies have been discouraging. By itself, ultrasound is only 64% to 75% sensitive for the identification of renal calculi and even less sensitive for the evaluation of acute hydronephrosis. Studies that combined kidney, ureter, and bladder radiographs and ultrasound in well-hydrated patients showed improved ability to identify kidney stones and hydronephrosis, but additional studies need to be done to address this issue further.

22. What are some future applications for emergency ultrasound?

The indications for emergency ultrasound are likely to grow as more physicians use it. Some examples are the ultrasound guidance of procedures such as central vascular access, bladder catheterization, or localization of abscesses. Ultrasound might be used to do serial examinations or to localize the site of solid organ injury in patients with blunt abdominal trauma. Testicular torsion and deep venous thrombosis are other types of pathology that are evaluated best by emergency Doppler ultrasound.

BIBLIOGRAPHY

1. Braffman BH, Coleman BG, Ramchandani P, et al: Emergency department screening for ectopic pregnancy: A prospective US study. Radiology 190:797–802, 1994.
2. Branney SW, Moore EE, Cantrill SV, et al: Ultrasound based key clinical pathway reduces the use of hospital resources for the evaluation of blunt abdominal trauma. J Trauma 42:1086–1090, 1997.
3. Kendall JL, Shimp RJ: Performance and interpretation of focused right upper quadrant ultrasound by emergency physicians. J Emerg Med 21:7–13, 2001.
4. Ma OJ, Kefer MP, Mateer JR, Thoma B: Evaluation of hemoperitoneum using a single- vs multiple-view ultrasonographic examination. Acad Emerg Med 2:581–586, 1995.
5. Mayron R, Gaudio FE, Plummer D, et al: Echocardiography performed by emergency physicians: Impact on diagnosis and therapy. Ann Emerg Med 17:150–154, 1988.
6. Nordenholz KE, Rubin MA, Gularte GG, Liang HK: Ultrasound in the evaluation and management of blunt abdominal trauma. Ann Emerg Med 29:357–366, 1997.
7. Ralls PW, Colletti PM, Chandrasoma P, et al: Real-time sonography in suspected acute cholecystitis. Radiology 155:767–771, 1985.
8. Schlager D, Lazzareschi G, Whitten D, et al: A prospective study of ultrasonography in the ED by emergency physicians. Am J Emerg Med 12:185–189, 1994.

6. GERIATRIC EMERGENCY MEDICINE

Kenneth C. Jackimczyk, M.D., and Winston Tripp, M.D.

1. Why dedicate a chapter to geriatric emergency medicine?

In 1990, approximately 31 million people were older than age 65 in the United States. By the year 2030, this number is expected to double, and over the next 20 years the number of individuals older than age 85 will grow three times faster than the general population. Geriatric patients (≥ 65 years old) account for 15% of all ED visits. Elderly patients frequently arrive in ambulances, stay in the ED longer, require more diagnostic studies, and have a higher admission rate than younger patients.

2. List the top 10 reasons elderly patients come to the ED.

1. Chest pain
2. Trauma
3. Pneumonia
4. Congestive heart failure
5. Abdominal pain
6. Electrolyte imbalance or dehydration
7. Stroke
8. Diabetes
9. Change in mental status
10. Sepsis

3. How can EMS personnel facilitate the care of elderly patients?

Elderly patients account for more than one third of EMS transports to the ED. EMS personnel can obtain information from family or health care workers at the scene regarding the patient's social and physical environment, their baseline functional and mental status, and the reason for EMS activation. Ambulance personnel can bring to the physician lists of medications the patient is using and any documentation regarding living wills or advance directives.

4. What are the four types of elder abuse?

1. **Physical abuse**: Nonaccidental force that results in bodily injury, pain, or impairment (e.g., hitting, biting, slapping, sexual assault, burns, or unreasonable restraint [physical, chemical]).

2. **Psychological abuse**: An act carried out with the intent of causing emotional pain or injury (e.g., threats to abandon, institutionalize, or harm physically).

3. **Exploitation**: Caretaker use of the resources of an elder for monetary or personal profit (e.g., stealing Social Security checks or retirement checks or coercion to change wills or other legal documents).

4. **Neglect**: Failure of the caretaker to provide the services necessary to avoid physical harm, mental anguish, or mental illness. This neglect can be *intentional* (e.g., willfully withholding food or medicine, abandonment for prolonged periods, or failure to provide proper hygiene) or *unintentional* (e.g., caretaker forgets to administer medicine or food or is physically unable to provide services for the patient).

5. List red flags that should alert the physician to the possibility of elder abuse.
History
- Delay in presentation with injury
- Discrepancies in history between patient and caregiver
- Vague or implausible explanation for injury

- Frequent ED visits for a chronic illness (despite a clear and previously defined medical plan)
- No caregiver accompanying an impaired patient to the ED

Physical examination
- Subdued or withdrawn behavior
- Unkempt or soiled appearance
- Poor nutrition or dehydration
- Multiple or unexplained bruises, cuts, or burns
- Gross decubiti
- Bites
- Rectal or vaginal bruises or tears
- Occult fracture

6. Why is it important to know the elderly patient's current medications?

Drug-drug interactions or side effects are a substantial cause of morbidity in elderly patients, resulting in 5% of elderly hospital admissions. It should be one of the top differential diagnoses in elderly patients presenting with a decline in mental or functional status. The elderly use 33% of all prescription drugs sold in the United States. The average elderly person uses more than four prescription medications and more than two over-the-counter medications daily. These numbers are even higher for institutionalized patients. Adverse reactions to medications occur twice as often in the elderly and are directly proportional to the number of medications they are taking. Be careful when prescribing new medications for the elderly patient. Avoid medications with sedative or anticholinergic properties because they commonly cause untoward side effects.

7. Should I worry if a geriatric trauma victim has normal vital signs with apparently minor injuries?

Yes. Elderly trauma victims have six times the mortality of younger patients. Elderly patients have a decreased cardiovascular reserve and an increased propensity for long-bone fractures. Even minor trauma may cause serious morbidity and mortality. Normal vital signs or a low injury severity score should never put the emergency physician at ease. Early but judicious resuscitation is the key to managing elderly trauma patients successfully. The more expeditiously patients can be moved to an ICU setting with invasive central monitoring, the better their chance of survival.

8. Which presentations in geriatric trauma are associated with an extremely high mortality rate?

- Automobile-pedestrian accidents
- Presenting systolic blood pressure less than 130 mm Hg
- Acidosis (pH < 7.35)
- Multiple fractures
- Head injury (67% of unconscious elderly trauma patients die)
- Pelvic fractures

9. Aren't falls a fact of life in the elderly?

No. Any fall in an elderly patient should raise concern. Although falls are more common in the elderly because of waning sensory input and gait disturbances, a more serious cause may be present. Falls are a significant cause of morbidity and mortality in elderly patients, and 50% of hospitalized patients die within 1 year of their fall. In addition to treating the physical trauma from the fall, the ED physician should determine the cause of the fall. Try to determine whether the fall occurred secondary to environmental causes or from a more concerning physiologic event. The differential diagnosis for physiologic causes includes syncope, arrhythmias, cerebrovascular accident, myocardial infarction, adverse drug effects, alcohol use, infection, and metabolic disorders. Environmental causes include items such as loose rugs or low-lying tables.

10. Don't elderly patients always have abnormal laboratory values?

No. In contrast to pediatric patients, most laboratory values in elderly patients do not require different reference ranges from traditional adult values. The fact that the patient is old should not be used to justify abnormal laboratory values. There are, however, some exceptions in patients older than age 65:

- Elevated serum alkaline phosphatase (may be 2.5 times greater than the normal)
- Elevated fasting blood glucose (135 to 150)
- Elevated erythrocyte sedimentation (40 mm/h)
- Decreased hemoglobin (11.0 g/dL in women or 11.5 g/dL in men)
- Elevated blood urea nitrogen (28 to 35 mg/dL)

11. Can procedural sedation be performed safely in the geriatric patient?

Yes. The physician must be aware of the altered pharmacokinetics and pharmacodynamics in the elderly. As the body ages, there is a reduction in lean body mass and total body water and an increase in total body fat. There also is a decrease in renal and hepatic blood flow. This has an effect on the metabolism and the distribution of medications administered to an elderly patient. Elderly patients have increased central nervous system sensitivity to analgesic and sedative medications. Remember: *start low and go slow*.

12. Why should I be concerned about atypical presentations of acute myocardial infarction (AMI) in the elderly?

Because AMI is the leading cause of death in the elderly. Half of all AMIs occur in the elderly and result in 80% of all deaths due to AMI. Nearly 40% of elderly patients diagnosed with AMI did not complain of chest pain on presentation, and, similarly, 50% had no evidence of ischemia or infarct on their presenting ECG. For these reasons, it is imperative that the ED physician know the atypical presentations of AMI in elderly patients. The mnemonic **GRAND-FATHERS** refers to atypical presentations of AMI in the elderly:

General malaise	**F**alls or **F**lu symptoms
Refers to a gastrointestinal complaint	**A**typical chest pain
Altered mental status	**T**rouble walking
Neurologic deficits	**H**ypotension
Dyspnea	**E**xhaustion
	Reverse in functional status
	Syncope or presyncope

13. Should I resuscitate the elderly patient in cardiac arrest?

Yes. Resuscitation studies document no difference in the percentage of successful outcomes across the age spectrum. Unless there is a well-defined advance directive, there should be no discrimination based on age in resuscitating elderly patients in cardiac arrest.

14. Is it safe to use thrombolytics in the elderly patient?

Yes. Most studies show benefits to using thrombolytics in the elderly. There is a twofold incidence of intracerebral hemorrhage in the elderly.

15. What is the most common surgical cause of acute abdominal pain in the elderly?

Cholecystitis. Acute abdominal pain in elderly patients is a serious complaint. Usually there is a delay in their presentation, which makes perforation more likely. Slightly more than 50% of elderly patients with acute abdominal pain have the *typical presentation* of their disease. Pay attention to vital signs, but do not be lulled into a false sense of security by normal vital signs. Do not delay surgical consultation waiting for laboratory results or radiographs. Keep a broad differential diagnosis, remembering the common causes such as appendicitis, but also including diseases specific to the elderly, such as diverticulitis, volvulus, mesenteric ischemia, abdominal aortic aneurysm, and carcinomas. Do not forget extraabdominal sources, such as pneumonia or AMI.

16. Which is more serious, dementia or delirium? How do I differentiate between them?

Delirium. Delirium is considered a medical emergency. A change in mental status is a common presentation to the ED for many elderly patients. It is common for patients already to have an underlying dementia. To attribute the change in mental status to worsening dementia is a serious error because delirium is reversible and carries with it a higher mortality.

DELIRIUM	DEMENTIA
Acute in onset	Insidious in onset
Decreased level of consciousness	Clear consciousness
Waxes and wanes	Progressive decline
Reversible cause	Usually irreversible cause
Irregular sleep-wake pattern	Regular sleep-wake pattern

17. Are there special concerns in discharging elderly patients?

What to Consider When Discharging the Elderly Patient

Cognitive function
_ Can the patient still live independently and self-administer medications?

Physical function
_ Can the patient perform the activities of daily living?
_ Does the patient require assistance devices such as wheelchairs?

Physical environment
_ Can the patient safely return with his or her current cognitive or functional status?
_ Did the current environment contribute to the ED presentation?

Social environment
_ Will the caregiver or spouse be able to care for the patient?
_ Is health care supervision available?

Resources
_ Is there a telephone available?
_ Is there money available for medicine or follow-up appointments?
_ Is there transportation to get to a follow-up appointment?

BIBLIOGRAPHY

1. Bosker G, Schwartz G, Jones JS, Sequeira M (eds): Geriatric Emergency Medicine. St. Louis, Mosby, 1990.
2. D'Andrea CC: Geriatric trauma. In Ferrera PC, et al (eds): Trauma Management: An Emergency Medicine Approach. St. Louis, Mosby, 2001, pp 533–545.
3. Jones JS: Elder abuse and neglect: Responding to a national problem. Ann Emerg Med 23:845–848, 1994.
4. Lachs MS, Pillemer K: Abuse and neglect of elderly persons. N Engl J Med 332:437–443, 1995.
5. Mandavia D: Geriatric trauma. Emerg Med Clin North Am 16:257–274, 1998.
6. McLeskey CH: Geriatric Anesthesia. Baltimore, Williams & Wilkins, 1997.
7. O'Keefe KP: Elderly patients with altered mental status. Emerg Med Clin North Am 16:701–715, 1998.
8. Sanders AB: Emergency Care of the Elder Person. St. Louis, Beverly Cracom Publications, 1996.

7. SAFETY ERRORS IN EMERGENCY MEDICINE

Patrick G. Croskerry, M.D., Ph.D., and Robert L. Wears, M.D., M.S.

1. The ED has been described as a *natural laboratory* for the study of safety. What makes it so?

EDs typically have a high number of error-producing conditions (EPCs) and violation-producing factors (VPFs). EPCs are primarily responsible for many of the errors that are made in the ED. VPFs arise more from the individuals who work in the ED and its culture.

2. Define some basic safety terms.

Error itself is a problematic concept, often dependent as much on the consequences of acts or omissions (which may not be under the physician's control) as the acts or omissions themselves. Working definitions have been proposed, however:

An *error* is the failure of a planned action to be completed as intended (i.e., error of execution) or the use of a wrong plan to achieve an aim (i.e., error of planning) without the intervention of some unforeseeable event.

Active errors are those whose effects are seen immediately. They most often are associated with individuals who perform on the front line, and the ED is as front line as it gets.

A *latent* error is one whose adverse consequences may lie dormant for some time, becoming evident only when it combines with other factors to breach the system's defenses. Individuals who designed the system often are responsible for latent errors.

Errors almost always are a retrospective understanding of behavior and are subject to ***hindsight bias***.

Slips are attentional or perceptual failures in the execution of an observable action sequence. Covert internal events (generally associated with memory failures) leading to a failure of execution are referred to as *lapses*. Slips and lapses are actions that deviate from the intended plan.

A *mistake* is a deficiency or failure in either the judgment or inferential process involved in the selection of an objective or in the specification of the means to achieve it, regardless of whether or not the actions directed by this decision scheme run according to plan.

A *medical error* is an undesirable event or omission that occurs in clinical practice that you would take steps to prevent happening again.

An *adverse event* or *adverse outcome* is an injury caused by medical management rather than the underlying condition of the patient. An adverse event attributable to error is a ***preventable adverse event***.

Negligent adverse events are a subset of preventable adverse events that satisfy legal criteria used in determining negligence (i.e., whether or not the care provided failed to meet the standard of care reasonably expected of an average physician qualified to take care of the patients in question).

3. I've heard the term *iatrogenic*—isn't that when physicians make mistakes?

Yes. The term *iatrogenic* originally was used to describe "disorders induced in the patient by autosuggestion based on the physician's examination, manner, or discussion" but later gained a broader definition as "the creation of additional problems or complications resulting from treatment by a physician or surgeon" (*Dorland's Medical Dictionary*, 25th edition, 1974). More recently, it has come to be used in a more general sense to describe adverse outcomes that result from a patient's treatment within the health care system.

4. What's the breakdown of safety problems in the ED?

We don't know because there have not been any systematic studies to date. Most of what is known comes from incidental observations made in major studies on hospitalized patients who

29

came through the ED, a few ED studies, and anecdotal observations. It seems that the error rate, especially of slips and lapses, is quite high, but that most of these are corrected before they result in an adverse outcome. One thing seems clear: The most costly and deadly errors generally result from mistakes associated with delayed or missed diagnoses.

5. **Am I likely to survive a career in emergency medicine without making a serious error?**
   No. When you work in the jungle, you get bitten by snakes.

6. **What's the ratio of detected to undetected failures?**
   About 1:50.

7. **What proportion of adverse events is preventable?**
   About 70%.

8. **What are EPCs? Give examples in the ED.**
   Any factor or condition that increases the probability of failure in a given system. The intrinsic properties of emergency medicine predispose it to error. There is no other area of medicine where this combination of EPCs exists.
   Examples:
   • Diagnostic uncertainty
   • High decision density
   • High cognitive load
   • VPFs
   • Novel or infrequently occurring situations
   • Time limitations for detection and correction of error
   • Low signal-to-noise ratio
   • Overcrowding/channel capacity overload (RACQITO; see question 14)
   • Mismatch between real and perceived risk
   • Poor feedback
   • Poor quality of person-to-person information transfer
   • Experience, training, or education limitations
   • Disruption of circadian rhythms by shift work
   • Compromised task pacing through interruptions or interventions
   • High physical and emotional stress levels

9. **Most of these conditions look self-evident, but what is meant by the *low signal-to-noise ratio* EPC?**
   Signals are crucial pieces of information that must not be missed. No signal is received in isolation. All signals are accompanied by noise, which consists of distracting stimuli or pieces of information that reduce the likelihood of detecting the signal. A **low signal-to-noise ratio** occurs when the base rate or incidence of the serious condition or diagnosis is low (e.g., subarachnoid hemorrhage) and well exceeded by the more common, usually benign diagnoses (tension and migraine headaches). The major problem in detection is that the signs and symptoms of the signal and the noise often can be similar to each other. Low signal-to-noise ratios exist for all serious conditions that present in the ED (e.g., abdominal aortic aneurysm as a cause of abdominal pain, pulmonary embolus as a cause of dyspnea, ectopic pregnancy as a cause of syncope, spinal column infection as a cause of low back pain, aortic dissection as a cause of chest pain).

10. **What is the significance of the *high cognitive load* EPC?**
    Cognitive load is the amount of thinking activity that an emergency physician must deal with at a given time. It requires varying degrees of memory, concentration, processing, and problem solving. Frequently, physicians are responsible for a variety of patients with a variety of illnesses, with a variety of acuities. It is akin to a juggler maintaining a number of objects in the air at the

same time. In no other branch of medicine is cognitive load so high and the burden of switching cognitive frames so great.

11. How can we reduce cognitive load and make fewer errors?

Any strategy or device that reduces the amount of cognitive work and cognitive time reduces cognitive load. Appropriate designation and delegation of tasks within the caregiver team distributes the cognitive load and reduces the individual burden.

Other examples:
- Mnemonics
- Hand-held computers
- Algorithms
- Decision rules
- Clinical practice guidelines/pathways
- Computerized physician order entry
- Computerized physician decision support
- Broselow-Luten pediatric resuscitation color-coding system

12. Don't all these aids lead to "medicine by numbers" and reduce my autonomy?

The practice of medicine is more complex than ever, and we need all the cognitive help we can get. There is ample room left for autonomy and clinical judgment.

13. How does the *poor feedback* EPC cause failures?

The efficient performance of any system depends on timely and reliable feedback. Good feedback results in good calibration, and physicians are no exception. In the absence of feedback, emergency physicians assume their diagnoses and management are acceptable, and there is no need to change behavior or recalibrate. The reliability and timeliness of feedback in the ED are generally poor.

14. What is RACQITO?

An acronym for **R**esource **A**vailability **C**ontinuous **Q**uality **I**mprovement **T**rade-**O**ff. It refers to conditions under which the vital signs of the ED become unstable. It is a tipping point at which a trade-off begins between the resources available to the ED and the ability of the people working there to maintain continuous quality improvement of care. Under conditions of RACQITO, the failure rate increases, and the quality of patient care declines.

15. What are VPFs? Give examples in the ED.

Violation-producing factors, which lead to error. They are associated with individual performance characteristics, having their origins in gender, cultural (local and general), and personality traits.

Examples:
- Underconfidence
- Overconfidence
- Perceived requirement to follow authority gradient
- Safety procedure compliance seen as an inconvenience
- Maladaptive group pressures
- Maladaptive copying behavior
- Risk-taking behavior
- Individual or group normalization of deviance

Some **necessary violations** are present in a complex system such as the ED. These are violations that are required to get the work done or meet production goals. For example, "working to rule" (i.e., refusing to engage in necessary violations) is a common job action strategy that can bring production to a halt.

16. What is normalization of deviance?

Deviance refers to the presence of individual or combinations of EPCs and VPFs. By definition, their presence is a deviation from a safe environment. Usually, they are identified, and the appropriate corrections are made to restore safety. In some EDs, however, insufficient resources or other limiting factors lead to persistence of these conditions. Eventually, people simply get used to working under these conditions (i.e., the deviance becomes normalized, and a chronic state of **RACQITO** is established).

17. What is the difference between safety management and continuous quality improvement?
Safety is a special case of quality. There is a great deal of overlap, but also significant differences. For example, delays in care are always low quality but may not always be unsafe.

18. Name the components of error management.
Error containment, error reduction, and error elimination.

19. Are we ever likely to eliminate error in the ED?
No, although it may be possible to make certain components of the system relatively error-free.

20. List examples of strategies for error management in the ED.
  • Designing good human factors engineering interfaces
  • Improved detection and assessment of latent error
  • Improved detection and reporting systems for error
  • Discovery, assessment, and elimination of specific EPCs
  • Cultural and individual awareness training to reduce VPFs
  • Recognizing RACQITO and the conditions that produce it
  • Improved awareness of error at departmental rounds
  • Training in containment and reduction of specific team errors
  • Specific training in the avoidance of procedural, affective, and cognitive errors
  • Improved response and support for individuals when adverse outcomes occur

21. What does the expression "geography is destiny" mean in the ED?
It refers to the **triage** process in the ED and the tendency to be treated according to where, or in whose territory, the patient happens to be. First, the triage system of EDs operates by trying to place the right patient in the right room. Eye complaints go to the eye room, cardiac complaints go to the cardiac room, and so on. Physicians and nurses tend to anchor on where the patient is placed initially (see question 37), which can be problematic and lead to error when the presenting symptoms are misleading (e.g., a complaint of constipation might be a dissecting abdominal aortic aneurysm). Emergency physicians need to maintain a state of willingness to undo geographical cues. Second, it refers to the natural tendency of experts to see particular problems within their own frame of reference. Right-sided abdominal pain in a woman may look like appendicitis to the surgeon, renal colic to the urologist, pelvic inflammatory disease to the gynecologist, and somatization to the psychiatrist. Experts are best engaged at the point at which the problem has become fairly well defined, and until it is, the emergency physician remains the best source of expertise.

22. What proportion of error in the ED is due to negligence?
Probably less than 5%. It is virtually meaningless to label bad outcomes as being the result of "bad apples." Human activity characterizes virtually all aspects of ED function, and whenever we see error and its consequences, it usually has been mediated by humans. Inevitably, physicians, nurses, technicians, and others are the human vector by which the error makes its appearance. This association of humans with error leads to a natural tendency to blame people when errors occur. This tendency is referred to as *fundamental attribution error*.

23. What is fundamental attribution error?
A term used by psychologists to describe the tendency to attribute blame to people when things go wrong. For example, if we see someone fall, we might characterize them as careless, clumsy, or accident-prone—we attribute the witnessed event to a failing, or dispositional qualities,

in that person. The person may have fallen, however, because the floor was slippery and they were on their way urgently to assist someone. In this case, less visible, situational factors might have been more responsible for the outcome. It is common to hear some emergency care providers abnegating responsibility for poor quality of care by virtue of the system and conditions under which they are obliged to work and over which they have limited control.

24. Do we make attribution errors in the management of our patients?

Yes (see question 30). This is the classic error made in the management of patients we do not like or whom we think could be exercising more control over their symptoms and disease. Several studies showed that emergency care providers may contribute iatrogenically to suicide through their attitudes toward psychiatric patients. Another example is the patient with borderline personality disorder who presents to the ED with self-inflicted cuts to the wrists. These wounds are perceived and often treated differently from accidental lacerations. Negative stereotyping has its basis in attribution error. We group classes of patients together (psychiatric patients, alcoholics, drug users, frequent flyers, somatizers) and attribute their behavior in the ED to dispositional factors. Physicians may be particularly prone to attribution error because they have so much autonomy and might be more likely to assume that others enjoy similar control over their behavior and lives.

25. Why are psychiatric patients especially vulnerable to error in the ED?

Historically, emergency physicians have failed to provide psychiatric patients with adequate medical clearance, have underestimated their concurrent physical illness, and have made attribution errors. Some studies suggested the attitudes of ED personnel can increase the risk of suicide in vulnerable patients. Part of the problem is that the psychiatric patient in the ED does not fit the type of model patient that physicians like to see.

Contrasting Features of Psychiatric and Nonpsychiatric Patients

FEATURE	NONPSYCHIATRIC PATIENT	PSYCHIATRIC PATIENT
Physical illness	Present	Absent
Behavior	Passive, compliant	Passive/aggressive, noncompliant
Attitude of patient	Grateful/appreciative	Neutral, ungrateful/resentful
Diagnosis	Mostly objective	Mostly subjective
Workup	Relatively fast	Usually slow
Laboratory/imaging studies	Contributory	Noncontributory
Management	Relatively clear	Difficult/deferred
Endpoint	Often definitive	Poor, revolving
Compliance	Usually good	Usually poor
Attitude of staff	Good, supportive	Often unsupportive

26. Do we make attribution errors in our perception of ourselves?

Yes. There is probably no one harder on physicians than physicians themselves. When we perceive ourselves as having committed an error, our reaction is often inappropriate, being overly harsh and punitive. By increasing our awareness and understanding of the nature of human error, we can develop a more appropriate response to it when it occurs.

27. This is beginning to sound like a psychology course.

Many of the terms that have come into usage in the new science of safety in health care have their origin in psychology. Much of the groundwork in this area was done by psychologists, ergonomists, sociologists, and others with a special interest in the area of human error. Some believe that cognitive psychology should be a required basic science for medical training.

28. Name the three major categories of mistakes made in the ED.

Procedural, affective, and cognitive.

29. What is procedural error? Give examples.

An error that occurs during the performance of a procedure. A procedural error involves some sort of psychomotor failure through a breakdown in or between motor function and visual and touch sensory modalities. Erorrs are often highly visible, their immediate consequences are apparent, and they are usually correctable by training.

Examples:
• Esophageal intubation
• Causing a pneumothorax putting in a central catheter
• Getting a venous sample while attempting an arterial blood gas
• Improper application of a cast
• Poor suturing technique
• Causing further injury while reducing a dislocation
• Injuring internal organs putting in a chest tube

30. Explain affective error.

Error occurs when the physician's affective state influences the quality and validity of clinical decision making. Affective error is usually occult, and physicians themselves may be unaware of the influence of their own affective state on decision making. The affective state can be independent of or related to patients in their care. An example of an independent instance is if the physician was experiencing a temporary mood disruption or even a depressed or hypomanic state. This mood change might result in the quality of decisions for all patients being compromised. Related instances occur when the physician develops feelings, either positive or negative, toward a specific patient or specific groups of patients. This is referred to as *countertransference*. **Negative countertransference** occurs when the physician develops negative feelings toward a patient, often on the basis of significant exemplars in the physician's past (i.e., the patient reminds the physician of a previous patient, class of patient, or some other figure with whom the physician has had a bad experience). As a result, the quality of decision making and care may be compromised. Patients with borderline personality disorder have an unusual capacity for generating negative countertransference in their caregivers. **Positive countertransference** also can compromise decision making and management. An example is overinvestigating a trivial complaint in a patient (through concern about not missing something significant) toward whom the physician has strong positive feelings. The **chagrin factor** is another example when physicians modify their investigations so that they do not expose themselves, or the patient, to the chagrin that might result from an undesirable finding. **Attribution error** (discussed in question 23) is an example of how negative judgmental behavior about patients may influence the quality of clinical decision making and outcomes.

31. Explain cognitive behavior.

Cognition is involved in all human behavior, from the simple **skill-based** levels; through the higher order, **rule-based** behaviors; to the most complex level of cognition, which is involved in **knowledge-based** behavior (see Table). There is some overlap in cognitive complexity between different levels. As experience accumulates, more behaviors can be relegated to lower levels of cognitive involvement. Paradoxically, novices operate at the knowledge-based level almost all the time, whereas experts operate at the skill-based level most of the time.

Complexity of Cognitive Behavior in the ED

LEVEL	ACTIVITY
Skill-based	Wound repair
	Dislocation reduction
	Intubation

(Table continued on next page.)

Complexity of Cognitive Behavior in the ED (cont.)

LEVEL	ACTIVITY
Rule-based	Radiographic decision rules Clinical practice guidelines Algorithms
Knowledge-based	Clinical decision making Management decisions Diagnostic reasoning

32. What is cognitive error?

Error at any level in the hierarchy of thinking processes. It is mostly at the highest level, **knowledge-based behavior**, where cognitive error leads to serious outcomes. The incidence of cognitive error increases under conditions of uncertainty, especially when thinking is hurried or pressured, and when heuristics are used. More common cognitive errors are referred to as *biases*, and some seem to be powerful and universal. Many biases are evident in the ED. Knowledge-based cognitive errors underlie preventable diagnostic errors, which can have serious consequences. Cognitive error, when viewed in retrospect, almost always is judged preventable.

33. In what areas of medicine are cognitive errors most likely?

Emergency medicine, family medicine, and internal medicine.

34. What are heuristics?

Strategies for thinking. The term usually refers to strategies that build economy and abbreviation into the thinking process. Essentially a well-established heuristic is a disposition or cognitive bias to respond in a particular way to a particular situation. For the most part, heuristics are useful in the ED, where physicians often are looking for short cuts.

35. Give examples of cognitive biases.

Many biases derive from three archetypal heuristics: **representativeness**, **availability**, and **anchoring**.

36. What is representativeness?

A subjective assessment or judgment of how similar a particular example is to its parent population. Patients who are experiencing angina classically present with gradual onset of a visceral quality of retrosternal pain, which may radiate to the arm, shoulder, neck, or jaw; lasts 5 to 15 minutes; and may be associated with nausea, diaphoresis, and dyspnea. These symptoms and signs generally are held to be representative of patients with angina. Some patients (geriatric, diabetic, female) are more likely, however, to present with atypical symptoms. The more unrepresentative the patient's presentation is, the greater the chances of the diagnosis being delayed or missed altogether. Because of unrepresentativeness, young patients also are more likely to experience a failed diagnosis. Representativeness error accounts for a significant proportion of the 4% or so of patients with chest pain caused by acute myocardial infarction being sent home from the ED. Insufficient experience or training increases the likelihood of making a representativeness error. Most medical textbooks tend to describe prototypical disease, and students unwittingly are trained to look for representativeness or prototypical manifestations of disease. Where diagnostic uncertainty is high, as in the ED, representativeness error is more likely.

37. Explain availability.

In the normal course of thinking, some memories are more available to us than others. If an emergency physician saw a patient a week ago who presented with a headache that turned out to be a subarachnoid hemorrhage, the image of that patient and the association of headache with subarachnoid hemorrhage is more available or recent than a headache that was seen a year ago.

The physician may have a greater tendency to look for a subarachnoid hemorrhage than otherwise would be dictated by the presentation of a particular patient. Availability similarly might be increased by a colleague's description of a clinical encounter, a recent presentation of a case at rounds, or if the physician had recently read a review of a particular disease. Availability would be *decreased* by long intervals since encountering or never having previously seen a particular disease. Availability is not determined solely by recency of experience. It also depends on the salience and emotional valence of previous encounters. If a physician had a vivid experience 10 years ago missing an acute myocardial infarction in a young person, the physician might be overcautious in managing all patients with chest pain, which might result in a bias toward overconsultation and poor use of resources. Availability influences decision making and can lead to error in overdiagnosing and underdiagnosing.

38. Discuss anchoring.
Anchoring can give rise to particularly devastating errors in the ED. These are the errors that occur when paramedics, nurses, or physicians attach, commit, or anchor to a particular diagnosis early on in the presentation. This usually occurs because certain sign and symptom patterns may strongly suggest a particular diagnosis, which is adopted without giving sufficient consideration to other possibilities on the differential. Consider a 60-year-old man with a history of renal stones presenting with flank pain, nausea and vomiting, and hematuria. The obvious diagnosis is ureteral colic, and inexperienced nurses and physicians would anchor on this. For most cases, the anchor would serve them well, but occasionally an aortic dissection would be missed, with sometimes fatal consequences. The order in which information is obtained strongly influences anchoring, with initial information being given greater importance than that gathered later. One way of avoiding anchoring is to try to stand back from initial impressions, or the diagnosis that is gathering momentum, and ask the question, "What else might this be?" Anchoring can be compounded seriously by the **confirmation bias**.

39. What is confirmation bias?
The tendency to look for evidence or information that can be used to bolster an hypothesis that already has been adopted (i.e., to look for things that rule in a diagnosis). Consider a patient who presents to the ED with a headache and fever, and the physician hypothesizes that the headache has a benign origin associated with a flulike syndrome. In the course of physical examination, the physician finds neck stiffness, which he attributes to myalgia and tension of the neck muscles. This is confirmation bias; the physician is fitting a significant finding (in this context of headache and fever) into the preformed diagnosis of a flulike illness. Instead, a more powerful strategy would be to look for disconfirming evidence that rejects a working hypothesis. In this case, a lumbar puncture would settle the issue quickly and rule out meningitis. If anchoring occurs early on in a presentation, and the clinician tends to work with a strong confirmation bias, the diagnosis may be missed completely.

40. What is search satisficing?
Another cognitive bias, one that probably has its origin in the representativeness and anchoring heuristics. Essentially, it refers to the tendency to call off a search when something has been found. It is illustrated by the following question: "What is the most commonly missed fracture in the ED?" The answer is not C7, the scaphoid, or Lisfranc (all occasionally missed), but the **second fracture** because physicians have a tendency to be satisfied when the first fracture is found and to call off the search for others. Search satisficing errors similarly arise when we call off the search for additional foreign bodies, concurrent diagnoses, or coingestants in a poisoning.

41. Are there other cognitive biases?
Yes. It is only relatively recently that we have come to appreciate just how much decision making in the ED can be influenced by cognitive biases. There is now a burgeoning literature on the topic.

42. What can I do to avoid the pitfalls associated with cognitive biases?

Awareness is crucial—simply knowing about cognitive biases can help. Many cognitive biases can be overcome by experience. Also, we can learn to anticipate the situations in which pitfalls and cognitive traps await us. When we learn to avoid reflexive thinking and action and instead take the time to think about how we think (a process called *metacognition*), we can minimize or avoid error. By reading this section you have already begun the process of reducing or eliminating the cognitive and other errors that occur in the ED.

BIBLIOGRAPHY

1. Bogner MS (ed): Human Error in Medicine. Hillsdale, NJ, Lawrence Erlbaum Associates, 1994.
2. Croskerry P: The cognitive imperative: Thinking about how we think. Acad Emerg Med 7:1223–1231, 2000.
3. Croskerry P: The feedback sanction. Acad Emerg Med 7:1232–1238, 2000.
4. Croskerry P, Sinclair D: Emergency medicine: A practice prone to error? Can J Emerg Med 3:271–276, 2001.
5. Kahneman D, Slovic P, Tversky A (eds): Judgment Under Uncertainty: Heuristics and Biases. New York, Cambridge University Press, 1982.
6. Kassirer JP. Kopelman RI: Learning Clinical Reasoning. Baltimore, Williams & Wilkins, 1991.
7. Kovacs G, Croskerry P: Clinical decision making: An emergency medicine perspective. Acad Emerg Med 6:947–952, 1999.
8. Leape L: Error in medicine. JAMA 272:1851–1857, 1994.
9. Reason J: Human Error. New York, Cambridge University Press, 1990.
10. Reason J: Managing the Risks of Organizational Accidents. Brookfield, VT, Ashgate Publishing, 1997.
11. Redelmeier DA, Ferris LE, Tu JV, et al: Problems for clinical judgment: Introducing cognitive psychology as one more basic science. Can Med Assoc J 164:358–360, 2001.
12. Sharpe VA, Faden AI: Medical Harm: Historical, Conceptual, and Ethical Dimensions of Iatrogenic Illness. Cambridge, Cambridge University Press, 1998.
13. Wears RL: Beyond error. Acad Emerg Med 7:1175–1176, 2000.
14. Wears RL, Janiak B, Moorhead JC, et al: Human error in medicine: Promise and pitfalls, part 1. Ann Emerg Med 36:58–60, 2000.
15. Wears RL, Janiak B, Moorhead JC, et al: Human error in medicine: Promise and pitfalls, part 2. Ann Emerg Med 36:142–144, 2000.
16. Wears RL, Leape LL: Human error in emergency medicine. Ann Emerg Med 34:370–372, 1999.
17. Wears RL, Wu AW: Dealing with failure: The aftermath of errors and adverse events. Ann Emerg Med 39:344–346, 2002
18. Wu AW: Medical error: The second victim. BMJ 7237:726–727, 2000.

8. HOW TO CRITICALLY REVIEW EMERGENCY MEDICINE LITERATURE

Debra Houry, M.D., M.P.H.

1. Can I skip this chapter if I don't plan to do research?

No! Reading the medical literature carefully and incorporating it into clinical practice are important for all physicians.

2. Why should I read medical journals?

1. To learn the clinical features and management of diseases seen in practice
2. To determine whether a new or existing diagnostic test or treatment would be beneficial for your patients
3. To stay abreast of recent medical developments and issues

3. How do I determine what articles to read?

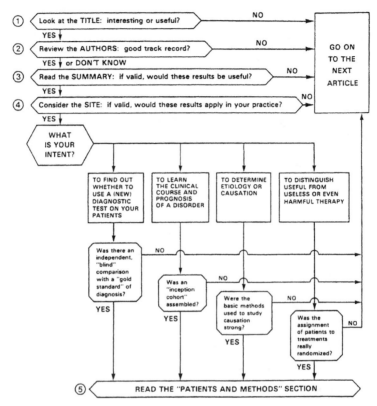

From Sackett DL: How to read clinical journals: Why to read them and how to start reading them critically. Can Med Assoc J 124:555–558, 1981, with permission.

4. Which study design is the best?

Randomized controlled trials are considered the strongest studies. Patients are randomly assigned to treatment groups, limiting bias. These studies are uncommon in the emergency medicine literature and often require large study populations. Other study designs may be more appropriate, such as in instances when performing a randomized trial would be unethical (withholding a lifesaving treatment or exposing patients deliberately to harm).

5. Are there any other types of study designs I should be familiar with?

Yes, cohort, case-control, and case series studies. **Cohort studies** divide groups by exposure status and prospectively follow the groups over time to determine who develops the disease. These studies are used to calculate the relative risks of various exposures. **Case-control studies** retrospectively compare cases (individuals with the disease) with controls (individuals without the disease) to determine the frequency of exposures. These research studies are subject to recall bias but can be used to determine odds ratios. **Case series** report characteristics of patients with a particular disease and can be valuable when looking at rare diseases or outcomes (HIV first was reported as a case series of *Pneumocystis carinii* pneumonia in homosexual populations).

6. What is blinding, and why is it important?

A technique in which patients, physicians, researchers, and anyone else involved in the research study are unaware of whether patients are in the experimental or control group. This helps eliminate potential bias, unequal distribution of groups, differential administration of interventions, and distorted results and outcome assessments.

7. Do sample size and power matter?
Power is the probability that the study will detect a treatment effect between the two experimental groups. The smaller the size of the treatment effect being studied, the larger the sample size should be. Many studies do not have a large enough sample size to detect a statistically significant difference and may report negative results when a significant difference may have been detected in an appropriate sample size. Without adequate power, the study results may be inconclusive.

8. What should I look for when evaluating a chart review study?
1. Trained chart abstractors
2. Explicit criteria for case selection and exclusion
3. Defined study variables
4. Standardized abstraction forms for data collection
5. Periodic meetings among researchers to resolve abstraction disputes
6. Monitored performance of abstractors
7. Blinded chart reviewers
8. Measures of interrater agreement

9. What does a *P* value refer to?
The probability that the results of a study or the differences between study subsets occurred by chance. The most commonly used value, $P < 0.05$, means that there is less than a 5% probability that the study results occurred by chance. This is *statistically* significant, but not necessarily clinically significant. A decrease by 1 minute in overall ED length of stay may be statistically significant ($P < 0.05$), but a 1-minute reduction in overall length of stay likely has no clinical relevance for physicians.

10. How do I interpret confidence intervals?
A confidence interval is the expected range of results in the study population. A **95% confidence interval** means that you would expect 95% of your results to fall within the specified range. A smaller range of values or less variance usually is found with larger sample sizes. A wide confidence interval could mean that some of the study results may not be clinically significant. Look at the upper and lower boundaries of the confidence interval and determine if both values still would hold clinical significance for you. If only the upper boundary value would have significance, there may not be an overall clinical benefit.

11. Does it matter who sponsors a study?
Yes. Any direct involvement in a study by a sponsor, particularly one with a financial interest in the outcomes of the research (e.g., pharmaceutical industry), has the potential to influence the study. Sponsors should not have any input in study design, data collection, or how to report the results. Many research studies do not adhere to these standards. Disclosure of financial support is important and should alert the reader that there is the potential for introduction of bias into the study. Industry-sponsored studies may provide valuable information but must be reviewed carefully.

12. Should I read reviews on clinical topics?
This depends on many factors:
- Are you looking for basic knowledge or understanding of a disease process? If so, a clinical review may be sufficient and can provide the foundation for you to continue your reading on the topic.
- Are you looking for the latest information? Clinical reviews may be outdated by the time of publication because the literature on which they are based was written before the review.

• Is it a narrative or systematic review? In narrative reviews, the author selects the articles to include in the review and summarizes the topic based in part on his or her experience. In a systematic review, the author identifies articles through a search and includes or excludes the articles based on predefined criteria and summarizes the topic based on strength of the evidence from the included articles.

13. How do I practice evidence-based medicine?

Critically reviewing the medical literature and applying the best evidence to your practice is evidence-based medicine. After reading this chapter, you should be able to read research studies and determine the strength of the study and their findings.

14. What are some of the statistical terms I should be familiar with?

<table>
<tr><td colspan="2"></td><td colspan="2" align="center">Disease</td></tr>
<tr><td colspan="2"></td><td align="center">Present</td><td align="center">Absent</td></tr>
<tr><td>Exposure/</td><td>Positive</td><td>A</td><td>B</td></tr>
<tr><td>Test Results</td><td>Negative</td><td>C</td><td>D</td></tr>
</table>

Relative risk: The risk of developing a disease after an exposure compared with individuals without an exposure. $A/(A+B) \div C/(C+D)$

Odds ratio: The odds of developing a disease after an exposure compared with those without an exposure. $(AD)/(BC)$

Sensitivity: The proportion of people with a positive test result who truly have the disease. $A/(A+C)$

Specificity: The proportion of people with a negative test result who do not have the disease. $D/(B+D)$

Positive predictive value: The likelihood that a person with a positive test result actually has the disease. $A/(A+B)$

Negative predictive value: The likelihood that a person with a negative test result does not have the disease. $D/(C+D)$

BIBLIOGRAPHY

1. Davidoff F, DeAngelis CD, Drazen JM, et al: Sponsorship, authorship, and accountability. JAMA 286:1232–1234, 2001.
2. Gallagher EJ: P<0.05: Threshold for decerebrate genuflection. Acad Emerg Med 6:1084–1087, 1999.
3. Gilbert EH, Lowenstein SR, Koziol-McLain J, et al: Chart reviews in emergency medicine: Where are the methods? Ann Emerg Med 27:305–308, 1996.
4. Jones JB: Research fundamentals: Statistical considerations in research design: A simple person's approach. Acad Emerg Med 7:194–199, 2000.
5. Sackett DL: How to read clinical journals: Why to read them and how to start reading them critically. Can Med Assoc J 124:555–558, 1981.

II. Primary Complaints

9. ALTERED MENTAL STATUS AND COMA

Kenneth C. Jackimczyk, M.D.

1. What is coma? What terms should be used to describe altered sensorium?

A depressed mental state in which verbal and physical stimuli cannot elicit useful responses. Other terms, such as *lethargic*, *stuporous*, or *obtunded*, mean different things to different observers and should be avoided. You may be "alert but confused" as you read this chapter. It is best to describe the mental functions the patient can perform (e.g., the patient is oriented to person, place, and time; knows the name of the President; and can count backward from 20).

2. What causes coma?

Mental alertness is maintained by the cerebral hemispheres in conjunction with the reticular activating system. Coma can be produced by diffuse disease of both cerebral hemispheres (usually a metabolic problem), disease in the brainstem that damages the reticular activating system, or a structural central nervous system (CNS) lesion that compresses the reticular activating system.

3. How can I remember the causes of coma and altered mental status?

TIPS–Vowels—that is, TIPS–AEIOU.

TIPS

T   Trauma, temperature
I   Infection (CNS and systemic)
P   Psychiatric
S   Space-occupying lesions, stroke, subarachnoid hemorrhage, shock

VOWELS

A   Alcohol and other drugs
E   Endocrine, exocrine, electrolytes
I   Insulin (diabetes)
O   Oxygen (lack of), opiates
U   Uremia

4. What important historical facts should be obtained from the patient with altered mental status or coma?

This seems like a stupid question because the patient with altered consciousness cannot give you a reliable history, and the comatose patient cannot give any history at all! You should question carefully prehospital personnel and attempt to contact the patient's friends or family. Ask about the onset of symptoms (acute or gradual), recent neurologic symptoms (headache, seizure, or focal neurologic abnormalities), drug or alcohol abuse, recent trauma, prior psychiatric problems, and past medical history (neurologic disorders, diabetes, renal failure, liver failure, or cardiac disease). If you are having trouble getting historical information, search the patient's belongings for pill bottles, check the patient's wallet for telephone numbers or names of friends, and review previous medical records.

5. How can I perform a brief, directed physical examination on a patient with altered consciousness?

The goal of the physical examination is to differentiate structural focal CNS problems from diffuse metabolic processes. Pay special attention to vital signs, general appearance, mental status, eye findings, and the motor examination. Vital signs and eye findings are discussed elsewhere in this chapter.

The **general appearance** should be noted before examining the patient. Are there signs of trauma? Is there symmetry of spontaneous movements?

Mental status should be assessed quickly. Ask four sets of progressively more difficult questions: (1) orientation to person, place, and time; (2) name the President of the United States; (3) count backward from 20 (if done correctly ask for serial 3s or 7s); and (4) recent recall of three unrelated objects.

Motor examination is done to determine the symmetry of motor tone or strength and response of deep tendon reflexes.

6. What is the Glasgow Coma Scale?

A simple reproducible scoring system used in trauma patients to define the level of coma. It is useful for standardizing assessments among multiple observers and for monitoring changes in the degree of coma. The score is determined by eliciting the best response obtained from the patient in three categories (see Table). It is not sensitive enough to detect subtle alterations of consciousness in the noncomatose patient.

Glasgow Coma Scale

OBSERVATION		POINTS
Eye opening	Spontaneous	4
	To verbal command	3
	To pain	2
	No response	1
Best verbal response	Oriented/converses	5
	Confused conversation	4
	Inappropriate words	3
	Incomprehensible sounds	2
	No response	1
Best motor response	Obeys	6
	Localizes pain	5
	Flexion withdrawal	4
	Decorticate posture	3
	Decerebrate posture	2
	No response	1
Total points		3–15

7. How important is measuring the temperature of the comatose patient?

Vital signs often provide clues to the cause of coma. A core temperature must be obtained. An elevated temperature should lead you to investigate the possibility of meningitis, sepsis, heatstroke, or hyperthyroidism. Hypothermia can result from environmental exposure, hypoglycemia, or, rarely, addisonian crisis. Do not assume that an abnormal temperature has a neurogenic cause until you eliminate other causes.

8. What is the significance of other vital signs?

Check the **cardiac** monitor. Bradycardia or arrhythmias can alter cerebral perfusion and cause altered sensorium.

Carefully count **respirations**. Tachypnea may indicate the presence of hypoxemia or a metabolic acidosis, and diminished respiratory efforts may require assisted ventilation.

Check the **blood pressure**. Do not assume that hypotension has a CNS cause. Look for hypovolemia or sepsis as a cause for hypotension, but remember that adults (in contrast to infants) cannot become hypovolemic from intracranial bleeding alone. Hypertension may be a result of increased intracranial pressure, but uncontrolled hypertension also may cause encephalopathy and coma.

Do not forget to obtain the fifth vital sign—measurement of **oxygen saturation** with a pulse oximeter.

9. What is Cushing's reflex?

An alteration of vital signs—increased blood pressure and decreased pulse—secondary to increased intracranial pressure.

10. Define decorticate and decerebrate posturing.

Posturing may be seen with noxious stimulation in a comatose patient with severe brain injury. **Decorticate posturing** is hyperextension of the legs with flexion of the arms and elbows. Decorticate posturing results from damage to the descending motor pathways above the central midbrain. **Decerebrate posturing** is hyperextension of the upper and lower extremities; this is a more grave sign. Decerebrate posturing reflects damage to the midbrain and upper pons. If you have trouble remembering which position is which, think of the upper extremities in flexion with the hands over the heart (*cor*) in de-*cor*-ticate posturing.

11. What information can be obtained from the eye examination of the comatose patient?

The eyes should be examined for **position**, **reactivity**, and **reflexes**.

When the eyelids are opened, note the **position** of the eyes. If the eyes flutter upward, exposing only the sclera, suspect psychogenic coma. If the eyes exhibit bilateral roving movements that cross the midline, you know that the brainstem is intact.

Pupil **reactivity** is the best test to differentiate metabolic coma from coma caused by a structural lesion because it is relatively resistant to metabolic insult and usually is preserved in a metabolic coma. Pupil reactivity may be subtle, necessitating use of a bright light in a dark room.

Testing of the eye **reflexes** is the best method for determining the status of the brainstem. Two methods can be used: (1) oculocephalic (doll's eyes) or (2) oculovestibular (cold calorics). Oculocephalic testing requires rapid twisting of the neck, which is a bad idea in the unconscious patient because occult cervical trauma may be present. Oculovestibular testing is easy to do and can be done without manipulating the neck. The ear canal is irrigated with 50 mL of ice water. A normal awake patient has two competing eye movements: rapid nystagmus away from the irrigated ear and slow tonic deviation toward the cold stimulus. Remember the mnemonic **COWS** (Cold **O**pposite, **W**arm **S**ame), which refers to the direction of the fast component.

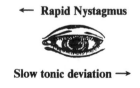
← **Rapid Nystagmus**

Slow tonic deviation →

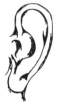
Cold water irrigation

A patient with psychogenic coma has normal reflexes and exhibits rapid nystagmus. A comatose patient with an intact brainstem lacks the nystagmus phase, and the eyes deviate slowly toward the irrigated ear. If the eyes do anything else (usually not a good sign), refer to Goetz to determine the location of the lesion (Goetz CG: Neurology. Philadelphia, W.B. Saunders, 1999).

12. I want to impress the attending physicians. Do you have any tips on physical examination that will let me assume my rightful position as star student?

- If a confused patient is suspected of being postictal, look in the mouth. A tongue laceration supports the diagnosis of a seizure.

- Put on gloves and inspect the scalp. Occult trauma is often overlooked, and you may find a laceration or dried blood. An old scar on the scalp may tip you off to a posttraumatic seizure disorder.
- Do not be fooled by a *positive blink test* in a patient with suspected psychogenic coma. When you rapidly flick your hand at a comatose patient who has open eyes, air movement may stimulate a corneal reflex in a patient who is truly comatose.
- Do not be misled by the odor of alcohol. Alcohol has almost no detectable odor, which is why alcoholics drink vodka at work. Other spirited liquors such as brandy have a strong odor. The comatose executive who "smells drunk" may have had a sudden subarachnoid hemorrhage and spilled brandy on his shirt.

13. Which radiographs should be obtained in the comatose patient?

A cervical spine series must be obtained in any comatose patient with suspected trauma because physical examination is unreliable. A chest radiograph may be helpful if hypoxemia or pulmonary infection is suspected. Skull series are rarely indicated and have been supplanted by CT scan.

14. Which diagnostic tests should be obtained in the patient with a significantly altered level of consciousness?

Obtain a rapid blood glucose (Dextrostix), and correct hypoglycemia if it is found. If alcohol intoxication is suspected, determine the alcohol level with either a Breathalyzer or serum blood alcohol. If the pupils are constricted or if narcotic ingestion is suspected, intravenous naloxone should be given. If hypoglycemia or alcohol intoxication is not found to be the cause of the patient's confusion, further tests are warranted. A complete blood count, electrolytes, blood urea nitrogen, glucose, and oxygen saturation should be obtained. Toxicologic screens may be done in a patient with a suspected ingestion, but they are expensive and do not detect routinely every possible ingested substance. Liver function tests, ammonia level, calcium level, carboxyhemoglobin level, and thyroid function studies may be helpful in selected patients.

15. When should I do a CT scan?

Although CT scans have revolutionized the practice of neurology, they are not indicated in every comatose patient. A good history, physical examination, and a few simple laboratory tests are adequate in most cases seen in the ED because drug and alcohol abuse are common. If a structural lesion is suspected, however, a CT scan should be ordered immediately. If the condition of a patient with a suspected metabolic coma worsens or does not improve after a period of observation, a CT scan should be obtained.

16. When should a lumbar puncture (LP) be done?

The indications and timing of LP depend on two questions: (1) Is CNS infection suspected? (2) Is there a suspicion of a structural lesion causing increased intracranial pressure?

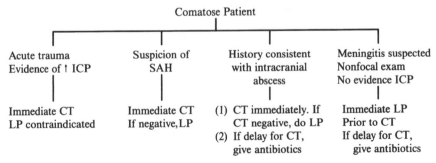

Timing and Indications for Lumbar Puncture

Comatose Patient

Acute trauma Evidence of ↑ ICP	Suspicion of SAH	History consistent with intracranial abscess	Meningitis suspected Nonfocal exam No evidence ICP
Immediate CT LP contraindicated	Immediate CT If negative, LP	(1) CT immediately. If CT negative, do LP (2) If delay for CT, give antibiotics	Immediate LP Prior to CT If delay for CT, give antibiotics

ICP = intracranial pressure

17. Okay. I have made the diagnosis of coma. How do I treat it?

Emergency medicine requires simultaneous assessment and treatment. A brilliant diagnosis is useless in a dead patient. Start with the **ABCs**: airway, breathing, circulation and cervical spine. Intubate patients with apnea or labored respirations, patients who are likely to aspirate, and any patient who is thought to have increased intracranial pressure. Maintain cervical spine precautions until the possibility of trauma has been excluded. Hypotension should be corrected so that cerebral perfusion pressure can be maintained.

When the ABCs have been addressed, check a Dextrostix; if the glucose is low, treat hypoglycemia with D50W. It is better to do a rapid blood glucose determination rather than to give glucose empirically. Next, give 100 mg of thiamine, and if opioid use is suspected, give 2 mg of naloxone intravenously. Empirical administration of flumazenil (benzodiazepine antagonist) or physostigmine (reverses anticholinergic agents) is not indicated in comatose patients. Antibiotic administration is considered in all febrile patients with coma of unknown origin. In suspected drug overdose, activated charcoal, 1 g/h, should be instilled via nasogastric tube.

A patient with increased intracranial pressure should be intubated and hyperventilated. Mannitol, 0.5 to 1 g/kg intravenously, is given.

18. I think my patient is faking it. How can I tell if this is psychogenic coma?

First, be grateful. A patient in psychogenic coma is better than one who is angry and combative. Approach the patient incorrectly, and you can awaken the patient to a hostile alert state.

Do a careful neurologic examination. Open the eyelids. If the eyes deviate upward and only the sclera show (Bell's phenomenon), you should suspect psychogenic coma. When the eyelids are opened in a patient with true coma, the lids close slowly and incompletely. It is difficult to fake this movement. Lift the arm and drop it toward the face; if the face is avoided, this is most likely psychogenic coma. If this does not work, you may want to check some simple laboratory tests, including a Dextrostix. If the patient remains comatose, irritating but nonpainful stimuli, such as tickling the feet with a cotton swab, may elicit a response. Remember that this test is not a test of wills between you and the patient. There is no indication for repeated painful stimulation because it can make the patient angry and ruin attempts at therapeutic intervention.

If all else fails, perform cold caloric testing. The presence of nystagmus confirms the diagnosis of psychogenic coma. What do you do then? It is time to pick up a copy of *Psychiatry Secrets*.

BIBLIOGRAPHY

1. Edlow JA, Caplan LR: Avoiding pitfalls in the diagnosis of subarachnoid hemorrhage. N Engl J Med 342:29–36, 2000.
2. Feske SK: Coma and confusional states: Emergency diagnosis and management. Neurol Clin 16:237–256, 1998.
3. Hoffman RS, Goldfrank LR: The poisoned patient with altered consciousness: Controversies in the use of a coma cocktail. JAMA 274:562–569, 1995.
4. Huff JS: Altered mental status and coma. In Tintinalli JE, et al (eds): Emergency Medicine: A Comprehensive Study Guide, 5th ed. New York, McGraw-Hill, 2000, pp 1440–1449.
5. O'Keefe KP, Sanson TG: Elderly patients with altered mental status. Emerg Med Clin North Am 16:701–715, 1998.
6. Wolfe R, Brown D: Coma. In Rosen P, Barkin RM (eds): Emergency Medicine: Concepts and Clinical Practice, 4th ed. St. Louis, Mosby, 1998, pp 2106–2118.

10. FEVER

Ryan P. Lamb, M.D., and Diane M. Birnbaumer, M.D.

> Give me the power to produce fever and I'll cure all disease.
>
> *Parmenides*, 500 BC
>
> Humanity has but three great enemies: fever, famine, and war: of these, by far the greatest, by far the most terrible, is fever.
>
> *Sir William Osler*

1. What is fever?

A true fever is an increase in core temperature caused by elevation of the hypothalamic set-point. This causes the body to attempt to generate heat (e.g., by shivering) to elevate the body's core temperature. In contrast, hyperthermia results in an elevated temperature without altering the set-point, so the body attempts to cool itself to achieve a normal temperature. Some examples of hyperthemia include heatstroke, hyperthyroidism, burns, and malignant hyperthermia.

2. Is fever a common chief complaint in the ED?

Yes, fever accounts for 6% of all adult and 20% to 40% of all pediatric visits to the ED.

3. Is a fever good for anything, or is it just to make me feel miserable?

As you can see from the above quotes, this is a matter of debate that has been ongoing for more than 2,500 years. Today, many investigators believe that fever is beneficial in fighting disease. Decades ago, before the discovery of antibiotics, experimentation revealed that syphilis could be cured by inducing fevers by infecting a patient with malaria. (Although successful, unless you want a letter from a lawyer, you probably shouldn't use this form of treatment.) Higher temperatures increase the activity of neutrophils and lymphocytes and decrease the levels of serum iron, a substrate that many bacteria need to reproduce. Other studies indicate that fever may be detrimental in patients with tetanus, streptococci, and pneumococci.

4. What temperature constitutes a fever?

We all wish we only had to remember one number; however, it varies depending on the patient:
1. In infants, 38°C (100.4°F) rectally constitutes a fever.
2. In adults, a temperature of 38.3°C (100.9°F) is a fever.
3. Certain patient populations may be exceptions, and this should be taken into account (e.g., elderly, IV drug users, and immunocompromised patients).
4. A temperature of 41.5°C (106.7°F) usually represents hyperthermia and not a true fever.

5. Does it matter which method I use to take a temperature?

Yes. **Rectal temperatures** are the most accurate representation of core temperatures. Oral, axillary, and tympanic temperatures have considerable variation, and these methods are frequently used and often inaccurate. There is not a correction factor for these alternate modalities to provide a reliable assessment of the core temperature.

6. What about subjective fevers? Can mothers accurately judge whether their child has a fever without using a thermometer?

Trust mothers—they know. Depending on the study, mothers are accurate in assessing the presence or absence of a fever 50% to 80% of the time. They seem to be more accurate at detecting when the child is febrile than they are at determining that the child is afebrile. Most pediatricians believe that fevers reported by mothers are probably real and need to be taken seriously.

With a measured home fever, 84% of children spike a temperature within 24 hours, even when afebrile in the ED.

7. Does the magnitude of the temperature indicate the severity of the illness?

No, there is no pathognomonic degree of fever that has been clearly associated with a specific risk of infection in patients, although before the widespread use of the *Haemophilus influenzae* vaccine, temperatures greater than 41.1°C were associated with a higher incidence of serious bacterial illness. In pediatrics medical decision making, the temperature should be used as only one piece of information in conjunction with many other factors.

8. Can a fever be dismissed if it responds to acetaminophen (Tylenol)?

No. Acetaminophen is treating the fever, not the illness. Temperature decline in response to acetaminophen is seen in patients with serious and benign causes of fever.

9. Are there causes of fever other than infection?

Yes. Although infections are definitely the most common causes of fever, there are numerous other causes. Neoplastic diseases (e.g., leukemia, lymphoma, solid tumors) and collagen vascular diseases (e.g., giant cell arteritis, polyarteritis nodosa, systemic lupus erythematosus, rheumatoid arthritis) are the second and third most common causes of fever. Other causes include central nervous system lesions (e.g., stroke, intracranial bleed, trauma), factitious fever, drugs, and environmental heat exposure.

10. Which drugs can cause fevers?

Although any drug is capable of producing a *drug fever*, the most common are listed in the Table. Of these, penicillin and penicillin analogues are the most frequent causative agents. The fever usually begins 7 to 10 days after initiation of drug therapy. There is an associated rash or eosinophilia in about 20% of cases. In addition to drug fevers, cocaine, amphetamines, tricyclic antidepressants, and aspirin may produce fevers after an acute ingestion, particularly in an overdose. Drug fever always should be a diagnosis of exclusion.

Drugs Commonly Associated with Drug Fevers

Antibiotics	Anticonvulsants	NSAIDs
INH	Carbamazepine	Ibuprofen
Nitrofurantoin	Phenytoin	Salicylates
Penicillins, cephalosporins	Cardiac drugs	Others
Rifampin	Hydralazine	Barbiturates
Sulfonamides	Methyldopa	Cimetidine
	Nifedipine	Iodides
Anticancer drugs	Phenytoin	
Bleomycin	Procainamide	
Streptozocin	Quinidine	

11. What is an FUO?

No, not an UFO, an FUO. FUO, or **fever of unknown origin**, is defined as a fever greater than 38.3°C (100.9°F), documented on several occasions during a period longer than 3 weeks, with an uncertain diagnosis after 1 week of evaluation in the hospital. If the patient presents for an initial evaluation of a fever, it is not an FUO. The most common causes of FUO are occult infection and malignancy, each accounting for approximately 30% of cases.

12. How do I evaluate a patient with a fever?

A thorough **history** and **physical examination** are paramount. Pay particular attention to associated symptoms (e.g., cough, shortness of breath, pain, dysuria), duration of fever, ill contacts, history or risk of immunocompromise (e.g., AIDS, diabetes, elderly, asplenic), travel, and current medications. In the physical examination, note the general appearance of the patient (does the patient look "sick" or "well"?). Pay particular attention to subtleties, such as mild mental status changes or rashes that might be indicative of more serious systemic diseases. Examine the patient for more occult sites of infection, such as the nose/sinuses and rectum (prostatitis, perirectal abscess), and consider doing a pelvic examination. Leave no stone unturned in a workup for fever.

13. What about the vital signs?

Why do you think they call them "vital"? Most importantly, vital signs help assess the degree of the patient's illness and provide guidance for the workup and treatment of a febrile illness. Patients with fever often have increased pulse and respirations, but it is important to look at the magnitude of the increase. The pulse should increase about 10 beats/min for each 0.6°C (1°F) increase in temperature. A **pulse-temperature dissociation** occurs when the patient has a fever but a heart rate that is lower than would be expected for the degree of fever. This dissociation occurs in typhoid, malaria, legionnaires' disease, and mycoplasma. In early septic shock, tachycardia that is inappropriate for the degree of fever often is seen. Tachypnea out of proportion to fever is characteristic of pneumonia and gram-negative bacteremia.

14. What laboratory tests should I order? How about radiographs?

There are no laboratory tests or radiographs that are always needed for every patient. It varies greatly depending on the patient. Usually the history and physical examination direct you toward which tests to order. Clinical judgment guides the need for diagnostic studies (e.g., in a patient who has recently received chemotherapy and presents with a fever, a white blood cell [WBC] count is needed to check for neutropenia).

15. How valuable is the WBC count?

The absolute WBC and band count are neither sensitive nor specific and, if measured at all, should be interpreted in light of the patient's clinical picture. Some believe that a normal WBC count and differential have a high negative predictive value for serious bacterial illnesses (i.e., normal values imply that serious disease does not exist). Some patients may present with serious infections but have a normal WBC and differential, such as the elderly or the immunocompromised. Low WBC counts may be indicative of immunocompromise, viral illnesses, or septicemia. Conversely, an elevated WBC count may be seen in nonbacterial illnesses, such as a viral syndrome, dehydration, or a sympathomimetic overdose.

16. What about antibiotics? Should everyone with a fever get antibiotics?

Absolutely not. Antibiotic use should be based on the patient's specific presentation and diagnosis after a thorough history and physical examination and directed laboratory and ancillary tests. Most clinicians advocate giving appropriate antibiotics immediately to any patient who appears toxic or has suspected bacterial meningitis, without delaying for cultures. Other patients who should be considered for early antibiotics are immunocompromised patients (e.g., neutropenic patients, transplant patients, AIDS patients) and elderly patients.

17. So, what's the bottom line on fever?

Solving the medical mystery of a patient's fever is challenging. The keys are the history, physical examination, general appearance, and vital signs of the patient. For each of these key points, certain patient populations have limitations in providing you with enough information (e.g., a healthy child with lots of cardiopulmonary reserve can look great and suddenly decompensate, a patient with an altered sensorium cannot provide a good history, elderly patients may not mount a fever even with a life-threatening infection).

18. How do I approach a child with a fever who is younger than 2 years old?

See Chapter 71, Fever in Children Younger than 2 Years.

CONTROVERSY

19. If my patient is febrile, should I always attempt to lower the temperature?
This is controversial. Fever may be beneficial in combating some infections. Antipyretics may mask a fever and delay a proper workup and treatment of a patient. Most physicians use antipyretics for patients who are uncomfortable because of fever, however. You should strongly consider using antipyretics in pregnant women, children at risk for febrile seizures, and patients with preexisting cardiac compromise who would not tolerate the increased metabolic demands of a fever. If the temperature is greater than 41.5°C (106.7°F), rapid cooling measures should be used, and the diagnosis and evaluation for hyperthermia should be considered.

BIBLIOGRAPHY

1. Alpert G, Hibbert E, Fleisher GR: Case-control study of hyperpyrexia in children. Pediatr Infect Dis J 9:161–163, 1990.
2. Baker MD, Fosarelli PD, Carpenter RO: Childhood fever: Correlation of diagnosis with temperature response to acetaminophen. Pediatrics 80:315–318, 1987.
3. Baraff LJ: Fever without a source in infants and children. Ann Emerg Med Dec 36:6, 2000.
4. Browne GJ, Ryan JM, McIntyre P: Evaluation of a protocol for selective empiric treatment of fever without localising signs. Arch Dis Child 76:129–133, 1997.
5. Crocetti M, Moghbeli N, Serwint J: Fever phobia revisited: Have parental misconceptions about fever changed in 20 years? Pediatrics 107:1241–1246, 2001.
6. Graneto JW, Soglin DF: Maternal screening of childhood fever by palpation. Pediatr Emerg Care 12:183–184, 1996.
7. Loveys AA, Dutko-Fioravanti I, Everly SW, et al: Comparison of ear to rectal temperature measurements in infants and toddlers. Clin Pediatr (Phila) 38:463–466, 1999.
8. Plaisance KI, Mackowiak PA: Antipyretic therapy: Physiologic rationale, diagnostic implications, and clinical consequences. Arch Intern Med 160:449–456, 2000.
9. Procop GW, Hartman JS, Sedor F: Laboratory tests in evaluation of acute febrile illness in pediatric emergency room patients. Am J Clin Pathol 107:114–121, 1997.
10. Sinkinson CA, Brusch JL, Fitzgerald FT: How to evaluate patients having fever without localizing signs or symptoms. Emerg Med Rep 10:177–184, 1989.

11. CHEST PAIN

Timothy Janz, M.D., James Brown, M.D., and Glenn C. Hamilton, M.D.

1. Why is the cause of chest pain often difficult to determine in the ED?
- Various disease processes in a variety of organs may result in chest pain.
- The severity of the pain is often unrelated to its life-threatening potential.
- The location of the pain as perceived by the patient frequently does not correspond with its source.
- Physical findings, laboratory assays, and radiologic studies are often nondiagnostic in the ED.
- More than one disease process may be present.
- The causes of acute chest pain often can be dynamic processes.

2. Why is the location of chest pain not diagnostic of its cause?
Somatic fibers from the dermis are numerous and enter the spinal cord at a single level, resulting in sharp, localized pain. Visceral afferent fibers from internal organs of the thorax and upper abdomen are less numerous. They enter the spinal cord at multiple levels from T1–T6, resulting in a pain that is dull, aching, and poorly localized. Connections between the visceral and somatic fibers may result in the visceral pain being perceived as originating from somatic locations, such as the shoulder or arm.

3. List life-threatening causes of acute chest pain that must be considered first when evaluating a patient in the ED.

Myocardial infarction	Pneumothorax
Unstable angina	Acute pericarditis
Aortic dissection	Esophageal rupture
Pulmonary embolism (PE)	

4. List some other conditions that may present as chest pain.

Stable angina	Peptic ulcer disease
Valvular heart disease	Cholecystitis
Pneumonia	Pancreatitis
Pleurisy	Herpes zoster
Reflux esophagitis	Anxiety
Esophageal spasm	Hyperventilation
Thoracic outlet syndrome	Sickle cell disease
Musculoskeletal pain	Cocaine use

5. What is the best initial approach to patients presenting with chest pain?

With few exceptions, all patients with acute chest pain should be approached with the assumption of a life-threatening cause. Before any diagnostic studies, supplemental oxygen, intravenous access, and cardiac monitoring should be initiated.

6. How do I begin to assess the patient with chest pain?

An accurate history is the most important component of the evaluation. Factors to be considered include the onset, quality, location, pattern of radiation, and duration of the pain and associated symptoms. Precipitating factors, such as exertion, movement, or inspiration, and relieving factors, such as rest, nitroglycerin, or body position, may provide clues to the origin of the pain.

Classic Patterns of Chest Pain

ETIOLOGY	QUALITY	LOCATION	RADIATION	DURATION	ASSOCIATED SYMPTOMS	ONSET
Myocardial infarction	Visceral	Retrosternal	Neck, jaw, shoulder, arm	> 15 min	Nausea, vomiting, diaphoresis, dyspnea	Variable
Angina	Visceral	Retrosternal	Neck, jaw, shoulder, arm	5–15 min	Nausea, diaphoresis, dyspnea	Gradual
Aortic dissection	Severe, tearing	Retrosternal	Interscapular	Constant	Nausea, dyspnea, diaphoresis	Sudden
Pulmonary embolism	Pleuritic	Lateral		Constant	Dyspnea, apprehension	Sudden
Pneumothorax	Pleuritic	Lateral	Neck, back	Constant	Dyspnea	Sudden
Pericarditis	Sharp, stabbing	Retrosternal	Neck, back shoulder, arm	Constant	Dyspnea, dysphagia	Variable
Esophageal rupture	Boring	Retrosternal, epigastric	Posterior thorax	Constant	Diaphoresis, dyspnea (late)	Sudden
Esophagitis	Aching, boring	Retrosternal	Interscapular	Minutes to hours	Dysphagia	Variable
Esophageal spasm	Visceral	Retrosternal	Interscapular	Minutes to hours	Dysphagia	Variable
Musculo-skeletal	Sharp, aching, superficial	Localized		Variable	Dyspnea	Variable

7. What are the major risk factors associated with ischemic heart disease, PE, and aortic dissection?

The risk factors associated with ischemic heart disease are age greater than 40, male gender, a family history of ischemic heart disease, cigarette smoking, hypercholesterolemia, hypertension, and diabetes mellitus. Of patients with PE, 80% to 90% have one or more risk factors related to Virchow's triad, including intimal damage to a blood vessel (trauma or surgery), venous stasis (immobility), or hypercoagulability (malignancy, coagulation disorders, or inflammatory conditions). One of the most significant risk factors for PE is a history of a previous venous thromboembolism. Hypertension is the cause in approximately 90% of patients with aortic dissection.

8. Is radiating chest pain significant?

Radiating chest pain is suggestive but not diagnostic of cardiac ischemia. Visceral pain, including aortic, esophageal, gastric, and pulmonary processes, may present with radiation of pain to the neck, shoulder, or arm. Chest pain that radiates to the arm and neck increases the likelihood of acute myocardial infarction. In one study of patients admitted with chest pain and subsequently diagnosed with myocardial infarction, 71% had pain radiating to the arms or neck. Similar radiation of pain occurred in only 39% of patients admitted with chest pain who did not have myocardial infarction. Chest pain radiating to both arms increases the likelihood of myocardial infarction sevenfold.

9. How does the patient's appearance correlate with the origin of chest pain?

Catastrophic illnesses often result in anxiety, diaphoresis, and an ill appearance. Splinting may be caused by PE, pleurisy, pneumothorax, or musculoskeletal chest pain. Levine's sign, which consists of a patient placing a clenched fist over the sternum to describe the pain, frequently is associated with ischemic heart disease. Kussmaul's sign is a paradoxical filling of the neck veins during inspiration, which suggests a right ventricular infarction, massive PE, or pericarditis.

10. How are vital signs helpful?

A blood pressure difference of more than 20 mm Hg between the upper extremities or a loss or reduction of lower extremity pulses indicates an aortic dissection. The presence of tachycardia should raise the suspicion of serious pathology or severe pain. Tachypnea may be caused by the hypoxia of PE, may be caused by pneumonia, or may be secondary to pain. An elevated temperature usually indicates an inflammatory or infectious process, such as pericarditis or pneumonia.

11. Which physical examination findings may help differentiate the causes of acute chest pain?

Isolated physical findings are rarely diagnostic of the origin of chest pain, but when used in context with the history, they may be extremely valuable. Palpation may reveal localized tenderness and reproduce musculoskeletal pain, but 5% to 10% of patients with chest pain partially or fully reproduced by palpation have ischemic heart disease. Cardiac auscultation may reveal a new murmur of aortic insufficiency suggestive of aortic dissection or a new murmur of mitral regurgitation secondary to papillary muscle dysfunction from an inferior wall myocardial infarction. A third heart sound increases the likelihood of myocardial infarction. A pericardial friction rub suggests pericarditis. Mediastinal air from an esophageal rupture results in a crunching sound called *Hammon's sign*. Decreased breath sounds or hyperresonance may indicate a pneumothorax. Localized rales suggest pulmonary pathology as the cause of the chest pain. Patients with unilateral leg swelling, pitting edema of one leg, tenderness over the deep venous system, or calf swelling greater than 3 cm in one leg are at increased risk for PE.

12. How is the ECG helpful in the evaluation of chest pain?

The ECG findings most often associated with myocardial ischemia are ST segment elevation, ST segment depression, inverted T waves, and new bundle-branch blocks. Initially the ECG may be normal in 20% to 50% of ED patients who later are diagnosed as having had an acute myocardial infarction. Comparison with previous ECGs may reveal subtle but significant changes. In pericarditis, the initial ECG changes may consist of diffuse ST elevation with depression of the P-R segment. The ECGs of patients with a PE often show a normal sinus rhythm. The most common ECG findings associated with acute PE are sinus tachycardia and ST-T wave abnormalities in the right precordial leads. Right heart strain secondary to a PE can result in a peaked P wave, right-axis deviation, or a prominent S wave in lead I, a Q wave in lead III, and a new T wave inversion in lead III (S1 Q3 T3 pattern); however, these findings are uncommon.

13. What abnormalities appear on the chest radiograph in diseases causing chest pain?

The chest radiographs of patients presenting with chest pain frequently are normal but may be diagnostic, as in a pneumothorax. Aortic dissection may show a widened mediastinum or a 4- to 5-mm or greater separation between the calcified intima and the lateral edge of the aortic knob. PE may show nonspecific signs, such as atelectasis or an elevated hemidiaphragm. Rare signs include Hampton's hump, a wedge-shaped, pleural-based infiltrate representing an area of infarction, and Westermark's sign, an absence of pulmonary shadows distal to a central embolism. Pneumonia typically produces one or more areas of pulmonary consolidation, which may show atelectasis and be accompanied by pleural effusion and cavitation. Esophageal rupture classically is associated with subcutaneous emphysema, pneumomediastinum, left-sided pleural effusion, or left-sided pneumothorax.

14. Are cardiac enzymes useful in the evaluation of chest pain in the ED?

Serial measurements documenting a rise of total creatine kinase (CK) and CK-MB can confirm the diagnosis of myocardial infarction. Single determinations in the ED are frequently nondiagnostic, however, because 3 to 4 hours may be required before elevation in the CK-MB level. Myoglobin may be detected within 1 to 2 hours after the onset of a myocardial infarction. Although the sensitivity of myoglobin approaches 90% in 4 to 6 hours, it is not specific for cardiac injury. The use of the CK-MB-to-CK ratio (also known as *index*; normal, < 0.05) is more sensitive and specific than an isolated CK-MB value. Troponin I shows high sensitivity and specificity for cardiac injury, even in the setting of musculoskeletal injury. Troponin I also requires several hours to elevate above the reference range. An advantage of troponin I is that it remains elevated for 7 days, allowing for the detection of myocardial damage in patients who present days after their ischemic event.

15. Are there any bedside tests that may help to identify the origin of acute chest pain?

Several bedside tests may be helpful, but they are rarely diagnostic in themselves. Relief with nitroglycerin occurs in angina and esophageal spasm, whereas acute myocardial infarction and unstable angina (acute coronary syndromes) may remain unrelieved. Antacids or a *GI cocktail*, consisting of viscous lidocaine and an antacid, frequently resolves esophageal pain but also relieves pain in 7% of patients with angina. The use of antacids as a diagnostic test should be avoided. Pain from pericarditis is frequently worse in the supine position and relieved when leaning forward. Pain from esophageal disease is worsened with changes in position, such as leaning forward or lying down. Musculoskeletal pain also is worsened with movement.

16. Are there any other useful radiologic studies?

Aortic dissection may be diagnosed by a thoracic arteriogram, a rapid-sequence CT scan, or a transesophageal echocardiogram. A suspected PE may be confirmed by a ventilation-perfusion scan, spiral CT scan of the thorax, or pulmonary angiography. Esophageal rupture may be diagnosed by an esophagogram with water-soluble contrast material.

17. Describe special considerations that must be taken into account when evaluating chest pain in geriatric, diabetic, or female patients.

Although the sources of chest pain in the elderly do not differ significantly from the general population, the presenting symptoms are often atypical. Instead of chest pain, ischemic heart disease may manifest as sudden progressive dyspnea, abdominal or epigastric fullness, extreme fatigue, confusion, or syncope. Patients with diabetes mellitus may have altered pain perception, resulting in an atypical presentation similar to that of the elderly. The risk of coronary heart disease in women increases with menopause, particularly in women not using estrogen therapy. Women with ischemic heart disease present in atypical patterns more frequently than men. This is because of the higher prevalence of less common causes of ischemia, such as vasospastic and microvascular angina.

18. Approximately 4% of patients with chest pain caused by acute myocardial infarction are discharged to home. List factors that have been associated with failure to make the diagnosis.
- Patient younger than typically seen
- Failure to obtain an accurate history
- Incorrect interpretation of the ECG
- Failure to recognize atypical presentations
- Hesitance to admit patients with vague symptoms
- Reliance on laboratory assays such as cardiac enzymes
- Insufficient experience or training

19. What is the disposition of acute chest pain?
The primary goal of the evaluation of acute chest pain is the determination of the presence of a life-threatening disease process. After assessing the likelihood of a life-threatening process, evaluation centers on the likelihood of non-acute coronary syndrome ischemic heart disease. If ischemic heart disease is unlikely, the evaluation focuses on nonischemic causes of chest pain. Management and disposition depends on the potential cause of the chest pain.

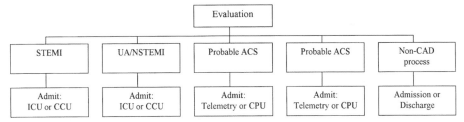

STEMI, ST segment elevation myocardial infarction; NSTEMI, non–ST segment elevation myocardial infarction; UA, unstable angina; ACS, acute coronary syndrome; CPU, chest pain observation unit

BIBLIOGRAPHY

1. Anderson DR, Wells PJ, Stiell I, et al: Thrombosis in the emergency department: Use of a clinical diagnosis model to safely avoid the need for urgent radiological intervention. Arch Intern Med 159:477–482, 1999.
2. Balk EM, Ioannidis JP, Salem D, et al: Accuracy of biomarkers to diagnose acute cardiac ischemia in the emergency department: A meta-analysis. Ann Emerg Med 37:478–494, 2001.
3. Brogan GX Jr, Vuori J, Friedman S, et al: Improved specificity of myoglobin plus carbonic anhydrase assay versus that of creatine kinase-MB for early diagnosis of acute myocardial infarction. Ann Emerg Med 27:22–28, 1996.
4. Douglas PS, Ginsburg GS: The evaluation of chest pain in women. N Engl J Med 334:1311–1315, 1996.
5. Gibler BW, Aufderheide TP (eds): Emergency Cardiac Care. St. Louis, Mosby, 1994.
6. Lee TH, Goldman L: Evaluation of the patient with acute chest pain. N Engl J Med 342:1187–1195, 2000.
7. Panju AA, Hemmelgarn BR, Guyatt GH, et al: Is this patient having a myocardial infarction? JAMA 280:1256–1263, 1998.
8. Pollack CV, Gibler WB: 2000 ACC/AHA guidelines for the management of patients with unstable angina and non-ST segment elevation myocardial infarction: A practical summary for emergency physicians. Ann Emerg Med 38:229–240, 2001.
9. Rusnak RA, Stair TO, Hansen K, Fastow JS: Litigation against the emergency physician: Common features in cases of missed myocardial infarction. Ann Emerg Med 18:1029–1034, 1989.

10. Schneider SM: Non-myocardial infarction chest pain: Differential diagnosis, clinical clues, and initial emergency management. Emerg Med Rep 16:25, 1995.
11. Selker HP, Zalenski RJ, Antman EM, et al: An evaluation of technologies for identifying acute cardiac ischemia in the emergency department: A report from a National Heart Attack Alert Program Working Group. Ann Emerg Med 29:13–87, 1997.

12. ABDOMINAL PAIN

Thomas B. Purcell, M.D.

1. What is the difference between visceral and somatic pain, and how is this of practical importance?

Evolving patterns of pain frequently reveal the source and give an idea of the extent to which the process has advanced. Early, the patient may describe a deep-seated, dull pain, which may be crampy (**visceral pain**) emanating from inflammation, ischemia, chemical irritation, or stretching of the smooth muscle of hollow viscera or the capsule of solid organs. This pain is poorly localized but generally falls somewhere along the midline of the abdomen, notable exceptions including kidney, ureter, ascending colon, and sigmoid colon. Later, as inflammation progresses to the parietal peritoneum, the pain becomes better localized, lateralized over the involved organ, sharper in intensity (**somatic** or **parietal pain**), and constant. Visceral pain that is superseded by somatic pain frequently signals the need for surgical intervention. A clear understanding of the process enables the clinician to identify more precisely cause and rate of progression of pathology.

2. What is the difference between localized and generalized peritonitis?

As the peritoneum adjacent to a diseased organ becomes inflamed, palpation or any abdominal movement causes stretching of the sensitized peritoneum and, consequently, pain localized at that site (localized peritonitis). If irritating material (pus, blood, gastric contents) spills into the peritoneal cavity, the entire peritoneal surface may become sensitive to stretch or motion, and any movement or palpation may provoke pain at any or all points within the abdominal cavity (generalized peritonitis).

3. Which tests for peritoneal irritation are best?

Rebound tenderness is the traditional physical examination finding for peritonitis. In a patient with likely generalized peritonitis (obvious distress, an excruciating pain every time the ambulance hits a bump), the standard tests for rebound tenderness are unnecessarily harsh. Asking the patient to cough generally supplies adequate peritoneal motion to give a positive test. When in every respect the examination is normal, one highly sensitive test for peritoneal irritation is the heel-drop jarring (Markle) test. The patient is asked to stand, rise up on tiptoe with knees straight, and forcibly drop down on both heels with an audible thump. Among patients with appendicitis, this test was found to be 74% sensitive, compared with 64% for the standard rebound test.

4. Why is it important to establish the temporal relationship of pain to vomiting?

Generally, pain preceding vomiting is suggestive of a surgical process, whereas vomiting before onset of pain is more typical of a nonsurgical condition. Epigastric pain that is relieved by vomiting suggests intragastric pathology or gastric outlet obstruction.

5. What is the relationship of peritoneal inflammation to loss of appetite?

Anorexia, nausea, and vomiting are directly proportional to the severity and extent of peritoneal irritation. The presence of appetite does not rule out a surgically significant inflammatory process, such as appendicitis. A retrocecal appendicitis with limited peritoneal irritation may be associated with minimal gastrointestinal upset, and one third of all patients with acute appendicitis do not report anorexia on initial presentation.

6. **Discuss the pitfalls in evaluating elderly patients with acute abdominal pain.**

Advanced age may blunt the manifestations of acute abdominal disease. Pain may be less severe; fever often is less pronounced; and signs of peritoneal inflammation, such as muscular guarding and rebound tenderness, may be diminished or absent. Elevation of the white blood cell (WBC) count is less sensitive in the elderly: In patients older than age 65 requiring immediate surgery, 39% have a WBC count greater than 10,000 compared with 71% of patients younger than 65. Nevertheless, the overall incidence of surgical pathology among patients older than 65 admitted for abdominal pain is high (from 33% to 39%) compared with patients younger than 65 (16%). Cholecystitis, intestinal obstruction, and appendicitis are the most common causes for acute surgical abdomen in the elderly. Of all elderly patients with peptic ulcer disease, 50% present with an acute surgical abdomen as their initial manifestation of this condition. Because of atypical clinical presentations, additional screening tests, such as amylase, liver function studies, and alkaline phosphatase, and the liberal use of ultrasound or CT scan may be useful in this age group.

7. **What other factors should be sought in the history that may alter significantly the presentation of patients with abdominal pain?**

Symptoms and physical findings in patients with schizophrenia and diabetes may be muted significantly. The use of narcotics, steroids, or antibiotics may alter signs and laboratory results substantially.

8. **State the significance of obstipation.**

Obstipation—the inability to pass either stool or flatus—for more than 8 hours despite a perceived need is highly suggestive of obstruction.

9. **What vital sign is associated most closely with the degree of peritonitis?**

Tachycardia is universal with advancing peritonitis. The initial pulse is less important than serial observations. An unexplained rise in pulse may be an early clue that early surgical exploration is indicated. This response may be blunted or absent in elderly patients, however.

10. **Does the duration of abdominal pain help in categorizing cause?**

Severe abdominal pain that persists for 6 or more hours is likely to be caused by surgically correctable problems. Patients with pain of less than 48 hours' duration have a significantly higher incidence of surgical disease than do patients with pain of longer duration.

11. **Name the two most commonly missed surgical causes of abdominal pain.**

Appendicitis and acute intestinal obstruction.

12. **Is there a place for narcotic analgesics in the management of acute abdominal pain of uncertain cause?**

For fear of masking vital symptoms or physical findings, conventional surgical wisdom proscribes the use of narcotic analgesics until a firm diagnosis is established. More recently, some authors have suggested that pain medication may be given to selected patients with stable vital signs because the analgesic effect may be reversed readily at any time after the administration of naloxone. Pace and Burke, in a prospective, double-blind study of 71 patients with acute abdominal pain, found that pain control with morphine (versus normal saline) had no deleterious effect on preoperative diagnostic accuracy. Although inconclusive, a growing body of data suggests that evaluation of acute abdominal disease may be facilitated when severe pain has been controlled and the patient can cooperate more fully. Surgical consultation should be obtained and all appropriate consent forms for anticipated treatment completed in patients needing surgery before the administration of large doses of narcotics. Patients who have received narcotics for pain control should be discouraged from leaving the ED against medical advice.

13. Which are the most useful preliminary laboratory tests to order?

A complete blood count with differential WBC count and urinalysis generally are recommended. The initial hematocrit helps to define antecedent anemia, and serial measurements may reveal ongoing hemorrhage. An elevated WBC count suggests significant pathology but is nonspecific. Elevated urinary specific gravity reflects dehydration, and an increased urinary bilirubin in the absence of urobilinogen points toward total obstruction of the common bile duct. Pyuria, hematuria, and a positive dipstick for glucose and ketones may reveal nonsurgical causes for abdominal pain. For patients with epigastric or right upper quadrant pain, lipase and liver function studies are advised. Amylase may be added but is nonspecific. In addition to indicating pancreatitis, amylase may be elevated with biliary obstruction, cholecystitis, posterior perforation of a peptic ulcer, bowel obstruction or inflammation, and salpingitis. Any woman with childbearing capability should receive a pregnancy test. Serum electrolytes, glucose, blood urea nitrogen, and creatinine are indicated if there is clinical hypovolemia resulting from copious vomiting or diarrhea, tense abdominal distention, or delay of several days after onset of symptoms and especially if the patient is likely to require emergency general anesthesia. An ECG should be obtained if the patient is older than age 40.

14. Are radiographs always indicated?

No. Plain films of the abdomen have the highest yield when used in the evaluation of patients with suspected bowel obstruction, intussusception, ileus, free air, intraabdominal mass, renal calculi, gallbladder disease, aortic aneurysm, past history of abdominal surgery or tumor, or severe generalized abdominal pain and tenderness. Conversely, among patients with uncomplicated peptic ulcer disease or massive hematemesis, pain present for more than 1 week, strangulated abdominal wall hernias, or other obvious clinical indications for laparotomy, plain radiographs probably add little.

15. Which plain films are most useful?

Traditional teaching holds that plain abdominal films should include a supine view plus either an upright view or a left lateral decubitus view (if unable to stand) or all three. The **supine view of the abdomen** is the most informative and worthwhile abdominal film. The upright film is superior for visualizing air-fluid levels associated with ileus and obstruction and biliary air. If the patient is unable to stand, the left lateral decubitus (left side down) view may be substituted when looking for either obstruction or free air. The **erect chest radiograph** is most sensitive for detection of free intraperitoneal air and may show basal pneumonia, ruptured esophagus, elevated hemidiaphragm, air-fluid levels associated with subdiaphragmatic or hepatic abscess, pleural effusion, and pneumothorax. In the evaluation of patients with abdominal pain, the upright chest film, taken alone, has been shown to be more useful than films of the abdomen itself.

16. Are air-fluid levels within the intestine always abnormal?

It is commonly taught that air-fluid levels when seen on an upright abdominal film are *pathognomonic* for small bowel obstruction. A study of 300 normal patients by Gammill and Nice showed, however, that the average number of air-fluid levels was 4 per patient, with some films showing 20. Although typically less than 2.5 cm in length, some were 10 cm. Most of the air-fluid levels were found in the large bowel; only 14 of 300 normal patients studied showed air-fluid levels in the small bowel. The authors suggested that before air-fluid levels are used as the sole criterion for the diagnosis of paralytic ileus or mechanical obstruction, one should see more than two air-fluid levels within the dilated loops of the small bowel.

17. A 7-year-old child presents with acute abdominal pain with a history of several similar bouts over the past 5 months. Physical examination is unremarkable. What is the most likely cause?

In children older than age 5, abdominal pain that is intermittent and of more than 3 months' duration is **functional** in greater than 95% of cases, especially in the absence of objective findings such as fever, delayed growth patterns, anemia, gastrointestinal bleeding, or lateralizing pain and tenderness.

18. A patient with severe abdominal pain is found to be in diabetic ketoacidosis (DKA). How do I decide whether the abdominal pain is a manifestation of the DKA or whether a surgical condition has precipitated DKA?

Patients with established DKA often present to the ED with severe abdominal pain. Physical examination reveals a dehydrated, hyperpneic patient with generalized abdominal tenderness and guarding, which may progress to boardlike rigidity. Bowel sounds usually are reduced or absent, and rebound tenderness may be noted. Although the precise mechanism of abdominal pain and ileus in patients with DKA is not well understood, hypovolemia, hypotension, and a total body potassium deficit probably contribute. An acute surgical lesion may initiate DKA; nevertheless, most patients have no such pathology. Symptoms characteristically resolve as medical treatment restores the patient to biochemical homeostasis. Treatment of the DKA must precede any surgical intervention because of the extremely high intraoperative mortality among patients not so stabilized. Similarly, among patients with alcoholic ketoacidosis, the most common complaints are gastrointestinal, including abdominal pain. Objective signs are typically absent, however, and when found reliably point to concomitant problems, such as pancreatitis, hepatitis, gastritis, or pneumonia.

BIBLIOGRAPHY

1. Brewer RJ, Golden GT, Hitch DC, et al: Abdominal pain: An analysis of 1,000 consecutive cases in a university hospital emergency room. Am J Surg 131:219–233, 1976.
2. Fischer JE, Nussbaum MS, Chance WT, Luchette F: Manifestations of gastrointestinal disease. In Schwartz SI, Shires GT, Spencer FC, et al (eds): Principles of Surgery, 7th ed. New York, McGraw-Hill, 1999, pp 1033–1079.
3. Markle GB: Heel-drop jarring test for appendicitis (letter). Arch Surg 120:243, 1985.
4. McHale PM, Lovecchio F: Narcotic analgesia in the acute abdomen—a review of prospective trials. Eur J Emerg Med 8:131–136, 2001.
5. Pace S, Burke TF: Intravenous morphine for early pain relief in patients with acute abdominal pain. Acad Emerg Med 3:1086–1092, 1996.
6. Parker LJ, Vukov LF, Wollan PC: Emergency department evaluation of geriatric patients with acute cholecystitis. Acad Emerg Med 4:51–55, 1997.
7. Rothrock SG, Green SM, Dobson M, et al: Misdiagnosis of appendicitis in nonpregnant women of childbearing age. J Emerg Med 13:1–8, 1995.
8. Silen W: Cope's Early Diagnosis of the Acute Abdomen, 19th ed. New York, Oxford University Press, 1996.
9. Wagner JM, McKinney WP, Carpenter JL: Does this patient have appendicitis? JAMA 276:1589–1594, 1996.
10. Wrenn KD, Slovis CM, Minion GE, Rutkowski R: The syndrome of alcoholic ketoacidosis. Am J Med 91:119–128, 1991.

13. NAUSEA AND VOMITING

Juliana Karp, M.D.

1. Vomiting? Do I really need to read this chapter when there are so many more interesting chapters in this book?

Yes! One of the most common and harmful mistakes made in the ED is assuming that nausea and vomiting is the result of gastroenteritis without thinking of and ruling out more serious causes. Besides, vomiting is one of the most common presenting complaints in the ED.

2. What causes vomiting?

The act of vomiting is a highly complex act involving a vomiting center in the medulla. This center may be excited in four ways:

1. Via vagal and sympathetic afferents from the peritoneum; gastrointestinal, biliary, and genitourinary tracts; pelvic organs; heart; pharynx; head; and vestibular apparatus
2. By impulses coming from sites higher in the central nervous system
3. Via the chemoreceptor trigger zone located in the floor of the fourth ventricle
4. Via the vestibular or vestibulocellular system (motion sickness and some medication-induced emesis)

3. Can vomiting itself lead to potential complications?

Yes. Some of these are life-threatening:

Severe dehydration
Metabolic alkalosis
Severe electrolyte depletion (particularly sodium, potassium, and chloride ions)
Pulmonary aspiration
Esophageal or gastric bleeding
Esophageal perforation or tear (Mallory-Weiss tear)

4. List the common gastrointestinal disorders that cause vomiting.

Gastroenteritis
Gastric outlet obstruction
Gastric retention
Alcoholic gastritis
Pancreatitis
Hepatitis
Small bowel obstruction
Appendicitis
Cholecystitis

5. Are there different gastrointestinal causes of vomiting in children?

Yes, particularly during the first year of life. These include gastrointestinal atresia, malrotation, volvulus, Hirschsprung's disease, gastroesophageal reflux, pyloric stenosis, intussusception, and inguinal hernia. (Vomiting in children presents considerations not covered in this chapter. See Chapter 75.)

6. List the common causes of vomiting other than gastrointestinal disorders.

Infections
  Pneumonia
  Meningitis
  Sepsis
Metabolic disturbances
  Diabetic ketoacidosis
  Uremia
  Hypercalcemia
Toxicologic
  Digoxin
  Theophylline
  Aspirin
  Iron
Neurologic
  Hydrocephalus
  Cerebral edema

Renal calculi
Ovarian or testicular torsion
Pregnancy
Ruptured ectopic pregnancy
Labyrinthitis
Myocardial ischemia

7. Can the character of the vomit help you to make a diagnosis?

Sometimes, especially with gastrointestinal disorders. In acute gastritis, vomit is usually stomach contents mixed with a little bile. In biliary or ureteral colic, the vomit is usually bilious. In sympathetic shock (acute torsion of abdominal or pelvic organ), it is common for the patient to retch frequently but vomit only a little. In intestinal obstruction, the character of vomit varies—first gastric contents, then bilious material, with progression to brown feculent material that is pathognomonic of small bowel obstruction. Vomiting of blood is a whole different story (see Chapter 34).

8. What else do I need to ask the patient?

1. **Associated signs and symptoms**, such as pain, fever, jaundice, and bowel habits. Think of hepatitis or biliary obstruction with jaundice. Always remember that gastroenteritis is uncommon without diarrhea.

2. **Relationship of vomiting to meals**. Vomiting that occurs soon after a meal is common with gastric outlet obstruction from peptic ulcer disease. Vomiting after a fatty meal is common with cholecystitis. Vomiting of food eaten more than 6 hours earlier is seen with gastric retention.

3. **Do not always focus on the gastrointestinal system**. Ask about medications and possible drug use, headache and other neurologic symptoms, and last menstrual period. Inquire about cardiac risk factors, especially in older patients.

9. What do I look for on the physical examination?

Physical examination is helpful but can be unreliable. Look for signs of dehydration, particularly in children. Check for bowel sounds, which are increased in gastroenteritis and absent with obstruction or serious abdominal infections. Abdominal tenderness may be present in a variety of disorders, but a rigid abdomen points to peritonitis, a surgical emergency. Women of childbearing age with vomiting and abdominal or pelvic pain require a pelvic examination. Always remember the neurologic examination.

10. Are laboratory tests indicated?

This question must be answered on an individual basis. In general, tests should be ordered based on the history and physical examination. Diabetics and elderly patients can "hide" serious infections and metabolic disturbances. Be careful with these patients.

11. When should I order radiographs?

This must be judged on an individual basis. Abdominal radiography is usually nonspecific but may show free air with perforation of an abdominal viscus or dilated bowel with obstruction. A chest film can be useful in cases of protracted vomiting to rule out aspiration or pneumomediastinum. Lobar pneumonia with diaphragmatic irritation may cause vomiting with abdominal pain and few respiratory symptoms.

12. How should I treat the vomiting patient?

1. Always remember to **protect the airway**. Patients with altered mental status should be placed on their side to prevent aspiration.

2. **IV fluids** usually are indicated for rehydration; normal saline or lactated Ringer's solution is preferred.

3. **Nasogastric suction** can be therapeutic and diagnostic and is always indicated when there is a suspicion of a gastrointestinal bleed or small bowel obstruction.

4. **Medications** to relieve nausea and vomiting must be used judiciously, especially in patients with altered mental status, hypotension, or uncertain diagnosis.

5. Determine and, if possible, treat the underlying cause.

13. What medications should I use?

Antiemetic Medications

GENERIC NAME	TRADE NAME	INDICATION	DOSE
Meclizine	Antivert	Vertigo and motion sickness	25 mg PO q.i.d.
Dolasetron mesylate	Anzemet	Vomiting associated with anesthesia or chemotherapy	12.5–100 mg PO or IV single dose
Hydroxyzine	Atarax	Nausea, vomiting, anxiety	25–100 mg PO or IM t.i.d. or q.i.d.
Diphenhydramine	Benadryl	Motion sickness	25–50 mg PO or IV q.i.d.
Prochlorperazine	Compazine	Nausea, vomiting, anxiety	10 mg PO, IM, or IV q.i.d. 25 mg PR b.i.d.
Phosphorated carbohydrate	Emetrol	Nausea and vomiting,	1–2 tbs PO q 15 min (not to exceed 5 doses)
Granisetron	Kytril	Nausea and vomiting with chemotherapy	10 µg/kg IV or 1 mg PO b.i.d. (only on day of chemotherapy)
Promethazine	Phenergan	Nausea vomiting, motion sickness, anxiety	12.5–50 mg PO or IV q.i.d.
Dronabinol	Marinol	Refractory nausea and vomiting with chemotherapy	5 mg PO t.i.d. or q.i.d.
Metoclopramide	Reglan	Nausea, vomiting, gastro-esophageal reflux, gastroparesis	5–10 mg PO or IV dosage varies
Chlorpromazine	Thorazine	Nausea, vomiting, anxiety	10–25 mg PO q.i.d. 25 mg IM q.i.d. 100 mg PR q.i.d.
Trimethobenzamide	Tigan	Nausea and vomiting	250 mg PO t.i.d. or q.i.d. 200 mg PR t.i.d. or q.i.d. 200 mg IM t.i.d. or q.i.d.
Thiethylperazine maleate	Torecan	Vomiting associated with anesthesia	10–30 mg PO q.d. 2 mL IM q.i.d. or t.i.d.
Scopolamine	Transderm Scop	Nausea, vomiting, motion sickness	1 patch q 3 days
Perphenazine	Trilafon	Severe nausea and vomiting	8–16 mg PO in divided doses q.i.d.
Hydroxyzine pamoate	Vistaril	Nausea, vomiting, anxiety	25–100 mg PO or IM t.i.d. or q.i.d.
Ondansetron	Zofran	Nausea and vomiting with chemotherapy	Dosage varies

BIBLIOGRAPHY

1. Davenport M: ABC of general surgery in children: Surgically correctable causes of vomiting in infancy. BMJ 312:236–239, 1996.
2. Ernst A: Prochlorperazine versus promethazine for uncomplicated nausea and vomiting in the emergency department: A randomized, double-blind clinical trial. Ann Emerg Med 36:89–94 2000.
3. Fuchs S, Jaffe D: Vomiting. Pediatr Emerg Care 6:162–170, 1990.
4. Harwood-Nuss AL, Linden C, Luten RC, et al (eds): The Clinical Practice of Emergency Medicine, 3rd ed. Philadelphia, Lippincott Williams & Wilkins, 2000.

5. Marx JA, Hockberger RS, Walls RM (eds): Rosen's Emergency Medicine: Concepts and Clinical Practice, 5th ed. St. Louis, Mosby, 2002.
6. Silen W (ed): Cope's Early Diagnosis of the Acute Abdomen. New York, Oxford University Press, 1987.

14. HEADACHE

Wyatt W. Decker, M.D., and Luis H. Haro, M.D.

1. How common are headaches? How often do people see a physician for one?
Of the U.S. population, 70% report having had a headache, and 5% have seen a physician for one. Greater than 1% of all office and ED visits are for headaches.

2. When someone has a headache, what exactly is it that hurts?
The brain, the pia and arachnoid mater, the skull, and the choroid plexus cannot feel pain. The structures in the head that can feel pain include the scalp; skin; vessels; scalp muscles; parts of the dura mater; dural arteries; intracerebral arteries; cranial nerves V, VI, and VII; and the cervical nerves. Irritation of any of these may result in a headache.

3. Name the most common headaches for which patients seek treatment.
Muscle contraction (tension) and vascular (migraine) headaches have a much higher incidence and are most common. Although painful, these disorders do not have life-threatening sequelae.

4. What true emergencies may present as a headache?
Headaches that are true emergencies include intracranial bleeding (subarachnoid hemorrhage, subdural or epidural hematoma, intracranial hemorrhage), ischemic cerebrovascular accident (CVA), dissection of a carotid or vertebral artery, hypertensive encephalopathy, brain tumor, giant cell arteritis (temporal arteritis), vasculitis, central nervous system infections (meningitis and abscess), cavernous sinus disease, pseudotumor cerebri, and dural venous thrombosis.

5. How do I approach a patient presenting to the ED with a headache?
In the ED, you must think first of headaches that have high morbidity and mortality and then of headache causes that are more common. If you don't, you may overlook serious pathology. To help sort out the serious headaches, several red flags should be kept in mind.

HEADACHE CHARACTERISTIC	DIFFERENTIAL DIAGNOSIS	POSSIBLE WORKUP
Headache begins after age 50	Mass lesion, temporal arteritis	Erythrocyte sedimentation rate, neuroimaging
Sudden onset of headache	Subarachnoid hemorrhage, pituitary apoplexy, hemorrhage into a mass lesion or vascular malformation, mass lesion (especially posterior fossa)	Neuroimaging, LP if CT is negative
Headaches increasing in frequency and severity	Mass lesion, subdural hematoma, medication overuse	Neuroimaging, drug screen
New-onset headache in patient who has risk factors for HIV, cancer	Meningitis (chronic or carcinomatous), brain abscess (including toxoplasmosis), metastasis	Neuroimaging, LP if neuroimaging is negative

(Table continued on next page.)

HEADACHE CHARACTERISTIC	DIFFERENTIAL DIAGNOSIS	POSSIBLE WORKUP
Headache with fever, meningismus, rash, or altered mentation	Meningitis, encephalitis, Lyme disease, systemic infection, collagen vascular disease	Neuroimaging, LP, serology
Focal neurologic symptoms or signs of disease (other than typical aura)	Mass lesion, vascular malformation, stroke, collagen vascular disease	Neuroimaging, collagen vascular evaluation (including antiphospholipid antibodies)
Papilledema	Mass lesion, pseudotumor, meningitis	Neuroimaging, LP
Headache after head trauma	Intracranial hemorrhage, subdural hematoma, epidural hematomas, posttraumatic headache	Neuroimaging of brain, skull, and possibly cervical spine

LP, lumbar puncture.

6. Are there clinical clues to distinguish tension and migraine headaches from headaches caused by more ominous conditions?

Yes. Tension and migraine headaches tend to be recurrent and similar from one episode to the next. A headache that is described as a "first" or "worst" headache or even just different from prior headaches requires close evaluation. A sudden, severe onset, commonly described as "the worst headache I have ever had," is classic for a subarachnoid hemorrhage. Likewise, the dull, boring headache that is unremitting over days to weeks and awakens one from sleep causes concern for an intracranial mass lesion or depression. Although focal neurologic signs are often present before the onset of a classic migraine, those that are atypical for the patient warrant concern. Associated fever requires evaluation for infection, tumor, or drug use.

7. The most important aspect of evaluating a patient with a headache complaint is the history. List the essential questions to ask in evaluating a patient with a headache.

1. Have you ever had a headache similar to this one before?
2. Is this headache different from the ones you've had before?
3. Have you had any recent head trauma?
4. What were you doing at the onset of the headache?
5. How did this headache start?
6. What treatment were you using at home?

8. Why are age and onset important in the history of a patient with a headache?

Headaches beginning after age 55 are much more likely to have a serious cause, such as a mass lesion, giant cell arteritis, or cerebrovascular disease. Knowing the age of onset of headaches also can aid in diagnosis. Migraines most commonly begin before age 30. Tension-type headaches usually begin before age 50. Headaches occurring in the peripartum period may be caused by cortical vein or sagittal sinus thrombosis. In general, if a patient has a long history of previous similar attacks, a serious cause is less likely. If a patient reports numerous identical attacks treated at home, it is important to understand why this particular one led to an ED visit.

9. Does the physical examination add any information?

The history should give you a good idea of what the problem is. The physical findings may support or refute your hypothesis. Vital signs are important. A fever may reflect infection. Hypertension may cause headache. Abnormal pulse or respiration may be due to infection or toxins. All vital signs may be altered, however, in the face of severe pain. On the head examination, palpate temporal arteries, sinuses, temporomandibular joints, and the scalp for tenderness. Check the neck for nuchal rigidity and photophobia. Perform a focused or complete neurologic examination as indicated by the patient's history and general physical examination.

10. How do I evaluate a patient who presents with a new sudden onset of a severe headache? What should be in my differential diagnosis?

Differential Diagnosis and Workup for Acute, Severe Headache

PATHOLOGIC PROCESS	CLINICAL CHARACTERISTICS	WORKUP
Subarachnoid hemorrhage	Headache worst of life Headache abrupt, effort related Normal neurologic examination to focal deficit or coma	CT; if normal, do LP

Vascular intracranial dissection
(carotid, vertebral, or middle
cerebral artery)
	History of trauma, Marfan's
	  syndrome, collagen disorders
	Carotid
	  Ipsilateral headache
	  Horner's syndrome
	  CVA
	Vertebral
	  Occipital-nuchal headache and
	    posterior circulation CVA
		Magnetic resonance angiography
		  preferred
		Vascular ultrasound and conven-
		  tional angiography if MRI not
		  an option

Intracerebral hemorrhage	History of hypertension
	History of brain tumor
	Severe headache with signs of
	  elevated intracranial pressure
	  and depressed mental status
		CT

Cerebral venous thrombosis
(superior sagittal sinus or
transverse sinus)
	Postpartum, hypercoagulable
	  states, and abrupt, dull, con-
	  stant headache
	Sixth nerve palsy, seizures
	Signs of raised intracranial
	  pressure
		MRI, magnetic resonance
		  venography, or conventional
		  angiography

Pituitary apoplexy	Abrupt severe headache,
	  progressive visual loss with
	  subsequent signs of pituitary
	  insufficiency
		CT with coronal views of the
		  pituitary

11. What is the sensitivity of a noncontrast head CT for detection of a subarachnoid hemorrhage?

Historically, 10% to 15% of subarachnoid hemorrhages were not seen on CT scans of the brain. Advances in imaging technology have led to improved accuracy of this study, however, and currently approximately 95% of subarachnoid hemorrhages are detected on CT scans of the head if done within 24 hours of the onset of symptoms. A lumbar puncture (LP) needs to be done to rule out subarachnoid hemorrhage in a patient with a normal CT scan with near 100% sensitivity.

12. How do I differentiate between a traumatic tap and a subarachnoid bleed?

By comparing the red blood cell counts in tube 1 and tube 3 or 4. With a traumatic tap, the blood should clear as it is collected, and an early tube is expected to have more cells than a later one. Xanthochromia, or heme pigment tinting, is always present if blood has been in the cerebrospinal fluid for 12 hours or longer and confirms an intracranial bleed.

13. What are migraine headaches?

Although people may refer to any severe headache as a migraine, a migraine is a specific type of headache. True migraines are familial and affect women twice as often as men. The first headache usually occurs in an individual in their teens or 20s. Headaches typically are described as unilateral, severe, and throbbing and commonly are associated with photophobia and nausea.

The headache may be nonthrobbing, however. Variations on all of the symptoms occur, but each patient tends to experience a similar constellation of symptoms with each headache.

14. What specific entities must be considered in patients with a headache and a history of immunosuppression?

In a patient known to have cancer, brain metastases or infections related to immunosuppression are more likely. In patients who are seropositive for HIV, opportunistic infections, such as cryptococcal meningitis or toxoplasmosis, brain abscess and primary lymphoma of the central nervous system should be considered.

15. What is special about a new-onset headache in a patient older than 55 with general malaise?

Temporal arteritis is a systemic arterial vasculitis that is rare before age 50 and dramatically increases in incidence afterward. Also known as *giant cell arteritis*, temporal arteritis should be suspected in any patient older than age 50 who has a new-onset headache or a change in an established pattern of headache. It is associated with localized scalp tenderness (anywhere in the scalp), malaise, myalgias, arthralgias, polymyalgia rheumatica, low-grade fevers, or other constitutional symptoms. Untreated, temporal arteritis can result in visual loss or stroke. Jaw claudication, if present, is strongly suggestive of the disorder. Erythrocyte sedimentation rate is greater than 50 mm/h, and biopsy is required to establish the diagnosis. Treatment should be initiated promptly based on the clinical presumption and results of the erythrocyte sedimentation rate and not delayed by biopsy. The initial doses of prednisone range from 60 to 80 mg daily.

16. What is a sentinel bleed?

Approximately 50% of patients who have subarachnoid hemorrhage experience a warning or sentinel hemorrhage before their catastrophic bleed. This warning hemorrhage tends to occur days to months before the major event and is characterized by a headache of unusual severity and location that is similar to but less intense than that occurring with the major bleed. These headaches caused by sentinel hemorrhages tend to resolve over 1 or 2 days but may last for 2 weeks. Sentinel hemorrhages are associated with nausea and vomiting in approximately 20% of subarachnoid hemorrhage patients, neck stiffness or neck pain in 30%, visual disturbances in 15%, and motor or sensory abnormalities in 15% to 20%. The warning headaches of sentinel hemorrhages are so atypical and alarming that 40% to 75% of the patients seek medical attention. Commonly, these headaches are misdiagnosed as migraine, sinusitis, or tension-type headache, however, and the patients are discharged from medical care.

17. How do I treat a migraine headache?

Patients who are unable to control their headache at home often present to the ED for better pain control or supportive therapy. The choice of treatment is based on case presentation, prior medications used, time elapsed since onset, patient's prior response to therapy, existence of comorbid conditions, and severity of the current attack.

Selected Medications for Acute Migraine Attacks

MEDICATION	DOSE AND ROUTE*	COMMENTS
Mild to moderate		
Acetaminophen	500–1000 mg	
Aspirin	650–1000 mg	GI upset
Ibuprofen	600–800 mg	GI upset
Naproxen sodium	275–550 mg	GI upset
Indomethacin	50 mg rectal suppository	
Moderate to severe		
Dihydroergotamine	1 mg IV or IM	May be repeated in 1 h but not if triptans used already; contraindicated in HTN, PVD, CAD, and pregnancy

(*Table continued on next page.*)

Selected Medications for Acute Migraine Attacks (cont.)

MEDICATION	DOSE AND ROUTE*	COMMENTS
Moderate to severe (cont.)		
Sumatriptan	6 mgs SQ	May be repeated in 1 h but not if ergots used already; contraindicated in HTN, PVD, CAD, and pregnancy
Metoclopramide	10 mg IV or IM	Sedation and dystonic reaction
Prochlorperazine	10 mg IV or IM	Sedation and dystonic reaction
Ketorolac	30–60 mg IV or IM	GI upset; caution in elderly and patients at risk for renal failure
Meperidine	25–100 mg IV or IM	Opioids less efficacious than other treatment modalities
Butorphanol	2 mg IV	Opioids less efficacious than other treatment modalities
Refractory attack, status migrainosus		
Dihydroergotamine	1 mg IV	Use in conjunction with antiemetic
Steroids	Various regimens	Controversial; based on anecdotal evidence

* Assumes average-size adult patient.
GI, gastrointestinal; HTN, hypertension; PVD, peripheral vascular disease; CAD, coronary artery disease.

18. How are cluster headaches different from migraines? How are they treated?

These are nonfamilial headaches predominantly affecting men. Excruciating unilateral pain lasting 30 to 90 minutes occurs multiple times a day for weeks, followed by a pain-free interval. During the attacks, autonomic signs of rhinorrhea and lacrimation frequently occur on the same side of the face. Attacks may be induced by smoking or alcohol. In the ED, oxygen relieves 90% of cluster headaches within 15 minutes. Other treatments include corticosteroids, calcium channel blockers, lithium, and methysergide.

19. How do I treat tension headaches?

When other causes of headache have been investigated, treatment starts with reassurance and education. Because these headaches are usually chronic, they should be treated with nonaddictive analgesics. Biofeedback and acupuncture may be beneficial. All patients with this diagnosis should be screened for mood disorders because depression is a common cause of tension headaches.

20. Which toxin may bring in entire families complaining of headache?

Improperly vented exhaust from stoves, furnaces, and automobiles may cause exposure to carbon monoxide. This colorless, odorless gas binds hemoglobin in preference to oxygen. Family members complain of recurring headache, dizziness, and nausea that are worst on awakening in the morning and improve after leaving the home. The treatment is high-flow oxygen for mild cases and hyperbaric oxygen for severe cases. Investigation of the source must not be overlooked.

21. What special diagnostic considerations must be given to a patient with AIDS and headache?

Headache is a frequent complaint among AIDS patients, occurring in 11% to 55% of patients, and may occur in many AIDS-related conditions. Aseptic meningitis associated with lymphocytic pleocytosis is seen in patients at the time of seroconversion. During acute HIV infections, patients may describe headache in association with fever, lymphadenopathy, sore throat, and myalgias. *Toxoplasma gondii* produces multiple brain abscesses and bilateral, persistent headaches. The diagnosis of toxoplasmosis is made by CT, MRI, or brain biopsy. Other central nervous system lesions include B-cell lymphoma and progressive multifocal leukoencephalopathy. Cryptococcal meningitis is a common cause of headache in AIDS patients, occurring in 10% of patients. Meningitis is characterized by fever, headache, and nausea. The presence of meningismus or mental status changes is uncommon. Patients who have HIV and who present to the ED with persistent headache usually require neuroimaging, and if imaging is normal, LP should be done.

22. What rapidly progressive infectious entity presents with fever, altered mental status, history of headache and on physical examination no signs of meningismus?

Herpes simplex encephalitis, the most common form of sporadic encephalitis. This is a necrotizing, hemorrhagic illness that results in brain destruction that mandates early aggressive treatment with antiviral therapy. Lumbar puncture with polymerase chain reaction and gadolinium-enhanced MRI are the diagnostic methods of choice.

23. Describe the presentation of idiopathic intracranial hypertension; what is the complication if not treated appropriately?

Formerly known as *benign intracranial hypertension* or *pseudotumor cerebri*, this entity presents classically in obese young women with recurrent headaches that are constant or intermittent and that may present with bilateral papilledema. Transient pulsatile tinnitus and visual phenomena are common. Occasionally, sixth nerve palsy may be seen in the physical examination. Usually CT is done to rule out a mass lesion, and if negative, LP is done; this not only is diagnostic, but also commonly therapeutic. High opening pressure (25 to 40 cm H_2O) and a suggestive clinical scenario are diagnostic. Without treatment, there is a risk of visual loss. Treatment is with serial LPs, acetazolamide, and diuretics such as furosemide. Optic nerve fenestration is indicated in refractory cases.

24. Which cranial nerves pass through the cavernous sinus?

Cranial nerves III, IV, V_{1-2}, and VI. Cavernous sinus disease may present as only a retroorbital headache. An abnormality of any of the nerves passing through the cavernous sinus is suggestive of the diagnosis, however, and warrants further evaluation.

25. How common are headaches in children?

By age 7, 35% of children have reported infrequent headaches, 2.5% have reported frequent nonmigraine headaches, and 1.4% have been diagnosed with migraine. By age 15, more than 50% have reported infrequent headaches, 15% have reported frequent nonmigraine headaches, and 5% have been diagnosed with migraine. Treatment can start with acetaminophen or ibuprofen. Ruling out significant pathology is crucial in children. Subarachnoid hemorrhage, primary cerebral tumors, cerebrovascular accidents, metabolic conditions, and toxicologic causes should be considered.

26. What is a blood patch?

One third of patients experience headaches within hours of a diagnostic LP. This can occur secondary to the leakage of cerebrospinal fluid from the dural rent that results in dilation of intracranial vessels and traction. Headache is usually worse when the patient sits up and gets better with bed rest. Treatment includes bed rest and analgesia. If all conservative methods fail, autologous blood clot is used, the so-called blood patch. Blood is drawn from the patient and injected into the soft tissue at the site of the LP (using smaller needle diameter for the LP decreases the incidence of spinal headache).

27. My 23-year-old patient with a history of migraines presents with a typical attack. She suggests the probability of a misdiagnosis and asks about the possibility of a brain tumor as the reason for her recurrent headaches. What can you tell her?

The most common presenting symptoms of patients with primary brain tumors in the ED are headache (56%), altered mental status (51%), nausea or vomiting (37%), seizures (37%), and visual changes (23%). At physical examination, motor weakness is present in 37%; ataxia, papilledema, and cranial nerve palsies are present in 20% to 30%. The lack of any of these signs and symptoms beyond a headache does not eliminate completely the possibility of a brain tumor.

In the absence of these findings and a typical migraine attack, the likelihood of a brain tumor is extremely low.

BIBLIOGRAPHY

1. Durand ML, Calderwood SB, Weber DJ, et al: Acute bacterial meningitis in adults: A review of 493 episodes. N Engl J Med 328:21–28, 1993.
2. Field AG, Wang E: Evaluation of the patient with nontraumatic headache: An evidence based approach. Emerg Med Clin North Am 17:127–152, 1999.
3. Fontanarosa PB: Recognition of subarachnoid hemorrhage. Ann Emerg Med 18:1199–1205, 1989.
4. Forsyth PA, Posner JB: Headaches in patients with brain tumors: A study of 111 patients. Neurology 43:1678–1683, 1993.
5. Freitag FG, Diamond M: Emergency treatment of headache. Med Clin North Am 75:749–761, 1991.
6. Henry GL: Headache. In Rosen P, Barkin RM (eds): Emergency Medicine: Concepts and Clinical Practice, 4th ed. St. Louis, Mosby, 1999, pp 2119–2131.
7. Linder SL, Winner P: Pediatric headache. Med Clin North Am 85:1037–1053, 2001.
8. Newman LC, Lipton RB: Emergency department evaluation of headache. Neurol Clin 16:285–303, 1998.
9. Snyder H, Robinson K, Shah D, et al: Signs and symptoms of patients with brain tumors presenting to the emergency department. J Emerg Med 11:253–258, 1993.
10. Ward TN, Levin M, Phillips JM: Evaluation and management of headache in the emergency department. Med Clin North Am 85:971–985, 2001.

15. SYNCOPE

William F. Young, Jr., M.D.

1. What is syncope?

A sudden temporary loss of consciousness with the inability to maintain postural tone. Because it is a symptom and not a disease, there are a wide variety of benign and life-threatening causes. Although many authorities and clinical research studies differentiate syncope from coma, head trauma, shock, and seizures, these entities initially may mimic syncope.

2. What are the odds of determining the cause of a syncopal episode?

Despite extensive and expensive workups, no cause is found in about 50% of cases.

3. What are some of the causes of syncope, and how can I remember them?

Guide your evaluation with the mnemonic **HEAD**, **HEART**, and **VESSELS**, representing central nervous system dysfunction (HEAD), cardiac pumping dysfunction (HEART), and loss of vascular tone or volume (VESSELS).

H	Hypoxia, hypoglycemia	**V**	Vasovagal
E	Epilepsy (major motor)	**E**	Ectopic pregnancy (hypovolemia, occult blood loss,
A	Anxiety, psychiatric		gastrointestinal bleed, abdominal aortic aneurysm rupture)
D	Dysfunction of brainstem	**S**	Situational
		S	Subclavian steal
H	Heart attack (ischemia)	**E**	Ear, nose, and throat (ENT) causes: glossopharyngeal
E	Embolism of pulmonary artery		neuralgia
A	Aortic obstruction	**L**	Low systemic vascular resistance
R	Rhythm disturbance	**S**	Sensitive carotid sinus
T	Tachydysrhythmias		

4. List the neurogenic (HEAD) causes of syncope.

Loss of vital nutrients such as oxygen (hypoxemia) or glucose (hypoglycemia)
Seizures (epilepsy)
Psychiatric issues (anxiety)
Vertebrobasilar ischemia (dysfunction of the brainstem)

5. What are the cardiovascular (HEART) causes of syncope?

Myocardial ischemia (heart attack), pulmonary embolism, aortic obstructions caused by idiopathic hypertrophic subaortic stenosis, aortic stenosis and atrial myxoma (aorta), rhythm disturbances such as sick sinus syndrome (rhythm), and tachyarrhythmias (tachycardia). Ventricular
tachycardia accounts for nearly 50% of the cardiac causes of syncope followed by sick sinus syndrome, bradycardia, and conduction blocks.

6. What are the vascular (VESSELS) causes of syncope?

Vascular causes include the common faint (vasovagal) and hypovolemia from blood or fluid
loss (ectopic pregnancy). Cough, defecation, and micturition syncope comprise the situational
causes, although these may be caused by arrhythmias or vasovagal reactions. Subclavian steal
may cause syncope by loss of posterior cerebral circulation. Glossopharyngeal neuralgia also
may cause syncope (ENT), such as from choking on a pretzel. Low systemic vascular resistance
can result from anaphylaxis, Addison's disease, drugs, or autonomic denervation such as that
seen in diabetes. Sensitive carotid sinus accounts for only 4% of syncopal episodes.

7. What determines blood pressure?

Blood pressure = systemic vascular resistance × stroke volume, where stroke volume is
the difference between ventricular filling (volume status) and emptying (contractility). A decrease in any of the components not compensated for by the others causes hypotension and syncope. Many medications cause orthostasis by decreasing systemic vascular resistance or
contractility and syncope.

8. Do strokes present as syncope?

Vertebrobasilar insufficiency may present as syncope with signs of brainstem dysfunction, such
as ataxia, diplopia, or vertigo. Strokes resulting from carotid artery disease rarely cause true syncope
because there is no rapid return to normal consciousness, and focal neurologic deficits occur.

9. Summarize the initial concerns when treating a patient with syncope.

Most patients with syncope rapidly return to a normal mental status and have stable vital
signs. There are treatment priorities, however.

1. Obtain vital signs and evaluate and treat for immediate life threats (the **ABCs** [airway,
breathing, circulation]).

2. Oxygen, intravenous access, and cardiac blood pressure monitoring should be initiated on
patients who have abnormal vital signs, a persistent altered level of consciousness, chest pain,
dyspnea, abdominal pain, or a significant history of cardiac disease.

3. Assess for any trauma secondary to fall. Elderly patients are more likely to suffer head
trauma secondary to syncope, and this may be a greater life threat initially than the cause of the
syncope.

10. Okay, I've ruled out the immediate life threats. Now what to I do?

Obtain a detailed history, do a directed physical examination, and obtain an ECG followed by
risk assessment. Then selectively obtain specific tests, and determine whether admission is indicated.

11. What components of the history are most important?

The most important historical clue is the patient's recollection of the events just before the
syncope. An abrupt onset of loss of consciousness with a brief (< 5 seconds) prodrome is a strong

indicator of a cardiac cause, especially a rhythm disturbance. Similarly, syncope associated with effort or while reclining or recumbent is associated with cardiac obstructive causes or arrhythmias. Patients who have vasovagal syncope often have premonitory symptoms of dizziness, yawning, nausea, and diaphoresis, and the event is during a period of some psychosocial stress. The physician should seek clues to hypovolemia, such as thirst, postural dizziness, decreased oral intake, melena, or unusually heavy vaginal bleeding. Syncope after micturition, cough, head turning, defecation, swallowing, or meals suggests situational syncope. Previous episodes of syncope, upper extremity exertion (e.g., subclavian steal syndrome), and the presence of cardiac risk factors should be determined. A family history of sudden death may suggest long Q-T syndrome. Many medications can cause syncope, so determine all of the patient's current medications, especially when treating the elderly. Using a program to examine for drug interactions might reveal unexpected causes (e.g., sildenafil [Viagra] and nitrates).

12. How do I know it was not a seizure?

A witness is invaluable but sometimes not available. Recovery from syncope is usually rapid, whereas a victim of a seizure awakens slowly with prolonged confusion or postictal state. Both may have trauma. Victims of arrhythmias and vasovagal faints often exhibit myoclonic jerks that many bystanders interpret as a seizure, so ask for specifics. The absence of an anion gap on blood drawn within 30 minutes of the event or no postictal state argues against a major motor seizure. Lateral tongue biting is highly specific for a major motor seizure.

13. What is a *directed physical examination*?

You are unlikely to detect an important physical finding unless you look for it. Be a detective, using HEAD, HEART, and VESSELS as a guide. Assume the patient with abrupt effort or exercise syncope has aortic stenosis or hypertrophic cardiomyopathy, and look for narrow pulse pressure, systolic murmur, or change in murmur with Valsalva. The presence of congestive heart failure places the patient at high risk. Examine the head carefully for trauma, bruits, and focal neurologic signs. Check blood pressure in both arms looking for subclavian steal. Search for occult blood loss or autonomic insufficiency. A complete neurologic examination is imperative.

14. Who needs carotid sinus massage, and how is it performed?

Some physicians consider carotid sinus massage to be an integral part of any syncope workup. This procedure has some risk, however, and should be tried only if the history is suggestive of carotid sensitivity and if there are no existing contraindications. This test is contraindicated in patients with sick sinus syndrome, in the presence of carotid bruits, in persons older than age 75, or in digitalis toxicity. In rare cases, this maneuver has caused transient or permanent neurologic deficits. After intravenous access and under cardiac monitoring with the availability of transcutaneous pacing and atropine, the right carotid sinus is massaged for 10 seconds while the patient counts to 10 in the supine position. Asystole for longer than 3 seconds or a blood pressure drop of more than 50 mm Hg constitutes a positive test.

15. Are tests needed to assist in diagnosis?

In most cases, no. The history is crucial, and historical clues can aid in directing your examination and determining a cause. A detailed history, a physical examination, and an ECG are sufficient to make the diagnosis in 50% of patients with syncope that could be categorized. The addition of a specific confirmatory test (e.g., echocardiography) should be guided by suspicion. CT, electroencephalogram, and radionuclide brain scanning have an extremely poor diagnostic yield without a suspicious history or examination.

16. What about laboratory testing?

In general, routine laboratory tests are of no help and should be ordered only if indicated by the history and physical examination. Serum electrolyte testing may be used to evaluate for seizure or hematocrit if anemia is suspected. Stool for occult blood might be more sensitive for early gastrointestinal blood loss. A pregnancy test is indicated in women of childbearing age.

17. Who needs an ECG?

Almost all patients with syncope should have an ECG. An abnormal ECG is found in 50% of victims of syncope but is diagnostic as a cause in only 5%. Nevertheless, unless an alternate cause is found during history and physical examination, an ECG should be done because it is not invasive, and if diagnostic, it may preclude more expensive and invasive testing.

18. What am I looking for on the ECG?

Check for markers of cardiac disease, such as ischemia, infarction, arrhythmias, preexcitation, long Q-T intervals, and conduction abnormalities. Left ventricular hypertrophy may be a clue to aortic stenosis, hypertension, or cardiomyopathy.

19. If the basic evaluation is not diagnostic, who should receive further testing?

Patients with unexplained syncope who have suspected organic heart disease based on an abnormal ECG, exertional symptoms, or sudden syncope or who are older than age 60 should have echocardiography and exercise treadmill testing considered. Holter or loop ECG monitoring also has reasonable yield.

20. What are the options concerning ambulatory cardiac monitoring?

Holter monitors continuously record data over a 24-hour period, which can be correlated to symptoms provided by a patient log. This brief window of monitoring finds about 4% of arrhythmias associated with symptoms and excludes arrhythmias as a cause of symptoms in another 15%. Extending the monitoring to 72 hours does not improve the yield. Loop ECG provides patient-activated recording of cardiac rhythm for 4 minutes before activation. These are useful in compliant patients with frequent episodes. In high-risk patients, this monitoring can be done in the hospital.

21. What factors help to assign a patient to a high-risk or low-risk group?

High risk: Significant cardiac risk factors, exertional syncope, age older than 60 years, recurrent unexplained syncope, aortic outflow obstruction, congestive heart failure, a history suggestive of cardiac arrhythmia or ischemia. Patients with a cardiac cause of syncope have a 5-year mortality of 50% and often die suddenly.

Low risk: Age younger than 30 years, a history of vasovagal syncope.

22. Shouldn't all patients with syncope be admitted to ensure that something doesn't "turn up" during admission?

That would be prohibitively expensive with low diagnostic yields. Patients for whom there is a high index of suspicion for a cardiac cause should be strongly considered for admission and expeditious workup. In low-risk patients, admission and comprehensive evaluation is unwarranted. Most causes of syncope either are evident on initial evaluation or are elusive, even with extensive testing with electrophysiologic studies, electroencephalogram, CT, and other modalities.

23. Who is the best candidate for electrophysiologic studies?

A patient with structural heart disease with recurrent unexplained syncope because the diagnostic yield is reasonable and the treatment of the discovered abnormalities is often successful.

CONTROVERSY

24. Are orthostatic vital signs helpful in the evaluation of syncope?

Yes: Orthostatic hypotension (defined as a blood pressure drop of ≥ 20 mm Hg on standing for 1 minute) is associated with volume loss or autonomic insufficiency and an increased risk of fall and syncope. A pulse rise of 30 beats/min or greater also indicates a 20% or greater blood loss, prompting a search for the cause. Reproduction of symptoms is a better predictor than any number change.

No: Parameters for orthostatic hypotension are neither sensitive nor specific enough to warrant their use. A blood pressure drop of 20 mm Hg has only 29% sensitivity and 81% specificity for 5% or greater fluid deficit. Of normal euvolemic patients older than age 65 years, more than 25% falsely test positive. Head-up, tilt-table testing (a passive position change), which has shown utility in selected cases, is not reproduced by orthostatic vital signs.

BIBLIOGRAPHY

1. American College of Emergency Physicians: Clinical policy: Critical issues in the evaluation and management of patients presenting with syncope. Ann Emerg Med 37:771–776, 2001.
2. Johnson DR, Douglas DD, Hauswald M, et al: Dehydration and orthostatic vital signs in women with hyperemesis gravidarum. Acad Emerg Med 2:692–697, 1995.
3. Kapoor WN: Evaluation and outcomes of patients with syncope. Medicine 69:160–175, 1990.
4. Kapoor WN: Evaluation and management of the patient with syncope. JAMA 268:2553–2560, 1992.
5. Linzer M, Yang EH, Estes NAM, et al: Diagnosing syncope: Part 1. Value of history, physical examination, and electrocardiography. Ann Intern Med 126:989–996, 1997.
6. Linzer M, Yang EH, Estes NAM, et al: Diagnosing syncope: Part 2. Unexplained syncope. Ann Intern Med 127:76–86, 1997.
7. Manolis AS, Linzer M, Salem D, et al: Syncope: Current diagnostic evaluation and management. Ann Intern Med 112:850–863, 1990.
8. Martin GJ, Adams SL, Martin HG, et al: Prospective evaluation of syncope. Ann Emerg Med 13:499–504, 1984.
9. Martin TP, Hanusa BH, Kapoor WN: Risk stratification of patients with syncope. Ann Emerg Med 29:459–466, 1997.
10. Meyer MD, Handler J:Evaluation of the patient with syncope: An evidence-based approach. Emerg Med Clin North Am 17:189–201, 1999.

16. VERTIGO AND DIZZINESS

Steven E. Doerr, M.D.

1. What is WADAO?

WADAO is an acronym for **weak and dizzy all over**. It is a common and potentially challenging presenting complaint in many ED patients.

2. Which three systems regulate equilibrium and spatial orientation?

1. The **visual system** (eyes and eye muscles)
2. The **proprioceptive system** (posterior columns, tendons, joints and muscles)
3. The **vestibular system** (labyrinth, eighth cranial nerve, brainstem, and cerebellum)

Disturbances within or between any of these systems can result in dizziness; however, abnormalities in the vestibular system alone usually cause vertigo.

3. How do I approach the workup of a patient with dizziness?

First, have the patient describe their sensation of dizziness, the circumstances in which it occurs, and the perception of their body's relationship to space. This patient description allows you to differentiate between vestibular (vertigo) and nonvestibular causes of dizziness.

Dizziness can be classified into six general categories: (1) vertigo (peripheral and central), (2) presyncopal dizziness, (3) hypoglycemic dizziness, (4) psychophysiologic dizziness, (5) drug-induced dizziness, and (6) dysequilibrium.

4. How is vertigo different from dizziness?

Vertigo is the illusion or sensation of motion when there is none. Patients may describe their vertiginous symptoms as spinning, rotating, whirling, rocking, or tilting. Vertigo is episodic, and associated symptoms may include nausea, vomiting, diaphoresis, auditory abnormalities (tinnitus, hearing loss, or ear pain), and abdominal cramping.

Dizziness is a nonspecific term used to describe various peculiar symptoms, such as faintness, giddiness, light-headedness, floating, swimming, or unsteadiness. Dizziness is usually persistent, and associated symptoms are less common.

5. What are causes of presyncopal, hypoglycemic, and psychophysiologic dizziness?

Presyncopal dizziness is caused by temporary pancerebral ischemia. Common causes include orthostatic hypotension, vasovagal attacks, cardiac abnormalities (dysrhythmias, aortic stenosis, cardiomyopathy), and hyperventilation.

Hypoglycemic dizziness is usually due to the complications of insulin or oral hypoglycemic medications in patients with diabetes mellitus but also can be caused by insulin-secreting tumors and alcoholism.

Psychophysiologic dizziness is due to the abnormal central integration of sensory signals as seen in patients with panic attacks, anxiety, and phobias.

6. What drugs are associated with dizziness?

Aminoglycosides, anticonvulsants, antimalarials, tranquilizers, salicylates, and alcohol may cause vertigo or dysequilibrium. Presyncopal dizziness may be caused by antihypertensives or diuretics, which induce orthostatic hypotension.

7. Define dysequilibrium.

The feeling of unsteadiness or imbalance without a sensation of illusionary movement or impending loss of consciousness. It is usually more pronounced when standing or walking. Loss of vestibulospinal, proprioceptive, or cerebellar function can cause dysequilibrium. Ototoxicity, cerebrovascular accidents, peripheral neuropathies, cerebellar degeneration, and advanced age are common causes.

8. What pertinent physical findings should I look for in a patient with dizziness?

A general physical examination should include particular attention to the pulse, blood pressure, cardiovascular system, and neurologic system. Orthostatic vital signs are essential. Examination of the eyes should note the presence and direction of nystagmus, whereas the ear examination should evaluate the external auditory canal, the tympanic membrane, and hearing. The cardiovascular examination should note any bruits, murmurs, or dysrhythmias. A rectal examination should be done to rule out occult gastrointestinal hemorrhage. A complete neurologic examination is warranted, with special attention to cranial nerves, cerebellar function, and gait.

Every patient with vertigo should be tested for positional nystagmus using the Dix-Hallpike test. This maneuver involves quickly changing the patient from the sitting to a supine position with the head turned 45° to one side, with the head ultimately resting slightly extended off the edge of the examination table. Lateral gaze nystagmus toward the undermost ear and associated symptoms (e.g., reproduction of vertigo, nausea, vomiting) should be evaluated promptly. The maneuver should be repeated turning the head to the opposite side. The affected ear is the side that elicits the greatest nystagmus or symptoms during the maneuver.

9. State the importance of nystagmus in the vertiginous patient.

If a patient's symptoms are due to an organic vestibular dysfunction, every episode of vertigo should be accompanied by nystagmus. If a patient complains of vertigo but lacks spontaneous nystagmus or positional nystagmus, a psychogenic origin is likely.

10. Why should I differentiate between peripheral vertigo and central vertigo?

Peripheral vertigo is caused by disorders of the labyrinth and peripheral eighth cranial nerve. Although often more symptomatically debilitating than central vertigo, the causes of peripheral vertigo are usually not life-threatening. Peripheral vertigo accounts for 85% of all cases of vertigo.

Central vertigo is caused by disorders of the brainstem or cerebellum. The causes of central vertigo may be life-threatening, possibly requiring immediate therapeutic intervention.

11. How does nystagmus help differentiate peripheral vertigo from central vertigo?

Patients with **peripheral vertigo** have horizontal or horizonto-rotatory nystagmus. The nystagmus is unidirectional and observed in both eyes. It is most pronounced at the onset and gradually subsides over several hours to several days. Visual fixation suppresses the nystagmus. Positional nystagmus induced by the Dix-Hallpike test shows latency (1 to 2 seconds) and transient suppressible nystagmus often associated with nausea, vomiting, and vertigo.

Conversely, patients with **central vertigo** may have nystagmus in any direction, and it may involve only one eye. Vertical and unilateral nystagmus typically signifies brainstem disease. The nystagmus may be continuous, and it is not visually suppressed. Central lesions occasionally may cause positional nystagmus; however, the nystagmus is sustained as long as the new position is maintained, and these patients rarely complain of vertigo while the nystagmus is present.

12. Are there other ways to differentiate peripheral vertigo from central vertigo?

Peripheral vertigo generally has an acute, sudden, often violent onset and frequently is associated with nausea and vomiting, diaphoresis, and auditory symptoms (hearing loss, tinnitus, a sensation of fullness in the ear, or ear pain). It is usually short-lived, episodic, and not associated with focal neurologic findings.

Central vertigo typically has a more insidious onset with milder associated symptoms and no auditory symptoms. It is usually more continuous in nature and may have associated focal neurologic findings.

13. List common causes of peripheral vertigo.

Benign paroxysmal positional vertigo
Obstruction of the external auditory canal
Ménière's disease
Acute labyrinthitis
Vestibular neuronitis
Acute or chronic otitis media
Trauma (labyrinthine concussion, perilymphatic fistula)

14. What is benign paroxysmal positional vertigo?

As the most common cause of vertigo, it most often occurs in the elderly and is characterized by recurrent brief episodes of vertigo provoked by positional changes, such as rolling over in bed, bending over, or looking upward. Free-floating particulate matter (otoliths) in the endolymph of the posterior semicircular canal is thought to be the source of the vertigo. The diagnosis is established based on the history and the presence of positional nystagmus with the Dix-Hallpike test.

15. What is the Epley maneuver?

This initial treatment for benign paroxysmal positional vertigo displaces the free-floating particulate matter from the posterior semicircular canal, providing immediate relief in 44% to 95% of patients. First, the Dix-Hallpike test is done toward the side of the affected ear. While still in the supine position and after the vertigo and nystagmus provoked have ceased, the patient's head is turned immediately to the opposite side with the opposite ear now facing down. The head and body are rotated further in that same direction until the patient's head is face down. The patient should be kept in this position for 10 to 15 seconds, then slowly brought into the seated position with the head still maintained turned opposite the affected ear. When seated, the head is tilted so that the chin is pointed downward. The Epley maneuver may need to be repeated until the patient is asymptomatic. If successful, patients are instructed to avoid lying flat for the next 24 to 48 hours.

16. What is Ménière's disease?

Ménière's disease is associated with a triad of symptoms: vertigo, tinnitus, and fluctuating sensorineural hearing loss. Patients also may experience a sense of fullness in the affected ear during an attack, and the hearing loss eventually may become permanent. It usually occurs between the ages of 30 and 60 years. The cause is unclear, but an increase in the volume of endolymph and distention of the endolymphatic system are thought to be the pathogenesis. Symptoms last 1 to 2 hours and are often recurrent.

17. What are acute labyrinthitis and vestibular neuronitis?

Acute labyrinthitis is an infection of the inner ear characterized by sudden-onset vertigo associated with nausea, vomiting, nystagmus, and some degree of hearing loss or tinnitus. The symptoms are often continuous and can last for several weeks. The infection can be viral or bacterial, and it can occur at any age.

Vestibular neuronitis is an infection of the vestibular nerve characterized by sudden-onset vertigo associated with nausea, vomiting, and nystagmus. Auditory symptoms are generally absent. Symptoms usually peak within 24 hours and resolve slowly over days to weeks. About 50% of patients report a preceding upper respiratory tract infection suggesting a viral origin. The highest incidence occurs between the ages of 30 and 50 years.

18. List causes of central vertigo.

Posterior fossa tumors
Vertebrobasilar artery insufficiency
Cerebellar infarct/hemorrhage
Acoustic neuroma
Temporal lobe epilepsy
Basilar artery migraine
Multiple sclerosis
Subclavian steal syndrome
Trauma (central vestibular nuclei injury)

19. What is an acoustic neuroma?

A slow-growing tumor that begins from sheath cells typically of the vestibular portion of the eighth cranial nerve in the internal auditory canal. Although it begins peripherally, it ultimately has central manifestations. Symptoms may include mild vertigo or unsteadiness, progressive unilateral sensorineural hearing loss, and tinnitus. As the neoplasm enlarges, cranial nerve or cerebellar dysfunction may ensue. If suspected, MRI is the diagnostic procedure of choice.

20. Are laboratory tests useful in patients with dizziness?

In general, they are not. If a patient has a history of diabetes or is older than age 45, blood glucose and an ECG should be obtained. Other tests include a pregnancy test in a young woman dizziness and a hematocrit in any patient with a history suggestive of anemia. If central vertigo is suspected, MRI or CT of the head should be performed. If vertebrobasilar artery insufficiency is strongly suspected, magnetic resonance angiography should be considered in consultation with a neurologist.

21. Which medications can I use for the symptomatic treatment of vertigo?

Treatment always should be directed at eliminating the underlying cause, if possible. Medications for the symptomatic treatment of peripheral vertigo and central vertigo may include antiemetics, sedatives, antihistamines, and anticholinergics. Prolonged outpatient use of these medications is discouraged because they may interfere with the normal process of central nervous system compensation of vertigo.

Pharmacotherapy for Vertigo

MEDICATION	DOSE
Antihistamines	
Dimenhydrinate (Dramamine)	50 mg PO Q 4–6 h
Meclizine (Antivert)	25–50 mg PO q 8 h
Promethazine (Phenergan)	12.5–25 mg PO/IM/PR q 6 h
Benzodiazepines	
Diazepam (Valium)	2–10 mg PO/IV q 6 h
Phenothiazines	
Prochlorperazine (Compazine)	5–10 mg IV/PO q 6 h
	25 mg PR q 12 h
Benzamides	
Metoclopramide (Reglan)	5–10 mg PO/IV q 4–6 h

22. Which patients with vertigo require admission?

Most patients with peripheral vertigo may be discharged home. Patients with acute bacterial labyrinthitis, intractable vomiting and dehydration, or severe disabling vertigo without a safe disposition home require admission. Conversely, many patients with central vertigo require admission, and this decision should be made in consultation with a neurologist or neurosurgeon.

BIBLIOGRAPHY

1. Baloh RW: Dizziness: Neurological emergencies. Neurol Clin North Am 16:305–321, 1998.
2. Baloh RW: Vertigo. Lancet 352:1841–1846, 1998.
3. Baloh RW: The dizzy patient. Postgrad Med 105:161–164, 167–172, 1999.
4. Derebery MJ: The diagnosis and treatment of dizziness. Med Clin North Am 83:163–177, 1999.
5. Furman JM, Cass SP: Benign paroxysmal positional vertigo. N Engl J Med 341:1590–1596, 1999.
6. Herr RD, Zun L, Mathews JJ: A directed approach to the dizzy patient. Ann Emerg Med 18:664–672, 1989.
7. Koelliker P, Summers RL, Hawkins B: Benign paroxysmal positional vertigo: Diagnosis and treatment in the emergency department: A review of the literature and discussion of canalith-repositioning maneuvers. Ann Emerg Med 37:392–398, 2001.
8. Olshaker J: Vertigo. In Rosen P, Barkin RM (eds): Emergency Medicine: Concepts and Clinical Practice, 4th ed. St. Louis, Mosby, 1998, pp 2165–2173.
9. Tusa RJ: Vertigo. Neurol Clin 19:23–55, 2001.

17. SEIZURES

Kent N. Hall, M.D.

1. What is a seizure?

Seizures are the result of excessive or chaotic discharge from cerebral neurons. Although most clinicians call the resulting effect (e.g., jerking movements, staring) a *seizure*, the seizure is the neuronal activity itself. The observable manifestation is called *seizure activity*.

The importance of seizures is obvious. Something is interfering with the normal functioning of a group of neurons. Studies that control for buildup of metabolic by-products show that it is the abnormal electrical activity itself, not the buildup of metabolic by-products, that causes neuronal damage and death. For an unknown reason, the hippocampus seems especially susceptible to this damage.

2. How do I recognize a seizure?

This is not as obvious as it may seem. Seizures can present in a variety of ways, depending on the size and location of the area of the brain involved. Generally, seizures fall into three categories: focal, generalized, and focal with secondary generalization. A focal seizure is confined to a particular area of the brain and affects only a given area of the body. A generalized seizure manifests itself by seizure activity involving the entire body. A focal seizure with secondary generalization initially involves a part of the brain but spreads to encompass the entire brain. The initial manifestation is isolated to a particular body area but spreads to involve the entire body. *Atypical* seizure activity is much more difficult to recognize. If a seizure has occurred but has stopped before your seeing the patient, you should look for secondary signs, including postictal confusion, incontinence of urine or feces, and biting of the tongue or buccal mucosa.

Classification of Seizures

TYPE	MANIFESTATIONS
Generalized	
Tonic-clonic (grand mal)	Loss of consciousness followed immediately by tonic contraction of muscles, then clonic contraction of muscles (jerking) that may last for several minutes. A period of disorientation (postictal period) occurs after the tonic-clonic activity.
Absence (petit mal)	Sudden loss of awareness with cessation of activity or body position control. The period usually lasts for seconds to minutes and is followed by a relatively short postictal phase.
Atonic (drop attacks)	Complete loss of postural control with falling to the ground, sometimes causing injury. Usually occurs in children.
Partial or Focal	
Simple partial	Multiple patterns are possible depending on the area of the brain affected. If the motor cortex is involved, the patient will have contraction of the corresponding body area. If nonmotor areas of the brain are involved, the sensation may include paresthesias, hallucinations, and déjà vu.
Complex partial	Usually there is loss of ongoing motor activity with minor motor activity, such as lip smacking, and walking aimlessly.
Partial with Secondary Generalization	Initial manifestations are the same as partial. However, the activity progresses to involve the entire body, with loss of postural control and possibly tonic-clonic muscle activity.

3. What is the initial approach to a patient who is having a seizure?

Start with the **ABCs** (airway, breathing, circulation), addressing *all* the vital signs. You first should direct your attention to the patient's airway. Multiple techniques are available for opening or obtaining an airway (see Chapter 3). Supplemental oxygen should be administered because of the increased oxygen demand caused by the excessive muscle contraction. Evaluation of the cardiovascular status with determination of blood pressure and capillary refill and subsequent correction with fluids (normal saline or lactated Ringer's solution) addresses circulation. Attention to the temperature and prompt response to an abnormality are important.

Most active intervention in the patient having a seizure is directed toward preventing injury or aspiration. The patient should be (gently) restrained and, if possible, turned onto one side to decrease the chances of aspiration. Suctioning of the patient's oral secretions should be done during the seizure. It is important not to put anything in the patient's mouth that might be aspirated or bitten off (this includes your fingers). Nasal cannula or mask supplemental oxygen should be administered, but the use of supplemental ventilation is rarely necessary in the patient with an uncomplicated seizure.

4. What is status epilepticus?

An "epileptic seizure that is so frequently repeated or so prolonged as to create a fixed and lasting epileptic condition." Traditionally, this definition applies if the seizure lasts longer than 30 minutes or in recurrent seizures with no interictal recovery. Current recommendations and descriptions are that seizure activity that lasts longer than 5 minutes and is unlikely to stop spontaneously should be considered status epilepticus. Treatment should be started within this 5-minute time frame.

Patients in whom status epilepticus is diagnosed require a thorough and extensive evaluation. This should include a complete evaluation to identify and treat any underlying reversible precipitating cause of the status epilepticus and rapid intervention to terminate the abnormal neuronal activity. Full medical support to prevent complications from the seizures or their therapy (i.e., respiratory depression, rhabdomyolysis, or hyperpyrexia) is important.

5. How are seizures stopped?

If a seizure lasts longer than 5 minutes, immediate intervention is indicated. In traditional medicine, the usual sequence is diagnosis, then treatment. Often in emergency medicine, it is necessary to diagnose and treat simultaneously. Do not wait until after taking a history, doing a complete physical examination, and ordering ancillary tests before addressing the seizure activity. **Seizures damage the brain; the longer they are allowed to continue, the more damage occurs.**

Benzodiazepines are the first-line drugs of choice for treating seizures that last longer than 5 minutes. Lorazepam is the preferred first-line benzodiazepine for treating seizures because of its apparent increased efficacy and its longer half-life in keeping seizures from recurring compared with diazepam. The adult dosage of lorazepam is 2 to 4 mg IV push to a total of 10 to 15 mg. If lorazepam is not available, diazepam in a dose of 5 to 10 mg IV push, not to exceed 30 mg in an 8-hour period, is indicated. If multiple doses of a benzodiazepine do not stop the seizure or benzodiazepines are contraindicated in the patient, a loading dose of a primary anticonvulsant (see later) should be administered.

If intravenous access is not available, midazolam can be used intramuscularly (IM) or per rectum. Although diazepam and lorazepam are not recommended for IM use because of erratic absorption, midazolam at a dose of 0.05 mg/kg IM has been used to treat status epilepticus successfully.

6. When the seizure has stopped, how do I keep it from recurring?

This question brings us to another class of drugs, the **anticonvulsants**. The drugs most often used to stop seizures or keep seizures from recurring, along with their doses and routes of administration, are listed in the Table. Anticonvulsants not only keep seizures from recurring in the ED, but also are used to stop seizures resistant to the benzodiazepines.

Anticonvulsants

NAME	DOSE	ROUTE OF ADMINISTRATION	COMMENTS
Phenytoin	18–20 mg/kg	IV	Should not be given faster than 50 mg/min; patient should be on a cardiac monitor; stop infusion if toxicity noted (prolongation of QRS > 50% of baseline, hypotension). If status epilepticus continues, may increase total dose to 30 mg/kg.
Fosphenytoin	15–20 PE/kg	IV, IM	Unit of measure is the phenytoin equivalent (PE), which is noted on the medication vial. This medication is a prodrug of phenytoin; as such it is safe to give as a rapid infusion with no adverse hemodynamic effects. A therapeutic level of this medication is reached much faster than with dilantin.

(Table continued on next page.)

Anticonvulsants (cont.)

NAME	DOSE	ROUTE OF ADMINISTRATION	COMMENTS
Phenobarbital	Up to 15 mg/kg	IV	Should not be given faster than 100 mg/min; dose can be repeated once at 30 minutes if no effect; maximum total dose is 600 mg acutely; beware of respiratory depression, especially if the patient has received diazepam.
Pentobarbital	12 mg/kg	IV	Use only when other agents (above) have failed
Lidocaine	1–1.5 mg/kg	IV	Has been reported to stop status epilepticus, but controlled trials not done.
Propofol	2 mg/kg	IV	Reports of its use in refractory status epilepticus exist, but no controlled trials. Should be used with intubation and mechanical ventilation. Beware of hypotension and be prepared to treat.

7. Name the most *common* causes of seizures.

The more common causes by age of patient are listed in the Table. Immediately reversible causes for which physicians should be especially vigilant include hypoglycemia and hypoxia (secondary to narcotic overdose). An initial Dextrostix and empirical administration of naloxone may be indicated. Note the similarity of causes of seizures in the very young and very old.

Causes of Seizures

Infant	Birth trauma (hypoxia, intracranial trauma)
	Infection (brain abscess, meningitis)
	Electrolyte abnormalities (hyponatremia, hypocalcemia, hypomagnesemia)
	Congenital malformations (intracerebral cysts, hydrocephalus)
	Genetic disorders (inborn errors of metabolism, pyridoxine deficiency)
Child	Febrile seizure
	Idiopathic seizure
	Trauma
	Infection (meningitis)
Adolescent	Trauma
	Idiopathic
	Drug or alcohol related (acute intoxication or withdrawal)
	Arteriovenous malformation
Young adult	Trauma
	Alcohol related (acute intoxication or withdrawal)
	Brain tumor
Older adult	Brain tumor
	Stroke
	Intracerebral hemorrhage
	Alcoholism
	Metabolic derangements (hyponatremia, hypernatremia, hypocalcemia, hypoglycemia, uremia, hepatic failure)

8. Is the history important?

The history is vitally important! You can use the mnemonic **COLD** to be sure you have covered the aspects of the seizure activity itself:

Character: What type of seizure activity occurred?
Onset: When did it start? What was the patient doing?
Location: Where did the activity start?
Duration: How long did it last?

In general, true seizures tend to occur abruptly, are stereotyped (the basic features of the seizures are maintained from one attack to the next), are not provoked by environmental stimuli, are manifested by movements that are purposeless or inappropriate, and, except for petit mal seizures, are followed by a period of confusion and lethargy (the postictal period). Other important points include the patient's past medical history (especially previous seizure history), alcohol use and other toxic ingestions, current medications, any history of central nervous system neoplasms, and history of recent or remote trauma.

9. Besides the neurologic examination, what other parts of the physical examination are important and why?

A complete head-to-toe examination is important. In addition to looking for causes of the seizure, the physician should look for trauma caused by the seizure. The examination is often normal but occasionally may give clues to an underlying problem. Specifically, examination of the skin might reveal lesions consistent with meningococcemia or other infectious problems. Examine the head for trauma. If nuchal rigidity is found, meningitis or subarachnoid hemorrhage should be suspected. A heart murmur, especially if records indicate none was heard before, might indicate subacute bacterial endocarditis, with resultant embolization as the cause of the seizure.

The neurologic examination is important. Focal neurologic findings, such as focal paresis after the seizure (Todd's paralysis) may indicate a focal cerebral lesion (tumor, abscess, cerebral contusion) as the cause of the seizure. Evaluation of the cranial nerves and the fundi can indicate increased intracranial pressure.

10. What ancillary test should I order for a seizure patient?

In general, the use of ancillary laboratory tests depends on the history and presentation of the patient. In the patient with a prior history of seizure disorder who presents with a single, unprovoked seizure, the only laboratory value that is useful is a serum anticonvulsant level. If the level is subtherapeutic, the patient should be given a loading dose of this medication to achieve a therapeutic level. The decision to evaluate the patient with other ancillary tests (laboratory and radiologic) should be based on the findings of the history and physical examination. If there is a question about whether the patient had a major motor seizure, order serum electrolytes on blood drawn by EMTs in the field and calculate the anion gap.

11. What is the significance of the anion gap in the diagnosis of grand mal seizure?

An increased transient (< 1-hour duration) anion gap is good evidence that a grand mal seizure has occurred. This is determined by blood samples drawn as close to the time of seizure as possible. Field blood samples are ideal for this study. If there is no anion gap acidosis, one may presume that the patient did not have a major motor seizure.

12. What if the patient has never had a seizure before?

If this is a new-onset seizure, ancillary tests are more important. The yield is still quite low, however. A screen for metabolic derangements (sodium, calcium, glucose, magnesium, elevated BUN, or creatinine) is important. Toxicologic screens targeted for substances that are known to cause seizures (cocaine, lidocaine, antidepressants, theophylline, and stimulants are among the most common) should be obtained if clinically indicated.

13. Do all patients with seizures need a CT scan of the head in the ED?

This is an area of ongoing study. The best answer that can be given at this time is that selective use of CT scans of the head is safe in appropriate situations. Patients who should have a head CT scan done in the ED include those in whom an acute intracranial event (i.e., subdural hematoma, subarachnoid hemorrhage) is suspected, those who have a prolonged abnormal mental status (prolonged postictal state) or an abnormal neurologic examination, and those who cannot assure rapid follow-up evaluation by a primary care physician or neurologist.

14. What is the appropriate disposition of a patient with a recurrence of seizures?

If there are no abnormal findings on history or physical examination, the patient can be discharged with follow-up by his or her primary care physician or neurologist. If the anticonvulsant level is normal or the history suggests a change in seizure activity (increased frequency, different type), the patient should be evaluated as a new seizure patient. This may include admission if follow-up is not assured or if findings during the workup indicate the need for hospitalization.

15. Does the fact that the patient has a first-time seizure make a difference in the management and disposition?

Patients with a first-time seizure are more likely to be admitted after ED evaluation. If the seizure was short-lived, the physical examination and ancillary testing are all normal, and close follow-up with a primary care physician or neurologist can be arranged before the patient is discharged from the ED, hospital admission may not be needed.

Similarly, not all first-time seizure patients need to be started on anticonvulsant medication. Specific recommendations about the use of these medications in these patients are difficult. If close follow-up is available with a primary care physician or neurologist, and the patient is reliable, discharge without starting anticonvulsants may be appropriate.

Discharge instructions should emphasize to the patient not to drive, operate machinery, or go to high, open places (e.g., construction platforms).

16. What is a pseudoseizure, and how is it diagnosed?

Pseudoseizures are seizure-like activity with no underlying abnormal electrical activity in the brain. They are difficult to diagnose in the ED. Maneuvers that have been shown to work in some cases include suggesting to the patient that the seizure will stop soon or attempting to distract the patient with loud noises or bright lights during the "seizure" activity. Aspects of the abnormal activity that make it more likely to be a pseudoseizure include asynchronous extremity movement, a forward thrusting movement of the pelvis, and the eyes being deviated toward the ground, no matter what position the head is placed in. The diagnosis can be made electrically if the patient is hooked up to an electrocephalography machine (not customary in the ED). During the pseudoseizure, no abnormal electrical activity is seen. Similarly, measurement of serum prolactin 20 minutes after the "seizure" helps differentiate a true seizure from a pseudoseizure. In true seizures, the prolactin level is elevated by at least two times, whereas in pseudoseizures the prolactin remains in the normal range. Neither of these methods is available in the ED. Pseudo-grand mal seizures usually do not result in an anion gap metabolic acidosis, and this determination is available in the ED.

BIBLIOGRAPHY

1. Barsan WG, Jastremsk MS, Syverud SA (eds): Emergency Drug Therapy. Philadelphia, W.B. Saunders, 1991.
2. Gabor AJ: Lorazepam versus phenobarbital: Candidates for drug of choice for treatment of status epilepticus. J Epilepsy 3:3–6, 1990.
3. Harwood-Nuss AL, Linden C, Luten RC, et al (eds): The Clinical Practice of Emergency Medicine, 2nd ed. Philadelphia, Lippincott-Raven, 1996.
4. Isselbacher KJ, Braunwald E, Wilson JD, et al (eds): Harrison's Principles of Internal Medicine, 13th ed. New York, McGraw-Hill, 1994.
5. Mitchell WG, Snodgrass SR, Crawford TO, et al: Lorazepam is the treatment of choice for status epilepticus. J Epilepsy 3:7–14, 1990.
6. Pollock CV, Pollock ES: Seizures. In Rosen P, Barkin RM (eds): Emergency Medicine: Concepts and Practice, 4th ed. St. Louis, Mosby, 1998.
7. Pritchard BP 3d: The effect of seizures on hormones. Epilepsia 32(suppl 6):S46–S50, 1991.
8. Tintinalli JE, Krome RL, Ruiz E (eds): Emergency Medicine: A Comprehensive Study Guide, 4th ed. New York, McGraw-Hill, 1996.
9. Treiman DM: The role of benzodiazepines in the management of status epilepticus. Neurology 40(suppl 2):32–42, 1990.
10. Turnbull TL, Vanden Hoek TL, Howes DS, Eisner RF: Utility of laboratory studies in the emergency department patient with new-onset seizure. Ann Emerg Med 19:373–377, 1990.

18. ANAPHYLAXIS

Vincent J. Markovchick, M.D.

1. What is anaphylaxis?

A systemic immediate hypersensitivity reaction of multiple organ systems to an antigen-induced, IgE-mediated immunologic mediator release in previously sensitized individuals.

2. What is an anaphylactoid reaction?

A potentially fatal syndrome clinically similar to anaphylaxis, which is not an IgE-mediated response and may follow a single first-time exposure to certain agents, such as radiopaque contrast media.

3. Name the most common causes of anaphylaxis

Ingestion, inhalation, or parenteral injection of antigens that sensitize predisposed individuals. Common antigens include drugs (e.g., penicillin), foods (shellfish, nuts, egg whites), insect stings (hymenoptera) and bites (snakes), diagnostic agents (ionic contrast media), and physical and environmental agents (latex, exercise, and cold). **Idiopathic anaphylaxis** is a diagnosis of exclusion that is made when no identifiable cause can be determined.

4. List the common *target* organs.

Skin (urticaria, angioedema)
Mucous membranes (edema)
Upper respiratory tract (edema and hypersecretions)
Lower respiratory tract (bronchoconstriction)
Cardiovascular system (vasodilation and cardiovascular collapse)

5. What are the most common signs and symptoms?

The clinical presentation ranges from mild to life-threatening. Mild manifestations that occur in most people include urticaria and angioedema. Life-threatening manifestations involve the respiratory and cardiovascular systems. Respiratory signs and symptoms include acute upper airway obstruction presenting with stridor or lower airway manifestations of bronchospasm with diffuse wheezing. Cardiovascular collapse presents in the form of syncope, hypotension, tachycardia, and arrhythmias.

6. What is the role of diagnostic studies?

There is no role for diagnostic studies in anaphylaxis because diagnosis and treatment are based solely on clinical signs and symptoms. There is a role for skin testing either before administration of an antigen or in follow-up referral to determine exact allergens involved.

7. What is the differential diagnosis?

Septic and cardiogenic shock, asthma, croup and epiglottitis, vasovagal syncope, and myocardial or any acute cardiovascular or respiratory collapse of unclear origin.

8. What is the most common form of anaphylaxis, and how is it treated?

Urticaria, either simple or confluent, is the most benign and the most common clinical manifestation. This is thought to be due to a capillary leak mediated by histamine release. It may be treated by the administration of antihistamines (orally, intramuscularly, or intravenously) or epinephrine (subcutaneous).

9. Summarize the initial treatment for life-threatening forms of anaphylaxis.

1. Upper airway obstruction with stridor and edema is treated with high-flow nebulized oxygen, racemic epinephrine, and intravenous epinephrine. If airway obstruction is severe or increases, perform endotracheal intubation or cricothyroidotomy.

2. Acute bronchospasm is treated with epinephrine. Mild-to-moderate wheezing in patients with normal blood pressure may be treated with 0.01 mg/kg of 1:1000 epinephrine administered subcutaneously or intramuscularly. If the patient is in severe respiratory distress or has a *quiet* chest, administer intravenous epinephrine via a drip infusion: 1 mg of epinephrine in 250 mL of D5W at an initial rate of 1 µg/min with titration to desired effect. Bronchospasm refractory to epinephrine may respond to a nebulized β-agonist, such as albuterol sulfate or metaproterenol, in recommended doses.

3. Cardiovascular collapse presenting with hypotension is treated with a constant infusion of epinephrine, titrating the rate to attain a systolic blood pressure of 100 mm Hg or mean arterial pressure of 80 mm Hg.

4. For patients in full cardiac arrest, administer 1:10,000 epinephrine, 0.1 to 0.2 mg/kg slow intravenous push or via endotracheal tube. Immediate endotracheal intubation or cricothyroidotomy should be performed.

10. What are the adjuncts to initial epinephrine and airway management?

If intubation is unsuccessful and cricothyroidotomy is contraindicated, percutaneous transtracheal jet ventilation via needle cricothyroidotomy should be considered, especially in small children. Intravenous diphenhydramine (1 mg/kg) should be given to all patients. Simultaneous administration of an H_2 blocker, such as cimetidine, 300 mg intravenously, may be helpful. Aerosolized bronchodilators, such as metaproterenol, are useful if bronchospasm is present. For refractory hypotension, pressors, such as norepinephrine or dopamine, may be administered. Glucagon, 1 mg intravenously every 5 minutes, may be helpful in *epinephrine-resistant* patients who are on long-term β-adrenergic blocking agents, such as propranolol. Corticosteroids have limited benefit because of the delayed onset of action, but they may be beneficial in patients with prolonged bronchospasm or hypotension.

11. What are the complications of bolus intravenous epinephrine administration?

When epinephrine 1:10,000 is administered via intravenous push in patients who have an obtainable blood pressure or pulse, there is significant potential for overtreatment and the potentiation of hypertension, tachycardia, ischemic chest pain, acute myocardial infarction, and ventricular arrhythmias. Extreme care must be exercised in elderly patients and in patients with underlying coronary artery disease. It is much safer to give intravenous epinephrine by a controlled titratable drip infusion with continuous monitoring of cardiac rhythm and blood pressure.

12. Is there a role for prophylactic treatment in anaphylaxis? How is this performed?

When the potential benefits of treatment or diagnosis outweigh the risks (e.g., administration of antivenom for life-threatening or limb-threatening snake bites), informed consent should be obtained if the patient is competent. Pretreatment with intravenous diphenhydramine (Benadryl) and corticosteroids should be carried out. An intravenous epinephrine infusion should be prepared. The patient should be in an ICU setting with continuous monitoring of blood pressure, cardiac rhythm, and oxygen saturation. Full intubation and cricothyroidotomy equipment should be at the bedside. Administration of the antigen (e.g., rattlesnake antivenom) should be started slowly with a physician at the bedside who is capable of immediately administering intravenous epinephrine and managing the airway. Nonionic contrast medium for diagnostic imaging studies should be given to patients with a history of anaphylaxis to ionic contrast material.

13. What about steroids?

Because corticosteroids have an onset of action of approximately 4 to 6 hours after administration, they have limited or no benefit in the initial acute treatment of anaphylaxis. The administration of hydrocortisone (250 to 1000 mg intravenously) or methylprednisolone (125 to 250 mg intravenously), followed by a tapering dose over 7 to 10 days, is an acceptable regimen after the resolution of the initial anaphylactic episode.

14. What is the disposition of a patient who initially responds to aggressive treatment?
Although most patients respond positively to early, aggressive treatment and may become asymptomatic, all patients with true anaphylactic reactions should be admitted to either an ED observation unit or the hospital for short-term observation. Patients who continue to have life-threatening symptoms (e.g., bronchospasm, hypotension, or upper airway obstruction) should be admitted to an ICU.

15. What is the prehospital or out-of-hospital treatment of anaphylaxis?
Patients who are known to be at high risk (e.g., previous anaphylactic reaction to hymenoptera) should be prescribed and educated in the self-administration of epinephrine with an autoinjector at the first sign of anaphylactic symptoms. Self-administration of oral diphenhydramine is indicated to treat mild reactions such as urticaria or concomitant with the administration of epinephrine.

BIBLIOGRAPHY

1. Horach A, et al: Severe myocardial ischemia induced by intravenous adrenaline. BMJ 286:519, 1983.
2. Kemp SF, et al: Anaphylaxis: A review of 266 cases, Arch Intern Med 155:1749–1754, 1995.
3. Lee ML: Glucagon in anaphylaxis (letter). J Allergy Clin Immunol 69:331, 1981.
4. Lucke WC, Thomas H: Anaphylaxis: Pathophysiology, clinical presentation and treatment. J Emerg Med 1:83–95, 1983.
5. Muellman RL, Tran PT: Allergy, hypersensitivity and anaphylaxis. In Rosen P (ed): Emergency Medicine: Concepts and Clinical Practice, 5th ed. St. Louis, Mosby, 2002, pp 1619–1634.
6. Runge JW, Martinex JC, Cavuti EM: Histamine antagonists in the treatment of acute allergic reactions. Ann Emerg Med 21:237–242, 1992.
7. Silverman JH, Van Hook C, Haponik EF: Hemodynamic changes in human anaphylaxis. Am J Med 77:341–344, 1984.
8. Volcheck GW, Li JT: Exercise-induced uticaria and anaphylaxis. Mayo Clin Proc 72:140–147, 1997.

19. LOW BACK PAIN

Robert S. Hockberger, M.D.

1. Can I skip this chapter?
Not if you anticipate a career that involves caring for adults. Low back pain (LBP) is the fourth most common adult ambulatory complaint in the United States, following the common cold, minor trauma, and headache. Four out of five people older than age 25 have at least one incapacitating episode of LBP during their life. LBP is the number one cause of restricted activity in patients younger than age 45 and ranks number three (after heart disease and arthritis) in patients older than age 45. The cost of diagnosis, treatment, disability, lost productivity, and litigation as a result of LBP exceeds $20 billion yearly, making it the third most expensive medical disorder in the United States (after heart disease and cancer).

2. What are the causes of LBP?
Most cases of LBP are **musculoskeletal**, involving principally an injury or strain of the ligaments or muscles of the lower back or lumbar disc disease. Other causes are renal disease, pancreatic disease, perforated peptic ulcer, retrocecal appendicitis, ruptured abdominal aortic aneurysm, and malignancies and infections involving the spinal column.

3. When should I suspect malignancy as a cause of LBP, and how should it be evaluated?

Patients younger than age 50 develop primary tumors of the spine (usually benign), and patients older than age 50 who develop malignancies (particularly thyroid, breast, lung, kidney, and prostate cancer) frequently develop metastases to the spinal column. At risk are patients with known malignancy or signs and symptoms suggestive of malignancy and patients who have had LBP for more than 1 month, particularly when treatment with nonsteroidal antiinflammatory medications (NSAIDs) has proved ineffective.

Evaluation of such patients should include lumbosacral spine radiographs and an erythrocyte sedimentation rate (ESR). If either test is abnormal, a more detailed imaging study (bone scan, CT, or MRI) should be obtained and the patient referred for further evaluation.

4. When should a spinal column infection be suspected, and how should it be evaluated?

Patients at greatest risk for vertebral body or disc space infections include children, immunosuppressed patients (particularly diabetics), intravenous drug abusers, and patients who recently have undergone back surgery. They usually present with LBP associated with fever and localized vertebral bony tenderness. Fever is absent in one third of cases, however. Lumbosacral spine radiographs are often normal (particularly if pain has been present for less than several weeks), but the ESR is usually elevated. Abnormal radiographs or an elevated ESR should result in hospitalization or emergent referral for a more detailed imaging study (bone scan, CT, or MRI) and definitive care.

5. What does it mean when a patient with LBP also has leg pain?

Patients with LBP may have pain that is referred down a leg as a result of inflammation of the sciatic nerve or that radiates down a leg as a result of nerve root impingement (usually from a herniated lumbar disc or narrowing of a vertebral foramen from spinal stenosis, but also occasionally from epidural metastases or abscesses in high-risk patients). Referred pain is usually dull and poorly localized, does not radiate distal to the knee, and is not associated with a positive straight-leg raising (SLR) test or neurologic impairment of the lower extremities. Alternatively, nerve root impingement results in sharp, well-localized radicular pain that frequently (but not always) radiates distal to the knee, invariably is associated with a positive SLR test, and may be associated with neurologic impairment.

6. How should the SLR test be performed? What does it mean?

With the patient lying supine on the examining table, the physician slowly raises the patient's involved leg off the bed (flexing the leg at the hip while keeping the knee straightened) until the patient complains of discomfort. Most healthy adults do not complain of discomfort or have only mild discomfort from the stretching of the hamstring muscles after the leg is elevated more than 60°. Some patients with low back strain complain of discomfort at the site of injury during the SLR test, but radicular symptoms do not occur. A **positive SLR test** occurs when leg elevation results in pain that radiates down the involved leg and infers nerve root impingement from a herniated lumbar disc or lateral spinal stenosis. A **positive crossed-SLR test** occurs when elevation of the uninvolved leg causes pain to radiate down the involved leg. When such pain is present, it is a sensitive and specific sign for disc herniation.

7. How extensive must the patient's history and physical examination be?

Include in the history the patient's age (infections and malignancies are more common in the very young and very old), known medical problems, and previous episodes of LBP; the nature of the injury; the duration of symptoms and response to treatment (if any); the presence or absence of radicular symptoms; and any history of bowel or bladder dysfunction (evidence of impingement on the cauda equina).

Physical examination should determine the degree of patient's distress and limitation of spinal movement, the presence of trigger points of maximal tenderness, evidence of paravertebral muscle spasm, and results of neurologic examination of the lower extremities (motor, sensory, and reflex evaluation).

8. Whom should I irradiate?

Radiographs are expensive (we spend approximately $1 billion per year on lumbosacral spine films in the United States), result in gonadal radiation, and rarely help in directing initial diagnosis and treatment. Lumbosacral spine films should be obtained in patients with acute LBP who are suspected of having a spinal column malignancy or infection, in patients who have experienced significant trauma or who are in marked physical distress, and in patients who exhibit a neurologic deficit. Otherwise, radiographs should be reserved for patients who fail to improve with initial management.

9. Who should receive a CT scan or MRI evaluation?

CT and MRI should be used acutely to evaluate patients with suspected disc herniation who present with lower extremity motor paralysis or bowel or bladder dysfunction (evidence of massive central disc herniation). Such patients should be hospitalized because they frequently require urgent neurosurgical intervention. CT or MRI should be used to evaluate patients with *any* evidence of neurologic impairment that possibly can be due to nerve impingement from a spinal epidural metastasis or an epidural abscess. The former requires high-dose radiation therapy; the latter, usually surgical drainage in addition to intravenous antibiotics.

10. Who should be hospitalized for treatment?

With the exception of previously discussed patients who require emergency CT or MRI, there are no standard indications for hospitalization. Hospitalize patients with suspected disc herniation who are in significant physical distress or exhibit evidence of motor impairment of the lower extremities; their failure to respond to aggressive conservative management may necessitate surgical intervention.

11. How should patients be treated in the ED?

Quickly. There is no need to await definitive diagnosis before providing pain relief. Patients who have trigger points frequently benefit from local injection with a steroid-local anesthetic combination. Other patients should be given oral or parenteral NSAIDs and a cold pack applied locally to injured muscles and ligaments. Occasionally, parenteral narcotics are necessary to provide adequate analgesia.

12. Describe the best initial outpatient treatment for LBP.

Most patients with mild-to-moderate discomfort do not require bed rest and do better if they continue with *limited* activity (i.e., no heavy lifting or prolonged sitting). Patients with moderate-to-severe discomfort profit from bed rest (except for bathroom privileges) for 2 to 3 days to rest injured muscles and ligaments. The period can extend to 7 to 10 days for patients with suspected disc herniation. A firm mattress is best.

Cryotherapy (cold application) should be administered four or five times a day. Instruct patients to use crushed ice placed in a self-sealed plastic bag and wrapped in a towel, maintaining the cold application for at least 30 minutes.

Most patients benefit from oral NSAIDs, but some require opioids to produce adequate analgesia during the first few days. Sedatives and muscle relaxants probably do little to *relax* injured muscles, but because of their sedating effects, they are helpful in improving patient compliance with instructions for bed rest.

13. Summarize appropriate aftercare instructions.

All patients with suspected disc disease and patients with low back strain who do not improve within 1 week should be seen by a physician for follow-up evaluation. All patients should be instructed to return immediately if they develop any bowel or bladder dysfunction or if they have increasing progressive weakness or radicular pain.

14. What happens to patients with LBP when they leave the ED?

The prognosis for patients having a first episode of LBP (when you have considered and eliminated the possibility of underlying disease) is good; 70% are better by 1 week, 80% by 2 weeks, and 90% by 1 month. Most studies comparing medical management, chiropractic manipulation, and other treatment modalities rarely find significant differences in outcome because almost everyone gets better no matter what you do. Patients who do not improve with conservative management may have underlying disease (inflammatory disorders, malignancy, infections, or disc disease) that was not apparent at the time of initial evaluation or, alternatively, may suffer from nonmedical conditions, such as psychiatric disorders, drug dependence, or job dissatisfaction.

BIBLIOGRAPHY

1. Borenstein DG: A clinician's approach to acute low back pain. Am J Med 102(suppl 1A):16S–22S, 1997.
2. Byrne TN: Spinal cord compression from epidural metastases. N Engl J Med 327:614–619, 1992.
3. Deen HG Jr: Diagnosis and management of lumbar disc disease. Mayo Clin Proc 71:283–287, 1996.
4. Deyo RA, Diehl AK: Cancer as a cause of back pain: Frequency, clinical presentation and diagnostic strategies. J Gen Intern Med 3:230–238, 1988.
5. Deyo RA, Rainville J, Kent DL: What can the history and physical examination tell us about low back pain? JAMA 268:760–765, 1992.
6. Deyo RA, Weinstein JN: Low back pain. N Engl J Med 344:363–370, 2001.
7. King PA: Evaluating the child with back pain. Pediatr Clin North Am 33:1489–1497, 1986.
8. Koes BW: Efficacy of nonsteroidal anti-inflammatory drugs for low back pain: A systematic review of randomized clinical trials. Ann Rheum Dis 56:214–220, 1997.
9. Malmivaara A, Hakkinen U, Aro T, et al: The treatment of acute low back pain: Bed rest, exercises, or ordinary activity? N Engl J Med 332:351–355, 1995.
10. Roland P, Gimbel R: Evaluation of the patient with spinal trauma and back pain: An evidence based approach. Emerg Med Clin North Am 17:25–39, 1999.
11. Suarez-Almazor ME, Belseck E, Russell AS, Mackel JV: Use of lumbar radiographs for the early diagnosis of low back pain. JAMA 277:1782–1786, 1997.
12. Von Korff M. Saunders K: The course of back pain in primary care. Spine 21:2833–2837, 1996.
13. Vroomen PC: Lack of effectiveness of bed rest for sciatica. N Engl J Med 340:418–424, 1999.

III. Nontraumatic Illness

20. NONTRAUMATIC OCULAR EMERGENCIES

Daniel F. Danzl, M.D.

1. What are some of the unique issues regarding ophthalmologic pharmacology?

Topical agents may have systemic effects, so exercise caution when prescribing β-blockers, vasoconstrictors, and anticholinergics. Ointments have a longer duration of action but blur vision.

Diagnostic medications include stains, such as fluorescein, that help identify corneal and conjunctival abnormalities, and topical anesthetics, which should never be dispensed. Nonsteroidal anti-inflammatory drugs, such as ketorolac, are useful for pain relief. Topical corticosteroids should be used with consultation.

Miotic eye drop bottles have green tops, and mydriatic/cycloplegic agents have red tops. Never allow Hemoccult drops (yellow or blue top) in an eye room because severe alkali burns have occurred.

2. Name some of the considerations involving pupillary dilation.

Phenylephrine (2.5%) is a direct sympathomimetic and mydriatic. Dilation may last 4 hours, and patients with a shallow anterior chamber may develop acute glaucoma after leaving the ED. Pupils generally do not require dilation in the ED. A PanOptic ophthalmoscope provides a five times larger view of the undilated fundus. For short-term cycloplegia, consider tropicamide (1 to 6 hours) or 1% to 5% homatropine (1 to 2 days); never use atropine (1 to 3 weeks).

3. What is conjunctivitis?

Inflammation of the bulbar and palpebral conjunctivae or mucous membranes. Most cases are viral or bacterial, and there is much overlap in presentation. **Viral conjunctivitis** is usually bilateral with clear epiphora or tearing. A preauricular node suggests epidemic keratoconjunctivitis (adenovirus). Two other viral pathogens are herpes simplex, with dendritic ulcers, and zoster, with involvement of the fifth cranial nerve. **Bacterial conjunctivitis** initially may be unilateral with purulent crusty drainage. Always consider an undiagnosed foreign body with unilateral conjunctivitis. *Chlamydia* or gonococcus should be considered in neonates or adults with sexually transmitted diseases. Allergies may cause papillae under the lids, chemosis, and itching.

4. How is conjunctivitis treated?

Common agents include tobramycin drops and sulfacetamide; the latter stings, which can decrease compliance. Erythromycin is available only in ointment form. Reserve the topical fluoroquinolones ciprofloxacin and ofloxacin for more severe infections and for contact lens wearers who are at risk for *Pseudomonas*. Avoid neomycin because hypersensitivity reactions are common.

5. What is endophthalmitis?

Infection or inflammation within the orbit. It usually is seen as a collection of pus in the anterior chamber (hypopyon) that resembles a dependent meniscus similar to the blood collection in a hyphema. Antecedent causes include corneal ulcers, direct inoculation or hematogenous spread, and conjunctivitis with organisms capable of penetrating the cornea (e.g., *Neisseria gonorrhoeae, Corynebacterium, Listeria, Haemophilus aegyptius*).

6. What is the difference between periorbital and orbital cellulitis?

Periorbital (preseptal) cellulitis is soft tissue infection of anterior eye structures usually localized to the eyelids and conjunctivae. **Orbital cellulitis** is a more serious infection (behind the septum) that involves posterior eye structures. Both tend to be unilateral and may be preceded by trauma and upper respiratory, sinus, or dental infections. Orbital cellulitis is most often the result of direct spread from ethmoid sinusitis, whereas periorbital cellulitis usually is caused by hematogenous spread of bacteria.

7. How do I differentiate clinically between periorbital and orbital cellulitis?

The two may be difficult to distinguish clinically, especially in children. **Periorbital cellulitis** tends to cause local eyelid symptoms and occasionally ocular discharge and may be associated with fever or leukocytosis. Visual acuity and pupillary reflexes are normal.

Orbital cellulitis may present with all of the above plus exophthalmos, fever, and pain with extraocular movements. Decreased visual acuity, loss of sensation over the ophthalmic and maxillary branches of the trigeminal nerve in V1 and V2 (division of cranial nerve V), and increased intraocular pressure are uncommon findings. Noncontrast CT scanning of the orbit is liberally indicated with periorbital swelling when there is a possibility of postseptal infection.

8. What is the common clinical presentation of cavernous sinus thrombosis?

Patients often progress from fever, headache, and chemosis to ophthalmoplegia, exophthalmos, and altered level of consciousness. Paralysis of cranial nerves III, IV, and VI usually is noted.

9. What if I don't have a slit lamp to evaluate the red eye?

Topical application of anesthetic drops should decrease or eradicate pain secondary to an abrasion or conjunctivitis (not so with iritis or glaucoma). Redness at the corneal-scleral junction (perilimbic flush) suggests iritis or glaucoma. Shining a light into the normal eye should make the opposite eye hurt if the patient has iritis (because of consensual movement of the inflamed affected contralateral iris). In addition to the consensual pupillary reflex test, the accommodative test is suggestive, which is simply pain precipitated by accommodation. Pain with either maneuver suggests ciliary spasm.

10. What typical findings help with the differential diagnosis of the red eye?

	CONJUNCTIVITIS	ACUTE IRITIS	ANGLE-CLOSURE GLAUCOMA
Incidence	Extremely common	Common	Uncommon
Discharge	Moderate to copious	Reflex epiphora	None
Vision	Normal	Slightly blurred	Very blurred (halos)
Pain	Gritty	Moderate	Severe
Conjunctival injection	Diffuse	Perilimbic	Perilimbic
Cornea	Clear	Keratotic precipitates	Steamy or hazy
Pupil size	Normal	Constricted	Dilated
Pupillary light response	Normal	Poor	Poor
Intraocular pressure	Normal	Normal	Elevated

11. Describe the clinical presentation of iritis.

Patients often present with perilimbic injection, ciliary spasm, and a constricted miotic pupil. Iritis can be bilateral and misdiagnosed as conjunctivitis. If a slit lamp is available, check the anterior chamber for cell and flare and for keratotic precipitates (white cells) on the back of the cornea.

12. What is acute angle-closure glaucoma?

In a patient with a narrow anterior chamber angle, reduced illumination causes mydriasis; folds of the peripheral iris can block the angle, which prevents aqueous humor outflow. The rapid elevation of intraocular pressure causes optic atrophy if not treated promptly. The diagnosis may be delayed by the misleading systemic complaints of nausea, vomiting, and pain.

13. How are iritis and acute angle-closure glaucoma treated?

Iritis is treated with systemic analgesics and a topical cycloplegic to paralyze accommodation and dilate the iris; this prevents adhesions between the iris and the lens (posterior synechiae). Consider steroids in consultation with an ophthalmologist.

Acute glaucoma is treated with intravenous mannitol or glycerol to decrease intraocular pressure by osmotic diuresis, topical 2% pilocarpine or 0.5% timolol to decrease pupil size and increase aqueous outflow, and acetazolamide intravenously to decrease aqueous production. Topical apraclonidine also reduces aqueous humor production. Emergent ophthalmologic consultation is indicated.

14. What is a subconjunctival hemorrhage?

Subconjunctival hemorrhage occurs when a blood vessel ruptures under the conjunctiva. Without trauma, it often results from a Valsalva maneuver associated with coughing or vomiting. Patients see the bright red sclera and frequently present with concerns of imminent blindness. Reassure the patient that vision will not be affected and that the blood will be absorbed over 10 to 14 days. Patients on anticoagulants should have their international normalized ratio measured and receive ophthalmologic follow-up.

15. What does the presence of an afferent pupillary defect (APD), also known as a Marcus-Gunn pupil, indicate?

If the patient has an APD, it confirms damage in the retina or optic nerve. To perform the *swinging flashlight test*, swing the light after several seconds from the normal eye to the other eye. After a brief pupillary constriction in the abnormal eye, the redilation in response to light reflects afferent deprivation. Patients with an APD usually have a central retinal artery occlusion, central retinal vein occlusion, or optic/retrobulbar neuritis. In contrast, retinal detachment, macular or vitreous hemorrhage, glaucoma, trauma, and hysteria do not have an APD.

16. In a patient with anisocoria, how does one determine which pupil is abnormal?

Begin the examination in a darkened room; if there is more anisocoria in the light, the large pupil is failing to constrict and is abnormal. More anisocoria that develops going into the dark indicates that the miotic pupil is failing to dilate. Never just assume that the larger pupil is abnormal.

17. What are common causes of a miotic pupil?

The two most common are Horner's syndrome and an Argyl-Robertson pupil. The clinical manifestations of **Horner's syndrome** include ptosis, miosis, and anhydrosis (in a cold ED, check for dilated conjunctival vessels). Bronchogenic carcinoma, stroke, and brachial plexus pathology may present with Horner's syndrome.

The **Argyl-Robertson pupil** is miotic, is irregular, and displays *light-near dissociation*: The pupil constricts to accommodation but not to light. This finding is common with diabetes and syphilis. A common testing error is to hold and shine a penlight directly in front of the eye, which can cause the pupil to constrict from accommodation, not light.

18. Is there another cause of light-near dissociation?

The only other cause is **Adie's pupil**, which results from idiopathic parasympathetic denervation in the ciliary ganglion in the eye. The patient is often a young woman with a mydriatic pupil that accommodates but does not react to light. Herpes zoster is another cause of Adie's pupil. There are no diseases that cause a pupil to react to light but fail to accommodate.

19. How can I be certain that a patient with no history of eye trauma has a pupil dilated from a medication?

If 1% pilocarpine fails to constrict the pupil, it is pharmacologically blocked, most commonly by phenylephrine, handling a scopolamine patch, or aerosolized anticholinergics.

20. What are some other causes of a unilateral dilated pupil?

This can be a normal finding or as a result of posttraumatic mydriasis or third nerve palsy.

21. What are some common causes of nontraumatic loss of vision?

Transient monocular	**Acute binocular**
Amaurosis fugax	Migraine
Temporal arteritis	Vertebral basilar insufficiency
Migraine	Cerebrovascular disease
Persistent monocular	Toxins (methanol, salicylates, quinine, ergot)
Central retinal artery occlusion	Optic or retrobulbar neuritis
Central retinal vein occlusion	Hysteria
Retinal detachment or hemorrhage	Malingering
Vitreous or macular hemorrhage	
Optic or retrobulbar neuritis	
Internal carotid occlusion	

22. Describe the presentation and treatment of central retinal artery and central retinal vein occlusion.

Occlusion of the retinal artery or its branches results in a dilated nonreactive pupil with an APD on the affected side. The retina is pale with a *cherry red spot* at the macula (macular blood supply is from the choroidal circulation). Occasionally, amaurosis fugax precedes central retinal artery occlusion.

The funduscopic examination of a central retinal vein occlusion is described as a "blood and thunder fundus" because of the presence of multiple large hemorrhages. Both occur in middle-aged atherosclerotic patients or elderly hypertensive patients and present as sudden painless loss of vision. Efforts to decrease intraocular pressure and dilate retinal vessels by increasing the PCO_2 (paper bag, carbogen) and globe massage are rarely useful acutely for arterial occlusions. Prognosis for both entities is poor.

23. What are other causes of sudden painless monocular loss of vision?

Suspect vitreous hemorrhage in diabetics with an obscured red reflex and retinal details. Nontraumatic retinal detachments are more common in patients with significant myopia. Most commonly, patients complain of seeing dark floating spots or *floaters*, which reflect benign vitreous separations and not a retinal detachment.

24. How do optic neuritis and papilledema differ?

Although these two processes appear similar on funduscopic examination, **optic neuritis** involves focal demyelination of the optic nerve, resulting in a hyperemic nerve head developing over hours to days. The average age of onset is in the 30s. An association with multiple sclerosis is common.

Papilledema is swelling of the optic disc caused by increased intracranial pressure. It is usually bilateral but may be asymmetric and may be the result of brain abscess or tumor, intracranial bleeding, meningitis/encephalitis, hydrocephalus, severe hypertension, or pseudotumor cerebri. The earliest sign of papilledema is the loss of spontaneous venous pulsations, which, if difficult to appreciate, can be elicited with ipsilateral jugular compression.

	Optic Neuritis	**Papilledema**
Pupil reactivity	Slow	Normal
Visual acuity	Decreased	Normal
Pain	Present	Absent
Usual localization	Unilateral	Bilateral
Fundus	Blurred disc margins	Blurred disc margins

25. What are a couple tricks to prove that a patient can see?
Induce nystagmus with an opticokinetic drum, or simply hold a mirror in front of the eyes and slowly move it-tracking requires vision.

BIBLIOGRAPHY

1. Davidson P, Shockley L: Bilateral eye pain and loss of vision. Acad Emerg Med 4:1068–1069, 1997.
2. Juang PS, Rosen P: Ocular examination techniques for the emergency department. J Emerg Med 15:793–810, 1997.
3. Leibowitz HM: The red eye. N Engl J Med 343:345–351, 2000.
4. Le Sage N, Verreault R, Rochette L: Efficacy of eye patching for traumatic corneal abrasions: A controlled clinical trial. Ann Emerg Med 38:129–134, 2001.
5. Shields SR: Managing eye disease in primary care: Part 3. When to refer for ophthalmologic care. Postgrad Med 108:99–106, 2000.
6. Shingleton BJ, O'Donoghue MW: Blurred vision. N Engl J Med 343:556–562, 2000.
7. Szucs PA, Nashed AH, Allegra JR, Eskin B: Safety and efficacy of diclofenac ophthalmic solution in the treatment of corneal abrasions. Ann Emerg Med 35:131–137, 2000.

21. NONTRAUMATIC ENT EMERGENCIES

Gwendolyn J. Hewitt, M.D., and Katherine Bakes, M.D.

EPISTAXIS

1. What are the most common causes of epistaxis?
Nosebleeds can appear spontaneously, usually in association with dry nasal mucosa (from a deviated septum or rhinitis sicca) or infection. Minor local trauma from nose picking or direct blows to the nose are frequent causes. Less commonly detected sources include foreign bodies, tumors, coagulopathies, exposure to anticoagulant drugs such as aspirin or warfarin (Coumadin), and exposure to toxic or caustic materials such as cocaine. Approximately 60% of people experience at least one episode of epistaxis in their lifetime, and 6% of those seek medical attention for it.

2. Doesn't hypertension cause epistaxis?
Not as an acute event. The hypertensive patient who presents with a nosebleed typically has hypertension as a chronic condition and has developed atherosclerosis, which makes the blood vessels relatively fragile and more likely to be disrupted when exposed to any of the above-mentioned conditions.

3. Does bleeding originate from any one particular source?
Approximately 90% of nosebleeds originate from the anterior portion of the nose, a rich vascular network on the anterior portion of the septum known as *Kiesselbach's plexus* or *Little's area*. The blood supply for most of this region is derived from the external carotid system. From a practical standpoint, a nosebleed with a source that can be seen directly or is controlled after proper placement of an anterior nasal pack is considered *anterior*. Posterior bleeds arise from either the external or the internal carotid artery branches and tend to be more difficult to control. The hemorrhage tends to be more severe and is seen more frequently in the elderly. Atraumatic bleeding almost always comes from an isolated, unilateral source, and when it appears from both nares, it is due to blood passing behind the nasal septum.

4. List the key historical questions to ask the patient.
1. Is there a prior history of nosebleeds?
2. How about a past medical history of hypertension, excessive alcohol use, bleeding disorders, or other underlying conditions?

3. Was any trauma (even nose picking) involved?
4. On which side did the bleeding start?
5. Any recent sinus infections or surgeries?
6. How about warfarin (Coumadin) or aspirin use?

5. Summarize the key points to successful management of nosebleeds.
There are two key considerations. The first is that of **preparation**. Because epistaxis rarely presents as a life-threatening condition that demands rapid institution of the ABCs of resuscitation, there almost always is time to assemble the necessary equipment and supplies for treatment (see Table). While obtaining the history, have the patient pinch the nose firmly or place a nasal clamp on the patient with firm pressure on the septum. The patient and the examiner should be gowned. The examiner should wear disposable gloves, mask, and eye protection. The second key point is to **identify the source** of the hemorrhage.

Supplies for Examination and Treatment of Nosebleeds

EXAMINATION	STABILIZATION	TREATMENT
Protective garb	Bayonet forceps	Silver nitrate cautery sticks
Head lamp or mirror	Cotton pledgets	Electrocautery (if available)
Nasal speculum	Lidocaine 4%	Gelfoam (or similar material)
Cotton swabs	Epinephrine 1:1000	$\frac{1}{2}$" Petroleum-impregnated gauze
Fraser tip suction	Tetracaine 0.5%	Antibiotic ointment
Emesis basin	Topical vasoconstrictor	Foley catheter or commercial balloon
4 × 4 Gauze		Rolled 4 × 4 gauze with silk suture

6. How do I treat epistaxis?
Using the nasal speculum, suction, and water-moistened cotton swabs, remove the existing clots until the bleeding site is seen. Insert a medicated pledget with topical anesthetic plus a vaso-constrictor for 5 to 10 minutes to allow vasoconstriction and anesthesia to occur. Remove the pledget and begin with simple methods. If the source is in Kiesselbach's plexus and is less than 1 cm², use silver nitrate or electrocautery with additional submucosal anesthetic infiltration (i.e., topical anesthesia was inadequate). Alternatively, a small piece of absorbable gelatin sponge (Gelfoam), Avitene, or similar substance may be moistened with a vasoconstrictor and applied to the bleeding site. If these methods are unsuccessful, an anterior nasal pack is used. In the past, stair-step application of $\frac{1}{2}$" antibiotic-coated petroleum gauze in an anterior-posterior direction was done with nasal speculum and bayonet forceps until the nasal cavity was filled from the floor, superiorly. Spongelike Merocel packs that are coated with antibiotic ointment and reconstituted with saline after insertion are easy to apply with minimal patient discomfort and are frequently effective. If inspection of the posterior pharynx reveals no continued bleeding after the vasoconstriction wears off (about 30 minutes), the patient may be discharged.

7. What are the important discharge instructions?
1. The pack should be removed in 24 to 48 hours. If the pack stays in place longer, systemic antibiotics (penicillin) should be initiated to prevent sinusitis.
2. The patient should avoid activities or ingestions that may transiently increase blood pressure (e.g., sneezing, bending over, caffeine).
3. If recurrences fail to respond to direct pressure at home for 10 minutes, the patient should seek medical attention.
4. Regular applications of petroleum or antibiotic ointment and use of room humidifiers can prevent bleeding from desiccated nasal mucosa.

8. How do I diagnose posterior epistaxis?
If a properly placed anterior pack fails, the patient has a posterior bleed, and more aggressive treatment is required. Posterior packs are accomplished with rolled 4 × 4-inch gauze, a Foley

catheter, or Nasostat or other commercially available balloon product. A unilateral anterior pack still is required in conjunction with a posterior pack.

9. Do I send a patient home with a posterior pack?

No. All patients who require a posterior pack require an ENT consultation. Although the mechanism is unclear, posterior packs can lead to hypoxia and apnea. These patients should be admitted for respiratory monitoring and supplemental oxygen if needed.

10. Didn't you forget to mention laboratory studies?

No, most patients don't need them. The exceptions are patients taking warfarin or with suspected coagulopathies and patients who are hemodynamically unstable or require admission.

FOREIGN BODIES

11. How should I remove a foreign body from the ear?

The following instruments can assist in extraction:

Foreign body (alligator) forceps	Fraser tip suction	Ear curette
Right-angle probe	Irrigation syringe	Water-Pik
Tissue forceps	Adson forceps	Skin hook
Cyanoacrylate glue	Fogarty biliary catheter	Day hook

If a live insect is in the external auditory canal (EAC), it first should be killed by instilling 2% lidocaine (which is quicker and less messy than mineral oil) before intact or segmental removal. If the tympanic membrane is intact and space exists between the EAC and the object, a stream of liquid can be directed behind the foreign body to force it out. A mixture of water and isopropyl alcohol as an irrigation solution tends to cause less swelling of organic matter and evaporates more quickly. Direct instrument manipulation or suction removes most other objects. Occasionally, cyanoacrylate glue on the end of a suture or a small balloon-tipped catheter can do the trick.

12. How do patients with nasal foreign bodies present?

Unless the patient or a witness reports the insertion of a foreign body, the chief complaint is that of unilateral, malodorous nasal discharge. The discharge may be thin and mucoid, serosanguineous, or, most often, purulent.

13. Is there any special trick to removing foreign bodies from the nose?

Prepare a 50/50 mixture of a topical vasoconstrictor and 4% topical lidocaine, and spray it into the involved nostril with an atomizer or spray bottle. Nebulized epinephrine also has been used as a vasoconstrictor with good results. This anesthetizes the sensitive nasal mucosa and reduces congestion to facilitate removal. When this is done, a simple measure, such as occluding the unaffected nostril and having the patient blow forcefully, can expel the object. If the patient is unable or unwilling to attempt this maneuver, positive-pressure insufflation can be attempted. The unaffected nostril is occluded, and a quick breath is delivered through a facemask connected to an Ambu-bag. Alternatively, a parent or caregiver can do this in *direct*, mouth-to-mouth fashion. If insufflation maneuvers are unsuccessful, an attempt should be made to remove the foreign body with suction or instruments such as a forceps. The general measures listed for foreign body removal from the ear can be applied in this situation. Because the nasal opening and cavity are larger, a greater number and larger instruments, such as a Kelly clamp, bayonet forceps, or Foley catheter, can be used, but instrument manipulation remains the mainstay for foreign body removal. Also, consider prescribing antibiotics because sinusitis or otitis media may coexist.

14. "I think I've got something stuck in my throat." How is the patient with this complaint managed?

The fact that the patient can talk is a good sign. Airway foreign body or compromise must be addressed and ruled out. The patient should be asked about the nature of the foreign body, the duration of the sensation, the ability to swallow liquids or solids, and the perceived location of the object. Patient estimates of location are surprisingly accurate. Direct visualization can identify sharp objects, such as fish bones, that may become impaled in the posterior pharynx or the base of the tongue. Indirect or fiberoptic laryngoscopy, in conjunction with local anesthesia, can pinpoint objects stuck in the vallecula, epiglottis, or pyriform sinus.

15. If the physical examination does not reveal the foreign body, what should be done next?
Soft tissue density lateral radiographs of the neck or chest radiographs should be obtained. Large and sharp, angulated objects tend to lodge in the esophagus. The next step involves the use of a water-soluble radiographic contrast material, with a water-soluble agent such as Gastrografin if esophageal perforation is a possibility. Barium should be avoided initially because it may interfere with subsequent endoscopy. Esophagoscopy should be considered in patients with persistent symptoms or when the diagnosis is in doubt.

16. If I can see a foreign body, how do I remove it?
After a topical spray anesthetic is administered, objects that can be seen can be removed with bayonet forceps or a Kelly clamp. Smooth objects in the esophagus can be removed by placing the patient in extreme Trendelenburg position, passing a Foley catheter beyond the object, expanding the balloon, and withdrawing the catheter. Intravenous glucagon (0.5 to 2.0 mg) may relax the lower esophageal sphincter, allowing a distal obstruction to pass. Because glucagon may elicit nausea and vomiting, it can cause esophageal perforation if unsuccessful. Papain-containing agents, which enzymatically dissolve meat, should *not* be used. Sharp objects should be removed endoscopically. Repeat esophagography should be done when the removal involves sharp or impaled objects or prolonged or aggressive manipulation or if perforation is a consideration.

17. Any parting words on the subject?
There's good news and bad news. Of foreign bodies, 80% to 90% pass through the gastrointestinal tract without significant problems. The remainder require surgical removal. These latter objects tend to be sharp or long (> 6.5 cm) and are among the 1% that cause perforation. A special case should be made for disk or button batteries. Because most are prone to leakage, every effort should be made to remove them if localized to the esophagus. Otherwise, the location in the gastrointestinal system should be followed until elimination is confirmed.

SINUSITIS

18. When do the sinuses form?
The maxillary and ethmoid sinuses form in the third and fourth months of gestation, whereas the sphenoid sinuses form by 5 years of age. The frontal sinuses begin to form at 7 years but are not complete until late adolescence.

19. What is sinusitis, and what are the common causes?
Sinusitis is an inflammation of the paranasal sinuses, including the maxillary, ethmoid, frontal, and sphenoid sinuses. It is the consequence of ostia occlusion, most commonly caused by local mucosal swelling from a viral upper respiratory infection. Allergies; trauma; and mechanical obstruction from tumors, foreign bodies, or abnormal anatomy also may cause occlusion that leads to bacterial overgrowth and excess mucus production. Of all viral upper respiratory infections, 0.5% to 5% are complicated by bacterial sinusitis. When symptoms last less than 3 weeks, the process is characterized as acute.

20. How do I make the diagnosis?
Maxillary dental pain, discolored or purulent nasal discharge, no improvement with decongestants, and a biphasic illness are four of the best indicators of acute sinusitis. Patients often have headache, fever, facial tenderness and pain, anosmia, and halitosis. Patients may relate a

history of nocturnal coughing, postnasal drip, and sore throat. Depending on the location of the infection, pain may intensify with bending forward or lying supine. The physical examination is often unrewarding, but one should attempt to elicit pain with palpation and percussion over the affected region. Anterior rhinoscopy with a headlamp and nasal speculum reveals the presence of pus, foreign bodies, masses, or anatomic abnormalities. Decreased transillumination of the maxillary and frontal sinuses with a strong point light source may indicate the need for further diagnostic studies because only negative studies (normal transillumination) are useful.

21. Which other diagnostic studies should I pursue?

The utility of plain radiographs is controversial. A single Waters' view is as sensitive as a full sinus series. Findings include mucosal thickening (> 6 mm), air-fluid levels, and opacification. For uncomplicated sinusitis, CT is not specific because 40% of asymptomatic and 87% of patients with a recent upper respiratory infection have abnormal findings on CT scan. CT can be useful to diagnose intrafacial or intracranial involvement. Nasal endoscopy is an excellent modality for identifying disease but is done only by an otolaryngologist and rarely on an emergent basis.

22. How is sinusitis treated?

There are two therapeutic goals: (1) to open the ostia to facilitate drainage and (2) to eliminate the infection. The former is accomplished with a variety of topical or systemic decongestants. The use of vasoconstrictor sprays, such as phenylephrine (Neo-Synephrine) or oxymetazoline (Afrin), can provide immediate relief but should be used no longer than 3 to 4 days because of the propensity for rebound edema. Oral agents allow for more prolonged treatment and affect deeper tissues not penetrated by the topical sprays. Antihistamines should not be used because they may worsen the course secondary to crusting and blockage of the ostia. Antibiotics should be aimed at the most likely organisms: *Streptococcus pneumoniae*, nontypable *Haemophilus influenzae*, *Moraxella catarrhalis*, other *Streptococcus* species, and anaerobes. Any of the following can be used either for 2 weeks or until symptoms resolve plus 7 days: amoxicillin, trimethoprim-sulfamethoxazole, penicillin VK, amoxicillin-clavulanate, doxycycline, cefaclor, azithromycin, and clarithromycin.

23. How does treatment differ in children?

The risk for resistance to amoxicillin is increased with daycare attendance and recent antibiotic use (< 90 days). These children should receive second-line antibiotics, such as amoxicillin-clavulanate, cefuroximine, cefpodoxime, cefdinir, azithromycin, and clarithromycin.

24. Which patients need referral and admission? What are the complications?

If there is no improvement after two complete courses of antibiotics, the patient should be referred to an otolaryngologist. Complications arising during therapy can be classified as local, orbital, and intracranial. Patients with sinusitis who show evidence of orbital or central nervous system involvement should be treated as medical emergencies. Locally, mucoceles and osteomyelitis can develop. Orbital complications are the most frequent, especially in children, and range from cellulitis to abscess formation. Cavernous sinus thrombosis, resulting from the direct spread of infection through valveless veins, is imminently life-threatening. It is heralded by a toxic appearance, high fever, cranial nerve palsies, retinal engorgement, and bilateral chemosis and proptosis. Other intracranial complications demanding aggressive intensive therapy include meningitis, subdural empyema, and brain abscesses.

25. Any other pearls?

Yes. Check a finger-stick glucose in the sick patient with sinusitis. *Mucor* in diabetic patients and *Aspergillus* in immunocompromised patients can be life-threatening, requiring hospital admission and specialist consultation.

EPIGLOTTITIS

26. How did George Washington die?
George Washington is believed to have died from epiglottitis. It is recorded that on December 14, 1799, the morning of his death, he had a severe sore throat and later developed stridor and hoarseness and was unable to lie supine.

27. List the signs and symptoms of epiglottitis in adults.
Symptoms:
    Sore throat (100%)
    Odynophagia/dysphagia (76%)
    Fever (88%)
    Shortness of breath (78%)
    Anterior neck tenderness
    Hoarseness or muffled voice
Signs:
    Lymphadenopathy
    Drooling
    Respiratory distress
    Extreme pain with palpation of the larynx

28. What is the thumbprint sign?
A finding on lateral neck radiographs caused by the presence of an edematous epiglottis. Lateral neck films are of limited use because they are only 38% sensitive and 76% specific.

29. Name the most common organisms identified in adult epiglottitis.
The two most common organisms found are *H. influenzae* and beta-hemolytic streptococci. In most cases, no organism is found, however, pointing toward a viral cause. With the introduction of the Hib vaccine in children, the reservoir for *H. influenzae* has decreased dramatically so that epiglottitis is seen more frequently in adults.

30. How do I manage epiglottitis? What signs and symptoms indicate the need for airway intervention?
Antibiotics should be started immediately. A second-generation or third-generation cephalosporin active against *H. influenzae* and beta-hemolytic streptococci is the drug of choice. The use of steroids is controversial and has not been shown to provide any benefit.

Patients with symptomatic respiratory distress, stridor, drooling, shorter duration of symptoms, and *H. influenzae* bacteremia are at increased risk for airway obstruction. Patients with a respiratory rate of less than 20 breaths/min and no respiratory distress should be observed closely in an ICU. Patients with a respiratory rate greater than 20 breaths/min and slight respiratory difficulty should be intubated in the operating room. Patients with a respiratory rate greater than 30 breaths/min, moderate-to-severe respiratory distress, PCO_2 of greater than 45 mm Hg, or cyanosis need immediate airway intervention.

CONTROVERSY

31. How is the definitive diagnosis of epiglottitis made?
The gold standard for definitive diagnosis of epiglottitis in **adults** is direct laryngoscopy and visualization of the inflamed epiglottis. In **children**, the appropriateness of direct visualization is more controversial. Some believe that any attempt at visualizing the inflamed epiglottis should take place in a controlled setting, such as the operating room. Others believe it is appropriate to use a tongue depressor to inspect the epiglottis of a small child sitting in his or her parent's lap. In either case, visualization should take place only by someone experienced in the management of pediatric airways.

OTITS EXTERNA

32. How does otitis externa present?
The classic finding is pain with manipulation of the external ear. Cardinal symptoms are itching, pain, tenderness to palpation, and less commonly hearing loss and fullness. Common signs are erythema and edema of the auditory canal, with crusting, pus, or weeping secretions. Predisposing factors for otitis externa, also called *swimmer's ear*, are excessive moisture in the ear canal and trauma (typically from overzealous cleaning).

33. How is it treated?
The goals for treatment are twofold: (1) to avoid precipitants and (2) to eradicate infection. To treat infection, 2% acetic acid combined with hydrocortisone should be placed in the ear canal. Alternatively, topical antibiotic drops can be used. If the external ear canal is extremely inflamed and narrowed, a wick can be placed to ensure drainage and instillation of medication. If otitis media coexists, be sure to add systemic antibiotics.

34. What is malignant otitis externa?
Malignant otitis externa is a potentially lethal extension of infection of the external ear canal into the mastoid or temporal bone. It is caused most commonly by *Pseudomonas aeruginosa* and occurs in patients with diabetes and immunocompromised states. The mortality rate can be greater than 50%. Malignant otitis externa should be considered when, despite adequate treatment, headache and otalgia persist or are greater than other clinical signs. CT or MRI confirms the diagnosis. Treatment includes admission, intravenous antipseudomonal antibiotics, and potentially surgical débridement.

PERITONSILLAR ABSCESS

35. State the typical signs and symptoms seen with peritonsillar abscess.
Symptoms: fever, unilateral sore throat, odynophagia, trismus, and occasionally referred otalgia. Patients typically have had pharyngitis for some time with recent antibiotic treatment.
Signs: limited opening of the mouth, drooling, speaking in a muffled "hot potato" voice, inability to open the mouth more than 2.5 cm, and rancid breath. Examining the oropharynx shows erythema with a deeper redness over the affected area. There is tense swelling of the anterior pillar and soft palate. Subsequently the tonsil is pushed downward and toward the midline. The uvula may be in an abnormal position, either shifted away from or lying flat against the affected side.

36. What are the treatment options for a peritonsillar abscess?
Needle aspiration followed by antibiotics is successful in 85% to 90% of patients. The patient should be seated and the tonsils visualized with a tongue depressor. Topical anesthetic should be applied using lidocaine or Cetacaine. A needle cover can be cut to provide a needle guard for an 18G to 20G needle, exposing no more than 0.5 cm of the needle. The guarded needle is inserted at the most purulent portion of the abscess. The physician should not penetrate deeper than 1 cm and stay medially to avoid the carotid artery. A positive aspiration is achieved if 1 mL or more of pus is obtained. If needle aspiration fails, referral to an ENT physician is necessary for surgical incision and drainage versus tonsillectomy.

RETROPHARYNGEAL ABSCESS

37. Describe the presentation of a retropharyngeal abscess.
Common presenting symptoms of retropharyngeal abscess include fever, odynophagia, and neck pain out of proportion to oropharyngeal findings. Patients are ill appearing and may hold the neck in extension and resist neck movement.

38. Why is this diagnosis so concerning?

The retropharyngeal space of the neck involves three facial layers between the paraspinal muscles and the pharynx. Infections and abscesses located here have the potential to cause airway compromise and offer a path of direct extension into the mediastinum.

39. How is a retropharyngeal abscess diagnosed?

It is sometimes visible on a soft tissue lateral neck radiograph, but definitive diagnosis is made by CT scan. Advanced airway management equipment should be at the bedside while an emergent consultation with an ENT physician is obtained. Intravenous antibiotics should be started, and the patient should be admitted to the ICU or taken directly to the operating room. Definitive management involves surgical incision and drainage. Mediastinal involvement mandates the involvement of a cardiothoracic surgeon.

BIBLIOGRAPHY

1. Bojrab DI, Bruderly T, Abdulrazzak Y: Otitis externa. Otolaryngol Clin North Am 29:761–782, 1996.
2. Carey MJ: Epiglottitis in adults. Am J Emerg Med 14:421–424, 1996.
3. Epperly TD, Wood TC: New trends in the management of peritonsillar abscess. Am Fam Physician 42:102–112, 1990.
4. Fagnan LJ: Acute sinusitis: A cost-effective approach to diagnosis and treatment. Am Fam Physician 58:1795–1801, 1998.
5. Fritz S, Kelen GD, Silvertson KT: Foreign bodies of the external auditory canal. Emerg Med Clin North Am 5:183–192, 1987.
6. Jones NS, Lannigan FJ, Salama NY: Foreign bodies in the throat: A prospective study of 388 cases. J Laryngol Otolaryngol 105:104–108, 1991.
7. Mayo-Smith MF, Spinale JW, Donsley CJ, et al: Acute epiglottitis: An 18-year experience in Rhode Island. Chest 108:1640–1648, 1995.
8. Lee SS, Schwartz RH, Bahadori RS: Retropharyngeal abscess: Epiglottitis of the new millennium. J Pediatr 138:435–437, 2001.
9. Poole MD: A focus on acute sinusitis in adults: Changes in disease management. Am J Med 106:38S–47S, 1999.
10. Shaw CB, Wax MK, Wetmore SJ: Epistaxis: A comparison of treatments. Otolaryngol Head Neck Surg 109:60–65, 1993.

22. DENTAL AND ORAL SURGICAL EMERGENCIES

Richard D. Zallen, D.D.S., M.D., Toby J. Feldman, D.D.S., and Richard L. McLain, D.D.S.

1. How are teeth numbered?

In adults, teeth are numbered starting from the upper right side: The third molar is tooth number 1, the upper right second molar is number 2, the upper right first molar is number 3, the next two bicuspids are numbers 4 and 5, the upper right canine is number 6, the upper right lateral incisor is number 7, the upper right central incisor is number 8, and the upper left central incisor is number 9. The rest of the upper left side is completed, with the upper left third molar being number 16. From here, you drop down to the lower left third molar, which is number 17, and continue on to the third molar on the right side, which is number 32.

Upper Right	Upper Left
1, 2, 3, 4, 5, 6, 7, 8, 9, 10, 11, 12, 13, 14, 15, 16	

Lower Right	Lower Left
32, 31, 30, 29, 28, 27, 26, 25, 24, 23, 22, 21, 20, 19, 18, 17	

In children with deciduous teeth (baby teeth), the upper right second molar is A, the first molar is B, the cuspid is C, the lateral incisor is D, the central incisor is E, and the upper left central incisor is F. The rest of the upper left side is completed, with the upper second molar being J. From here, you drop down to the lower left second molar, which is K, and continue on to the second molar on the right side, which is T.

Upper Right   Upper Left

A, B, C, D, E, F, G, H, I, J

Lower Right   Lower Left

T, S, R, Q, P, O, N, M, L, K

Children between the ages of 6 and 13 are in a mixed dentition stage with some adult and some deciduous teeth. Their teeth are numbered and lettered as the previous two diagrams illustrate.

2. Describe the types of tooth fractures and the treatment required.

The two basic types are fractures of the crown and fractures of the root. Ellis classified tooth fractures for anterior teeth as class I, II, III, and IV (modified). An Ellis class I fracture involves the enamel only and does not require emergent treatment. An Ellis class II fracture involves the enamel and dentin and requires placement of calcium hydroxide paste over the fracture. An Ellis class III fracture involves the enamel, dentin, and pulp and requires placement of calcium hydroxide. An Ellis class IV fracture involves the root of the tooth and may require extraction, root canal therapy, or splinting with dental resin, ligature wire, or Erich arch bars.

3. How should an avulsed tooth be transported?

The best transport medium is Hank's balanced salt solution or Viaspan. Hank's balanced salt solution comes in Save-A-Tooth 3M containers. If neither solution is available, milk can be used or a wet handkerchief. The patient's saliva should not be used because it can damage the periodontal ligament that is adherent to the root surface.

4. When should an avulsed tooth be replanted, and how is it stabilized?

The tooth should be replanted as soon as possible within the first 2 hours. Primary teeth should not be replanted. Stabilization of replanted teeth is necessary, provided that there is not any extensive caries, periodontal disease, or large alveolar housing fractures. Teeth are stabilized by physiologic splinting with dentin resin and ligature wire for 7 to 10 days.

5. What are alveolar housing fractures, and how are they treated?

Fractures of the alveolar ridge encompassing the dentition in either the maxilla or mandible. The treatment involves the reduction of the fracture usually manually and rigid splint fixation with an Erich arch bar for 4 to 5 weeks.

6. Should antibiotics be prescribed for an alveolar housing fracture or a reimplanted tooth?

Yes. A 5-day course of penicillin is recommended. The oral dose of penicillin V is 500 mg for adults and 25 to 50 mg/kg/d in four divided doses for children. In penicillin-allergic patients, clindamycin is preferred. The oral dose of clindamycin is 300 mg four times a day for adults and 10 to 20 mg/kg/d in four divided doses for children.

7. What are the concerns with electrical burns to the mouth?

Electrical burns are deceptive. The ultimate extent of tissue damage is greater than is present on initial examination, and the full extent of the injury may not be appreciated for 4 to 7 days. Wound contracture may produce microstomia. Close observation is warranted because of the possibility of delayed arterial hemorrhage.

8. How should a tongue laceration with profuse bleeding be treated?

Initially, packing with gauze and applying pressure should allow visualization of the source of bleeding. Injection of a local anesthetic with 1:100,000 epinephrine aids with vasoconstriction.

Clamping, ligating, or using electrocautery helps to control the larger bleeders when the bleeding site can be identified clearly. If minor bleeding persists, the laceration should be closed in a layered fashion using resorbable sutures for deep approximation and polyglactin 910 (Vicryl) for surface approximation.

9. How should a through-and-through lip laceration be closed?

Initial débridement of the wound may require surgical and saline débridement. Mucosal preparation with hexachlorophene (pHisoHex) is recommended. The mucosa is sutured with resorbable suture. Repreparation from the outside is recommended. A layered closure is done, using resorbable sutures for deep tissue approximation and nylon for skin. If the laceration involves the vermillion border, this should be approximated first. Prophylactic antibiotic coverage with penicillin for 5 days is recommended.

10. How should human or animal bites of the mouth be treated?

Human bites are managed best with copious irrigation, surgical débridement, and prophylactic antibiotics. The drug of choice is amoxicillin with clavulanic acid. Wounds should be closed primarily if possible, although delayed primary closure is an option in some cases. Animal bites are handled in a similar way. Antibiotics are recommended and may vary depending on species. Patients bitten by animals with suspected rabies must be treated aggressively, including irrigation with 10% povidone-iodine solution followed by normal saline, rabies postexposure prophylaxis, and tetanus prophylaxis.

11. When should antibiotics be used in management of dental infections?

An acute dentoalveolar abscess usually requires antibiotic therapy, with penicillin being the drug of choice. Adjunctive therapy should include endodontic treatment or extraction of the offending tooth and incision and drainage. The patient should be followed closely, usually within 24 hours.

12. List some nondental causes of orofacial pain.

Temporomandibular joint
Muscles of mastication
Salivary glands
Nose and paranasal sinuses
Blood vessels (arteritis)
Nerves
Oral ulcers

13. When should a patient with a dental abscess be admitted to the hospital?

Criteria for admission should be based on history and physical findings: size and location of swelling; rapidity of onset; dysphagia; dyspnea; fever; malaise; trismus; and age, state of hydration, laboratory evaluation, and immune status of the patient.

14. Name the risks of regional dental anesthesia.

Toxicity, allergy, syncope, muscle trismus, needle tract infection, intraarterial or intravenous injection, hematomas, and transient Bell's palsy from accidental injection into the area of the parotid gland. Broken needles rarely occur.

15. What is ANUG, and how is it treated?

Acute necrotizing ulcerative gingivitis (ANUG) is an acute infection of the gingiva that can be precipitated by psychological stress, smoking, and poor oral hygiene. ANUG typically presents with blunted interdental papilla, which represents areas of necrosis, gingival bleeding, pain, fetor oris, gingival swelling, and lymphadenopathy. ANUG responds well to local débridement and irrigation. Antibiotics should be used only in refractory cases, and penicillin is the drug of choice.

16. Why is a lateral pharyngeal abscess of great concern?
This infection is potentially life-threatening because of airway obstruction and requires urgent incision and drainage. This abscess occurs between the pharyngeal mucosa and the superior constrictor muscle. Presenting symptoms usually include dysphagia, pain, trismus, and fever. Medial bulging of the lateral pharyngeal wall frequently occurs, causing displacement of the uvula to the opposite side.

17. What is Ludwig's angina?
An infection of the submandibular, sublingual, and submental spaces bilaterally. A dental cause is present in 90% of cases. Treatment consists of maintaining the airway, removal of the cause, incision and drainage, intravenous antibiotics (high-dose penicillin or clindamycin), and hydration.

18. How are aphthous ulcers and herpetic lesions differentiated in the oral cavity?
Recurrent **aphthous ulcers**, also known as *canker sores*, occur as a single circular ulcer and usually are less than 1 cm in diameter. The lesion has a central yellow area surrounded by a prominent band of erythema. **Herpetic lesions** usually present as clusters of small vesicles that eventually coalesce. Recurrent aphthous ulcers may occur anywhere in the oral cavity except the lips, hard palate, and attached gingiva. Recurrent herpes occurs exclusively in these areas. Both types of lesions can be quite painful.

19. How are oral cavity ulcers treated?
Recurrent aphthous ulcers are treated symptomatically with therapy that ranges from topical corticosteroids, to antibiotics, to anesthetic mouth rinses. An attapulgite (Kaopectate), diphenhydramine (Benadryl), and lidocaine (Xylocaine) suspension has been shown to provide relief in cases of multiple recurrent aphthous ulcers. The treatment of **herpes simplex virus** is aimed at palliation of pain. Topical acyclovir, when used during the prodromal stage, has been shown to decrease size and time to resolution of the lesions.

20. How is postextraction hemorrhage evaluated and treated?
The patient's past medical history and current medications should be reviewed thoroughly. Evaluation must include good lighting and suction to evaluate the alveolus for a bleeding source. Application of a gauze dressing over the extraction site stops most bleeding episodes. Other available agents are absorbable gelatin sponges (Gelfoam), absorbable knitted fabric (Surgicel), bone wax, and topical thrombin. A carefully placed suture often helps to stop the bleeding. Refractory bleeding should be evaluated further with appropriate laboratory studies.

21. What is the classification of mandibular fractures?
The best clinical classification is by anatomic region: symphysis (midline and parasymphyseal), body, angle, ascending ramus, condyle, and alveolar housing. Another classification describes the specific type of fracture: simple, compound, comminuted, multiple, greenstick, or pathologic.

22. How do you radiologically examine a patient for a mandibular fracture?
Panographic, Towne's, posteroanterior, lateral oblique right and left, dental periapical, CT scan (rarely), and temporomandibular (rarely).

23. How do you clinically examine a patient for a mandibular fracture?
The main diagnostic criteria are a history of trauma; abnormal mandibular movements elicited by bimanual palpation; step deformities or changes in the occlusion; and soft tissue trauma, including laceration, hematoma, and loose teeth.

24. What is a lasso ligature?
A 24-, 25-, or 26-gauge wire that is placed around one or two teeth adjacent to a fracture. A lasso ligature is used when a mandibular fracture is located between two teeth. The wire is tightened

so as to bring the fracture into closer alignment. This helps to relieve pain, stop bleeding, and prevent the continued flow of saliva into the fracture site.

25. When are antibiotics indicated for a mandibular fracture?
Antibiotics are indicated in all mandibular fractures except subcondylar fractures that are not compounded into the external auditory canal. Penicillin is the drug of choice.

26. What is a mandibular contrecoup fracture?
A fracture away from the site of trauma. A classic example is trauma to the parasymphysis area with unilateral or bilateral subcondylar fracture.

27. List the immediate clinical problems associated with a fractured mandible.
Airway compromise
Bleeding
Pain
Fracture displacement
Displaced or aspirated teeth
Lacerations
Trismus
Subcutaneous emphysema

28. What is a dry socket, and how is it treated?
A painful postextraction tooth socket usually in the mandibular third molars but also may affect other sockets. It starts 2 to 3 days after the extraction and may persist for 5 to 10 days. It is treated by irrigating any debris out of the socket and placing a sedative dressing in the socket.

BIBLIOGRAPHY

1. Alling C, Osbon D (eds): Maxillofacial Trauma. Philadelphia, Lea & Febiger, 1988.
2. Flynn T: Odontogenic infections. Oral Maxillofacial Surg Clin North Am 3:311–329, 1991.
3. Fonseca R, Walker R (eds): Oral and Maxillofacial Trauma, 3rd ed. Philadelphia, W.B. Saunders, 2000.
4. Johnson B, Engel D: Acute necrotizing ulcerative gingivitis. J Periodontol 57:141–150, 1986.
5. Josell S, Abrams R: Managing common dental problems and emergencies. Pediatr Clin North Am 38:1325–1342, 1991.
6. Kaban L, Pogrel M (eds): Complications in Oral and Maxillofacial Surgery. Philadelphia, W.B. Saunders, 1997.
7. Morgan J, Haug R: Management of facial dog bite injuries. J Oral Maxillofac Surg 53:435–441, 1995.
8. Topazian R, Goldberg M (eds): Oral and Maxillofacial Infections, 3rd ed. Philadelphia, W.B. Saunders, 1994.
9. Ziccardi V, Goldfarb W: Oral and maxillofacial surgical considerations in the management of burn victims. J Oral Maxillofac Surg 52:607–613, 1994.

IV. Central Nervous System

23. TRANSIENT ISCHEMIC ATTACK AND CEREBROVASCULAR ACCIDENT

Richard L. Hughes, M.D., and Michael P. Earnest, M.D.

1. What do you mean we're number 3?

Despite significant reductions in morbidity and mortality, stroke remains the third most common cause of death and the third most common diagnosis on admission to hospitals. Stroke is not always triaged and approached as aggressively as are other life-threatening emergencies. The physician must assess the stroke victim quickly to ensure that his or her brain is receiving an optimal supply of the three key metabolic substrates: glucose, oxygen, and blood flow. Severe hypoglycemia and hyperglycemia have a negative impact on the ischemic brain. Hypoxemia and hypotension are worse. Hypertension also must be managed aggressively. The goal for acute treatment of severe hypertension and a stroke is to maintain a blood pressure of approximately 200 mm Hg systolic or 110 mm Hg diastolic unless other indications exist that require further reductions.

2. What is the difference between a transient ischemic attack (TIA) and a cerebral vascular accident (CVA)?

TIA and CVA refer to ischemia in the brain that results in neurologic deficits. If the **clinical deficit** resolves within 24 hours, the ischemia is referred to as a *TIA*. If the deficit is persistent at 24 hours, even if it resolves over a few days, it is called a *CVA* or *stroke*. The nomenclature becomes more complicated because 30% to 50% of patients with **clinically** defined TIA have a permanent abnormality on CT scan or in the brain at autopsy. TIAs can be the clinical expression of small areas of cell death in the brain, even though there is no permanent neurologic deficit.

3. Nothing can be done for most strokes, so what good is emergency therapy?

Although emergency resuscitation is possible and appropriate in only a few patients, complications of stroke and early stroke recurrence should be addressed in the ED. This is philosophically similar to the approach taken with myocardial infarction (MI). The highest risk for a recurrent stroke is within the first few days and weeks after an initial stroke or TIA. It is crucial that patients have an appropriate evaluation to determine the cause of their stroke so that a second ischemic event can be prevented. Because the exact mechanism of stroke is usually not apparent in the ED, aspirin therapy or anticoagulation (heparin) therapy on a short-term basis should be initiated during the hospital stay. At discharge, a long-term plan can be devised to aid in the prevention of another stroke.

The use of tissue plasminogen activator (TPA) was approved in June 1996 for use in patients having ischemic stroke. In the one study resulting in Food and Drug Administration (FDA) approval, patients who were given TPA within 3 hours of stroke onset had better outcomes and showed no increase in death or severe disability. For patients who arrive in the ED early (i.e., ≤ 2 hours), stroke is a medical emergency.

4. How can my hospital use thrombolytics safely in the treatment of stroke?

First, basic support, such as CT scanning, laboratory testing, and an ICU level of care, must be available. Second, emergency physicians and neurologists must develop a rapid response protocol to stroke. Third, the basic indications and contraindications for thrombolytics based on the most current clinical trials must be followed. Fourth, a reasonable plan for stroke complications, including hemorrhage, should be in place. For many hospitals, this includes transfer to a Neuro-ICU or neurosurgical center.

- The CT scan has become an important aspect of care selection for thrombolytic therapy. Although a completely normal scan is best, the presence of old (months) strokes or early ischemic changes in small areas, less than one third of the middle cerebral artery territory, does not contraindicate administration of a thrombolytic.
- The safe use of TPA requires an understanding of the hemorrhage risks. Most notable is the use of TPA after the 3-hour limit. Many thrombolytic trials were done with a 6-hour limit from stroke onset and were uniformly negative. Thrombolytics are contraindicated if there is any hemorrhage, signs of recent trauma, or a large (more than one third of the middle cerebral artery) area of obvious stroke.
- Blood pressure is often high in the first minutes after stroke but steadily falls over the first hour. An initial reading of 220/120 mm Hg often drops to an acceptable level (185/110 mm Hg) by the second or third hour. Some centers set fixed amounts that the blood pressure can be lowered (i.e., 15/7 mm Hg) with medication to allow the use of thrombolytics. Severe or sustained hypertension that requires a continuous intravenous infusion of antihypertensive agents is another contraindication.
- The hemorrhage risk is higher in the largest strokes. This explains the lower death rate in the treated group because the patients suffering fatal or severe stroke have poor outcomes whether or not they receive TPA. Even in this subgroup, you are better off with treatment. An increased glucose level is a strong predictor of hemorrhage. This does not mean that patients with increased glucose should not be treated, but more caution should be exercised, and a greater risk should be expected.
- Remember, it took a few years for thrombolytics to gain acceptance as a treatment for MI. The same process and additional clinical outcome data are needed for thrombolytics and stroke.

5. What if I treat something that turns out not to be a stroke?

After the CT scan excludes hemorrhages, the things that mimic stroke are not harmed by thrombolytics. Complicated migraine, psychogenic weakness, postictal weakness, and TIA are not likely to be affected.

6. Don't you need a detailed consent for TPA?

Obtaining informed consent can be difficult or impossible in patients with *TPA-sized* stroke, who commonly are aphasic (dominant hemisphere) or neglectful (nondominant hemisphere). Either condition makes obtaining meaningful consent questionable or impossible. Family members similarly can be so shocked that they balk at any decision making. Because intravenous TPA is approved by the FDA, a long and detailed consent is not needed. A general approach is to obtain whatever level of consent is possible from the patient and family. Failing that, approach the use of TPA as any other emergency procedure, with a thoughtful note that justifies treatment choice (either to treat or not to treat with TPA) in the individual circumstance.

7. Is intraarterial thrombolytic treatment better than intravenous TPA?

Until a clinical trial compares these methods of thrombolytic treatment, there can be no clear answer. Data from the PROACT trial of intraarterial prourokinase showed better racanalization and better outcomes even though they started treatment after 4 to 5 hours in most cases. It seems that intra-arterial techniques can achieve better recanalization, but it takes longer to initiate the treatment. Because "time is brain," this delay may counter any benefit.

8. Why obtain a CT scan when the patient is stable and obviously has had a stroke?

For the most part, a CT scan in a patient with *obvious* stroke adds very little information. In 5% to 10% of cases, the deficit is caused by hemorrhage, tumor, trauma, or abscess. Because anticoagulant or antiplatelet therapy in these patients can be catastrophic, it is advisable to obtain a CT scan in all patients with strokes and TIAs before such therapies are instituted.

9. What is the role of MRI in the stroke patient?

In general, MRI is indicated only when it can answer a specific question that CT cannot. Ischemic strokes usually do not show up on either CT or MRI within the first few hours. Scanning is used within these first few hours to exclude other processes (hemorrhage, tumor, abscess); CT can do this as well as MRI. CT and MRI can image a stroke adequately by 5 to 7 days. Smaller (i.e., milder) strokes may be viewed better with MRI, but specificity is a problem. MRI is the test of choice to image a stroke (or anything else) in the posterior fossa (brainstem and cerebellum).

MRI has the advantage of being better able to image small vessel infarctions (e.g., lacunar infarcts). MRI tends to have poor specificity because patients with typical vascular risk factors often have many high signal abnormalities in the white matter from stroke or age-related changes. A thorough knowledge of neuroanatomy often can identify the symptomatic abnormality from MRI scans with multiple abnormalities.

As MRI and CT technology improves, we may be able to use either modality as a single test to look at the brain, intracranial vasculature, extracranial vasculature, and cerebral blood flow. These modalities need to prove that the information is worth the extra time and cost before they become routine for all strokes.

10. Should I give steroids to a patient with a stroke?

No. Despite the efficacy of steroids in cerebral edema associated with tumor and abscess, they do not work in ischemic stroke. The edema that is produced by stroke is more complicated than tumor edema. Because of anecdotal reports of success, steroids sometimes are used in large, life-threatening strokes as an act of desperation. Similar attempts to use barbiturates, general anesthesia, naloxone, calcium channel blockers, or hemodilution to reduce the severity of the stroke have been disappointing.

11. Which patients should be monitored?

In general, patients without a known cause for TIA or stroke or patients with uncertain cardiac risks can benefit from short-term (i.e., 1 day) monitoring:

1. Monitoring increases the likelihood of identifying a cardiac arrhythmia or cardiac ischemia.
2. ICU monitoring allows close neurologic observation.

Patients with a well-defined mechanism of stroke and a stable cardiac physiology do not usually require ICU or cardiac monitoring. Some institutions have dedicated stroke units, similar to step-down ICUs, to allow closer observation of stroke patients at less expense than a conventional ICU.

12. Do all stroke patients need a cardiac echocardiogram?

No, but all patients need to have the **mechanism** of their stroke defined. Cardiac ultrasound, either transthoracic or transesophageal, has shown a larger number of potential cardiac sources for emboli. This includes common sources, such as atrial fibrillation, prosthetic valves, endocarditis, and mural thrombi, and newer considerations, such as paradoxic emboli through patent foramen ovale. Young stroke victims (< 45 years old) have a two to three times greater prevalence of patent foramen ovale than do normal age-matched controls, suggesting that these abnormalities have an important role in causing strokes.

13. How can I prevent strokes from occurring in my ED?

In the ED, two groups of patients are potentially identifiable before a stroke.

1. The first group includes patients with acute MI. Most emboli associated with MI occur soon after MI. Patients with anterior wall MIs are at highest risk. Appropriate intervention with anticoagulation or antiplatelet therapy in the ED may prevent a stroke a few hours later.

2. The second group includes patients with multiple traumatic injuries. These patients are notorious for having a stroke in the hospital after their "life has been saved." The highest risk of trauma-related stroke is in patients with direct trauma to the carotid or vertebral arteries. The vertebral artery is particularly prone to injury from rapid head motions. Facial fractures have been associated with a higher risk of carotid injury, leading to carotid occlusion, dissection, or artery-to-artery embolism. Recognition of high-risk patients and early angiography allows preventive measures, such as anticoagulation therapy, to be instituted if there are no contraindications.

14. Should stroke and TIA patients be allowed to eat?

Most stroke and TIA patients are able to swallow without difficulty. Patients with obviously garbled speech or reduced alertness or patients who have had very large strokes should be kept NPO until tested. Neurologic dysphagia is tested better with liquids than solids. Although feeding can be deferred until patients are admitted to a hospital bed, patients often need to take routine oral medications during their wait.

15. How much aspirin is enough to prevent stroke?

Although initially it was 4 per day, then later 3 per day, evidence has shown that 1 aspirin per day is as effective as the higher doses. It may be possible to reduce this dosage further so that even lower dosages of aspirin (e.g., 80 mg/d, 1 aspirin 3 days a week) eventually may become the standard. Reducing the dosage of aspirin can reduce the risk of gastrointestinal hemorrhages and perhaps cerebral hemorrhages. A few patients with hyperaggregable platelets need higher doses of aspirin to block platelet aggregation effectively. There are no specific guidelines on who might need a higher dose of aspirin or platelet aggregation testing. Reserve higher doses or platelet aggregation testing for patients who have failed low-dose aspirin, young patients, or patients without typical risk factors for stroke.

16. What good are these newer antiplatelet agents?

Everyone wishes there were more direct comparisons. Looking at all studies in all ischemic areas, the **thienopyridines (clopidogrel and ticlopidine)** work better than aspirin by about 10%. They are a great choice for aspirin-intolerant patients. Clopidogrel (Plavix) is a bit safer than ticlopidine (Ticlid) and requires no routine blood testing, so it is the popular choice. Because of data from cardiac stent patency, the combination of either agent with aspirin, instead of aspirin alone, has become popular in stroke patients perceived to be a high risk or who have failed aspirin alone. This use needs to be verified in the specific stroke population.

Dipyridamole, a popular *add-on* to aspirin in the 1970s, was abandoned in the 1980s because studies failed to show it helped at all. Two more recent European trials (ESPS-1 and ESPS-2) have revived hope that the aspirin/dipyridamole combination may have some merit in either the standard release form (available as a generic) or as a sustained-release form. Because these data are so inconsistent from trial to trial, the dipyridamole/aspirin combination needs to be verified.

CONTROVERSIES

17. Does carotid surgery really work?

For **symptomatic** patients, *yes*. Three prospective, randomized, multicenter carotid endarterectomy trials reported their results in dealing with symptomatic patients. Patients with carotid stenosis of 70% or greater have a relative risk reduction of 71% at 24 months (North American Symptomatic Carotid Endarterectomy Trial [NASCET]). These results were confirmed by the European Carotid Surgery Trial and the Veterans' Administration Cooperative Study. The NASCET study determined that there is a role for surgery in patients with moderate carotid stenosis (50% to 69%), but the benefits are modest.

There is considerable controversy over the utility of carotid endarterectomy in **asymptomatic** carotid stenosis or in moderate (50% to 69%) symptomatic stenosis. Four major prospective trials were completed: the Asymptomatic Carotid Atherosclerosis Study (ACAS), the Veterans' Administration Cooperative Study, the Carotid Artery Surgery Asymptomatic Narrowing Operation vs. Aspirin (CASANOVA), and the Mayo Asymptomatic Carotid Endarterectomy (MACE) trial. ACAS showed a benefit (11% to 5%) for surgery over 5 years. The other trials were not helpful.

Our personal approach is first to have a long discussion with the patient about the pros and cons of surgery. Some patients understand the uncertainty but prefer to undergo a small operative risk for a better long-term outlook. Others would rather die than have a surgery (and some do). Some die with surgery. Overall, patients do well if they are compliant with a comprehensive risk factor reduction program, with or without surgery. The benefits of this procedure are long-term, so patients with a short life expectancy (3 to 5 years) are ill-advised to consider surgery.

18. Does anticoagulation still work?

It is unclear if it ever really worked. Nonetheless, intravenous heparin and warfarin have remained popular to prevent the formation and embolization of large red thrombus or thromboemboli.

Heparin

More recent studies of intravenous heparin, subcutaneous heparin, or low-molecular-weight heparin have been disappointing but commonly have not used heparin in the manner that traditional stroke neurologists have popularized. Many are less inclined to use heparin except in the high-risk patient. Perpetuation of heparin use is fueled largely by deep venous thrombosis prevention and the negligible benefits of aspirin, the standard alternative to heparin.

Warfarin

The benefits of warfarin in atrial fibrillation remain outstanding, with 70% risk reductions, including reductions in large and fatal strokes. Warfarin for prosthetic valve, dissection, and hypercoagulable states remains reasonable, although data on some conditions could be better. The enthusiasm for warfarin in general atherosclerosis has faded with the WARSS trial, which tested aspirin against warfarin in patients who typically were given aspirin after stroke. Even the presence of antiphospholipid antibodies and patent foramen ovale failed to make warfarin a winner. One subgroup of patients with embolic signatures to their event seemed to benefit, but further analysis is needed to determine how to identify such patients.

BIBLIOGRAPHY

1. American Heart Association: 1991 Heart and Stroke Facts. Dallas, TX, American Heart Association, 1991.
2. Antiplatelet Trialists' Collaboration: Collaborative overview of randomized trials of antiplatelet therapy: I. Prevention of death, myocardial infarction, and stroke by prolonged antiplatelet therapy in various categories of patients. BMJ 308:87–106, 1994.
3. Atrial Fibrillation, Aspirin, Anticoagulation Study Group; Boston Area Anticoagulation Trial for Atrial Fibrillation Study Group; Canadian Atrial Fibrillation Anticoagulation Study Group; Veterans Affairs Stroke Prevention in Nonrheumatic Atrial Fibrillation Study Group: Risk factors for stroke and efficacy of antithrombotic therapy in atrial fibrillation. Arch Intern Med 154:1449–1457, 1994.
4. Caplan LR: Diagnosis and treatment of ischemic stroke. JAMA 266:2413–2418, 1991.
5. CAPRIE Steering Committee: A randomised, blinded, trial of clopidogrel versus aspirin in patients at risk of ischemic events (CAPRIE). Lancet 348:1329–1338, 1996.
6. Executive Committee for the Asymptomatic Carotid Atherosclerosis Study: Endarterectomy for asymptomatic carotid stenosis. JAMA 273:1421–1428, 1995.
7. Haley EC Jr, Lewandowski C, Tilley BC, NINDS rt-PA Stroke Study Group: Myths regarding the NINDS rt-PA stroke trial: Setting the record straight. Ann Emerg Med 30:676–682, 1997.
8. Hass WK, Easton JD, Adams HD, et al: A randomized trial comparing ticlopidine hydrochloride with aspirin for the prevention of stroke in high-risk patients. N Engl J Med 321:501–507, 1989.
9. Hughes RL: Carotid endarterectomy for the asymptomatic patient. J La State Med Soc 348:1329–1338, 1996.
10. Kasner SE, Grotta JC: Emergency identification and treatment of acute ischemic stroke. Ann Emerg Med 30:642–653, 1997.
11. Kumpe DA, Hughes RL: Thrombolytic therapy for acute stroke. In Whittemore AD (ed): Advances in Vascular Surgery, Vol 4. Chicago, Mosby-Year Book, 1996.

12. NASCET Collaborators: Beneficial effect of carotid endarterectomy in symptomatic patients with high-grade carotid stenosis. N Engl J Med 325:445–453, 1991.
13. Wyer PC, Osborn HH: Recombinant tissue plasminogen activator: In my community hospital ED, will early administration of rt-PA to patients with the initial diagnosis of acute ischemic stroke reduce mortality and disability? Ann Emerg Med 30:629–638, 1997.

24. MENINGITIS

Andrew B. Ziller, M.D.

1. What is meningitis?

A disease of the central nervous system involving inflammation of the membranes surrounding the brain and spinal cord.

2. What are the causes of meningitis?

Infectious
   Bacteria
   Viruses
   Fungi
   Parasites
   Tuberculosis
Noninfectious causes
   Neoplastic
   Collagen vascular

Streptococcus pneumoniae and *Neisseria meningitidis* are the most common causes of bacterial meningitis.

3. Why is it important to know about meningitis?

Mortality from bacterial and fungal meningitis is 10% to 50%. This is an important issue because prompt recognition and treatment of bacterial meningitis can lessen morbidity and mortality. In EDs, failure to diagnose meningitis ranks second in total malpractice dollars paid per case.

4. Which patients are at risk for meningitis?

Very young and older patients are most at risk. Others at risk include immunocompromised patients (e.g., splenectomized patients); immunosuppressed patients; alcoholics; patients with recent neurosurgical procedures; and patients who have underlying infections, such as endocarditis, pneumonia, sinusitis, and otitis media. Outbreaks of meningitis from *N. meningitidis* occur in high schools, in colleges, and among new military recruits.

5. List the common presenting symptoms.

Fever
Change in mental status
Headache
Photophobia
Stiff neck
Lethargy
Irritability
Malaise
Confusion
Seizures

6. Describe the physical findings in meningitis.

Nuchal rigidity, Kernig's sign, and Brudzinski's sign are seen in some patients. Kernig's sign is pain or resistance of the hamstrings when the knees are extended with the hips flexed at 90°. Brudzinski's sign is flexion of the hips caused by passive flexion of the neck. These physical findings often are absent in very young and older patients—the ones most likely to get meningitis. In infants, a tense or bulging fontanelle may be helpful but may not be manifest if there is associated dehydration.

7. If the symptoms are not specific and the physical findings often are absent, what are the indications for lumbar puncture (LP)?

LP should be done whenever meningitis is suspected because analyzing spinal fluid is the only way to diagnose meningitis.

8. What tests should be done before doing an LP?

When possible, the patient should be checked for papilledema and spontaneous venous pulsations. A head CT scan should be done if papilledema is present, if spontaneous venous pulsations are absent, if the patient has an altered mental status, if there is a focal neurologic examination or a new-onset seizure, or if there is clinical suspicion for recent trauma or subarachnoid hemorrhage. If a bleeding disorder is suspected based on history or physical examination, coagulation studies and platelet count should be checked before doing an LP.

9. What is the most common error in the ED management of meningitis?

Delaying administration of antibiotics until the LP is done. Antibiotics can and should be given to a patient who clinically has bacterial meningitis. Intravenous antibiotics given 2 hours or less before the LP (and ideally after blood and urine cultures are obtained) will not affect the results of the cerebrospinal fluid (CSF) analysis.

10. Discuss the risks of LP.

Almost every physician has encountered patients who believe that an LP will cause paralysis. Paralysis is highly unlikely because the needle is inserted below the level of the spinal cord at L4 or L5 in adults. This misconception probably arises from the fact that occasionally patients experience transient leg paresthesias during LP from irritation of nerve roots by the needle. There are rare reports of cauda equina syndrome from hematoma formation, but only in patients with a coagulopathy. Headache is the most common sequela, occurring in 5% to 30% of patients. Headache is believed to be minimized by using a small-gauge needle (e.g., 20G or 22G in adults) and by having the patient lie flat for several hours after the LP. Most agree that tonsillar herniation is a potential complication after LP in a patient with increased intracranial pressure; however, the risk is eliminated if the patient has a normal head CT scan before the LP.

11. What is the secret to performing LP successfully?

The proper positioning of the patient is crucial. If the LP is done with the patient lying down, be sure the shoulders and hips are in a straight plane perpendicular to the floor. The patient should be in the *tightest* fetal position possible. If the LP is done with the patient sitting up, have the upper body rest on a bedside table and have the patient push his or her back toward you as if he or she is an angry cat.

12. Which laboratory studies should I order for the CSF?

In an adult, four tubes are usually collected, each containing 1to 1.5 mL. More CSF is needed if special tests are required.

Tube 1. Cell count and differential.

Tube 2. Gram stain and culture and sensitivity. Special tests in certain patients (e.g., immunocompromised patients) include viral cultures, tuberculosis cultures and acid-fast stain, fungal antigen studies and India ink stain (most commonly cryptococcosis), and serologic tests for neurosyphilis. Countercurrent immunoelectrophoresis is used occasionally to detect specific bacterial antigens in the CSF.

Tube 3. Glucose and protein.

Tube 4. Cell count and differential.

In pediatric patients, three tubes are usually collected: tube 1 for microbiology studies, tube 2 for glucose and protein, and tube 3 for cell count and differential.

13. Which results from the CSF analysis indicate meningitis?

In adults, a CSF white blood cell count greater than 5 suggests meningitis. A white blood cell count less than 30 is considered normal in neonates. Polymorphonuclear leukocytes suggest a bacterial cause. Elevated CSF protein is seen in meningitis. A CSF-to-serum glucose ratio of less than 0.5 occurs in patients with bacterial meningitis, and in patients with diabetes, a CSF-to-serum ratio glucose of less than 0.6 is considered low. Gram stain is useful in diagnosing bacterial meningitis; 20% of the time, the causative organism can be identified. The CSF laboratory studies may be normal early in meningitis; if clinical suspicion is high, a repeat LP may be indicated in 24 hours.

14. Which antibiotics should be prescribed when the causative organism is unknown?

For children, see Chapter 71. For adults, refer to the following table.

Antimicrobial Therapy for Bacterial Meningitis*

ORGANISM	TREATMENT
N. meningitidis	Penicillin G, 3–4 million IU IV every 4 hr *or* ampicillin, 2 gm IV every 4 hr
S. pneumoniae	Penicillin G, 3–4 million IU IV every 4 hr *or* ampicillin, 2 gm IV every 4 hr
H. influenzae	Cefotaxime,[†] 2 gm IV every 4 hr
S. aureus	Nafcillin, 2 gm IV every 4 hr
E. coli and other gram-negative enterics except *P. aeruginosa*	Cefotaxime,[†] 2 gm IV every 4 hr
P. aeruginosa	Ceftazidime, 4 gm IV every 8 hr, *plus* gentamicin, 2 mg/kg IV at once then 1.7 mg/kg IV every 8 hr (adjusted according to renal function) plus intrathecally every 12 hr if required
L. monocytogenes	Ampicillin, 2 gm IV every 4 hr, *plus* gentamicin (as for *P. aeruginosa*)

[*] All does assume normal renal function.
[†] Or equivalent third-generation cephalosporin (e.g., ceftriaxone, 2–3 gm IV every 12 hr, or ceftizoxime, 3 gm IV every 8 hr).
Adapted from Walls RM, et al: Central nervous system infections. In Marx JA, et al (eds): Rosen's Emergency Medicine: Concepts and Clinical Practice, 5th ed. St. Louis, Mosby, 2002.

15. What about steroids?

This is always a good question regardless of the disease or the rotation. Steroids (dexamethasone, 0.15 mg/kg) have been shown to reduce the incidence and severity of hearing loss in infants and children with meningitis caused by *H. influenzae*. To date, no study has shown a benefit from steroids in other pediatric or adult patients with bacterial meningitis.

16. Do people exposed to a patient with meningitis need to take antibiotics?

Individuals who have had close contact with someone who has, or is suspected to have, meningococcal meningitis should take rifampin, 600 mg twice a day for 2 days, or ciprofloxacin,

500 mg orally for adults A 4-day course of rifampin is recommended for most individuals who have been in close contact with someone with *H. influenzae* type b meningitis. Individuals exposed to someone with another type of meningitis, especially viral, do not need prophylactic antibiotics.

BIBLIOGRAPHY

1. Attia J, Hatala R, Cook DJ, Wong JG: Does this adult patient have acute meningitis? JAMA 282:175–181, 1999.
2. Hasbun R, Abrahams J, Jekel J, Quagliarello VJ: Computed tomography of the head before lumbar puncture in adults with suspected meningitis. N Engl J Med 345:1727–1733, 2001.
3. Kookier JC: Spinal puncture and cerebrospinal fluid examination. In Roberts JR, Hedges JR (eds): Clinical Procedures in Emergency Medicine, 2nd ed. Philadelphia, W.B. Saunders, 1991, pp 969–984.
4. Lavoie FW, Saucier JR: Central nervous system infections. In Marx JA (ed): Rosen's Emergency Medicine: Concepts and Clinical Practice, 5th ed. St. Louis, Mosby, 2002, pp 1527–1541.
5. McIntyre PB, Berkey CS, King SM, et al: Dexamethasone as adjunctive therapy in bacterial meningitis: A meta-analysis of randomized clinical trials since 1988. JAMA 278:925–931, 1997.
6. Quagliarello VJ, Scheld WM: Treatment of bacterial meningitis. N Engl J Med 336:708–716, 1997.
7. Shuchat A, Robinson K, Wenger JD, et al: Bacterial meningitis in the United States in 1995. N Engl J Med 337:970–976, 1997.
8. Talan DA: New concepts in antimicrobial therapy for emergency department infections. Ann Emerg Med 34:503–516, 1999.

V. Respiratory System

25. BREATHING AND VENTILATION

John L. Kendall, M.D.

1. How useful is the respiratory rate in the evaluation of a patient?

The respiratory rate is invaluable as a vital sign. Normal respiratory rate in children varies with age, whereas adults typically breathe 12 to 16 times per minute. As a testament to its usefulness, the respiratory rate can be helpful in many conditions other than primary pulmonary pathology. It is elevated in patients with anemia, arteriovenous fistula, pregnancy, cyanotic heart disease, metabolic acidosis, febrile illness, central nervous system pathology, anxiety, exercise, and at high altitude. It is important that the respiratory rate be counted carefully for at least 30 seconds. Often the respiratory rate is grossly estimated from a short period of observation.

2. Which breathing patterns are associated with pathologic conditions?

Kussmaul respirations are deep, rapid breaths that are associated with metabolic acidosis. **Cheyne-Stokes** breathing comprises respirations that wax and wane cyclically so that periods of deep breathing alternate with periods of apnea. Causes include congestive heart failure, hypertensive crisis, hyponatremia, high-altitude illness, and head injury. **Ataxic** breathing is characterized by unpredictable irregularity. Breaths may be shallow or deep and may stop for short periods. Causes include respiratory depression and brainstem injury at the level of the medulla.

3. Which pulmonary function tests are commonly used in the ED?

Other than respiratory rate, the most useful pulmonary function tests for ED patients are the forced end-expiratory volume at 1 second and the peak expiratory flow rate. The latter is used more commonly. It is achieved by having a patient exhale at a maximum rate through a peak flowmeter. Normal values range from 350 to 600 L/min. Lower levels are characteristic of increased airway resistance as commonly seen in asthma and chronic obstructive pulmonary disease (COPD) exacerbations. Patients who present with values of 75 to 100 L/min have severe airflow obstruction. Serial measurements are helpful for objectively quantifying response to treatment.

4. How does pulse oximetry work?

Pulse oximetry is based on a combination of spectrophotometry and plethysmography. **Spectrophotometry** is based on the Beer-Lambert law, which holds that optical absorbance is proportional to the concentration of the substance and the thickness of the medium. Using this principle, two wavelengths of light are used to distinguish between the absorption of oxyhemoglobin (O_2Hb) and reduced hemoglobin (Hb). **Plethysmography** measures the tissue displacement caused by an arterial pulse. This allows for assessment of the increase in light absorption caused by local arterial flow compared with the background of composite tissues and venous blood.

Pulse oximeters function by placing a pulsatile vascular bed between a light-emitting diode (LED) and a detector. Light is transmitted through the tissue at two wavelengths, 660 nm (red, primarily absorbed by O_2Hb) and 940 nm (infrared, primarily absorbed by Hb), which allows differentiation of O_2Hb from Hb. A microprocessor algorithm is used to discriminate arterial saturation from artifact. With the signal transmission during diastole providing a reference point, the changes observed during periods of pulsation are used as measurement intervals for O_2Hb saturation. This also allows for determination of heart rate. The arterial oxygen saturation measurements are timed to changes in light absorption caused by the arterial pulse.

5. How can pulse oximetry be useful, and in which situations can it yield false readings?
Pulse oximetry is useful when monitoring arterial O_2Hb saturation in cardiopulmonary disorders; monitoring oxygen saturation during conscious sedation, airway management, or in patients with a decreased level of consciousness; or quantifying the arterial O_2Hb saturation response to therapeutic interventions. Situations in which the usefulness of pulse oximetry is limited include excessive movement, vasoconstriction, low O_2Hb saturations ($< 83\%$), abnormal hemoglobins (carboxyhemoglobin, methemoglobin), intravascular dyes, exposure of the measuring sensor to ambient light sources, skin pigmentation, and when nail polish is present. Oxygen saturation measurements may be falsely elevated in the presence of carboxyhemoglobin and falsely decreased in the presence of methemoglobin.

6. What percentage of fraction of inspired oxygen (FiO_2) corresponds with the various types of oxygen delivery systems?
The three primary means of oxygen delivery are (1) nasal cannula, (2) facemask, and (3) facemask with oxygen reservoir. Nasal cannula can be used to deliver oxygen at rates of 1 to 6 L/min. For every 1 L/min of flow increase, the FiO_2 increases by 4%. This corresponds to 25% to 40% FiO_2 of oxygen delivery. A facemask relies on an oxygen flow of 8 to 10 L/min with an FiO_2 ranging from 40% to 60%. The nonrebreather mask has a constant flow of oxygen so that higher concentrations of oxygen can be achieved. A flow rate of 6 L/min gives an FiO_2 of approximately 60%. At 10 L/min, the FiO_2 is about 90%.

7. What is noninvasive ventilation?
A means of delivering positive-pressure ventilation without placing a nasotracheal or endotracheal tube. As such, the patient is still awake, able to protect his or her airway, and able to initiate an adequate respiratory rate.

8. What forms of noninvasive ventilation are available to emergency physicians?
The two most useful forms are mask continuous positive airway pressure ventilation and bilevel positive airway pressure. Each method involves placing a tight-fitting mask over the patient's face and delivering breaths by positive pressure. **Continuous positive airway pressure** delivers a continuous amount of positive airway pressure during and after inspiration and expiration. **Bilevel positive airway pressure** not only provides a set positive pressure during exhalation, but also delivers a set inspiratory pressure when the patient initiates a breath. The inspiratory pressure is always set higher than the expiratory pressure, can be sustained for various periods, and stops when the patient ceases to inhale or begins to exhale.

9. In what circumstances would noninvasive ventilation be preferred over standard invasive ventilation?
Noninvasive ventilation has been shown to be useful in many conditions, including pulmonary edema, pneumonia, asthma, COPD, and nocturnal hypoventilation. When the equipment and personnel are available, most patients with the aforementioned conditions should be considered for noninvasive ventilation. The benefit of noninvasive ventilation is that its use may prevent the subsequent need for invasive ventilation and the difficulty of weaning a COPD patient from the ventilator.

10. How do I determine the initial ventilator settings in someone who has just been intubated?
Ventilator settings must take into account the patient's oxygenation status and his or her ventilation or acid-base status. The primary method for affecting the oxygenation of a patient is to alter the FiO_2. Initially, intubated patients should be given 100% oxygen or an FiO_2 of 1.00.

Subsequently, if arterial blood gas analysis reveals that the PaO_2 is high, the FiO_2 may be lowered incrementally.

The main factors determining a patient's ventilatory status are tidal volume and respiratory rate. Changes in each are reflected by the carbon dioxide from arterial blood gas analysis. High respiratory rates and large tidal volumes decrease the carbon dioxide, whereas the converse elevates the carbon dioxide. Initially the tidal volume can be estimated to be 10 to 12 mL/kg; for a 70-kg patient, that is 700 to 800 mL.

The initial respiratory rate varies depending on the clinical situation. On average, the rate should be set between 12 and 18 breaths/min.

11. Are ventilator settings always the same?

No. Each clinical condition merits attention to the initial ventilatory settings. A patient with an obstructive condition such as asthma does best with small tidal volumes, high respiratory rates, and low levels of positive end-expiratory pressure (PEEP). In contrast, a patient with a COPD exacerbation requires lower respiratory rates, higher tidal volumes, no PEEP, and a prolonged expiratory time. Other common ventilator settings are for patients with closed head injury, congestive heart failure (CHF), or metabolic acidosis. Guidelines for each are given in the following table.

CONDITION	FiO_2	TIDAL VOLUME	RESPIRATORY RATE	PEEP
Asthma	100%	5–10 mL/kg	8–12/min.	2.5–10
COPD	100%	8–12 mL/kg	6–8/min.	2.5–5.0
Head Injury	100%	12–15 mL/kg	14–20/min.	None
CHF	100%	8–12 mL/kg	8–12/min.	5–10

12. What are the different ventilator modes?

The main modes of ventilation are controlled mechanical ventilation (CMV), assist control (AC), intermittent mandatory ventilation (IMV), and synchronized intermittent mandatory ventilation (SIMV). In the CMV mode, the ventilator delivers a certain volume or pressure at a preset rate, regardless of any ventilatory effort by the patient. AC is similar to CMV in that the tidal volume or inspiratory pressure and minimum respiratory rate are set. It differs from CMV by allowing patients to trigger the ventilator over a set minimum respiratory rate. IMV allows the patient to breathe spontaneously without having a preset tidal volume or pressure. A set rate similar to the CMV mode is in place. This allows the patient to breathe spontaneously, while ensuring a set respiratory rate and tidal volume. SIMV differs from IMV in that the ventilator senses the patient's spontaneous respirations and does not deliver a breath if the patient has already triggered the ventilator. This prevents stacking of respirations, which can be a component of the IMV mode.

13. What is PEEP?

Positive pressure applied during expiration. In so doing, the alveoli fail to collapse, and functional residual capacity increases. The end result is improved ventilation-perfusion matching in the pulmonary circulation. PEEP is usually set at 2.5 or 5.0 cm H_2O.

14. What is auto-PEEP?

Auto-PEEP develops when a positive-pressure breath is delivered before complete exhalation of the previous breath. As a result, air becomes trapped, and pressure within the lungs increases. This can lead to complications, such as decreased cardiac output, hypotension, barotrauma, pneumothorax, and inaccurate pulmonary artery catheter measurements.

15. What are the most common complications of mechanical ventilation?

The most common complication is **barotrauma**. High pressure can lead to rupture of the alveolar wall, which can lead to pneumomediastinum, pneumothorax, tension pneumothorax, pneumoperitoneum, and subcutaneous emphysema. Other common complications include increased intracranial pressure, fluid retention, renal failure, hyponatremia, local trauma to the nares and mouth, tracheal necrosis, sinusitis, and pneumonia.

16. What is heliox therapy?

Heliox is the mixture of oxygen and helium. A patient breathing air takes in 21% oxygen and about 89% nitrogen. In heliox, helium essentially replaces the nitrogen. The significance of this is that helium is seven times lighter than nitrogen so that it flows less turbulently and requires less respiratory effort for ventilation. In the standard mixture, the percentage of oxygen is the same as in air so that if significant hypoxia is present, supplemental oxygen may be needed. As the concentration of oxygen goes up, the concentration of helium goes down, which limits the effectiveness of heliox to decrease the work of breathing.

17. When should I use heliox?

Heliox can be used in many respiratory conditions, including upper respiratory obstruction, severe COPD, and asthma exacerbation. An important point to stress is that heliox is not primary treatment for any of these conditions, but rather it is a temporizing measure while waiting for the primary treatment to take effect.

BIBLIOGRAPHY

1. AARC Clinical Practice Guidelines: Pulse oximetry. Respir Care 36:1406–1409, 1991.
2. Cummins RO: Adjuncts for airway control, ventilation and oxygenation. In Cummins RO (ed): Advanced Cardiac Life Support. Dallas, TX, American Heart Association, 1994.
3. Murphy MF: Monitoring the emergency patient. In Rosen P, Barkin RM (eds): Emergency Medicine: Concepts and Clinical Practice, 4th ed. St. Louis, Mosby, 1998, pp 119–123.
4. Pilbeam SP (ed): Mechanical Ventilation: Physiologic and Clinical Applications. St. Louis, Mosby, 1998.
5. Shaughnessy TE: Pulse oximetry and capnography. In Parsons PE, Wiener-Kronish JP (eds): Critical Care Secrets. Philadelphia, Hanley & Belfus, 1998, pp 10–15.
6. McGee DL, Wald DA, Hinchliffe S: Helium-oxygen therapy in the emergency department. J Emerg Med 15:291–296, 1997.

26. ASTHMA AND CHRONIC OBSTRUCTIVE PULMONARY DISEASE

Shirley H. Kung, M.D.

ASTHMA

1. What is asthma?

A chronic inflammatory disorder characterized by bronchiolar obstruction and narrowing of airways caused by hyperreactive smooth muscle contraction, cellular infiltrates, and mucus production.

2. Describe the classic presentation of acute asthma.

The classic triad consists of cough, wheezing, and dyspnea. Other symptoms of asthma include rhinitis, chest tightness, breathlessness, and gastroesophageal reflux. Although not always a good correlate to symptoms, the degree of obstruction determines exacerbation severity. Asthmatics with recurrent exacerbations often have a blunted perception of dyspnea.

3. **Asthma: "To wheeze or not to wheeze?"**

An exacerbation of asthma can occur without wheezing. Wheezing is produced by turbulent airflow and concomitant airway obstruction. Patients who have little air movement secondary to significant obstruction may not have wheezing. A certain subset of patients, mostly children or elderly, have cough-variant asthma and present with cough and shortness of breath alone.

4. **What is the differential diagnosis of wheezing?**

Chronic obstructive pulmonary disease (COPD), congestive heart failure, foreign body aspiration, anaphylaxis, epiglottitis, tracheobronchitis, reactive airway disease, and asthma.

5. **Which aspects of the asthmatic's history are important to the current exacerbation?**

Ask questions regarding exposure to common precipitants, such as viral upper respiratory tract infections, allergens, cold, exercise, and possible aspirin or nonsteroidal antiinflammatory drug use. Also important are duration and severity of symptoms, past history and frequency of sudden exacerbations, prior hospitalizations and intubations, number of recent ED visits, current medications, worsening of symptoms while on or if weaning off corticosteroids, and other comorbidities.

6. **What is the most helpful clinical indicator of bronchoconstriction?**

The most accurate measurement of bronchoconstriction is spirometry to determine forced expiratory volume in 1 second (FEV_1) or peak expiratory flow rate (PEFR). Calculate the percentage of the patient's predicted or personal best effort. Asthma exacerbations can be divided into three categories: (1) mild (PEFR $\geq$ 80%), (2) moderate (PEFR 50% to 80%), and (3) severe (PEFR $\leq$ 50%). FEV_1 or PEFR (the best of three attempts) should be obtained on presentation and after initial treatment to determine the need for more aggressive therapy or hospitalization.

7. **Are there any other helpful laboratory tests?**

Most laboratory tests, including arterial blood gases, are not useful in the management of asthma except in cases of active or impending respiratory failure. A complete blood count may be useful if the patient is febrile and has productive sputum. Theophylline levels should be ordered if the patient is taking theophylline to rule out medication toxicity.

8. **When should I order a chest radiograph?**

Chest films may be helpful if the patient does not respond to initial treatment or if a pulmonary complication, such as foreign body obstruction, pneumonia, pneumomediastinum, pneumothorax, or congestive heart failure, is suspected.

9. **What is the first-line treatment for acute asthma in the ED?**

The main goals in the ED are to prevent hypoxia and reverse bronchiolar obstruction. Patients should be placed on oxygen (keeping oxygen saturation $\geq$ 90% to 95%). Inhaled β_2-agonist therapy, either through metered-dose inhaler (MDI) or through aerosolized solutions, is the mainstay of acute asthma treatment. Albuterol (Proventil) nebulization, 2.5 to 5.0 mg every 20 to 30 minutes $\times$ 3 doses or continuous nebulization for 1 hour, is used most commonly for initial management of moderate-to-severe exacerbations. Albuterol is more β_2 selective, is longer acting, and has fewer side effects than other β_2-agonists. Metaanalyses showed increased benefit in adults from the addition of inhaled anticholinergic medications to standard albuterol treatment. Ipratropium bromide (Atrovent) nebulization, 0.5 mg every 20 to 30 minutes $\times$ 3 doses mixed with the β_2-agonist, has been shown to increase pulmonary function modestly and decrease need for hospitalization. Atrovent (0.25 mg) also has been shown to be effective acutely in children in the ED.

10. Which medications can be used in patients unable to tolerate nebulized bronchodilators?

Subcutaneous administration of terbutaline or epinephrine may be helpful. Terbutaline (0.25 mg), a long-acting β_2-agonist, can be administered every 20 minutes × 3 doses. Epinephrine, with α-adrenergic and β-adrenergic effects, has an increased risk for adverse reactions and should be administered as a 1:1000 solution 0.2 to 0.5 mL every 20 to 30 minutes × 3 doses.

11. When should corticosteroids be given?

Early steroid therapy currently is considered part of the initial treatment of asthma exacerbations, although there is still controversy over their efficacy in the acute setting. In general, patients not responding well to initial treatment or any patient already on inhaled or parenteral steroids should be given an initial dose of oral prednisone (40 to 60 mg) or intravenous methylprednisolone (60 to 125 mg). Initial steroid dosing for children is 1 mg/kg. Oral and intravenous steroids are equally as effective in equivalent doses, and their onset of action requires 6 to 24 hours. Evidence-based evaluation of systemic corticosteroid therapy shows no immediate improvements in airway obstruction and does not affect decisions on patient hospitalization. High-dose inhaled corticosteroids may have some benefit in the acute setting and can be continued safely by patients already on inhaled steroids.

12. Is the use of magnesium sulfate effective in managing acute asthma?

Magnesium can help reverse bronchospasm in conjunction with standard therapy for adults and children with severe acute asthma. Doses of 2 to 3 mg of intravenous magnesium sulfate for adults and 20 to 25mg/kg for children seem to be safe and beneficial for patients with PEFR 25% or less. Intravenous magnesium should not be used in patients with mild-to-moderate exacerbations because the adverse effects outweigh the benefits. Some improvement in pulmonary function has been seen with nebulized isotonic magnesium sulfate, which may be used with or without aerosolized albuterol.

13. Which medications are not recommended?

Methylxanthines, such as intravenous aminophylline and oral theophylline, generally are not recommended in the acute care of an asthmatic patient; however, they may be used if patients are hospitalized or require long-term asthma management. **Antibiotics** are not recommended unless the patient presents with fever and productive sputum. Other nonrecommended medications include sedative or anxiolytic medication, which may decrease respiratory rate dangerously, and mucolytics, which have not been shown to be effective.

14. What if patients continue to worsen despite standard inhaled and systemic medications?

Noninvasive strategies for critically ill patients include the use of heliox, continuous positive airway pressure (CPAP), and intravenous ketamine. Heliox (a mixture of helium and oxygen) reduces turbulent flow in obstructed airways, which allows a decrease in work of breathing and increases PEEP. Not all studies support its use in the acute setting. CPAP increases oxygenation, improves gas exchange, and decreases the use of inspiratory muscles. Intravenous ketamine, a dissociative anesthetic, has bronchodilating properties, which may help to mitigate impending respiratory failure.

15. When does an asthmatic need intubation?

Although there are no absolute indications except for respiratory arrest and coma, increasing exhaustion, worsening respiratory distress, persistent or increasing hypercarbia, and changes in mental status should be considered as possible indications for intubation. General anesthesia may be helpful for patients in status asthmaticus who continue to be refractory to treatment while intubated.

16. Disposition of patients in the ED: "Should they stay or should they go?"

Disposition of patients is determined by clinical response after the third dose of inhaled β_2-agonist therapy in addition to other described treatments. If patients have clear breath sounds and no longer are dyspneic or are back to baseline, they may be discharged home. FEV_1/PEFR can be measured and percent predicted or best personal effort calculated.

% PREDICTED % PERSONAL BEST	DISPOSITION OF PATIENT	TREATMENT OPTIONS
PEFR ≤ 50%	Admission to ICU for aggressive treatment and management of mechanical intubation	Patients severely dyspneic at rest with impending respiratory failure should be intubated, treated with oxygen, hourly or continuous bronchodilators, intravenous steroids, possible heliox, or CPAP and reassessed periodically for improvement
PEFR 50–70%	Admit to ED observation unit or discuss with patient regarding need for hospitalization	Patients with mild-to-moderate exacerbations, not pregnant or with other comorbid illness needing extended care can be treated in ED observation. If patients have significant improvement, discharge home should be considered
PEFR ≥ 70%	Discharge home	Continue inhaled bronchodilators and regular medications. Add cortico-steroids as needed. Patients should have close follow-up with their primary physician in 3–5 days

17. What medication changes should be considered at time of discharge?

Patients who received corticosteroids acutely should continue oral steroid therapy at home for 3 to 5 days. Dosing parameters are controversial, so choose a moderate regimen; no tapering is required. Patients on inhaled corticosteroids should be advised to double their current dose. If no inhaled corticosteroid is being used, high-dose budesonide, 400 µg 2 puffs twice a day, can be started. Consider adding leukotriene modifiers, such as zafirlukast and montelukast, which may decrease hospitalization and relapse rates and increase asthma control. Patients should be continued on their β_2-agonist MDI or nebulizer.

18. Is nebulization of medication more effective than MDIs?

No. If MDIs are used properly with equivalent doses given (10:1 standard nebulization dose to single puff from MDI), both are equally effective.

19. What is the correct way to use an MDI?

MDIs should be assembled and held upright 3 to 4 cm away from the mouth. Patients should exhale completely, actuate the inhaler, and breathe in slowly over 5 to 6 seconds. The inspired breath is held for 10 full seconds. If patients have difficulty with this technique, often a spacer helps with medication delivery. Patients should be advised to rinse their mouth after each use.

20. Does pregnancy change the management of acute asthma?

No. It is important to treat pregnant asthmatics aggressively to prevent maternal hypoxia and subsequent fetal death. Patients should not be undertreated because of fear of teratogenicity; the risks from respiratory failure and severe acute asthma are greater than from therapy with standard medications.

CHRONIC OBSTRUCTIVE PULMONARY DISEASE

21. What is COPD?

A combination of three disease processes, including emphysema and chronic bronchitis with an element of reactive airway disease (asthma). These three components contribute in varying degrees to the severity of COPD. Smoking is the most common cause of COPD.

22. How does emphysema contribute to COPD?

Emphysema is caused by irreversible airway collapse secondary to gradual destruction of airway septations and capillary beds. Patients subsequently have obstructed expiration and decreased pulmonary blood flow.

23. How does bronchitis contribute to COPD?

Bronchitis is the reversible component of COPD caused by continuous airway inflammation of small and large bronchi. Increased edema of bronchial mucosa with hyperactivity of the mucus-producing goblet cells causes damage to the endothelium and an impaired response to normal mucociliary action.

24. What is the classic presentation of patients with COPD?

Similar to asthmatics, wheezing can be obvious during an exacerbation. Patients with pure emphysema or a large emphysematous component often present with pursed-lip expirations. They are generally thin, are anxious, and have marked dyspnea and tachypnea. Classically, patients with pure bronchitis or a large bronchitic component have severe cough that worsens over time, hypoxemia secondary to chronic respiratory failure, and evidence of cor pulmonale.

25. Which diagnostic tests are helpful in the management of COPD?

Pulse oximetry should be used in every patient with COPD. Oxygen saturation less than 90% indicates severe hypoxia. Arterial blood gas measurements often can identify patients with increased and continuing hypoxia, hypercarbia, and respiratory acidosis, especially if compared with the patient's baseline values. Check theophylline levels if indicated. Chest radiographs are appropriate in COPD exacerbations to help manage complications and concomitant disease. In patients with cor pulmonale, continuous cardiac monitoring may identify any associated arrhythmias. In contrast to asthma, pulmonary function tests are less helpful because of the irreversible nature of airway destruction.

26. Is there any danger in treating COPD patients with high-flow oxygen?

Patients with COPD often develop hypoxemia and hypercarbia over time, which normally causes respiratory acidosis, tachypnea, and hyperventilation. If patients lose their hypercarbic drive to breathe, they may have slow respirations driven by hypoxemia alone. Excessive supplemental oxygen in this small subset of patients can cause respiratory arrest secondary to loss of their hypoxemia-induced ventilatory drive. This possibility should not preclude you, however, from giving as much oxygen as needed to keep the oxygen saturation greater than 90% to 95%.

27. How should COPD be managed?

β_2-Agonist bronchodilators and systemic corticosteroids are the mainstays of treatment. Studies support the use of ipratropium bromide as first-line therapy with albuterol for acute COPD exacerbations and in chronic COPD management. These two medications, given in either MDI or nebulization form, have powerful bronchodilating properties.

28. What about antibiotics?

Routine antibiotic coverage is controversial, but some recommend antibiotic therapy for patients with pneumonia, increased sputum production, fever, and worsening dyspnea. Sputum cultures usually are not helpful in choosing therapy. Macrolides and fluoroquinolones are generally appropriate for outpatient therapy of acute bronchitis, and guidelines for treatment of pneumonia, if present, should be considered.

29. When should a patient with COPD be intubated?

For respiratory failure. Noninvasive modalities such as CPAP and bilevel positive airway pressure often can obviate the need for intubation by improving gas exchange, decreasing hypoxia, and, reducing work of breathing. Any patient with changes in mental status, increased respiratory distress with cyanosis, acute deterioration, or exhaustion should be intubated and mechanically ventilated immediately.

30. Which factors should be considered in the decision to admit or discharge patients with COPD?

Patients with significant COPD exacerbations often take longer to recover and require hospitalization. They have less respiratory reserve and function not quickly reversible. Failure to improve while in the ED, failed outpatient management, and pulmonary infections are reasons for hospitalization. Patients who return to near baseline with some improvement from ED treatment may be discharged home with close follow-up and a 2-week taper of oral steroids.

31. When is ipratropium bromide contraindicated in the management of patients with asthma or COPD?

Ipratropium bromide contains derivatives of soya lecithin and related food products. Patients with soybean or peanut allergies may develop anaphylaxis if exposed to this medication in either MDI or nebulized forms.

BIBLIOGRAPHY

1. Campbell S: For COPD a combination of ipratropium bromide and albuterol sulfate is more effective than albuterol base. Arch Intern Med 159:156–160, 1999.
2. Kerstjens H, Postma D: Chronic obstructive pulmonary disease: Short and long term effects of maintenance drug treatment. Clinical Evidence 5, 2001; available at www.clinicalevidence.org.
3. MICROMEDEX Healthcare Series Volume 111. Expires 3/2002; available at http://micromedex.exempla.org.
4. Mondavia DP, Dailey RH: Chronic obstructive pulmonary disease. In Marx JA, Hockberger RS, Walls RM (eds): Rosen's Emergency Medicine: Concepts and Clinical Practice, 5th ed. St. Louis, Mosby, 2002, pp 956–969.
5. Nannini J Jr, Pendino JC, Corna RA, et al: Magnesium sulfate as a vehicle for nebulized salbutamol in acute asthma. Am J Med 108:193–197, 2000.
6. National Institutes of Health, National Heart, Lung, and Blood Institute: Expert panel report 2: Guidelines for the diagnosis and management of asthma. NIH Pub No 97-4051. Bethesda, MD, NIH, 1997.
7. Nowak R, Tokarski G: Asthma. In Marx JA, Hockberger RS, Walls RM (eds): Rosen's Emergency Medicine: Concepts and Clinical Practice, 5th ed. St. Louis, Mosby, 2002, pp 938–956.
8. Rodrigo G, Rodrigo C: Corticosteroids in the emergency department therapy of acute adult asthma: An evidence-based evaluation. Chest 116:285–295, 1999.
9. Rodrigo G, Rodrigo C, Burschtin O: Ipratropium bromide in acute adult severe asthma: A metaanalysis of randomized control trials. Am J Med 107:363–370, 1999.
10. Rowe BH, Bretzlaff JA, Bourdon C, et al: Magnesium sulfate for treating exacerbations of acute asthma in the emergency department. Cochrane Database of Systemic Reviews 2:CD001490, 2000.

27. PNEUMONIA

Robert G. Chin, M.D.

1. What is the clinical impact of pneumonia?

Pneumonia is the sixth leading cause of death and the leading cause of death from infectious disease in the United States. There are approximately 5 million identified cases of community-acquired pneumonia annually, resulting in an estimated 500,000 hospitalizations. Most cases of community-acquired pneumonia are treated in the outpatient setting with a mortality of less than 1%. Pneumonia requiring hospitalization has an associated mortality of 15%. The emergency physician's role is to diagnose pneumonia accurately, recognize the indications for hospitalization, and initiate respiratory support and empirical antibiotic therapy.

2. How does pneumonia develop?

Pneumonia is an infection of the alveolar spaces of the lung. Pulmonary infections most often result from aspiration of oropharyngeal secretions. Approximately 50% of healthy adults aspirate small amounts of these secretions during sleep. The development of clinical pneumonia depends on the virulence of the organisms aspirated, the size of the inoculum, and the ability of host defenses to respond effectively. Pneumonia may develop when pathogens are spread hematogenously from another infected site such as the urinary tract or skin.

3. List factors that predispose to the development of pneumonia.

- Endotracheal and nasogastric intubation (aspiration)
- Cigarette smoking (impairs mucociliary and macrophage function)
- Viral infections (damage respiratory epithelium)
- Advanced age (decline in mucociliary clearance, immune function)
- Immunosuppression (human immunodeficiency virus [HIV], hematologic malignancy, chemotherapy)

4. Describe the clinical features of pneumonia.

Typical pneumonia presents as a cough productive of purulent sputum, dyspnea, and fever. Less than 50% with a community-acquired pneumonia are able to produce sputum, and no single clinical finding is sufficiently reliable to establish or exclude the diagnosis. Bacterial pneumonia usually can be excluded in older children and adults based on the history and the absence of abnormalities in vital signs and chest auscultation. Infants may present with fever associated with irritability, tachypnea, tachycardia, intercostal retractions, nasal flaring, or grunting. Cough may be absent. Elderly or debilitated patients may present with nonspecific complaints and findings such as confusion or deterioration of baseline function, rather than the classic symptoms.

Atypical pneumonia is caused by *Mycoplasma pneumoniae*, *Chlamydia pneumoniae*, and *Legionella*. Atypical pneumonia is more insidious in onset and includes the absence of sputum production, leukocytosis, and consolidation on chest radiography. Cough and sore throat are prominent symptoms, and these patients are more likely to have extrapulmonary manifestations, such as dermatitis, neurologic complications (headache, aseptic meningitis), cardiac complications (pericarditis, myocarditis), hepatitis, and renal disease. Numerous studies have found no consistent clinical or radiographic criteria to distinguish typical from atypical pneumonia, and a syndromic approach to therapy is gradually being discarded.

5. Who is at greatest risk for developing pneumonia?

The very old and the very young are at greatest risk. Patients with impaired gag reflex or altered mental status caused by head injury, alcohol or drug intoxication, cerebrovascular accidents, or seizures are at great risk. Underlying pulmonary disease, such as pulmonary embolus, contusion, foreign body or tumor, chronic obstructive pulmonary disease, and atelectasis, predisposes patients to pulmonary infection. Patients with chest wall disorders, such as rib fractures, surgical wounds, or myopathies, often are unable to cough and clear secretions well. Impaired mucociliary clearance mechanisms from smoking, smog, alcohol, viral infections, or chronic obstructive pulmonary disease increase risk significantly. Impaired immune function from cancer and chemotherapy, malnutrition, HIV infection, and sickle-cell disease are commonly associated with pneumonia. Patients with a history of diabetes, alcoholism, recent antibiotic therapy, or hospitalization may be colonized with more virulent organisms and may suffer from serious pulmonary infection.

6. Discuss the key aspects of the physical examination in assessing suspected pneumonia.

The physical examination of patients with respiratory complaints begins with a review of vital signs. Findings supporting the diagnosis of pneumonia include fever, tachypnea, and tachycardia. With severe infection, patients appear toxic and may have mental status changes secondary to hypoxia. Examination of the chest includes inspection, palpation, percussion, and auscultation. The respiratory pattern should be observed for evidence of pleuritic pain that prevents deep inspiration, use of accessory muscles, weak respiratory effort, or decreased respiratory drive.

When alveoli become filled with fluid (pus), the lung examination changes. Sound is transmitted more efficiently through consolidated areas of lung tissue. By palpating the chest while the patient speaks, the examiner notes the increase in vibration over the consolidated lobe, which is called *vocal fremitus*. By the same mechanism, whispered words are better transmitted (*whispered pectoriloquy*). The chest should be percussed to identify areas of dullness caused by consolidation or the development of an empyema. The finding of localized rales on auscultation suggests pneumonia.

Although the presence of many of these findings increases the likelihood of the diagnosis being pneumonia, none of these findings should be considered absolute proof. The absence of any one finding does not rule out pneumonia. The sum of these historical and physical examination findings leads the experienced practitioner to the appropriate confirmatory tests and treatment.

7. What are the most common causative agents in community-acquired pneumonia?

The causative organism is unknown in 40% to 50% of all patients. In cases in which an organism is identified, the pathogens found reflect the population studied and the type of diagnostic test used. When sputum culture is used, *Streptococcus pneumoniae* is the most commonly detected organism, accounting for 9% to 20% of all episodes. Among these isolates, the prevalence of drug-resistant strains has risen steadily and is now approximately 30% in the United States. When serologic testing is used, *M. pneumoniae* is the most commonly identified pathogen (13% to 37% of all cases). Other common pathogens include *C. pneumoniae* (17% of outpatients) and *Legionella* (0.7% to 13% of all cases). The presence of viruses is highly variable but was 36% in one case series.

8. What are the most common causative agents in hospitalized patients?

S. pneumoniae was identified most commonly (20% to 60% of all cases), followed by *H. influenzae* (3% to 10%), then *Staphylococcus aureus*, enteric gram-negatives, *Legionella*, *M. pneumoniae*, *C. pneumoniae*, and viruses (each < 10% of cases). Several studies suggest *M. pneumoniae* and *C. pneumoniae* may be present in 40% to 60% of cases as part of a mixed infection.

9. What are the most common causative agents of aspiration pneumonia?

Pneumonia resulting from oropharyngeal aspiration is typically polymicrobial and caused by anaerobic organisms, including *Peptostreptococcus*, *Bacteroides*, *Fusobacterium*, and *Prevotella*. Risk factors for aspiration include central nervous system depression (often from alcohol) and swallowing dysfunction.

10. List tests that are useful for diagnosis or treatment.
Pulse oximetry
Chest radiography
Complete blood count
Blood chemistries
Arterial blood gas analysis

11. In which patients is arterial blood gas analysis indicated?
Patients who are significantly tachypneic, cyanotic, confused, or hypoxic. Elderly patients may be particularly difficult to evaluate, and arterial blood gases should be considered whenever a significant pulmonary infection is present.

12. What treatment should be administered in the ED?
Supportive care, including oxygen, should be given as required. The antibiotic of choice varies with the clinical situation and changes constantly. Broad-spectrum empirical therapy for the most likely pathogens is begun after reviewing the latest Centers for Disease Control recommendations (available at www.cdc.gov/ncidod/guidelines/guidelines_type.htm), pending specific identification of the organism and its sensitivities.

Therapy of Community-Acquired Pneumonia

CLINICAL SETTING*	ANTIBIOTIC REGIMEN	COMMENTS
Decision to treat as outpatient (no cardiopulmonary disease)	Advanced generation macrolide (azithromycin or clarithromycin) or doxycycline.	Erythromycin is not active against *H. influenzae*. Azithromycin and clarithromycin better tolerated
Decision to treat as outpatient (with cardiopulmonary disease)	β-lactam (oral cefpodoxime, cefuroxime, amoxicillin-clavulanate, or parenteral cefpodoxime) *plus* macrolide *or* doxycycline or antipneumococcal fluoroquinolone[†] (used alone)	Doxycycline provides adequate coverage for *H. influenzae*
Decision to treat as inpatient (no cardiopulmonary disease)	Intravenous azithromycin alone *or* doxycycline and a β-lactam *or* antipneumococcal fluoroquinolone[†] (used alone)	
Decision to treat as inpatient (with cardiopulmonary disease or residing in a skilled nursing facility)	Intravenous β-lactam (cefotaxime, ceftriaxone, ampicillin-sulbactam) *plus* intravenous or oral macrolide *or* intravenous antipneumococcal fluoroquinolone[†] alone	Doxycycline may be substituted for macrolide
Decision to treat in ICU	Intravenous antipseudomonal β-lactam (cefepime, imipenem, meropenem, piperacillin-tazobactam) *plus* intravenous antipseudomonal quinolone (ciprofloxacin)	Intravenous aminoglycoside *plus either* intravenous macrolide *or* intravenous nonpseudomonal fluoroquinolone may be substituted for ciprofloxacin

* Consider treatment for *P. carinii* pneumonia if HIV risks are present.
† Gatifloxacin, levofloxacin, moxifloxacin, trovafloxacin, and sparfloxacin

13. Should all patients be treated for atypical pathogens?
Atypical pathogens cannot be treated by β-lactam therapy but require a macrolide, tetracycline, or quinolone. Numerous studies indicate that atypical pathogens are common causes of

pneumonia and often cause coinfection with a bacterial pathogen. Additionally, evidence suggests that coinfection with an atypical agent potentiates the severity of pneumococcal infection. In light of these findings, the most recent guidelines from the American Thoracic Society, Canadian Thoracic Society, and Infectious Disease Society of America (available at www.uphs.upenn.edu/bugdrug/antibiotic_manual/table%20of%20contents.htm#atscap) all recommend empirical treatment for atypical pathogen infection.

14. Who can be treated as an outpatient?
No firm guidelines exist regarding hospital admission. Many factors associated with an increased mortality or complicated clinical course have been recognized, and their presence or absence can guide the admission decision. Patients at lowest risk and recommended for outpatient therapy are those younger than age 50 who lack significant comorbid disease (neoplasm, congestive heart failure, cerebrovascular disease, renal disease, liver disease, and HIV infection) and who lack the following physical findings: altered mental status, pulse greater than 125 beats/min, respiratory rate greater than 30 breaths/min, systolic blood pressure less than 90 mm Hg, and temperature less than 35°C (95°F) or greater than 40°C (104°F). Admission should be considered for patients with immunodeficiency, patients who already have failed outpatient antibiotic therapy, patients who are unable to take oral antibiotics, patients who have a room-air pulse oximetry less than 90%, patients who lack adequate home support, and patients who are unable to follow up with a physician.

15. How does pneumonia differ in the elderly?
The incidence of pneumonia increases with age and has been reported to be 3.6 times greater in individuals 65 years old and older compared with individuals 45 to 65 years old. The elderly have increased oropharyngeal colonization with *Staphylococcus aureus* and aerobic gram-negative bacilli. This combined with a decline in the cough reflex and alteration of mental status resulting from central nervous system disease or medication may predispose them to aspiration pneumonia with these organisms. Age-related declines in mucociliary transport and cell-mediated immunity also may contribute to the increase in incidence. Elderly patients may lack the usual symptoms and instead present with nonspecific complaints, such as confusion, lethargy, weakness, episodes of falling, and deterioration from baseline function. The pathogens that commonly cause pneumonia in the elderly are similar to those prevalent in younger patients except that atypical organisms are thought to play a less prominent role. Mortality from pneumonia also is increased in the elderly and is estimated at 20% for community-acquired infection.

16. How does pneumonia differ in patients with HIV disease?
Pulmonary infections are the most common opportunistic infection in patients with acquired immunodeficiency syndrome (AIDS). In the early years of the HIV epidemic, *Pneumocystis carinii* pneumonia accounted for two thirds of initial AIDS diagnoses, but this has declined to 40% as a result of prophylactic therapy. *P. carinii* is still the most common cause of pneumonia in this population, the most common AIDS-defining diagnosis, and the most common identifiable cause of death in patients with AIDS. The infection is rare in patients with CD4 cell counts greater that 200/mL. Patients typically present with nonproductive cough, fever, and dyspnea that develop over several weeks, but fever may be absent in 20% of cases. Chest radiography classically shows bilateral interstitial infiltrates that begin in the perihilar region, although it may be normal in 30%. Empirical treatment with trimethoprim-sulfamethoxazole usually is initiated in patients with typical presentations, with the addition of prednisone for patients with a partial pressure of oxygen that is less than 70 mm Hg. The diagnosis can be verified with induced sputum or bronchoscopy in patients with atypical presentations, severe symptoms, or lack of clinical response within 4 to 5 days.

The incidence of pneumococcal pneumonia is 7 to 10 times higher, whereas that for *Haemophilus influenzae* pneumonia is 100 times higher than in the non-HIV population. The presentation and treatment of these infections are similar to those among non-HIV patients.

The relative risk of developing active disease among patients with latent tuberculosis is 113-fold higher in patients with HIV infection. Patients with CD4 cell counts greater than 200/mL present with typical radiographic findings of cavitary disease, whereas patients with lower counts are more likely to have infiltrates in midlung zones without cavity formation. Rifampin is contraindicated in patients treated with most protease inhibitors and nonnucleoside reverse transcriptase inhibitors because it reduces their efficacy.

17. What are the special considerations in other immunocompromised patients?

The number of patients taking immunosuppressive drugs related to the treatment of malignancy, transplantation, or autoimmune disease is increasing. The distribution of pathogens in community-acquired pneumonia is similar in normal and compromised hosts, but the latter group shows an increase in uncommon pathogens. *Pseudomonas* pneumonia can occur in persistently leukopenic patients but is rare in normal hosts. *Nocardia, Aspergillus,* and *Cryptococcus* also are seen primarily in compromised patients and present with a subacute or chronic course. Transbronchial or lung biopsy may be necessary to establish the diagnosis. Physicians also need to be vigilant for changes in the predominant organism causing an infection because compromised patients are prone to sequential infections. The approach to empirical antibiotic therapy is the same in normal and compromised hosts. If a nonbacterial pneumonia is suspected based on history or atypical findings on chest radiography, a specific tissue diagnosis should be pursued as part of an inpatient evaluation to guide therapy further.

18. What are the clinical features of pulmonary anthrax?

The term *anthrax pneumonia* is misleading because true bronchopneumonia does not occur. Inhalation of anthrax spores results in a hemorrhagic thoracic lymphadenitis and hemorrhagic mediastinitis resulting in the chest radiograph finding of a widened mediastinum but no pulmonary infiltrates. Within 2 to 60 days after inhalation of infectious spores, the patient may develop fever, dyspnea, cough, chest pain, headache, vomiting, chills, and abdominal pain. In some, there is a brief period of apparent recovery followed by abrupt onset of respiratory failure and hemodynamic collapse. The mortality rate for occupationally acquired cases in the United States is 89%.

CONTROVERSY

19. What is the role of a sputum Gram stain and culture?

The value of the Gram stain for expectorated sputum is controversial because it is often uncertain how accurately expectorated sputum reflects lower respiratory tract secretions. A widely used criterion for an acceptable specimen is that it should have fewer than 10 squamous epithelial cells and more than 25 polymorphonuclear leukocytes per low-power (10×) field, but this criterion has not been validated. Wide variability in the sensitivity and specificity of this test has been reported because of contamination of the specimen by oral flora, a lower likelihood to show gram-negative organisms, and lower accuracy when the test is done by less experienced physicians outside the microbiology laboratory. Gram stain does not detect atypical pathogens. The sputum Gram stain may be helpful in the management of patients with severe pneumonia, patients who fail to respond to empirical therapy, and immunosuppressed patients.

BIBLIOGRAPHY

1. American Thoracic Society: Guidelines for the management of adults with community-acquired pneumonia: Diagnosis, assessment of severity, antimicrobial therapy, and prevention. Am J Respir Crit Care Med 163:1730–1754, 2001.
2. Bartlett JG: Pneumonia in the patient with HIV infection. Infect Dis Clin North Am 12:807–820, 1998.
3. Cunha BA: Pneumonias in the compromised host. Infect Dis Clin North Am 15:591–612, 2001.
4. Feldman C: Pneumonia in the elderly. Med Clin North Am 85:1441–1459, 2001.
5. Fine MJ, Auble TE, Yealy DM, et al: A prediction rule to identify low-risk patients with community-acquired pneumonia. N Engl J Med 336:243–250, 1997.

6. Gupta SK, Sarosi GA: The role of atypical pathogens in community-acquired pneumonia. Med Clin North Am 85:1349–1365, 2001.
7. Inglesby TV, Henderson DA, Bartlett JG, et al: Anthrax as a biological weapon: Medical and public health management. JAMA 281:1735–1745, 1999.
8. Marik PE: Aspiration pneumonitis and aspiration pneumonia. N Engl J Med 344:665–671, 2001.
9. Marx JA, Hockberger RS, Walls RM (eds): Emergency Medicine: Concepts and Clinical Practice, 5th ed. St. Louis, Mosby, 2002.
10. Niederman MS: Guidelines for the management of community-acquired pneumonia: Current recommendations and antibiotic selection issues. Med Clin North Am 85:1493–1509, 2001.
11. Smith PR: What diagnostic tests are needed for community-acquired pneumonia? Med Clin North Am 85:1381–1396, 2001.

28. DEEP VENOUS THROMBOSIS AND PULMONARY EMBOLISM

Katherine Bakes, M.D., and Polly E. Parsons, M.D.

1. List some of the risk factors for the development of deep venous thrombosis (DVT).

- Age > 70 years
- Active cancer or within 6 months of treatment
- Pelvic or lower extremity surgery or trauma
- Any surgery requiring general anesthesia for > 30 minutes
- Travel > 1000 miles in previous 12 weeks
- Estrogen/progesterone therapy
- Postpartum state
- *Hypercoagulable states*, including circulating lupus anticoagulant, antithrombin III deficiency, and protein C or S deficiency
- Bed rest ≥ 3 days or surgery within previous 4 weeks

2. Are there classic symptoms and physical examination findings for a lower extremity DVT?

Physicians are taught that patients with DVT complain of leg swelling and pain and on physical examination have a swollen red leg, a palpable cord, and a positive Homan's sign. In reality, only half of patients have these complaints or findings on physical examination, so a high index of suspicion in patients at risk is paramount.

3. What other disease processes can present with similar signs and symptoms?

Superficial thrombophlebitis, contusion, hematoma, Baker's cyst, cellulitis, and muscle strain.

4. What noninvasive methods are available for the diagnosis of DVT?

Radiofibrinogen leg scanning: Good for detecting distal clots, including clots in the calf, popliteal ligament, and distal thigh vein, but relatively poor for more proximal clots.

Impedance plethysmography: The diagnostic sensitivity and specificity depend on the technical expertise of the person doing the study, but in many centers this test detects more than 95% of acute proximal lower extremity DVT.

Duplex ultrasound: The sensitivity and specificity are operator dependent, but this test can detect more than 95% of acute proximal DVT.

Spiral CT venography: Although rarely used and not extensively studied, reports show promise for this modality, with a sensitivity and specificity comparable to ultrasound.

MRI venography: Can be useful, particularly for patients with inconclusive ultrasound studies or a contraindication to radiation or contrast dye (i.e., pregnant patients). It has proved accurate not only for lower extremity DVT, but also for pelvic DVT.

5. **What is the gold standard test for the diagnosis of DVT?**
   Venogram. Contrast venography is highly sensitive but associated with multiple complications, including dye extravasation, allergic reaction, and postvenography DVT in 2% of patients. Because this test is invasive, requires specialized resources, and is associated with an increased risk DVT, it is rarely performed.

6. **Are D-dimer measurements useful in the diagnosis of acute venous thromboembolism?**
   D-dimer, a degradation product of cross-linked fibronectin, is found in increased levels of the circulation of patients with acute venous thromboembolism. The enzyme-linked immunosorbent assay (ELISA) and whole-blood agglutination D-dimer assay are useful to exclude thromboembolic disease. The rapid ELISA and latex agglutination tests cannot be used in these algorithms because of poor negative predictive values. Although useful in ruling out venothromboembolic disease in select populations, owing to a lack of specificity, D-dimer has not proved useful at ruling *in* the diagnosis.
   The combination of a low pretest probability and a negative whole-blood agglutination D-dimer safely ruled out DVT in 177 consecutive outpatients. Similarly, an algorithm for diagnosing pulmonary emboli (PE) based on a combined pretest probability scoring system and whole-blood agglutination D-dimer assay showed a negative predictive value of 99.5% in patients with a low pretest probability and negative D-dimer.

7. **Where do PE come from?**
   Most (> 90%) come from lower extremity DVT.

8. **What percentage of patients with DVT have PE?**
   The incidence is higher than you think. In one study of 101 patients with proven DVT without pulmonary symptoms, 51% had a high-probability lung scan at the time of the diagnosis of DVT.

9. **Are there any diagnostic signs or symptoms for PE?**
   No. The common clinical symptoms—shortness of breath and chest pain—and clinical signs—tachypnea and tachycardia—are nonspecific. Patient presentations can range from mild shortness of breath to cardiovascular collapse.

10. **What studies should be considered if PE is suspected?**
    Arterial blood gases. The most common findings are a mild acute respiratory alkalosis and hypoxemia (i.e., an abnormal AaO_2 gradient), although the arterial blood gas may be completely normal. Arterial blood gas is not useful to rule in or out the diagnosis of PE. It may be used to approximate severity of disease when the diagnosis of PE has been made.
    Chest radiograph. The chest radiograph is often normal. Subtle abnormalities such as focal atelectasis, slight elevation of a hemidiaphragm, or focal hyperlucency of the lung parenchyma, may be present.
    ECG. The findings classically associated with PE (S_1, Q_3, T_3 pattern, new right bundle-branch block) occur in less than 15% of patients. The more common findings are sinus tachycardia and nonspecific ST segment and T wave changes.

11. **What studies are diagnostic for PE?**
    Ventilation/perfusion scan. A normal lung scan essentially rules out a diagnosis of PE, although there are rare incidences of patients with a normal lung scan who subsequently had PE documented by pulmonary angiogram. A high-probability scan is diagnostic for PE. The problems

arise when the lung scan is read as indeterminate, which is frequently the case when the chest radiograph is abnormal or the patient has underlying cardiopulmonary disease. An indeterminate scan probably should be followed up with a pulmonary angiogram.

Pulmonary angiogram: The gold standard for the diagnosis.

Spiral CT: In the setting of an abnormal chest radiograph, spiral CT can be useful not only in diagnosing PE, but also in defining other pathology. This modality is rapid and requires no additional technical support. It cannot be used in patients with a contraindication to contrast dye injection and requires radiologic expertise to interpret. Although shown to be highly sensitive in diagnosing central emboli, spiral CT is not sensitive enough to rule out peripheral clots. With the advent of fourth-generation CT scanners, the ability to detect PE down to the subsegmental level may be possible. Further investigation is necessary before this modality can be used safely to rule out the diagnosis.

Magnetic resonance angiogram (MRA): Limited studies have shown MRA has sensitivities and specificities comparable to standard pulmonary angiogram. Although often not immediately available, MRA is a useful modality when contraindications to conventional studies, such as pregnancy, exist.

12. What happens if the diagnosis of PE is missed?

PE is listed as one of the most common causes of death in the United States, and yet only about 25% of cases are diagnosed. Of the undiagnosed 75%, a small number die within 1 hour of presentation, so it is unlikely that diagnosis and intervention could improve outcome in that group. In the rest, however, the mortality from untreated PE is approximately 30%.

13. What is a massive PE?

A massive PE can be either anatomically defined as the occlusion of greater than 50% of the pulmonary vasculature or physiologically defined as an embolus that is complicated by systemic hypotension and severe hypoxemia. These two definitions are not synonymous because a normal individual can lose 50% of pulmonary circulation without significant hemodynamic compromise, whereas a patient with significant underlying cardiopulmonary disease could suffer major hemodynamic compromise with a much smaller clot.

14. What is the treatment for thromboembolic disease?

Anticoagulation for diagnosed thromboembolic disease should begin in the ED with heparin or low-molecular-weight heparin (LMWH). Investigations suggest that patients with proximal DVTs and temporary risk factors can be anticoagulated with heparin or warfarin for 3 months, whereas patients with calf DVTs need to be treated for only 6 weeks. Patients with permanent risk factors potentially need lifelong treatment but should be anticoagulated for at least 6 months. **LMWH** is at least as effective as heparin for the treatment of DVT and probably should be considered the treatment of choice based on efficacy, low side effect profile, and cost-effectiveness. Outpatient management of DVT with LMWH is becoming commonplace and has proved safe and effective. Subgroup analysis indicates that LMWH probably will be adopted for the treatment of PE as well, although further conclusive studies are needed.

15. When should inferior vena caval filter placement be considered?

When a patient cannot be anticoagulated because of acute bleeding or recent trauma or when a patient has a documented recurrent PE on a therapeutic anticoagulation regimen, inferior vena caval filter placement should be considered.

CONTROVERSY

16. Should thrombolytic therapy be used in patients with massive PE?

For: There are three major goals in the treatment of PE: (1) to prevent further thrombus formation; (2) to promote resolution of existing thrombus; and (3) to prevent the sequelae of PE, including recurrent emboli. The standard therapy, heparin, does prevent further thrombus formation but is not effective in the other two areas. Thrombolytic therapy has been shown to increase the rate of resolution of PE, and some suggest in the literature that the long-term sequelae of PE may decrease slightly in patients who receive thrombolytic therapy.

Against: In large clinical trials, there were no differences in morbidity or mortality when heparin and thrombolytic therapy for PE were compared. Because thrombolytic therapy may be associated with a higher complication rate, heparin therapy may be preferred.

BIBLIOGRAPHY

1. Becker DM, Philbrick JT, Bachhuber TL, Humphries JE: D-dimer testing and acute venous thromboembolism. Arch Intern Med 156:939–946, 1996.
2. Ginsberg JS: Management of venous thromboembolism. N Engl J Med 335:1816–1828, 1996.
3. Goldman LR, Lipchik RJ: Diagnosis of acute pulmonary embolism: Time for a new approach. Radiology 199:22–27, 1996.
4. Kearon C, Ginsberg JS, Douketis J, et al: Management of suspected deep venous thrombosis in outpatients by using clinical assessment and D-dimer testing. Ann Intern Med 135:108–111, 2001.
5. Kline JA, Johns KL, Colucciello SA, et al: New diagnostic tests for pulmonary embolism. Ann Emerg Med 35:168–180, 2000.
6. Meaney JFM, Weg JG, Chenevert TL, et al: Diagnosis of pulmonary embolism with magnetic resonance angiography. N Engl J Med 336:1422–1427, 1997.
7. Pinede L, Ninet J, Duhaut P, et al: Comparison of 3 and 6 months of oral anticoagulant therapy after a first episode of proximal deep vein thrombosis or pulmonary embolism and comparison of 6 and 12 weeks of therapy after isolated calf deep vein thrombosis. Circulation 103:2453, 2001.
8. Rosen CL, Tracy JA: The diagnosis of lower extremity deep venous thrombosis. Emerg Med Clin N Am 19:895–912, 2001.
9. Rowe BH: Use of low molecular weight heparins in patients with acute venous thromboembolism. Ann Emerg Med 39:555–557, 2002.
10. Stein PD, Terrin ML, Hales CA, et al: Clinical, laboratory, roentgenographic, and electrocardiographic findings in patients with acute pulmonary embolism and no pre-existing cardiac or pulmonary disease. Chest 100:598–603, 1991.
11. Wells PS, Anderson DR, Rodger M, et al: Excluding pulmonary embolism at the bedside without diagnostic imaging: Management of patients with suspected pulmonary embolism presenting to the emergency department by using a simple clinical model and D-dimer. Ann Intern Med 135:98–107, 2001.

VI. Cardiovascular System

29. CONGESTIVE HEART FAILURE AND ACUTE PULMONARY EDEMA

Rodney W. Smith, M.D., and Christopher R.H. Newton, M.D.

1. What is congestive heart failure (CHF)?

Cardiac dysfunction that leads to an inability of the heart to work as a pump to meet the circulatory demands of the patient. As a result, pulmonary congestion occurs, and when the problem is severe enough, pulmonary edema results.

2. What causes CHF?

Myocardial disease, which may be primary (cardiomyopathies) or secondary (myocardial infarction secondary to coronary artery disease). Cardiac response to volume overload (as in mitral regurgitation) or pressure overload (as in hypertension or aortic stenosis) also can lead to CHF.

3. Describe the symptoms of CHF.

Common symptoms are **dyspnea** (the subjective feeling of difficulty with breathing) and **fatigue**. Early in the course of CHF, the patient reports exertional dyspnea; the heart is able to supply enough cardiac output for sedentary activities but does not have the reserve to increase cardiac output during exercise. As heart failure worsens, even minimal activity may be difficult. Patients also report orthopnea (dyspnea relieved by assuming an erect posture), paroxysmal nocturnal dyspnea (sudden onset of dyspnea at night), and nocturia.

4. What causes these symptoms?

When the patient with CHF assumes the supine posture, fluid is redistributed from the abdomen and lower extremities to the pulmonary vasculature, causing increased pulmonary hydrostatic pressure and increased ventricular filling pressures. The patient has difficulty lying flat and sleeps with several pillows or sitting in a chair to relieve these symptoms. Redistribution of fluid may lead to increased urine output and nocturia. In severe CHF, volume redistribution may be sufficient to lead to acute pulmonary edema.

5. Name the four main determinants of cardiac function in CHF.

- Preload
- Afterload
- Myocardial contractility
- Heart rate

6. What is preload?

Within limits, the amount of work cardiac muscle can do is related to the length of the muscle at the beginning of its contraction. This relationship is shown graphically by the **Frank-Starling curve**, in which left ventricular end-diastolic volume (LVEDV) represents muscle length, and the stroke volume (SV) represents cardiac work. (It is easier to measure pressure than volume, so we graph LVEDP versus SV). Preload refers to LVEDP. As LVEDP increases, SV increases. At higher LVEDP, the increase in SV is less for a given increase in LVEDP. Note from the figure that the heart can function on different Frank-Starling curves, depending on the contractility.

Frank-Starling Curves

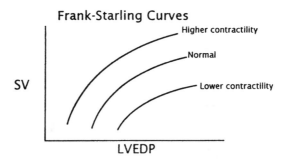

7. **What about afterload and heart rate?**
    Afterload refers to the pressure work the ventricle must do. The important components here are ventricular wall tension and systemic vascular resistance. Ventricular wall tension is related directly to intraventricular pressure and ventricular radius and inversely related to ventricular wall thickness. Because cardiac output = SV × heart rate, the **heart rate** is an important determinant of cardiac output. At high heart rates, there may be insufficient time to fill the ventricle during diastole, leading to decreased LVEDP and SV, so that cardiac output may become compromised despite the tachycardia.

8. **How does this physiology relate to treatment?**
    The goal of treatment of CHF is to improve cardiac output. This can be accomplished by modifying each of these parameters. Diuretics, dietary salt, and water restriction decrease preload and improve volume work. Digoxin improves contractility. Vasodilators are helpful in reducing afterload and the pressure work required of the heart.

9. **Describe the role of natriuretic peptides in CHF.**
    Natriuretic peptides are hormones produced by the heart in response to increased wall stress and are secreted into the circulation as a marker of failure. B-type natriuretic peptide is an independent predictor of increased LVEDP, and levels correlate with symptoms and severity of disease. It has been suggested as a screening tool and for the diagnosis of CHF in the ED. Natriuretic peptides also have been used to treat CHF and may affect mortality.

10. **Discuss acute pulmonary edema.**
    The most dramatic presentation of CHF is acute pulmonary edema. To understand pulmonary edema, we must return to the physiologist Starling, who described the interaction of forces at the capillary membrane that lead to flow of fluid from capillaries to the interstitium. Simply put, there is a balance between hydrostatic pressure and osmotic pressure. Under normal circumstances, this leads to a small net movement of fluid from the capillaries into the lung interstitium. This fluid is carried away by lymphatics. In CHF, the capillary hydrostatic pressure increases to the point that the lymphatics no longer can handle the fluid. Interstitial edema initially results, then alveolar edema.

11. **How do patients with acute pulmonary edema usually present?**
    Patients develop acute shortness of breath and generally are fighting for air. These patients sit upright to decrease venous return (preload); they cough up frothy, red-tinged sputum. Auscultation of the lungs reveals wet rales throughout and sometimes wheezes (owing to bronchospasm). This presentation is a true emergency and requires immediate aggressive therapy.

12. **What is the treatment of acute pulmonary edema?**
    First, follow the ABCs (airway, breathing, circulation). In severe hypoxia, airway and breathing may be compromised, and the patient needs to be intubated. Nasal intubation is often the best

procedure because it can be accomplished with the patient in an upright position. Intubation may be avoided with aggressive medical treatment. If you choose this route, however, constant attention to the patient is needed, and you need to set your decision point early. For example, you might decide, "I will intubate if the patient is not better in 15 minutes or worsens during that time." Administer oxygen to maintain sufficient oxygen saturation (> 90%), either by nasal cannula or nonrebreather mask. The use of continuous positive airway pressure has decreased the need for intubation of patients with pulmonary edema; however, this has not significantly affected in-hospital mortality. Continuously monitor oxygen saturation with pulse oximetry.

13. What about drug therapy?

Drug therapy is aimed at decreasing preload. Furosemide is given as a 40-mg intravenous bolus (larger amounts if the patient is on diuretics). Within 5 to 15 minutes of the injection, venodilation occurs and accounts for the rapid response to this drug. This action is followed within 30 minutes by diuresis. In addition to furosemide, morphine is given, 5 to 10 mg intravenously, to decrease anxiety and the work of breathing. It also is a venodilator, decreasing preload. With decreased anxiety, there is decreased sympathetic response and decreased afterload. Nitrates are useful in the form of sublingual nitroglycerin (NTG), topical NTG paste, or intravenous NTG drip. NTG is predominantly a venodilator, reducing preload, but also dilates coronary arteries, so it may be especially helpful in the setting of coronary artery disease. Sublingual captopril is a potentially useful adjunct in the treatment of acute pulmonary edema.

14. Are there other drugs that are useful in the treatment of acute pulmonary edema?

Yes. For the patient who is hypertensive, it is often helpful to lower the blood pressure (afterload). Hypertension and tachycardia generally result from reflex mechanisms because of the acute decompensation and often correct themselves with the initial treatment outlined previously. With severe hypertension, nitroprusside is the treatment of choice. It is a venodilator and arterial dilator, reducing preload and afterload. Start the infusion at 10 μg/min and titrate upward every 5 minutes. It is important to monitor the blood pressure closely. If the patient becomes hypotensive, stopping the infusion causes a prompt increase in blood pressure because nitroprusside has such a short half-life. Generally, doses of 0.5 to 2 μg/kg/min are sufficient.

15. What about giving positive inotropic drugs?

Digoxin, which is used in the treatment of chronic CHF, has little role in the treatment of acute pulmonary edema. Inotropic agents that are helpful include dobutamine, dopamine, and milrinone. Dobutamine and dopamine are positive inotropic agents. Dopamine has more alpha effect, especially at higher doses, and should be reserved for hypotensive patients. In cardiogenic shock that is refractory to these agents, milrinone infusion may be given. The ideal situation for administering these agents is in an ICU with pulmonary artery monitoring to measure filling pressures, cardiac output, and other hemodynamic parameters.

16. When the initial treatment has begun, what else needs to be done?

After the patient is stabilized, routine tests are done, the most important being chest radiograph and ECG. Cardiac monitoring is begun, pulse oximetry is monitored continuously, and vital signs are recorded frequently. It is generally necessary to insert a Foley catheter for close monitoring of urine output. The search is on to try to discover the underlying reason for acute decompensation.

17. Do all patients with CHF need to be admitted to the hospital?

Patients with a new diagnosis of CHF need an inpatient workup that includes serial cardiac enzymes and an assessment of the global function of the heart. Patients with known CHF who have mild symptoms or signs may be managed on an outpatient basis, assuming that they are compliant with medications, have an appropriate social network, and follow up with their primary care physician.

18. What are the usual precipitating causes of acute pulmonary edema?

The most common cause is undermedication, either as a result of patient noncompliance with medication orders or dietary salt restrictions or as a result of a change in medication under a physician's supervision. Other causes include pulmonary embolism, acute myocardial infarction, infection, anemia, arrhythmias, and severe hypertension. After precipitating factors are identified, specific therapy should be initiated.

19. What is the outpatient treatment of CHF?

Angiotensin-converting enzyme (ACE) inhibitors are the mainstay of long-term treatment of CHF, leading to a decrease in mortality and an increase in functional capacity. Other drugs that act on the renin-angiotensin system (angiotensin receptor antagonists and spironolactone) also are effective. β-Blockers are useful in that they block the cardiac effects of long-term adrenergic stimulation. Diuretics also are beneficial, especially in patients with volume overload. Digoxin causes an improvement in symptoms but no overall decrease in mortality. Combined therapy with hydralazine and isosorbide dinitrate has shown a decrease in mortality and is particularly useful in patients who have contraindications to other classes of drugs.

20. How do ACE inhibitors work in CHF?

In response to cardiac decompensation, the renin-angiotensin system is activated. Angiotensin is a potent vasoconstrictor, leading to increased afterload. Stimulation of aldosterone leads to sodium retention and extracellular fluid volume expansion and increased preload. ACE inhibitors help to decrease afterload by decreasing angiotensin II-mediated vasoconstriction and decrease preload by blocking sodium retention and volume expansion.

21. What is the long-term prognosis for patients with CHF?

Prognosis depends on the cause and severity of the heart failure. The prognosis is good when the underlying cause can be corrected, as in valvular heart disease. Patients with mild disease that can be controlled with ACE inhibitors with or without low doses of diuretics generally do well. Overall, however, patients with CHF have a 10% to 20% yearly death rate, and fewer than half survive 5 years.

BIBLIOGRAPHY

1. Carson P: Beta-blocker therapy in heart failure. Cardiol Clin 19:267–278, 2001.
2. Dao Q, Krishnaswamy P, Kazanegra R, et al: Utility of B-type natriuretic peptide in the diagnosis of congestive heart failure in an urgent-care setting. J Am Coll Cardiol 37:379–385, 2001.
3. DeNofrio D: Natriuretic peptides for the treatment of congestive heart failure. Am Heart J 138:597–598, 1999.
4. Digitalis Investigation Group: The effect of digoxin on mortality and morbidity in patients with heart failure. N Engl J Med 336:525–533, 1997.
5. Gomberg-Maitland M, Baran DA, Fuster V: Treatment of congestive heart failure: Guidelines for the primary care physician and the heart failure specialist. Arch Intern Med 161:342–352, 2001.
6. Graff L, Orledge J, Radford MJ, et al: Correlation of the Agency for Health Care Policy and Research congestive heart failure admission guideline with mortality: Peer Review Organisation Voluntary Hospital Association Initiative to Decrease Events (PROVIDE) for congestive heart failure. Ann Emerg Med 34:429–437, 1999.
7. Hamilton RJ, Carter WA, Gallagher EJ: Rapid improvement of acute pulmonary edema with sublingual captopril. Acad Emerg Med 3:205–212, 1996.
8. Miller AB, Srivastava P: Angiotensin receptor blockers and aldosterone antagonists in chronic heart failure. Cardiol Clin 19:195–202, 2001.
9. Pang D, Keenan SP, Cook DJ, et al: The effect of positive pressure airway support on mortality and the need for intubation in cardiogenic pulmonary edema. Chest 114:1185–1192, 1998.
10. Wigder HN: Pressure support noninvasive positive pressure ventilation treatment of acute cardiogenic pulmonary edema. Am J Emerg Med 19:179–181, 2001.

30. ISCHEMIC HEART DISEASE

Edward P. Havranek, M.D.

1. How is acute ischemic heart disease classified?
1. Chronic stable ischemic heart disease
2. Acute coronary syndromes
   a. Unstable angina
   b. Acute non-ST segment elevation myocardial infarction (MI)
   c. Acute ST segment elevation MI

2. How do patients with acute ischemic heart disease present?
The most common presenting symptom is central **chest discomfort**. The discomfort also may be felt (in descending order of frequency) in the right or left chest, the right or left shoulder or arm, the throat or jaw, the epigastrium, and, rarely, the ear. Less commonly, patients may present with episodic dyspnea. Some patients may have ischemia and even acute MI with no symptoms.

3. To define the discomfort better, what information should be obtained?

• Chronology	• Frequency
• Location	• Precipitating factors
• Radiation	• Alleviating factors
• Duration	• Quality
• Intensity	• Associated symptoms

4. Describe the typical features of the chest discomfort in ischemic heart disease.
Typically, patients with stable angina have episodes of discomfort during exertion that are relieved within minutes by rest. The amount of exertion bringing on the discomfort can be variable. The discomfort is often vague; is described most often as a tightness or heaviness; and is substernal in location with radiation to the jaw, shoulder, or upper extremity common.

Unstable angina patients usually have similar pain, but it occurs at rest or with progressively less exertion (crescendo angina). Patients with unstable angina who have pain at rest also should have pain with exertion. **Prinzmetal's angina**, which is caused by coronary artery spasm, is an exception to this rule. Patients with Prinzmetal's angina typically have pain at rest, usually in the early morning hours, and often do not have exertional discomfort. True vasospastic angina is uncommon.

The pain of MI is typically more severe than any preceding angina. It may be described as crushing, but usually not ripping or tearing, pain. The presence of diaphoresis or radiation to the jaw or arm should raise the suspicion of acute MI markedly.

5. What other symptoms are associated with the chest discomfort of ischemic heart disease?
Shortness of breath commonly accompanies angina. Many conditions other than angina that cause chest discomfort, such as pulmonary disease and anxiety disorder, also are accompanied by shortness of breath. Diaphoresis occurs less frequently with angina but should raise one's level of suspicion of angina because it does not occur often with other disorders that cause chest pain.

6. Is there anything different about evaluating elderly patients?
The symptoms associated with ischemic heart disease in patients older than age 75 years are more likely to be atypical. The older the patient, the more atypical the symptoms become.

7. How should demographic features and the presence or absence of coronary risk factors be used?

They are not reliable. A young woman with no risk factors but with typical symptoms and ECG changes should be suspected of having ischemic disease. Conversely, a middle-aged man with diabetes and hypertension whose pain has no typical features should not be treated as having the disease.

8. List the key elements of the initial evaluation of a patient with a suspected acute coronary syndrome.

- The patient should have an **ECG** as soon as possible, preferably within 5 minutes of presentation.
- **Vital signs** are vital. The presence of hypertension, hypotension, or tachycardia must be dealt with early.
- A **history** directed at the key elements described previously and a **cardiovascular examination** come next; the examination is useful for ruling out other diagnoses, such as pericarditis and aortic dissection.
- While the history and physical examination are being done, it is generally a good idea to start an intravenous line, administer oxygen by nasal cannula, place the patient on a cardiac monitor, and give an aspirin.

9. What is the significance of abnormal ST segment changes on an ECG?

Abnormal ST segment changes may or may not represent ischemic cardiac injury. The *current of injury* that accompanies ST segment elevation MI is typically a convex-downward elevation of the ST segment. It may be confused with pericarditis or early repolarization. ST elevation also may be due to left ventricular hypertrophy, acute pericarditis, acute cor pulmonale, hyperkalemia, hypothermia, cardiac tumor, or aneurysm. ST depression not only may be caused by cardiac ischemia, but also by such things as ventricular hypertrophy, drugs (e.g., digoxin), atrioventricular junctional rhythm with a retrograde P wave, or electrolyte abnormalities.

10. What is the typical time course of ECG changes in ischemic cardiac injury?

The initial changes are T wave prolongation and increased T wave magnitude, either upright or inverted. Next the ST segment displays elevation or depression. A Q wave may be seen in the initial ECG or may not develop for hours to days. As the ST segment returns to baseline, symmetrically inverted T waves evolve. This classic evolution is documented in approximately 65% of patients with acute MI.

11. Can the ECG be normal while a patient is having cardiac ischemia or an acute MI?

Although serial ECGs showing evolving changes are diagnostic for acute MI in greater than 90% of patients, 20% to 50% of initial ECGs are normal or show only nonspecific abnormalities. The initial ECG may be diagnostic for acute MI in only half of patients. An early repeat ECG may be helpful.

12. Are cardiac markers useful in the ED?

Not really. Myoglobin levels begin to rise within 1 to 2 hours after the onset of pain, but elevations of this protein are nonspecific. Troponin and creatine phosphokinase levels may begin to rise at 4 to 6 hours, but single determinations are generally not sufficiently specific to make a diagnosis. Conversely, patients may have unstable angina necessitating ICU admission but still have normal levels.

13. How can echocardiography be useful in ED patients with suspected acute coronary syndrome?

It is particularly useful when the ECG is nondiagnostic, such as when there is a left bundle-branch block or minimal ST elevation. The presence of a wall motion abnormality is strong evidence to support the diagnosis of ischemia. Echocardiography also may provide information about complications, such as mitral regurgitation and pericardial effusion. A negative echocardiogram in the setting of a typical history and ECG does not rule out the diagnosis of an acute coronary syndrome.

14. What other diagnoses should be considered in a patient with chest pain?

The patient's history is paramount:
- Pleuritic chest pain may be caused by pleuritis, pericarditis, pneumothorax, or pulmonary embolism.
- Nonanginal pain may be found with the onset of herpes zoster or with cervical or thoracic nerve root compression.
- Esophagitis, esophageal spasm, and esophageal rupture may mimic pain of cardiac origin.
- Patients with anxiety or depression syndromes often complain of chest pain.
- A life-threatening condition, **dissecting aortic aneurysm**, also may cause sustained chest pain or typical angina.

15. State the indications for reperfusion therapy in acute MI.

1. ST elevation greater than 1 mm in two leads.
2. Pain not immediately responsive to nitroglycerin.
3. Pain lasting less than 6 hours. In many patients, it still may be of benefit 12 hours after the onset of pain.

16. What is the preferred therapy for cardiogenic shock?

The only therapy shown to decrease the historically high mortality associated with this syndrome is primary angioplasty. This should be performed without delay. An exception to this is cardiogenic shock caused by **right ventricular infarction**. This problem should be suspected whenever shock accompanies an acute inferior MI. The presence of jugular venous distention is an important clue to the diagnosis of this syndrome, and volume expansion usually reverses the hypotension.

17. List contraindications to thrombolytic therapy.

Contraindications:
1. Active bleeding
2. Major surgery or trauma in the past 3 weeks
3. Neurosurgery or stroke in the past 3 months
4. Prolonged (> 10 minutes) or traumatic cardiopulmonary resuscitation (CPR)
5. Hypertension (systolic > 180 mmHg, diastolic > 110 mmHg).

Relative contraindications:
1. Major trauma or surgery more than 3 weeks ago
2. Neurosurgery or stroke more than 3 months ago
3. Active peptic ulcer
4. Hemorrhagic ophthalmic condition, especially diabetic retinopathy

Patients with a known allergy to streptokinase or anisoylated plasminogen streptokinase activator complex (APSAC) should be treated with another agent. Exposure to streptokinase or APSAC in the previous 6 months or streptococcal infection in the previous 6 months are reasons to use another agent.

18. What other diagnoses should be considered before giving thrombolytic therapy?

Aortic dissection and **acute pericarditis** can mimic acute MI. Both have had fatal outcomes when thrombolytics were given. Dissection can be excluded with a careful history, examination of peripheral pulses, and chest radiograph. Pericarditis can be excluded by carefully listening for a rub and examining the ECG for widespread, concave-upward ST elevation.

19. What is the risk for fatal complications of thrombolytic therapy for acute MI?

Mortality, which almost invariably results from intracranial hemorrhage, occurs in about 0.5% of treated patients.

20. What are reperfusion arrhythmias?

Approximately 45 minutes after initiation of a thrombolytic agent, blood flow is restored in most patients. This event may be accompanied by arrhythmias, especially ventricular tachycardia or accelerated idioventricular rhythm. In patients with inferior MI, sinus bradycardia or heart block may occur. These arrhythmias are transient (generally lasting < 30 seconds). Reperfusion may be accompanied by a brief increase in pain.

21. What other medications are useful adjuvants to thrombolytic therapy?

1. **Morphine**. MI can cause excruciating pain and severe fear and anxiety. Intravenous morphine sulfate should be administered in increments of 2 to 4 mg to alleviate these symptoms.

2. **Aspirin**. Aspirin should be given immediately because it reduces mortality independent of thrombolytic therapy.

3. **β-Blockers**. Given intravenously during thrombolytic therapy, metoprolol, atenolol, or esmolol reduce mortality and infarct size further. They are better tolerated than one may think and are underused.

4. **Heparin**. With t-PA, initiation of heparin is imperative at least 1 hour before the completion of the thrombolytic infusion. With streptokinase or APSAC, administration of heparin should be delayed 4 to 6 hours. There is currently controversy over whether low-molecular-weight heparin is superior to unfractionated heparin for reducing recurrent events.

5. **Nitroglycerin**. If control of blood pressure is an issue, nitroglycerin is the preferred agent.

22. What other arrhythmias occur with acute MI?

Ventricular irritability, with frequent premature ventricular contractions, nonsustained ventricular tachycardia, and ventricular fibrillation, may occur and should be treated with lidocaine. Sustained ventricular tachycardia (lasting >30 seconds) is uncommon in acute MI. Accelerated idioventricular rhythm (heart rate, 60 to 100 beats/min) should not be treated.

Bradyarrhythmias also may occur. Second-degree or third-degree heart block that accompanies inferior MI is usually transient, and a temporary pacemaker generally is not required. When heart block accompanies an anterior MI, a temporary pacer *is* required. A prophylactic temporary pacer probably is indicated when severe conductive system disease (bifascicular block or left bundle-branch block plus first-degree block) accompanies an anterior acute MI.

23. Which patients with unstable angina are at highest risk for MI and benefit from more aggressive treatment?

Patients with transient or fixed ST segment depression or T wave inversion, especially when these changes are in leads V_1 through V_3, and patients with elevated troponin levels are at higher risk. These patients are thought to benefit more from more aggressive medical treatment (see question 24) and early catheterization. Age greater than 65, known coronary artery disease, presence of three or more coronary risk factors (smoking, hypertension, diabetes, elevated cholesterol, family history), and severe angina within the prior 24 hours also are factors that increase risk.

24. How should unstable angina be managed in the ED?

- Always administer **aspirin**. Evidence suggests that addition of clopidogrel to aspirin may reduce risk of death and MI better than aspirin alone.
- Virtually all patients with unstable angina should be treated with **β-blockers**. It may be desirable to start this therapy in the ED.
- For patients with ongoing pain, always treat with **nitroglycerin**. Start with the sublingual route of administration, and move to intravenous nitroglycerin if that does not work. Nitroglycerin is the preferred agent when the patient has concurrent hypertension.
- **Heparin** should be started. For low-risk or intermediate-risk patients, heparin may be reserved for patients refractory to aspirin, nitrates, and β-blockers. It is currently unclear if

low-molecular-weight heparin reduces subsequent risk of MI or death more than unfractionated heparin does. Some low-molecular-weight heparin preparations may reduce these end points better than others.

- High-risk patients (see question 23) benefit from use of the intravenous antiplatelet agents **tirofiban** or **eptifibatide**. The other agent in this class of antiplatelet drugs (glycoprotein IIB/IIIA inhibitors), abciximab, is not effective in acute coronary syndromes (although it is an effective adjuvant during percutaneous coronary interventions).

- Add **calcium channel blockers** when symptoms recur despite aspirin, nitrates, and β-blockers. *Never* use short-acting dihydropyridines, such as nifedipine, without β-blockers. In the setting of unstable angina, use without concurrent β-blockade increases the risk of myocardial infarction.

CONTROVERSY

25. What is the preferred method of reperfusion therapy in acute MI?
Thrombolytic therapy versus primary angioplasty: Optimally delivered angioplasty in the setting of acute MI probably reduces mortality to a greater degree than does thrombolytic therapy. Primary angioplasty has the added advantages of lower rates of reocclusion in the subsequent few days and probably lower risks of intracranial bleeding. The problem is that studies from community settings show that optimally delivered angioplasty is not often accomplished. Unless a skilled catheterization laboratory team can do an angioplasty in less than 2 hours after presentation, thrombolytic therapy is probably preferable. There are passionate advocates for both sides of this argument.

Choice of thrombolytic therapy: The GUSTO study compared streptokinase and tissue plasminogen activator (t-PA) for the treatment of acute MI and found lower mortality with t-PA (7.3% versus 6.3%). Many have argued, however, that this small decrement in mortality is not worth the much higher cost of t-PA. In the United States, t-PA has become the most popular agent, but its use is not universal.

BIBLIOGRAPHY

1. Aufderheide T, Gibler WB: Acute ischemic coronary syndromes. In Rosen P, Barkin RM (eds): Emergency Medicine: Concepts and Clinical Practice, 4th ed. St. Louis, Mosby, 1998, pp 1655–1716.
2. GISSI collaborators, GISSI-2: A factorial randomized trial of alteplase versus streptokinase and heparin versus no heparin among 12,490 patients with acute myocardial infarction. Lancet 336:65–71, 1990.
3. Goldman L, Cook EF, Johnson PA, et al: Prediction of the need for intensive care in patients who come to emergency departments with acute chest pain. N Engl J Med 334:1498–1504, 1996.
4. Green GB, Hansen KN, Chan DW, et al: The potential utility of a rapid CK-MB assay in evaluating emergency department patients with possible myocardial infarction. Ann Emerg Med 20:954–960, 1991.
5. GUSTO Investigators: An international randomized trial comparing four thrombolytic strategies for acute myocardial infarction. N Engl J Med 329:673–682, 1993.
6. Hauser AM: The emerging role of echocardiography in the emergency department. Ann Emerg Med 18:1298–1303, 1989.
7. Karlson BW, Herlitz J, Wiklund O, et al: Early prediction of acute myocardial infarction from clinical history, examination and electrocardiogram in the emergency room. Am J Cardiol 68:171–175, 1991.
8. Lamas GA, Muller JE, Turi ZG, et al: A simplified method to predict occurrence of complete heart block during myocardial infarction. Lancet 336:65–71, 1990.
9. Lau J, Antman EM, Jimenez-Silva J, et al: Cumulative meta-analysis of therapeutic trials for myocardial infarction. N Engl J Med 327:248–254, 1992.
10. U.S. Department of Health and Human Services, Agency for Health Care Policy and Research: Clinical Practice Guideline No. 10: Diagnosing and managing unstable angina. AHCPR Publication No. 94-0602. Silver Springs, MD, USDHHS, 1994.
11. Verstraete M, Bory M, Collen D, et al: Randomized trial of intravenous recombinant tissue-type plasminogen activator versus intravenous streptokinase in acute myocardial infarction. Lancet 336:65–71, 1990.

31. CARDIAC ARRHYTHMIAS

Christopher B. Colwell, M.D., and Alden H. Harken, M.D.

1. Is it necessary to identify an arrhythmia to treat it?
No.

2. How do I know whether a patient's arrhythmia is causing hemodynamic compromise?
Typically, if a patient's ventricular rate is between 60 and 100 beats/min, any hemodynamic instability is caused by something else. It is unusual, although not impossible, for a tachyarrhythmia with a rate of less than 150 beats/min to be the primary cause of hemodynamic instability. It is unusual that a heart rate of less than 150 beats/min requires electrical cardioversion.

3. What is synchronized cardioversion?
Synchronization of delivered energy to match the QRS complex. This reduces the chance that a shock will induce ventricular fibrillation, which can occur when electrical energy impinges on the relative refractory portion of the cardiac electrical activity (downslope of the T wave).

4. How do I perform synchronized cardioversion?
Select a lead on the monitor that clearly reveals an R wave of greater amplitude than the T wave. Turn on the defibrillator. Engage the synchronization mode by pressing the sync control button, and look for markers on the R waves indicating the sync mode is functioning and capturing the QRS complex and not the T wave. You may need to adjust the R wave gain until the sync markers occur with each QRS complex. Then select the appropriate energy level, position the paddles appropriately, apply 25 lb of pressure on both paddles, and press the discharge buttons simultaneously. Always remember to use adequate sedation in any awake patient. Options include diazepam, midazolam, barbiturates, and ketamine, with or without analgesic agents such as fentanyl, morphine, or meperidine.

5. How do I treat bradyarrhythmias?
Do not treat a bradycardia if the patient is hemodynamically stable and asymptomatic. Always treat the patient, not a number. If the patient has a heart rate less than 60 beats/min and is hemodynamically unstable:
  1. Give 0.5 mg (0.01 mg/kg in a child) intravenous atropine (may repeat as needed).
  2. Initiate pacemaker (do not forget the external pacemaker). The transvenous pacemaker (especially without fluoroscopy) always takes much longer than you think it will.

6. Is there a limit above which tachycardia no longer increases cardiac output?
A reasonable rule of thumb is that you can increase cardiac output by increasing the heart rate up to 200 beats/min minus the age of the patient.

7. What is a sinus beat?
At the end of each heartbeat, all myocardial cells are depolarized and experience a refractory period. At this point, certain cardiac cells (sinoatrial and atrioventricular [AV] nodes and some ventricular cells) float back up through phase IV depolarization toward *threshold potential*. It is like a race, and typically the sinoatrial node cells win this race, achieve threshold, fire, and assume the pacemaker *sinus beat* function of the heart.

8. Define premature ventricular contraction.
A premature ventricular contraction occurs when a ventricular site wins the "race" among myocardial cells and ventricular depolarization originates from an ectopic ventricular site.

9. What is a narrow-complex tachycardia?

The AV node attaches directly to the Purkinje system, which courses over the endocardial surface of the ventricles. An electrical impulse travels over the Purkinje fibers fast: 2 to 3 m/sec. If an impulse enters the ventricles from the AV node, it can activate electrically the entire ventricular muscle mass rapidly—in 0.12 sec, 120 msec, or three little boxes on ECG paper. *Narrow complex* refers to the width of the QRS complex. A narrow-complex tachycardia must originate above the AV node and is a supraventricular tachycardia (SVT).

10. What is the AV node?

The AV node is not simply a passive connection between the atria and ventricles. It is "smart." Normally, all atrial impulses are conducted to the ventricles. When the ventricular rate becomes sufficiently rapid that cardiac output is compromised, conduction velocity begins to slow in the AV node. This progressive slowing filters the rapid atrial impulses so that serial atrial impulses are not conducted at all (otherwise known as **Wenkebach block**). This progressive AV nodal conduction block is a protective mechanism to prevent dysfunctionally rapid ventricular rate.

11. Do I need to distinguish the multiple varieties of narrow-complex tachycardia (i.e., rapid atrial fibrillation [AF], SVT, atrial flutter) to treat effectively?

No, as long as it is unstable. You do not want to convert stable AF or atrial flutter if there is any chance it has been going on for more than 48 hours because of the risk of embolizing clot. Electrical conversion is always the treatment if the tachycardia is unstable.

12. How do I treat narrow-complex tachycardia in a hemodynamically stable patient?

A narrow-complex tachycardia must be supraventricular, originating above the AV node (see question 9). To control the ventricular rate, you need to block the AV node pharmacologically. Verapamil, 5 to 10 mg intravenously over 1 to 2 minutes, terminates or controls the ventricular response rate in 80% to 90% of cases. Alternatively, adenosine, 6 mg intravenous rapid bolus followed by 12 mg (which may be repeated), has a response rate of 85% to 90%. Although more expensive than verapamil, adenosine has no serious side effects. Adenosine exhibits little effect on infranodal conduction, which has led some authors to recommend its use as a diagnostic agent in wide-complex tachycardias.

13. What is a wide-complex tachycardia?

When an impulse originates from a typically damaged or ischemic bit of ventricular muscle, it takes a while to access the Purkinje superhighways, permitting electrical activation of the entire ventricular mass. The QRS is measured from its initial deflection (at the ectopic site) to the completion of all ventricular activity. When the major conduction pathways are not used primarily, it takes a long time (> 0.12 sec, 120 msec, or three little boxes on the ECG paper) to inscribe the QRS complex. This ectopic, ventricular origin complex is referred to as *wide*.

14. What is the most common cause of wide-complex tachycardia?

Ventricular tachycardia (VT). Of patients presenting to the ED with a wide-complex tachycardia, 80% to 90% have VT, and only 10% to 20% have SVT with aberrancy. VT is even more likely if the patient has a history of a prior myocardial infarction or congestive heart failure.

15. How do I treat wide-complex tachycardia?

Immediately cardiovert an unstable patient. Medical management may be considered in a stable patient with a wide-complex tachycardia. Advanced Cardiac Life Support (ACLS) 2000 algorithms suggest procainamide or amiodarone for wide-complex tachycardia of unknown type in a patient with preserved cardiac function (no clinical congestive heart failure). If the patient has clinical congestive heart failure, amiodarone is suggested. If the rhythm is known to be ventricular in origin, lidocaine, procainamide, or amiodarone should be considered. The dose of procainamide is 17 mg/kg at a rate of 20 mg/min (to be stopped if the arrhythmia is suppressed, hypotension occurs, or the QRS complex widens by 50% of its original width). The dose of lidocaine is 1.0 to 1.5 mg/kg repeated every 5 minutes to a maximum of 3 mg/kg. Intravenous amiodarone is given over 10 to 15 minutes at a dose of 0.75 mg/kg (or 150 mg for most adults).

16. What is a supraventricular rhythm with aberrancy?

Usually a supraventricular rhythm traverses the AV node and courses through the large endoventricular conduction fibers, activating the ventricles rapidly and resulting in a narrow QRS complex (< 0.12 sec). A wide-complex tachycardia typically represents a tachycardia of ventricular origin. Although less frequent, a supraventricular origin impulse that travels through the ventricle in an aberrant fashion also can be wide and is called supraventricular rhythm with aberrancy.

17. How do I treat tachyarrhythmias?

Any unstable patient with a tachyarrhythmia that either is or may be the cause of the instability requires cardioversion. An unstable patient is any patient with hypotension (systolic blood pressure < 90 mmHg) plus altered level of consciousness or complaining of chest pain or shortness of breath. SVT and atrial flutter often respond to low voltages (50 J), whereas most other tachyarrhythmias typically require at least 100 J to convert to a sinus rhythm. One may consider vagal maneuvers or pharmacotherapy before cardioversion in stable patients.

18. Does it make sense to cardiovert asystole?

Strictly speaking, no. Theoretically, electrical cardioversion synchronously depolarizes all myocardial cells simultaneously. All cells then should repolarize synchronously and spontaneously reinitiate sinus rhythm. With asystole, there is nothing to depolarize and nothing to cardiovert. Clinicians in favor of attempting to cardiovert apparent asystole point out, however, that you have nothing to lose. Conceivably the major QRS vector is perpendicular to the axis of the ECG lead, making ventricular fibrillation appear as asystole. In this instance, cardioversion of apparent asystole could help.

19. How do I make the diagnosis of AF when the ventricular rate is fast?

Rapid AF may be impossible to differentiate from SVT on a cardiac rhythm strip. The diagnosis of AF is made by palpating a peripheral pulse and simultaneously auscultating the heart or visualizing the cardiac rhythm. Atrial fibrillation is the only arrhythmia that results in a pulse deficit (fewer beats palpable than observed or auscultated) and that has an irregularly irregular pulse with varying intensity of the pulse. When rapid AF is present on ECG or monitor, it is difficult to differentiate it from paroxysmal atrial tachycardia or atrial flutter because it appears regular.

20. What drug is contraindicated in the treatment of any wide-complex tachycardia?

Verapamil. Because all wide-complex tachycardias must be considered to be of ventricular origin, verapamil is likely to cause hypotension and may cause degeneration of the rhythm to ventricular fibrillation or asystole. Procainamide may induce hypotension, particularly in patients with impaired left ventricular function.

21. Is VT always hemodynamically unstable?

No. Hemodynamic status should not be used to determine the nature of a wide QRS tachycardia: Do not assume a wide-complex tachycardia is not VT if the patient is hemodynamically stable.

22. Summarize some of the methods of differentiating VT from SVT with aberrancy.

- **History**: A history of coronary artery disease or congestive heart failure strongly suggests VT.
- **Physical examination**: Evidence of AV dissociation (cannon A waves) suggests VT.
- **ECG**: Heart rate is of no value in distinguishing VT from SVT. AV dissociation during tachycardia strongly suggests VT. The presence of fusion or capture beats also suggests

VT. Left-axis deviation, right-axis deviation, a QRS width of more than 140 msec, and concordance of QRS complexes in the precordial leads all suggest VT over SVT as the cause. Monophasic or biphasic QRS in lead V_1 and an rS or QS in lead V_6 also favor VT. In general, if it does not seem to be a typical bundle-branch block pattern, it is probably VT.

23. When is it necessary to anticoagulate a patient with AF?

In a stable patient who presents to the ED in AF, rate control is the primary goal. β-Blockers (metoprolol, 5 to 10 mg over 2 minutes) and calcium channel blockers (diltiazem, 20 mg over 2 minutes) are effective AV nodal blocking agents and can achieve adequate rate control in most patients with AF. Anticoagulation in patients who have AF for less than 48 hours is unnecessary because the risk of thromboembolism is lower. If the duration of AF has been greater than 48 hours and the patient is stable, cardioversion should be delayed until the patient is fully anticoagulated.

24. What does amiodarone do, and should we be using it in the ED?

Amiodarone (Cordarone) is a class III antiarrhythmic that prolongs the action potential duration and refractory period, slows automaticity in pacemaker cells, and slows conduction in the AV node. It is approved for the treatment of ventricular and supraventricular arrhythmias, including AF, atrial flutter, and accessory pathway syndromes. Amiodarone is a good option to consider in a hemodynamically stable patient with known VT or a wide-complex tachycardia of unknown mechanism, particularly in patients in whom lidocaine and procainamide have been ineffective. Primary side effects are hypotension, bradycardia, and heart failure. The loading dose is 0.75 mg/kg given over 10 to 15 minutes. Amiodarone exhibits a slow onset of action and an even slower clearance. Amiodarone is also considerably more expensive than most other antiarrhythmics. Current ACLS guidelines suggest amiodarone can be used instead of lidocaine for monomorphic VT, but its use as a primary agent probably should wait until the results of direct comparative trials with long-term survival outcomes measured become available.

25. Should we be using monophasic or biphasic waveform defibrillation in the ED?

Theoretical advantages to biphasic waveforms include less energy required to achieve effective defibrillation and less postshock myocardial damage and dysfunction at equivalent energy levels. There are no data at this point, however, that show a benefit in terms of long-term survival when biphasic waveforms are used. As in the case with amiodarone, we should wait for outcome data to show a clear survival to discharge benefit before we declare this new technology the standard. Biphasic defibrillation may or may not be beneficial and cost-effective for patients; the jury is still out at this point. It is unnecessary to replace well-functioning monophasic defibrillators with new expensive biphasic defibrillators.

26. What is the one message I should come away with from this chapter?

An unstable patient with *any* tachyarrhythmia, regardless of the mechanism, requires cardioversion.

BIBLIOGRAPHY

1. Angelos MG, Menegazzi JJ, Callaway CW: Bench to bedside: Resuscitation from prolonged ventricular fibrillation. Acad Emerg Med 8:909–924, 2001.
2. Connolly SJ: Evidence-based analysis of amiodarone efficacy and safety. Circulation 100:2025–2034, 1999.
3. Harken AH, Honigman B, Van Way C: Cardiac dysrhythmias in the acute setting: Recognition and treatment (or) anyone can treat cardiac dysrhythmias. J Emerg Med 5:129–134, 1987.
4. Li H, Easley A, Barrington W, et al: Evaluation and management of AF in the emergency department. Emerg Med Clin North Am 16:389–403, 1998.
5. Shah CP, Thakur RK, Xie B, Hoon VK: Clinical approach to wide QRS complex tachycardias. Emerg Med Clin North Am 16:331–360, 1998.
6. Weigner MJ, Caulfiel TA, Danias PG, et al: Risk for clinical thromboembolism associated with conversion to sinus rhythm in patients with AF lasting less than 48 hours. Ann Intern Med 126:615–620, 1997.

32. HYPERTENSION AND HYPERTENSIVE CRISES

Neide Fehrenbacher, M.D.

1. Define hypertension (HTN).

The textbook definition is blood pressure (BP) greater than 160/95 mmHg. **Borderline HTN** ranges from a systolic blood pressure (SBP) of 140 to 159 mmHg and a diastolic blood pressure (DBP) of 90 to 95 mmHg. The upper limit of normal is 140/90 mmHg. Patients may have **isolated systolic HTN** with SBP greater than 160 mmHg but normal DBP. This condition is common in the elderly secondary to the progressive large vessel atherosclerosis that occurs with aging. A patient must have had at least three elevated BP readings documented at three separate office visits to be labeled as a hypertensive.

2. Name several common causes of BP elevation in a patient without true HTN.

Anxiety, pain, illicit drug use (e.g., cocaine, amphetamines, PCP, LSD), over-the-counter medications containing sympathomimetics, and alcohol withdrawal.

3. What are the two general classifications of HTN?

Essential or **primary HTN** and **secondary HTN**. More than 90% of patients have essential HTN, and the cause is unknown. Factors known to contribute to increased BP include age, race, obesity, heredity, smoking, and high sodium ingestion. In contrast to essential HTN, secondary HTN has an identifiable cause. It may result from an abnormality of the neurologic, hormonal, renal, or vascular system. The most common causes are renal vascular disease, renal parenchymal disease, and endocrine abnormalities (e.g., Addison's disease, pheochromocytoma).

4. Describe the pathologic changes that occur with prolonged HTN.

It is well known that the contractile properties of smooth muscle in the arterial walls become altered in hypertensive patients. What is not known is whether this is the primary cause of HTN or the response to chronically elevated pressures resulting from failed autoregulatory mechanisms. Chronically elevated peripheral vascular resistance leads to left ventricular hypertrophy and increases the subsequent risk of congestive heart failure, angina, and myocardial infarction. Chronic HTN also increases the risk of stroke, retinal disease, and renal disease.

5. What signs and symptoms might you see in a patient with chronic HTN and end-organ damage?

Cardiac: Dyspnea on exertion, paroxysmal nocturnal dyspnea, nocturia, cough, dyspnea, and right upper quadrant pain from passive congestion of the liver. On examination, you may find a laterally displaced point of maximal impulse, an S_3 or S_4, jugular venous distention, rales, dependent pitting edema, and hepatomegaly.

Retinal changes: Visual field cuts or blurred vision. Funduscopic examination may reveal retinal vessel spasm with arteriovenous-nicking; *copper-wiring*; and progression to hemorrhage, exudates, and papilledema.

Central nervous system: Morning occipital headaches, dizziness, lightheadedness, and tinnitus. The signs of central nervous system involvement vary according to the vascular distribution affected.

Renal: Generalized weakness, malaise, nausea, and oliguria (symptoms of acute renal failure). If related to renal artery stenosis, abdominal bruits may be heard.

6. Are any laboratory tests necessary in the ED?

Asymptomatic patients found to have elevated BP do not need specific testing to rule out end-organ damage in the ED. These screening tests can be done on an outpatient basis and include an ECG (looking for evidence of left ventricular hypertrophy, ischemic changes, and infarction patterns), urinalysis (looking for proteinuria, hematuria, and glycosuria), and a chemistry panel (looking at the electrolytes, blood urea nitrogen, and creatinine). If secondary causes of HTN are suspected, more extensive testing would be indicated. The answer to this question changes, however, if there are any signs or symptoms of associated end-organ damage because this defines a **hypertensive emergency**.

7. Describe conventional HTN therapy.

Unless immediate BP reduction is indicated, therapy is best initiated in a primary care setting. Management usually begins with diet, exercise, weight loss, stress reduction, and behavior modification. If medication is required, diuretics are usually the first-line agents. Specific medication regimens usually are chosen based on the patient and any associated comorbidities. Frequently used medications include diuretics in combination with potassium-sparing agents, central α-agonists, α-blockers, β-blockers, vasodilators, calcium channel blockers, and angiotensin-converting enzyme inhibitors. Success of a medication class may vary among patients of different ethnic backgrounds, doses may need to be adjusted, and new medications may need to be added over time.

8. Define hypertensive crisis.

A hypertensive crisis is a true medical emergency. It is a sudden increase in BP that leads to acute end-organ damage, specifically of the brain, cardiovascular system, and kidneys. Blood pressure in this situation must be lowered within 1 hour, ideally a 20% to 25% decrease in mean arterial pressure (MAP), to avoid permanent life-threatening damage. Feared complications of hypertensive crises include hypertensive encephalopathy, ischemic cardiac syndromes with or without pulmonary edema, dissecting aortic aneurysm, and renal failure.

9. What is the difference between hypertensive emergency and hypertensive urgency?

Hypertensive urgency involves severely elevated BP, but by definition, **does not** have associated end-organ damage.

10. What are other important causes of hypertensive emergencies to consider in a patient with no known history of essential HTN?

Any condition leading to elevated circulating catecholamines can lead to a hypertensive crisis. Examples include presence of a pheochromocytoma, patients taking monoamine oxidase inhibitor antidepressants who ingest tyramine-containing compounds, and the use of sympathomimetic drugs (i.e., cocaine, amphetamines, PCP, LSD, and diet pills), which may precipitate a prompt hypertensive response.

11. What must be considered in a patient with a history of essential HTN who presents with hypertensive emergency?

Ask if the patient has been prescribed a short-acting sympathetic blocker such as clonidine or a β-blocker. Ask whether the patient abruptly stopped or ran out of HTN medications because clonidine and β-blocker withdrawal can cause significant rebound HTN.

12. What class of antihypertensive medications is contraindicated in a catecholamine-induced hypertensive emergency?

β-blockers. β-Receptor-induced vasodilation results in unopposed α-adrenergic vasoconstriction and elevates BP further. In patients with concomitant cocaine ingestions, β-blockers enhance cocaine-induced coronary artery vasoconstriction, increase BP, fail to decrease heart rate, decrease the seizure threshold, and increase mortality. Labetalol, an α-blocker and β-blocker, has detrimental effects in patients with cocaine ingestion or pheochromocytoma. Acceptable agents for treatment of a catecholamine-induced hypertensive emergency include nicardipine, fenoldopam, phentolamine, and nitroprusside.

13. What is the difference between accelerated HTN and malignant HTN?

Accelerated HTN consists of elevated BP and funduscopic changes consisting of flame hemorrhages and cotton-wool spots. **Malignant HTN** has the same funduscopic changes and papilledema. Some sources include the presence of either encephalopathy or nephropathy in the definition of malignant HTN.

14. What is hypertensive encephalopathy?

A form of hypertensive emergency that occurs when BP becomes so high that cerebral autoregulation fails. When this occurs, blood flow to the brain no longer is controlled, and elevated intracranial pressure (ICP) ensues. Hypertensive encephalopathy is characterized by acute onset of symptoms associated with an abrupt elevation in BP. Symptoms are reversible with BP reduction and include headache, vomiting, drowsiness, confusion, seizures, vision changes, focal neurologic findings, and decreased level of consciousness. If left untreated, coma and death occur within hours.

15. Why is it important to understand cerebral autoregulation?

Cerebral autoregulation works only within a certain range of MAP; overtreating hypertensive emergencies can be just as damaging as not treating them at all. Cerebral blood flow (CBF) depends on cerebral perfusion pressure (CPP), the pressure gradient across the brain. CPP is the difference between MAP and ICP: CPP = MAP – ICP. To maintain CBF and CPP at relatively constant levels, cerebral arteries vasoconstrict when MAP increases and vasodilate when MAP decreases. Cerebral autoregulation maintains constant CBF between a MAP of 60 and 120 mmHg in normotensive individuals.

When MAP exceeds 160 mmHg or decreases to less 60 mmHg, autoregulation fails. In patients with chronic HTN, this lower limit is reset to a higher level than in normotensive individuals. If the goal of therapy is to reach a *normal* BP, this may lead to inadequate CBF and subsequent ischemia and infarction. When treating hypertensive emergencies, it is recommended that MAP not be lowered by more than 20–25% or that the DBP not be lowered to less than 110 mmHg over 30 minutes to 1 hour. Careful monitoring of therapy is essential to avoid precipitous drops in BP.

16. How do I treat a patient with hypertensive encephalopathy?

All patients with any form of hypertensive emergency should be on a monitor with supplemental oxygen and at minimum two peripheral intravenous lines. An arterial line for continuous BP monitoring is also essential. Several medications work well for treatment of hypertensive encephalopathy. They work by different mechanisms but have three important properties in common: (1) They are given as an intravenous drip, enabling easy titration; (2) they have rapid onset; and (3) they have a short duration of action. Traditionally the drug of choice has been nitroprusside, which has immediate onset of action and causes powerful vasodilation of the resistance and capacitance vessels. Nitroprusside is relatively contraindicated in pregnancy, can cause elevated ICP, has cyanide as an intermediate metabolite, and is a light-sensitive compound that must remain covered at all times by an opaque material. For equally effective treatment with potentially fewer limitations, consider fenoldopam mesylate, labetalol, or esmolol.

17. What other neurologic syndromes are associated with HTN?

Thromboembolic and hemorrhagic strokes are associated with HTN, but HTN is not the direct cause. When patients present to the ED, they may have an elevated BP. This is probably an adaptive response of the brain to try to maintain CPP and blood flow to the ischemic brain. Lowering or *normalizing* BP is potentially dangerous in patients with ischemic stroke and is not recommended. BP decreases gradually over the following 10 days in most patients. With hemorrhagic strokes and radiologic evidence of major intracranial bleeding, cautious lowering of BP is suggested if SBP is greater than 200 mmHg or DBP is greater than 120 mmHg. Rapid lowering of BP within the first 24 hours is associated with increased mortality. Potential treatment options include intravenous nitroprusside, labetalol, nicardipine, fenoldopam, or esmolol. Decision making should be done in close consultation with a neurologist or neurosurgeon.

18. How do I treat a patient with severe HTN and evidence of pulmonary edema?
Start with standard treatment for pulmonary edema: afterload reduction, nitrites, oxygen, and diuretics. If this is inadequate, add nitroprusside to decrease peripheral vascular resistance further.

19. How do I treat a patient with severe HTN and chest pain?
Acute ischemia of the left ventricle with associated chest pain often is accompanied by severe HTN. Reduction of peripheral vascular resistance is crucial and decreases the work of the myocardium, preventing ongoing ischemia. First-line treatment is intravenous nitroglycerin combined with intravenous labetalol or esmolol. If this fails to control BP, intravenous nicardipine or fenoldopam can be added. Nitroprusside had been advocated as second-line treatment, but more recently it was shown to cause a coronary-steal phenomenon in patients with coronary artery disease, causing increased mortality in the presence of an acute myocardial infarction.

20. Is ischemia the only cause of chest pain to worry about in a hypertensive patient?
No. Always think about the possibility of acute aortic dissection because this can be a rapidly fatal cause of chest pain. The goal of therapy is to lessen the pulsatile load and shear forces on the aorta. If this diagnosis is being strongly considered, therapy should be instituted immediately before doing any diagnostic study. Therapy should aim for rapid reduction of SBP to a range of 100 to 110 mmHg. A surgeon should be informed of the patient before definitive diagnosis because dissection of either the arch or the proximal portion of the aorta requires emergent surgical repair. Dissection of the descending aorta is managed medically. Traditional therapy has employed the intravenous nitroprusside, to decrease preload and afterload, and an intravenous β-blocker such as esmolol, which should be started first. This prevents the reflex tachycardia associated with nitroprusside and subsequent propagation of the dissection. Alternative treatment regimens include intravenous labetalol used as a single agent and intravenous nicardipine or fenoldopam in place of nitroprusside.

21. What are the agents of choice in a patient with severe HTN and acute renal failure?
Intravenous fenoldopam has been approved by the Food and Drug Administration for use in the United States for hypertensive emergencies and is a dopamine-1-receptor agonist. It is short acting and has advantages over traditional nitroprusside therapy in that it increases renal blood flow, creatinine clearance, sodium excretion, and diuresis. It has equivalent efficacy to nitroprusside in lowering BP and no reported adverse effects. Another reasonable alternative to traditional therapy with equal efficacy is nicardipine, an intravenous calcium channel blocker.

22. What must you always think about in a pregnant woman with severe HTN?
Preeclampsia. Definitive treatment requires delivery of the fetus and the placenta, but magnesium should be started immediately for seizure prophylaxis and to prevent evolution of preeclampsia to eclampsia. Hydralazine classically has been used for the treatment of HTN during pregnancy but can cause reflex tachycardia, often requires concomitant β-blockade, and does not enable easy titration. Patients with preeclampsia generally require ICU admission, and intravenous labetalol or nicardipine is preferred.

23. What is the current opinion on using oral agents to treat hypertensive emergencies?
Oral agents are acceptable for use in patients with hypertensive **urgencies** and no symptoms or evidence of end-organ damage. Treating hypertensive emergencies with oral agents is strongly

discouraged because they yield unpredictable responses, cannot be titrated, and cannot be discontinued immediately if the patient's BP drops to unsafe levels.

24. Is it ever necessary to treat a patient who has an elevated BP with no signs or symptoms of end-organ damage?
No. There are no data to support acutely lowering someone's BP in the ED if they have no signs or symptoms of end-organ damage. Instituting HTN therapy usually should be left to the primary care physician but can be initiated from the ED if the patient has a known history of elevated BP and has appropriate follow-up. If you choose to give an oral antihypertensive in the ED under the aforementioned circumstances, there is no need to monitor the patient until the BP comes down. The patient can be discharged safely without an observational period with appropriate follow-up for ongoing antihypertensive therapy.

25. Summarize common parenteral antihypertensive medications and their indications and contraindications.

DRUG	DOSAGE	ONSET OF ACTION	DURATION OF ACTION	INDICATIONS	CONTRAINDICATIONS
Nitroprusside	0.3–10 μg/kg/min IV	1–2 min	1–2 min	CHF, aortic dissection, catecholamine excess	Pregnancy, need for prolonged therapy in patients with hepatic/renal insufficiency
Nitroglycerin	10–100 μg/min IV	2–5 min	3–5 min	AMI, CHF	CVA, renal failure
Fenoldopam	0.1-1.7 μg/kg/min IV	5–15 min	1–4 h	CHF, renal insufficiency, sympathetic crisis, AMI, hypertensive encephalopathy, aortic dissection	Glaucoma because it increases intraocular pressure
Hydralazine	10–20 mg IV bolus; repeat q 4–6 h as needed (max 40 mg)	10–20 min	3–8 h	Eclampsia	AMI, aortic dissection, CVA
Nicardipine	5–15 mg/h IV drip	15 min	6 h	AMI, hypertensive encephalopathy, eclampsia, renal failure, sympathetic crisis	CHF, second- or third-degree AVB
Esmolol	500 μg/kg bolus over 1 min, then 50–300 μg/kg/min	1–2 min	10–20 min	CAD, aortic dissection	CHF, second- or third-degree AVB
Labetalol	20 mg IV bolus, then 40–80 mg q 10 min as needed to 300 mg or 2 mg/min IV	2–10 min	2–4 h	CAD, hypertensive encephalopathy, aortic dissection, eclampsia	CHF, second- or third-degree AVB, asthma

(Table continued on next page.)

DRUG	DOSAGE	ONSET OF ACTION	DURATION OF ACTION	INDICATIONS	CONTRAINDICATIONS
Phentolamine	5 mg IV, repeat as needed (max 20 mg)	1–2 min	10–30 min	Catecholamine excess	AMI

CHF, congestive heart failure; AMI, acute myocardial infarction; CVA, cerebrovascular accident; AVB, atrioventricular block; CAD, coronary artery disease.

BIBLIOGRAPHY

1. Bales A: Hypertensive crisis: How to tell if it's an emergency or an urgency. Postgrad Med 105:119–126, 1999.
2. Gray RO, Mathews JJ: Hypertension. In Marx JA, Hockberger RS, Walls RM (eds): Rosen's Emergency Medicine: Concepts and Clinical Practice, 5th ed. St. Louis, Mosby, 2002, pp 1158–1171.
3. Tumlin JA, Dunbar LM, Oparil S, et al: Fenoldopam, a dopamine agonist, for hypertensive emergency: A multicenter randomized trial. Acad Emerg Med 7:653–662, 2000.
4. Varon J, Marik PE: The diagnosis and management of hypertensive crises. Chest 118:214–227, 2000.
5. Vaughn CJ, Delanty N: Hypertensive emergencies. Lancet 356:411–417, 2000.
6. Vidt DG: Emergency room management of hypertensive urgencies and emergencies. J Clin Hypertens 3:158–164, 2001.

33. PERICARDITIS AND MYOCARDITIS

John L. Kendall, M.D., and Christopher B. Colwell, M.D.

PERICARDITIS

1. Describe a normal pericardium.
The pericardium is 1 to 2 mm thick and envelops the heart. It has two layers. Between the two layers is the pericardial space, which normally contains 25 to 50 mL of fluid.

2. What is pericarditis?
Inflammation of the pericardium.

3. What causes pericarditis?
Infectious agents, such as viruses and bacteria, can cause pericarditis as a result of direct spread of infections to the pericardium. Pericarditis also may be caused by the antibody-mediated autoimmune reaction that occurs 2 to 4 weeks after a viral illness. This postviral pericarditis, termed *idiopathic* because a viral source has not been isolated, is probably the most common form of pericarditis. An autoimmune reaction to cardiac antigens may occur after cardiac instrumentation or acute myocardial infarction (MI). The likelihood of postinfarction pericarditis is reduced by half (from approximately 12% to 6%) when a thrombolytic agent is used.

Causes of Pericarditis

Infection	Immunologically mediated diseases	Trauma
Viral	Postinfectious	Blunt
Coxsackie B	Postcardiac injury syndrome	Penetrating

(Table continued on next page.)

Causes of Pericarditis (cont.)

Infection (cont.)	Immunologically mediated diseases (cont.)	Drugs
Cytomegalovirus	Postpericardiotomy	Procainamide
Echovirus	Postinfarction (Dressler's syndrome)	Cromolyn sodium
HIV	Autoimmune disorders	Hydralazine
Bacterial	Acute rheumatic fever	**Uremia**
Tuberculosis	Rheumatoid arthritis	**Radiation**
Staphylococcus	Connective tissue diseases	**Neoplasm**
Fungal	Lupus erythematosus	
Parasitic		

4. Who is most susceptible to infectious pericarditis?

Viral and idiopathic pericarditis occur most commonly in healthy persons 20 to 40 years old. Bacterial pericarditis occurs in patients with a bacterial infection of the lungs, endocardium, or blood. Patients with HIV are susceptible to pericarditis caused by opportunistic infections.

5. Describe the clinical presentation of pericarditis.

The most common symptom is chest pain, described as midline and sharp. The pain is worse with movement and breathing, and relief is obtained from sitting up and leaning forward. It may radiate to the neck, back, or left shoulder. Dyspnea, malaise, and fever may occur. The pathognomonic clinical finding is a friction rub, which is a scratchy noise, similar to creaking leather. The optimal patient position for a rub to be auscultated is sitting up, leaning forward, and in full expiration. The diaphragm of the stethoscope should be pressed firmly to the chest at the lower left sternal border. A little luck is needed to detect a rub because it occurs intermittently.

6. How does the ECG appear in pericarditis?

The ECG typically evolves through four stages. **In stage 1,** The first hours to days of illness may show ST segment elevation and P-R segment depression in all leads except aVR and V_1, where reciprocal changes occur. **In stage 2,** the ST and P-R segments normalize, and the T waves flatten. **In stage 3,** deep T wave inversion occurs. **In stage 4,** the ECG reverts to normal. Occasionally, stage 4 does not occur, which results in permanent generalized or focal T wave inversions and flattenings. The ST segment displacement seen in stage 1 is attributed to the associated subepicardial myocarditis, whereas the P-R segment depression is attributed to subepicardial atrial injury.

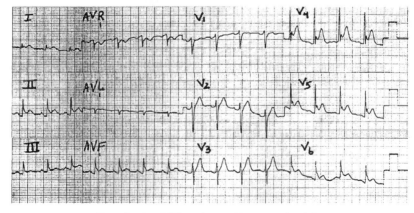

Example of an ECG consistent with acute pericarditis.

7. How can acute pericarditis be distinguished from acute MI?

ST segment elevations in stage 1 of acute pericarditis tend to be upwardly concave rather than convex, and simultaneous T wave inversions are not typically seen. The progression to T wave inversions in stage 2 tends to occur after the ST segments have returned to baseline, whereas in acute MI, the T wave inversion is more likely to accompany ST segment elevation. The ST segment elevations in acute pericarditis typically are diffuse as opposed to an anatomic distribution, which typically is seen in acute MI.

Clinically, patients with acute pericarditis are more likely to be younger, to be otherwise healthy, and to have a history of a preceding viral illness and pleuritic-type chest pain. Patients with acute MI are more likely to be older with risk factors for coronary disease. Ventricular arrhythmias are not associated with isolated pericardial disease and suggest the presence of underlying cardiac disease.

8. How can acute pericarditis be distinguished from musculoskeletal chest pain?

Musculoskeletal chest pain generally is not relieved by sitting up, and the characteristic friction rub and ECG abnormalities of pericarditis are not present.

9. Is pericardial effusion a concern in patients with pericarditis?

Yes. Pericardial effusion occurs most commonly in patients with acute viral or idiopathic, neoplastic, postradiation, or posttraumatic pericarditis. Its effects range from insignificant to life-threatening if tamponade occurs.

10. How much pericardial effusion is significant?

The answer depends entirely on the clinical situation. A patient with a stab wound to the heart may be able to accommodate only 80 to 200 mL of pericardial fluid before tamponade develops. Patients with long-standing pericardial fluid collections may tolerate 2000 mL without hemodynamic compromise.

11. How can a pericardial effusion be diagnosed?

The physical examination is unreliable in detecting or excluding a pericardial effusion. Similarly the cardiac silhouette is not enlarged on chest radiograph until at least 250 mL of fluid has accumulated. **Echocardiography** has excellent sensitivity and specificity; it can detect 15 mL of pericardial fluid.

12. What is cardiac tamponade?

Cardiac tamponade exists when excess pericardial fluid leads to increased pericardial pressure to the point that it prevents the atria and ventricles from filling adequately during diastole, decreasing the volume of blood available to be pumped during systole and causing hemodynamic compromise. Although any form of pericarditis may lead to cardiac tamponade, acute tamponade usually is caused by trauma. Subacute tamponade occurs most commonly in neoplastic pericarditis.

13. How is cardiac tamponade diagnosed?

The first step is to confirm the presence of a pericardial effusion by echocardiography. Absence of a pericardial effusion rules out cardiac tamponade. If an effusion is present, a combination of physical examination and echocardiographic findings can confirm of the diagnosis of tamponade. Physical examination findings suggestive of tamponade include tachycardia, hypotension, cyanosis, dyspnea, jugular venous distention, pulsus paradoxus, and elevated central venous pressure (> 15 mmHg). Echocardiographic findings are more specific, and they develop sequentially as pericardial pressure increases: right atrial collapse, right ventricular collapse, and bowing of the interventricular septum. Another helpful finding is to perform the *sniff test*. Instruct the patient to inhale quickly through the nose while the examiner visualizes the inferior vena cava. Incomplete collapse of the inferior vena cava correlates well with elevated central venous pressure measurements.

14. What is pulsus paradoxus?

An abnormally large (> 10 mmHg) drop in the systolic blood pressure with inspiration. Kussmaul termed this phenomenon *paradoxical* because of the disappearance of the pulse during inspiration when the heart was obviously beating. Pulsus paradoxus is a pulse, not a pressure, change and is an exaggeration of the normal inspiratory fall in arterial flow and systolic pressure. Inspiration favors right-sided heart filling by decreasing pericardial pressure, whereas expiration favors left-sided heart filling. Pulsus paradoxus usually signals large reductions in ventricular volumes and equilibration of mean pericardial and all cardiac diastolic pressures. The detection of pulsus paradoxus on physical examination suggests (and may be one of the earliest clues to) the existence of cardiac tamponade.

15. What is the appropriate ED management of pericarditis?

Antiinflammatory agents, such as indomethacin (Indocin), 25 to 75 mg four times a day; aspirin, 650 mg every 3 to 4 hours; or ibuprofen, 600 mg four times a day, should be administered. The use of corticosteroids is controversial. Although corticosteroids are effective antiinflammatory agents, 10% to 20% of patients develop recurrent pericarditis as tapering occurs. Echocardiography is indicated to rule out pericardial effusion. If cardiac tamponade is present, percutaneous pericardiocentesis must be done to relieve intracardiac pressure. Intravenous fluids should be infused rapidly to increase arterial pressure and cardiac output.

16. What is the prognosis for patients with pericarditis?

Most patients recover fully, although 15% to 20% have a recurrence, probably because of an autoimmune mechanism. Nonsteroidal antiinflammatory drugs are used for recurrences. If these agents are ineffective, corticosteroid therapy is initiated. Colchicine holds promise as an adjunctive therapy in recurrent pericarditis. If medical interventions fail, pericardiectomy usually is done.

MYOCARDITIS

17. What is myocarditis?

An inflammation of the myocardium in the absence of ischemia.

18. What causes myocarditis?

In the **United States**, myocarditis is caused most commonly by viruses. Enteroviruses, especially the coxsackie B virus, predominate as causative agents. Infectious agents cause myocardial damage by three basic mechanisms: (1) the direct invasion of the myocardium, (2) production of a myocardial toxin (e.g., diphtheria), or (3) immunologically mediated myocardial damage. The immunologically mediated destruction of cardiac tissue from infiltration of host cellular immune components is probably the more common mechanism in adults, whereas in neonates, damage from direct viral invasion is more likely.

Worldwide, Chagas' disease is the leading cause of myocarditis. Other organisms that are known to infiltrate the myocardium include influenza A and B, adenovirus, hepatitis A and B, tuberculosis, *Chlamydia pneumoniae*, *Borrelia burgdorferi* (Lyme disease), *Legionella pneumophila*, cytomegalovirus, *Toxoplasma gondii*, and *Trichinella spiralis*.

19. When should a diagnosis of myocarditis be considered in the ED?

Diagnosing myocarditis in the ED can be a challenge, and because the presenting symptoms and signs are typically nonspecific, this is often a diagnosis of exclusion. Nonspecific symptoms include fatigue, myalgias, dyspnea, palpitations, and precordial discomfort. Chest pain often reflects associated pericarditis. Patients may present with dilated cardiomyopathy without evidence of ischemia or valvular disease. Myocarditis probably should be considered in any previously healthy person who develops dyspnea, orthopnea, decreased exercise tolerance, palpitations, or syncope when no other obvious cause is found. Patients should be asked about concomitant or recent upper respiratory or gastrointestinal illness.

20. What clinical findings may be present?

Flulike complaints, such as fatigue, myalgias, nausea, vomiting, diarrhea, and fever, are usually the earliest symptoms and signs of myocarditis. Tachycardia is common and can be disproportionate to the temperature or apparent toxicity. This may be the only clue that something more serious than a simple viral illness exists. Clinical evidence of congestive heart failure occurs only in more severe cases. Typical findings in patients with congestive heart failure include tachypnea, rales, and pedal edema. A pericardial rub may be auscultated if myopericarditis is present. Complications of myocarditis include ventricular arrhythmias and left ventricular aneurysms.

21. Are there any chest radiograph or ECG abnormalities?

The **chest radiograph** may be abnormal, depending on the extent of disease. The cardiac silhouette may be enlarged, which can be due to a dilated cardiomyopathy or a pericardial effusion.

The **ECG** commonly shows a sinus tachycardia and low electrical activity. Nonspecific ST segment and T wave abnormalities, a prolonged corrected Q-T interval, atrioventricular block, or acute MI pattern also may occur. Atrial arrhythmias have been described.

22. How is myocarditis diagnosed?

Making the diagnosis clinically can be difficult. Endocardial biopsy currently is considered the gold standard, although it has highly variable sensitivity and specificity. In contrast to patients with pericarditis, cardiac enzymes frequently are elevated in patients with myocarditis. White blood cell count and erythrocyte sedimentation rate may be elevated but are nonspecific. Indium-111 antimyosin antibodies show myocardial necrosis by binding to exposed myosin in damaged myocardial cells. In situations in which myocarditis is suspected clinically, indium-111 antimyosin imaging may be helpful. Viral titers have been suggested but have a low yield. Echocardiography often shows global dysfunction that does not correspond to a specific coronary artery distribution.

23. How can acute myocarditis be distinguished from acute MI?

Myocarditis occurs primarily in young healthy patients without significant cardiac history or risk factors for coronary artery disease. Chest pain, dyspnea, ECG abnormalities, and cardiac enzyme elevation may occur in both conditions. In the ED, it may be impossible to distinguish between these two entities. Treatment for acute MI should be initiated.

24. Is myocarditis a concern in AIDS?

Yes. The incidence of myocarditis found at autopsy of AIDS patients has been reported as 52%, compared with almost 10% in the population as a whole. The increased risk of myocarditis in patients with AIDS may be due to an abnormal autoimmune reaction, opportunistic infections, or HIV itself.

25. Describe the appropriate ED management of a patient with myocarditis.

The current recommended treatment consists of supportive therapy. The only uniformly accepted beneficial therapy is bed rest. All patients with suspected myocarditis should be admitted to a monitored bed in the hospital. Dilated cardiomyopathy is treated with diuresis, afterload reduction, and digoxin. In severe cases, temporary pacing and external circulatory support may be needed. Patients with a fulminant clinical course may require cardiac transplantation. Immunosuppressive therapy has been studied, but controlled studies have not established efficacy. High-dose gamma globulin has been studied and may be associated with improved left ventricular function and better survival during the first year after initial presentation.

26. What is the prognosis for patients with acute myocarditis?

Mortality for patients with myocarditis has been reported to be 20% at 1 year and 56% at 4 years, although many patients do recover completely.

BIBLIOGRAPHY

1. Brown CA, O'Connell JB: Myocarditis and idiopathic dilated cardiomyopathy. Am J Med 99:309–314, 1995.
2. Jouriles NJ: Pericardial and myocardial disease. In Marx JA (ed): Rosen's Emergency Medicine: Concepts and Clinical Practice, 5th ed. St. Louis, Mosby, 2002, pp 1130–1149.
3. Liu P, Martino T, Opavsky MA, Penninger J: Viral myocarditis: Balance between viral infection and immune response. Can J Cardiol 12:935–943, 1996.
4. McCarthy RE 3rd, Bochmer JP, Hruban RH, et al: Long-term outcome of fulminant myocarditis as compared with acute (non-fulminant) myocarditis. N Engl J Med 342:690–695, 2000.
5. Spodick DH: Mechanisms of acute pericardial and myocardial injury in pericardial disease. Chest 13:855–856, 1998.
6. Spodich DH: Pericardial diseases. In Braunwald E, Zipes DP, Libby P (eds): Heart Disease: A Textbook of Cardiovascular Medicine, 6th ed. Philadelphia, W.B. Saunders, 2001, pp 1823–1876.
7. Wynne J, Braunwald E: The cardiomyopathies and myocarditides. In Braunwald E, Zipes DP, Libby P (eds): Heart Disease: A Textbook of Cardiovascular Medicine, 6th ed. Philadelphia, W.B. Saunders, 2001, pp 1783–1806.

34. AORTIC ANEURYSMS AND AORTIC DISSECTION

Thomas R. Drake, M.D.

1. Are aortic dissections and aortic aneurysms the same disease?

No. The processes occurring in the two diseases are different. Aortic dissection by definition involves intimal separation with formation of a pseudoaneurysm. A true aneurysm involves dilation of all layers of the arterial wall.

2. What are the risk factors for aortic aneurysms?

Hypertension is the most important predisposing factor for the development of aortic dissection. Atherosclerosis, diabetes, hyperlipidemia, smoking, hypertension, genetic predisposition, and, more rarely, congenital defects are major predisposing factors. Other rare causes are syphilis, other infections, and aortitis. Men are 10 times more likely to develop an aneurysm than women.

3. Describe the typical patient with an abdominal aneurysm.

An elderly man who has had manifestations of atherosclerosis, such as coronary artery disease or peripheral vascular disease.

4. What are the usual presenting signs and symptoms of abdominal aortic aneurysms?

Aortic aneurysms often may be found fortuitously on routine physical examination or through radiologic studies ordered for other reasons. The most common symptom with an acutely expanding or leaking aneurysm is constant **abdominal pain**, often localizing to the left middle or lower quadrant with radiation to the back. Depending on the degree of blood loss, the patient may have variable signs or hypovolemia, such as hypotension, syncope, or falling hematocrit.

5. Which studies should be ordered if an abdominal aneurysm is suspected?

No further studies should be done in an unstable patient who has the clinical picture of a leaking aneurysm if performing the study delays operative intervention. If the patient is hemodynamically stable, the best screening examination is an ultrasound, which may be done quickly in the ED, where constant supervision of the patient is possible. If the aorta is normal, other potential conditions can be evaluated, such as biliary colic, nephrolithiasis, or pancreatitis. Disadvantages include potential obscuring of the aorta by bowel gas and the lack of demonstration of extravasation. CT is also an excellent way of visualizing the abdominal aorta and presence of retroperitoneal or free peritoneal blood. CT is time-consuming, however, and requires moving the patient from the ED in most institutions. Angiography, considered by many to be the gold standard for evaluation of the aorta, gives excellent anatomic evaluation of the aorta and its branches but is invasive and time-consuming. The study chosen most often is determined by judging the stability of the patient in relation to the specific anatomic questions to be answered.

6. What are the common reasons for missing the diagnosis of aortic aneurysm or aortic dissection?

Although physical examination is the best way of identifying an abdominal aneurysm (palpation possible in 80% to 90%), it may be difficult in the obese patient. Other more common and benign diagnoses that aortic aneurysm may mimic include pancreatitis, renal colic, biliary disease, and musculoskeletal back pain. Aneurysms may present atypically as gastrointestinal bleeding from a fistulous connection of the aorta with the small bowel. This presentation most commonly occurs in patients with previous aortic surgery. A large aneurysm may cause unusual symptoms related to mass effect, such as bowel or ureteral obstruction. Radicular pain may occur if retroperitoneal bleeding causes a femoral or sciatic neuropathy. Peripheral embolization of mural plaque may cause peripheral ischemia as a presenting symptom. Patients may present with episodic pain that is caused either by the dissection or by expansion. If the patient is in a pain-free period, the conditions can be missed because of the benign appearance of the patient. An abrupt episode of severe atraumatic back, chest, or abdominal pain should be considered a worrisome symptom.

7. List the most common mistakes in the management of ruptured abdominal aneurysms in the ED.

1. Ascribing a patient's symptoms to a more benign condition.
2. Underaggressive fluid or blood volume resuscitation because of concerns about the patient's age or cardiac status.
3. Delaying operative intervention while waiting for diagnostic studies.
4. Allowing hypothermia to occur from use of cold fluids and blood products. This causes many problems, most notably a significant coagulopathy.

8. Is the lateral abdominal radiograph useful?

It may be useful if the aorta is calcified. A nonvisualized aorta has no diagnostic use.

9. What is the natural history of true aneurysms of the aorta?

Although smaller aneurysms fare better than larger ones, the natural history of this disease is progressive expansion and eventual rupture. The 1-year mortality rate of patients with initially asymptomatic abdominal aneurysm is about 50%. The elective operative mortality is 6% or less. The operative mortality for a ruptured abdominal aneurysm is approximately 50%.

10. Do thoracic aortic dissections present in a different fashion?

Yes. Thoracic aortic dissections most commonly involve the proximal aorta and are more likely to cause chest and thoracic back pain that is typically excruciating. The patient usually looks acutely ill, requires large doses of narcotics to relieve pain, and is likely to be significantly hypertensive. Myocardial infarction may be present if the dissecting process involves the coronary arteries. A classic presentation is that of an elderly man with severe chest or back pain with the appearance of an acutely ill patient having a myocardial infarction, but in whom the ECG is normal or has nonspecific findings.

11. Do all patients present with pain?

No. About 5% to 10% of patients with aortic dissection do not have pain as a major complaint. Aortic dissection may be painless in a few patients or, because of involvement of the carotids, may cause a stroke and render the patient incapable of communicating the pain. Unusual manifestations of dissection may relate to the process of involving almost any peripheral artery. The patient may present with abdominal pain from mesenteric artery involvement, with renal failure from renal artery obstruction, or with peripheral ischemia of an arm or leg. Rupture of a bronchial artery may cause hemoptysis, or hoarseness may result from compression of the recurrent laryngeal nerve. Other mass effects may cause dysphagia or a chronic cough. Congestive heart failure may be caused by involvement of the aortic valve. Syncope and pericardial tamponade may be caused by rupture into the pericardial space.

12. What diagnostic studies prove thoracic aortic dissection?

The most important diagnostic steps in the evaluation of suspected aortic dissection are:
- Confirmation of the diagnosis
- Differentiation of type A from type B (descending aorta) dissection because of different surgical approaches to the corrective procedure (ascending aorta and aortic arch)
- Determination of involvement of the aortic valve or other vascular structures

Plain radiographs are abnormal in about 80% of patients. The chest film may show dilation of the ascending aorta, mediastinal widening, loss of the aortic knob, left pleural effusion, deviation of the trachea or nasogastric tube, apical *pleural capping*, or displacement of intimal calcium in the aorta. These signs are mostly indirect evidence and require confirmation by a more definitive study. The clinical suspicion of aortic dissection should not be altered by a lack of findings on the plain chest radiograph. CT, MRI, and transesophageal echocardiography are used successfully in the evaluation of aortic dissection. Each modality has its limitations, however. MRI is highly sensitive and specific for the detection of dissection, but visualization of entry and exit points is difficult. It requires long evaluation times, limits access to the patient, and has limited availability in many institutions. Transesophageal echocardiography, done by placing the ultrasound transducer in the esophagus, can provide an excellent view of the aorta and heart. It also can assist in the evaluation by determining involvement of the aortic valve and coronary arteries and by detecting pericardial effusion or tamponade. It is highly user dependent and invasive, however, and it causes an undesirable hypertensive response in inadequately sedated patients. Also, availability is limited in many facilities. CT is readily available, relatively operator independent, and highly accurate in the evaluation of suspected dissection. Spiral CT has advantages over incremental CT, including short examination times, less motion artifact, and the ability to evaluate other vascular structures. Ultimately the study used depends on availability, stability of the patient, and specific anatomic questions to be answered in any particular situation. Angiography may have a role in selected instances but is no longer the diagnostic method of choice.

13. What is the optimal ED treatment of aortic dissection?

Presumptive treatment of aortic dissection, which should be started before specific radiologic confirmation, includes aggressive control of blood pressure and pulse with nitroprusside and β-blockers. Some authorities recommend using esmolol, a short-acting, intravenous β-blocker, because of its titratability. Narcotics should be used to relieve pain, but the goal of blood pressure and pulse control is to relieve pain by aborting or retarding the dissecting process.

14. Do all thoracic dissections require surgery?

Indications for surgery include all dissections involving the ascending aorta or aortic valve, rupture, enlargement, end-organ ischemia, or progression despite medical therapy. Type B dissections that are controlled with blood pressure and heart rate reductions that do not show distal vascular compromise may be treated medically. Patients who are poor surgical candidates often are treated medically, albeit with a high mortality. The perioperative mortality for patients older than 80 with type A dissection is exceedingly high, and some suggest that these patients are not appropriate candidates for surgery.

15. Are there any therapeutic options now available for patients with acute aneurysms and dissection who are not surgical candidates?

Yes. New, less invasive endovascular procedures have been developed to treat aortic aneurysms. A self-expanding stent graft is placed through a distant arterial access site to support the aortic wall and prevent rupture. Initial series are encouraging, and this technique holds great promise for future treatment of this disease.

BIBLIOGRAPHY

1. Grabenwoger M, Hutschala D, Ehrlich MP, et al: Thoracic aortic aneurysms: Treatment with endovascular self-expandable stent grafts. Ann Thorac Surg 69:445, 2000.
2. Hagan PG, Nienabe CA, Isselbacher EM, et al: The International Registry of Acute Aortic Dissection (IRAD): New insight into an old disease. JAMA 283:897–903, 2000.
3. Jehle D, Davis E, Evans T, et al: Emergency department sonography by emergency physicians. Am J Emerg Med 7:605–611, 1989.
4. Kronzon I, Demopoulos L, Schrem SS, et al: Pitfalls in the diagnosis of thoracic aortic aneurysm by transesophageal echocardiography. J Am Soc Echocardiogr 3:145–148, 1990.
5. Pierce GE (ed): Abdominal aortic aneurysms. Surg Clin North Am vol 69, 1989.
6. Slonim SM, Nyman U, Semba CP, et al: Aortic dissection: Percutaneous management of ischemic complications with endovascular stents and balloon fenestration. J Vasc Surg 23:241–253, 1996.
7. Sommer T, Fehske W, Holzknecht N, et al: Aortic dissection: A comparative study of diagnosis with spiral CT, multiplanar transesophageal echocardiography, and MR imaging. Radiology 199:347–352, 1996.
8. Swinton NW, Jewell ER, Tsapatsaris NP: Abdominal aortic aneurysms. Cardiol Clin 9:433–438, 1991.
9. Taams M, Gissemjpvem WK, Schippers LA, et al: The value of transesophageal echocardiography for diagnosis of thoracic aorta pathology. Eur Heart J 9:1308–1316, 1988.

35. CARDIAC PACEMAKERS AND AUTOMATIC IMPLANTABLE CARDIOVERTER DEFIBRILLATORS

Shamai A Grossman, M.D., M.S.

1. What is a pacemaker?

An external source of energy used to stimulate the heart. It consists of a pulse generator (i.e., power source), an output circuit, a sensing circuit, a timing circuit, and pacing leads. The battery most commonly used in permanent pacers is a lithium-iodide type and has a life span of 5 to 8 years. Temporary pacemakers use an external generator with transvenous, transcutaneous, or transthoracic leads. Temporary transvenous pacers use a household 9-volt battery.

2. What are the indications for temporary pacemakers?

Most hospital and prehospital studies report no long-term survivors from asystole using external pacing. Hemodynamically unstable bradycardias have 50% to 100% survival-to-discharge rates. Pacemakers also can be used for overdrive pacing in an attempt to terminate ventricular tachycardia by placing a ventricular extrasystole during the vulnerable period of the cardiac cycle. Temporary emergency pacing is indicated for therapy of significant and hemodynamically unstable bradyarrhythmias and prevention of bradycardia-dependent malignant arrhythmias Prophylactic temporary pacing is indicated for insertion of a pulmonary artery catheter in a patient with an underlying left bundle-branch block or use of medications that may cause or exacerbate hemodynamically significant bradycardia.

3. Pacemakers are indicated for what specific arrhythmias?

Sinus node dysfunction
    Symptomatic sinus bradycardia
    Sinus pauses > 3 sec
Atrioventricular (AV) nodal block
    Symptomatic second-degree AV block
      (Mobitz I)
    Symptomatic complete heart block
AV, atrioventricular.

Infranodal block
    New bifascicular block associated
      with acute myocardial infarction
    Alternating bundle-branch block
      with changing P-R interval
    Second-degree AV block (Mobitz II)
    Complete heart block

4. Where are external/transcutaneous pacemakers placed, and how are they operated?

Pacing pads and monitor leads are placed preferably in the midanterior chest and just below the left scapula. The desired heart rate is chosen, and the current is set to 0 mA. The external pacemaker is turned on, and the current is increased as tolerated until capture is achieved.

5. State the limiting factors in the use of external pacemakers.

Skeletal muscle contraction can be uncomfortable and often limits use of external pacemakers. Placing electrodes over areas of least skeletal muscle may minimize the discomfort. The physician should use the lowest effective current. Sedation should be considered if these measures are inadequate.

6. What are the complications of long-term external cardiac pacing?

Continued patient discomfort is the only significant problem because no enzymatic, electrocardiographic, or microscopic evidence of myocardial damage has been found after pacing for 60 minutes.

7. Can an external pacemaker be used if a permanent pacemaker malfunctions?

Yes, but be careful to place the external pacer on a *pace only* (fixed-rate) mode and not the sensing mode; otherwise, it may sense spikes from the permanent pacemaker and not fire.

8. What are the advantages of transvenous versus transcutaneous pacemakers?

Transcutaneous leads are the easiest to use for rapid initiation of temporary pacing. Transvenous leads are the more reliable and more comfortable because external pacing requires 30 to 100 times the current needed for internal transvenous pacing.

9. How are transvenous and transthoracic pacemakers placed?

Semifloating or flexible balloon-tipped catheters can be placed with central venous access into the subclavian or internal jugular veins. In the ED, using ECG guidance, an alligator clip is connected to a precordial lead such as V1 with another clip attached to the pacing wire. When a current of injury (ST elevation) is seen on the monitor, the wire should be withdrawn slightly, leaving it in pacing position. If available, fluoroscopy is preferred to ensure proper placement. Transthoracic catheters are inserted directly into the right ventricle through a left parasternal or subxiphoid approach and can be used in a cardiac arrest situation. This procedure, generally reserved for cardiac arrest, has many complications and rarely produces effective mechanical cardiac contraction.

10. Can CPR be performed with a pacemaker?

CPR can be performed safely with the external pacing pads in place. Turning the external pacemaker off during CPR is advisable, in particular when defibrillating or cardioverting a patient. Defibrillator paddles should be placed at least 2 to 3 cm away from pacing pads to prevent arching of current.

11. List the indications for a permanent pacemaker.

Absolute indications:

Sick sinus syndrome

Symptomatic sinus bradycardia

Tachycardia-bradycardia syndrome

Atrial fibrillation with a slow ventricular response

Complete heart block

Chronotropic incompetence (inability to increase the heart rate to match a level of exercise)

Long Q-T syndrome

Relative indications:

Cardiomyopathies (hypertrophic or dilated)

Severe refractory neurocardiogenic syncope

Paroxysmal atrial fibrillation

12. Describe the complications of permanent pacemaker implantation.

Routine placement of a pacemaker generator into a subcutaneous or submuscular pocket carries the risk of pocket hematoma, which if large enough to palpate often needs surgical drainage. Pocket infection, manifest as local inflammation, fluctuance, and abscess formation or local cellulitis, is common. Rarely the pocket itself may erode with extrusion of the generator, secondary to infection, trauma, or local tissue ischemia. Infection usually is caused by *Staphylococcus aureus* acutely and *Staphylococcus epidermidis* in chronic infections. Treatment is empirical antibiotics and ultimately removal of the device and reimplantation at a remote site. Wound dehiscence may require admission for débridement and reapproximation of wound edges.

13. What are the complications of lead placement?

Placement of transvenous leads can lead to pneumothorax or hemothorax, venous thrombosis, or lead infection. Thrombosis may occur at the lead implant, the tricuspid valve, or the subclavian vein and may cause superior vena cava syndrome.

14. What does a pacer setting of *DDD* mean?

The letters represent a pacing code. The code consists of three to five letters that describe the different types of pacer function. The first letter indicates the chamber paced, the second indicates the chamber in which electrical activity is sensed, and the third indicates the response to a sensed event. A fourth and fifth letter may be added to describe whether the pacemaker is programmable and whether special functions to protect against tachycardia are available. A DDD pacer is able to pace and sense atria and ventricles ([D]ual chambers) and has a (D)ual response to the sensed ventricular and atrial activity (i.e., can pace either the atrium or the ventricle). Spontaneous atrial and ventricular activity inhibits atrial and ventricular pacing; atrial activity without ventricular activity triggers only ventricular pacing.

Pacing Code

FIRST LETTER: CHAMBER PACED TO A SENSED EVENT	SECOND LETTER: CHAMBER SENSED	THIRD LETTER: RESPONSE
A(trial)	A(trial)	O (no response)
V(entricle)	V(entricle)	I(nhibition)
D(ual chamber)	D(ual chamber)	T(riggering)
		D(ual response)

15. How can the type of permanent pacemaker be identified in the ED?

Patients should carry a card with them providing information about their particular model. Most pacemaker generators have an x-ray code that can be seen on a standard chest radiograph.

The markings, along with the shape of the generator, may assist with determining the manufacturer of the generator and pacemaker battery.

16. What are the complications of permanent pacemakers?

Pacemaker complications include oversensing, undersensing, operative failures, and failure to capture. **Oversensing** occurs when a pacer incorrectly senses electrical activity and is inhibited from correctly pacing. This may be due to muscular activity, particularly oversensing of the diaphragm or pectoralis muscles; electromagnetic interference; or lead insulation breakage. **Undersensing** occurs when a pacer incorrectly misses intrinsic depolarization and paces despite intrinsic activity. This may be due to poor lead positioning, lead dislodgment, magnet application, low battery states, or myocardial infarction. **Operative failures** include malfunction resulting from mechanical factors, such as pneumothorax, pericarditis, infection, skin erosion, hematoma, lead dislodgment, and venous thrombosis. **Failure to capture** occurs when a pacing spike is not followed by either an atrial or a ventricular complex. This may be due to lead fracture, lead dislodgment, a break in lead insulation, an elevated pacing threshold, myocardial infarction at the lead tip, drugs, metabolic abnormalities, cardiac perforation, poor lead connection at the takeoff from the generator, and improper amplitude or pulse width settings.

17. What is the most common cause of permanent pacemaker malfunction?

Today, most pacemaker failures are the result of problems with the electrodes or the wires, not the battery or the pulse generator. Because of greater technologic sophistication, patients with pacemaker problems present to the ED much less commonly now than in the past.

18. What is pacemaker syndrome?

A clinical spectrum of lightheadedness, fatigue, palpitations, syncope, dyspnea on exertion, and hypotension that usually is attributed to asynchronous atrioventricular contraction and loss of atrial functional support.

19. Name the most common reason for early pacemaker malfunction.

Lead dislodgment.

20. How do I assess a patient with potential pacemaker malfunction?

1. Take a focused history on symptoms related to pacemaker malfunction, including palpitations, weakness, fatigue, shortness of breath, hiccups, syncope, or pain or erythema at the generator site.

2. The physician examination should focus on vital signs, mental status, cardiovascular system, and inspection of the generator site.

3. An ECG should be obtained to evaluate pacemaker function, and anteroposterior and lateral chest radiographs should be obtained to check pacemaker lead placement and lead and connector integrity.

21. What is *twiddler's syndrome*?

The most common cause of late lead dislodgment. It results from the twisting or *twiddling* of a pulse generator in its pouch to the point of twisting leads around the generator box, shortening and dislodging them from their proper position. The pulse generator may erode through the skin.

22. What is pacemaker-mediated tachycardia?

A normally functioning pacemaker may initiate a tachyarrhythmia. Retrograde conduction of a ventricular beat may cause the atrium to trigger a second ventricular contraction that falls during the pacemaker's refractory period. Because this contraction is not sensed by the pacemaker, the pulse generator fires, initiating a reentrant tachycardia.

23. How is pacemaker-mediated tachycardia treated?

Treatment consists of lengthening the atrioventricular time by any of the following methods:
1. Programming an increase in the atrial refractory time
2. Administering adenosine or verapamil
3. Increasing atrial sensory threshold
4. Applying a magnet to stop atrial sensing by the pacemaker

24. What is a runaway pacemaker?

Malfunction of the pacemaker that is manifested by tachycardias secondary to rapid ventricular pacing. The problem is recognized when rates are greater than the upper rate limit settings of the pacemaker and may require drastic measures, such as cutting the pacer leads.

25. What happens as pacemakers lose battery power?

Pacemakers usually show a decline in the rate of magnet-mediated pacing, usually to a predetermined manufacturer's rate. Pacer response varies with manufacturer; some models may change pacer mode also (e.g., DDD to VVI).

26. What is the most reliable indicator of pacer malfunction?

Rates that are usually inappropriate for paced hearts. A nonpaced ventricular rate less than 60 beats/min or a paced rate greater than 100 beats/min is probably secondary to pacemaker malfunction.

27. What does a magnet do?

Placing a pacemaker magnet over the pulse generator stops the pacemaker from sensing or responding to a sensed event. The pacemaker reverts to one of three fixed rate modes: the AOO (atrium paced), the VOO (ventricle paced), or the DOO (atrium and ventricle paced) mode. The purpose is to check the pacing rate, which should be done quickly because the pulse generator no longer is prevented from firing during the T wave or from inhibiting serious arrhythmias.

28. Can a patient with a permanent pacemaker be defibrillated?

Yes, but it is important to place the paddles away from the pulse generator, preferably in the anteroposterior position.

29. Can defibrillation damage the pulse generator when current passes through?

Yes. Temporary and even permanent loss of ventricular or atrial capture may occur secondary to elevation of the capture threshold of the pacer leads.

30. What is an AICD?

An **automatic implantable cardioverter defibrillator (AICD)** is a specialized device designed to treat a cardiac tachyarrhythmia. If the device senses a ventricular rate that exceeds the programmed cutoff rate of the implantable cardioverter defibrillator, the device performs cardioversion/defibrillation. Alternatively the device may attempt to pace rapidly for a number of pulses, usually around 10, to attempt pace termination of the ventricular tachycardia. Newer AICDs are a combination of implantable cardioverter defibrillator and pacemaker in one unit.

31. Discuss complications associated with an AICD.

AICD complications include operative failures, sensing or pacing failures, inappropriate cardioversion, ineffective cardioversion/defibrillation, and device deactivation. Operative failures and sensing problems are similar to those found in regular pacemakers. An example of appropriate failure to treat is when a device is set at 180 beats/min, and ventricular tachycardia occurs at 160 beats/min, the device fails to cardiovert the patient because the rate of the arrhythmia is below the programmed rate. Inappropriate cardioversion may occur if a patient presents in atrial fibrillation or has received multiple shocks in rapid succession. If a patient develops atrial fibrillation with a ventricular response of greater than 180 beats/min, and the device is set at 160 beats/min, the device delivers therapy. Ineffective cardioversion may be seen because of T wave oversensing, lead fracture, lead insulation breakage, electrocautery, MRI, and electromagnetic interference. Failure to deliver cardioversion is caused by failure to sense, lead fracture, electromagnetic interference, and inadvertent AICD deactivation. Ineffective cardioversion may be due to inadequate energy output, rise in the defibrillation threshold secondary to antiarrhythmic medications, myocardial infarction at the lead site, lead fracture, insulation breakage, or dislodgment of the leads of cardioversion patches.

32. Name the most frequent complication associated with AICDs.
Inappropriate cardioversion.

33. What will a magnet do when placed over an AICD?
Use of a magnet over the AICD inhibits further shocks, but it does not inhibit bradycardiac pacing should the patient require it. In older devices, application of a magnet produces a beep for each QRS complex. If the magnet is left on for 30 seconds, the AICD is disabled, and a continuous tone is produced. To reactivate the device, the magnet is removed and replaced. After 30 seconds, a beep returns for every QRS complex.

BIBLIOGRAPHY

1. Bocka JJ: External transcutaneous pacemakers. Ann Emerg Med 18:1280–1286, 1989.
2. Cardall TY, Chan TC, Brady WJ, et al: Permanent cardiac pacemakers: Issues relevant to the emergency physician: Part I. J Emerg Med 17:479–489, 1999.
3. Cardall TY, Brady WJ, Chan TC, et al: Permanent cardiac pacemakers: Issues relevant to the emergency physician: Part II. J Emerg Med 17:697–709, 1999.
4. Ellenbogen KA: Clinical Cardiac Pacing. Philadelphia, W.B. Saunders, 1995.
5. Garson A Jr: Stepwise approach to the unknown pacemaker ECG. Am Heart J 119:924–941, 1990.
6. Gillis AM: The current status of the implantable cardioverter defibrillator. Annu Rev Med 47:85–93, 1996.
7. Glikson M, Hayes DL: Cardiac pacing: A review. Med Clin North Am 85:369–421, 2001.
8. Hayes DL: Evolving indications for permanent pacing. Am J Cardiol 83:161D–165D, 1999.
9. Higgins GL 3rd: The automatic implantable cardioverter-defibrillator: Management issues relevant to the emergency care provider. Am J Emerg Med 8:342–347, 1990.
10. McComb JM, Gribbin GM: Effect of pacing mode on morbidity and mortality: Update of clinical pacing trials. Am J Cardiol 83:211D–213D, 1999.
11. Sarko JA, Tiffany BR: Cardiac pacemakers: Evaluation and management of malfunctions. Am J Emerg Med 18:435–440, 2000.

VII. Gastrointestinal Tract

36. ESOPHAGUS AND STOMACH DISORDERS

Philip L. Henneman, M.D.

1. How are gastrointestinal (GI) problems differentiated from acute myocardial infarction?

Esophageal or gastric pain can present with visceral-type chest pain or upper abdominal pain and nausea that are difficult to differentiate from pain and nausea related to myocardial ischemia or infarction. Description of the pain, determination of cardiac risk factors, and appropriate use of an ECG in adult patients with visceral-type pain or cardiac risk factors minimize clinical errors. Nitroglycerin, antacids, and GI cocktails are therapeutic interventions, not diagnostic tests. Patients with esophageal spasm may respond to nitroglycerin and antacids, or GI cocktails may provide a placebo-like benefit to patients with cardiac ischemia.

2. What is a GI cocktail?

The two most commonly used GI cocktails contain antacids (30 mL), viscous lidocaine (10 mL), and either Donnatal (10 mL) or dicyclomine (Bentyl) (20 mg). These cocktails may provide temporary symptomatic relief of minor esophageal and gastric irritation.

3. What is heartburn?

Retrosternal burning discomfort that may radiate to the sides of the chest, neck, or jaw. The description of the pain may be similar to the pain of cardiac ischemia. Heartburn is characteristic of reflux esophagitis and often is made worse by bending forward or lying recumbent or after meals. It may be relieved by upright posture, liquids (including saliva or water), or, more reliably, antacids. Heartburn is probably due to heightened mucosal sensitivity and can be reproduced by infusion of dilute hydrochloric acid (Bernstein test) into the esophagus.

4. How is reflux esophagitis treated?

In addition to antacids, general measures include elevation of the head of the bed (e.g., 4 inches), weight reduction, and elimination of factors that increase abdominal pressure. Patients should avoid alcohol, chocolate, coffee, fatty foods, mint, orange juice, smoking, ingestion of large quantities of food and drink, and certain medications (e.g., anticholinergics or calcium channel blockers). Antacids after meals and H_2-blockers (e.g., cimetidine) before bedtime are often helpful. Resistant cases may respond to sucralfate before meals and metoclopramide (10 mg four times daily). Treatment may need to be continued for 6 months, and the disease may recur quickly.

5. What are the esophageal causes of odynophagia?

Odynophagia, or painful swallowing, is a characteristic of nonreflux esophagitis. Infectious esophagitis is a common cause and usually occurs in immunocompromised patients and can be due to fungal (e.g., monilial), viral (e.g., herpes, cytomegalovirus), bacterial (e.g., lactobacillus, β-hemolytic streptococci), or parasitic organisms. Other types of nonreflux esophagitis include radiation, corrosive, pill-induced, and certain systemic diseases (e.g., Behçet's, Crohn's, pemphigus vulgaris, Stevens-Johnson syndrome). Odynophagia is unusual in reflux esophagitis but may occur with a peptic ulcer of the esophagus (Barrett's ulcer).

6. How does esophageal obstruction present?

Except in infants, there is usually a history of eating or swallowing something that is followed by the onset of chest pain, odynophagia, or inability to swallow. Foreign bodies usually lodge at one of four locations: cervical esophagus, upper esophageal sphincter, aortic arch, and lower esophageal sphincter. Obstruction by food may occur wherever there is narrowing of the lumen because of stricture, carcinoma, or a lower esophageal ring. Round, blunt objects may be removed using a Foley catheter that is inserted beyond the object; the balloon is inflated, then the catheter is withdrawn gently with the patient in a steep head-down position. This procedure most often is done under fluoroscopy. Foreign bodies, especially those that are sharp (e.g., needle); impacted food; or objects that cannot be removed with the Foley method are best removed endoscopically. Meat tenderizer should not be used to facilitate passage of obstructed meat. Glucagon (0.5 to 2 mg intravenously) may relieve distal esophageal food obstruction in about one third of patients.

7. What is Mallory-Weiss syndrome?

A mucosal tear that usually involves the gastric mucosa near the squamocolumnar mucosal junction; it also may involve the esophageal mucosa. It usually is caused by vomiting and retching. Patients may present with upper GI bleeding.

8. What causes esophageal perforation, and how is it diagnosed and treated?

Esophageal perforation, a true emergency, can be caused by iatrogenic damage during instrumentation, trauma (most often penetrating), increased intraesophageal pressure associated with forceful vomiting (Boerhaave's syndrome), or diseases of the esophagus (e.g., corrosive esophagitis, ulceration, neoplasm). Esophageal perforation causes chest pain that is often severe and may be worsened by swallowing and breathing. Chest radiograph may reveal air within the mediastinum, pericardium, pleural space (pneumothorax), or subcutaneous tissue. Esophageal perforation may lead to leakage of gastric contents into the mediastinum and secondary infection (i.e., mediastinitis). The diagnosis is confirmed by swallow and leakage of radiopaque contrast material. Treatment includes broad-spectrum antibiotics, gastric suction, and surgical repair and drainage as soon as possible.

9. What are causes of abdominal pain that are gastric or duodenal in origin?

An estimated 10% of cases of abdominal pain seen in the ED are due to gastric or duodenal disease. Gastritis and peptic ulcer disease (PUD) (i.e., ulcer of the stomach or duodenum owing to gastric acid) account for most patients with abdominal pain secondary to gastric or duodenal disease. Perforated PUD and gastric volvulus are the two most serious conditions requiring immediate diagnosis and treatment.

10. What are the common causes of gastritis and PUD?

Gastritis is associated with alcohol, salicylates, nonsteroidal antiinflammatory drugs (NSAIDs), and hiatal hernia. PUD is related to family history, associated disease (e.g., chronic obstructive pulmonary disease [COPD], cirrhosis, chronic renal failure), male gender, advanced age, and smoking. The use of certain drugs, such as aspirin or NSAIDs, and the psychological profile may be related to PUD, but diet (e.g., caffeine and spicy foods) and alcohol are not. *Helicobacter pylori* has been shown to be the probable cause of many duodenal ulcers.

11. How does perforated PUD present?

Perforated PUD (and gastric volvulus) presents with sudden onset of abdominal pain that may or may not be related to eating. The pain is usually steady and refractory to antacids; it often radiates to the back but also may radiate to the chest or upper abdomen. Vomiting is present in approximately 50%.

On **physical examination**, patients appear in acute distress and often have tachycardia. Blood pressure may be elevated secondary to pain or decreased secondary to extensive fluid loss from generalized peritonitis. Patients usually lie still and avoid movement. Involuntary guarding, rebound tenderness, and abdominal rigidity are common. Bowel sounds are usually absent or significantly decreased.

Laboratory work may reveal nonspecific leukocytosis (40% have a white blood cell count > 14,000 per mm^3). If vomiting has been significant, hypochloremic, hypokalemic, metabolic alkalosis may be seen. A small percentage of patients have mild elevation in amylase or lipase. Free air is present on upright chest radiograph or abdominal left lateral decubitus view in more than 70% of patients.

12. How should a patient suspected of having a perforated ulcer be managed?
Patients with severe abdominal pain should be undressed, placed on a cardiac monitor, and have a large-bore intravenous catheter placed for fluid resuscitation with crystalloid (normal saline or lactated Ringer's solution). Patients at risk for cardiac disease should be given supplemental oxygen. A prompt but thorough physical examination should be done, including pelvic and rectal examinations. Blood should be drawn for complete blood count, electrolytes, blood urea nitrogen (BUN), creatinine, amylase, lipase, and type and screen. An ECG should be obtained on patients older than 40 years. A Foley catheter should be placed and urinalysis done. A portable upright chest radiograph or abdominal left lateral decubitus view often helps to show free intraperitoneal air. A nasogastric tube should be placed and prompt surgical consultation obtained. Broad-spectrum antibiotics should be given and the patient prepared for emergency laparotomy. When the decision has been made to operate on the patient, intravenous analgesics (opiates) should be given for patient comfort.

13. What differentiates upper from lower GI hemorrhage?
Upper GI hemorrhage is bleeding that is proximal to the ligament of Treitz, and lower GI bleeding is distal. In the ED, this is evaluated by placement of a nasogastric or orogastric tube and aspiration of gastric and proximal duodenal contents. Physical appearance of the aspirate (*coffee grounds*, red-tinged fluid, or fresh blood) is the best way of determining the presence of significant upper GI bleeding; testing of gastric content for blood with various cards (e.g., Hemoccult) is not reliable.

14. List the causes of upper GI bleeding.

CAUSE	%
Peptic ulcer disease	45
Gastric erosions	23
Varices	10
Mallory-Weiss tear	7
Esophagitis	6
Duodenitis	6

Adapted from Henneman PL: Gastrointestinal bleeding. In Rosen P, Barkin RM (eds): Emergency Medicine and Clinical Practice, 4th ed. St. Louis, Mosby, 1998, pp 1903–1917.

15. Discuss the emergency management of upper GI bleeding.
Management begins with a rapid assessment and management of the patient's airway, breathing, and cardiovascular status. Patients should be undressed, placed on a cardiac monitor, and given supplemental oxygen. Patients with compromised or unprotected airway should be promptly intubated. The history of GI bleeding (i.e., vomiting blood or passing black or bloody stool) is sufficient to lead to the placement of a large-bore, peripheral intravenous catheter with infusion of normal saline. A focused physical examination should be done, checking for signs of shock (e.g., altered mental status, tachycardia, hypotension, cool extremities, delayed capillary fill). The evaluation should include skin signs; pulmonary, cardiac, and abdominal examination;

and testing of stool for blood. Patients who have abnormal vital signs or signs of shock should have two or more intravenous lines placed and be given rapid infusion of crystalloid (5 to 30 mL/kg). During the initial examination and resuscitation, a history should be obtained. Patients with stable vital signs should be cautiously evaluated for postural changes in blood pressure or pulse. Blood should be drawn for type and crossmatching, hematocrit, platelet count, prothrombin time, electrolytes, BUN, creatinine, and lipase. Elderly patients, patients with a history of cardiovascular disease, and patients who are severely anemic should have an ECG to evaluate for signs of cardiac ischemia (i.e., ST depression). Obtain a chest radiograph (portable, upright to rule out subdiaphragmatic air or aspiration. A nasogastric (or orogastric) tube should be placed to determine the presence of blood in the stomach, then removed. Applying an anesthetic spray to the nose and posterior pharynx decreases the discomfort of placing the nasogastric tube. Gastric lavage is not necessary unless emergent endoscopy is to be done immediately after the lavage.

GI bleeding usually stops spontaneously, and no further ED management is necessary other than admission and perhaps transfusion if there is significant anemia (i.e., hematocrit < 25%). In 20% or less of patients, continued GI hemorrhage requires prompt management and treatment.

16. How should a patient with continued GI hemorrhage be managed?

Blood replacement should begin in patients who continue to show signs of shock or cardiovascular instability. Patients who do not respond promptly (i.e., remain hypotensive) to a 30 mL/kg infusion of crystalloid should be given O-negative blood if type-specific blood is not yet available. Crossmatched blood takes approximately 45 to 60 minutes to become available. If patients continue to show signs of shock or require more than 3 or 4 U of blood, a surgery and gastroenterology consultation should be obtained promptly. Upper GI bleeding may be stopped through the endoscope, but emergency operative repair often is required in patients with persistent GI bleeding.

17. Is placement of a nasogastric or orogastric tube contraindicated in someone with esophageal varices?

There is no evidence that a properly placed nasogastric or orogastric tube results in a significantly increased risk of tearing varices or increased size of a Mallory-Weiss tear. Nasogastric or orogastric tubes can perforate the esophagus or posterior pharynx if they are placed too aggressively. Diagnostic nasogastric or orogastric tubes are unnecessary if the patient vomits gastric contents in the ED because this may be inspected for the presence of blood.

18. Does iced saline lavage decrease gastric bleeding?

No. The use of iced fluid to lavage patients with upper GI hemorrhage no longer is recommended because it may result in hypothermia.

19. When should gastric lavage be used in patients with upper GI bleeding?

Gastric lavage is necessary only in patients who have no aspirate after the tube is placed. Lavage fluid need not be saline or sterile; regular tap water is fine. The only other indication for gastric lavage in patients with upper GI bleeding is immediately before endoscopy to improve visualization.

20. Should all patients with upper GI bleeding undergo endoscopy?

Endoscopy is the most accurate diagnostic tool available in the evaluation of patients with upper GI bleeding, identifying a lesion in 78% to 95% of patients if it is done within 12 to 24 hours of hemorrhage. Accurate identification of the bleeding site allows risk stratification with respect to predicting rebleeding and mortality. Risk stratification facilitates a proper disposition decision.

21. How does one risk stratify patients with GI bleeding?

Initial ED Risk Stratification for Patients With GI Bleeding

LOW RISK	MODERATE RISK	HIGH RISK
Age < 60	Age > 60	
Initial SBP ≥ 100 mmHg	Initial SBP < 100 mmHg	Persistent SBP < 100 mmHg
Normal vitals for 1 h	Mild ongoing tachycardia for 1 h	Persistent moderate-to-severe tachycardia
No transfusion requirement	Transfusion required ≤ 4 U	Transfusion required > 4 U
No active major comorbid diseases	Stable major comorbid diseases	Unstable major comorbid diseases
No liver disease	Mild liver disease—PT normal or near normal	Decompensated liver disease— coagulopathy, ascites, encephalopathy
No moderate or high-risk clinical features	No high-risk clinical features	

SBP, systolic blood pressure; PT, prothrombin time.
Adapted from Lindenauer PK, Terdiman JP: Acute gastrointestinal bleeding. In Wachter RM, Goldman L, Hollander H (eds): Hospital Medicine. Philadelphia, Lippincott Williams & Wilkins, 2000.

Final Risk Stratification for Patients with Upper GI Bleeding After Endoscopy

ENDOSCOPY	CLINICAL RISK STRATIFICATION		
	LOW RISK	MODERATE RISK	HIGH RISK
Low risk	Immediate discharge[*]	24-h inpatient stay (floor)[†]	Close monitoring for 24 h[‡]; ≥ 48-h hospitalization
Moderate risk	24-h patient stay[†]	24–48 h inpatient stay (floor)[†]	Close monitoring for 24 h; ≥ 48-h hospitalization
High risk	Close monitoring for 24 h; 48–72 h hospitalization	Close monitoring for 24 h; 48–72 h hospitalization	Close monitoring ≥ 72-h hospitalization

[*] Patients with low-risk clinical and endoscopic findings can be discharged home with appropriate treatment based on diagnosis, scheduled follow-up evaluation within 24 hours, and proper patient education to ensure immediate return if signs of rebleeding.
[†] Patients may be discharged after 24 to 48 hours of in-hospital observation if there is no evidence of rebleeding, vital signs are normal, there is no need for further transfusion, and the hemoglobin or hematocrit has remained stable. They should be provided with appropriate treatment based on diagnosis, scheduled follow-up evaluation within 24 hours, and proper patient education to ensure immediate return if signs of rebleeding.
[‡] Patients with high-risk clinical or endoscopic findings should be admitted and closely monitored for evidence of rebleeding.
Adapted from Lindenauer PK, Terdiman JP: Acute gastrointestinal bleeding. In Wachter RM, Goldman L, Hollander H (eds): Hospital Medicine. Philadelphia, Lippincott Williams & Wilkins, 2000.

22. What are the low risk criteria that allow a patient who is complaining of GI bleeding to be sent home?

- No comorbid diseases
- Normal vital signs
- Normal or trace positive stool guaiac
- Negative gastric aspirate, if done
- Normal or near-normal hemoglobin and hematocrit
- No problem home support
- Proper understanding of signs and symptoms of significant bleeding
- Immediate access to emergent care if needed
- Follow-up arranged within 24 hours

BIBLIOGRAPHY
1. Drugs for treatment of peptic ulcers. Med Lett Drugs Ther 39:1–4,1997.
2. Henneman PL: Gastrointestinal bleeding. In Marx J, Hockberger R, Walls R (eds): Rosen's Emergency
   Medicine and Clinical Practice, 5th ed. St. Louis, Mosby, 2002, pp 194–200.
3. Lindenauer PK, Terdiman JP: Acute gastrointestinal bleeding. In Wachter RM, Goldman L, Hollander H
   (eds): Hospital Medicine. Philadelphia, Lippincott Williams & Wilkins, 2000, pp 599–610.
4. Lowell M, Bowen WG: Esophagus, stomach, and duodenum. In Marx J, Hockberger R, Walls R (eds):
   Rosen's Emergency Medicine Concepts and Clinical Practice, 5th ed. St. Louis, Mosby, 2002, pp
   1234–1250.

37. APPENDICITIS

Salvator J. Vicario, M.D.

1. What is the function of the human appendix?
The human appendix is a vestigial organ that contains lymphoid tissue. Removal of the appendix produces no detectable defect in the function of the immune system. The appendix is thought to be a useful, but nonessential, immunologic organ.

2. What is the incidence of appendicitis?
Appendicitis is the most common cause of the acute surgical abdomen. It has a reported incidence of approximately 0.1% of the population per year. It can occur at any age but is most prevalent in the teens and 20s (this corresponds to maximum proliferation of lymphoid follicles in the appendix). The male-to-female ratio is 2:1 between the ages of 15 and 25 years but is 1:1 in all other age groups.

3. When should acute appendicitis be suspected?
This diagnosis must be considered in any patient presenting with abdominal pain who has not already had an appendectomy, including the gravid patient.

4. What is the cause and pathogenesis of acute appendicitis?
The most common cause of appendicitis is obstruction of the lumen. This usually is caused by fecaliths (40% to 90%) but also may be caused by lymphoid tissue hypertrophy, inspissated barium from radiologic studies, fruit and vegetable seeds, and intestinal worms. As the mucosal secretions continue to collect in the appendiceal lumen, accompanied by rapid proliferation of resident bacteria, a symptomatic closed-loop obstruction develops. Secretion of 0.5 mL of fluid distal to a block raises the intraluminal pressure to about 60 cm H_2O. Distention results in dull, vague, and diffuse mid and lower abdominal pain mediated by visceral afferent pain fibers. As venous pressure is exceeded, arteriolar inflow causes vascular congestion, resulting in reflex nausea. A shift of more severe and localized pain to the right lower quadrant results from serosal engorgement and inflammation of the parietal peritoneum. As distention progresses, an antimesenteric infarct and perforation may occur. With perforation, the patient may be transiently pain-free, developing peritonitis several hours later.

5. Describe the classic symptoms of acute appendicitis.
The patient's initial complaint is of vague, diffuse epigastric or periumbilical pain that is moderate to severe and usually constant. The pain localizes into the right lower quadrant within 1 to 12 hours (mean, 4 to 6 hours). This symptom often is accompanied by anorexia, nausea, and vomiting. Some patients report obstipation or diarrhea, but these findings are so variable that they are of little diagnostic value. The sequence of events is often suggestive of appendicitis. In almost

90% of adult patients, anorexia is the first symptom, followed by abdominal pain, nausea, and vomiting. In infants, anorexia, irritability, and lethargy may be the only symptoms.

6. How does the location of the appendix alter this classic presentation?

Normal variations in the location of the appendix may account for unusual locations of the somatic phase of pain. A retrocecal appendix may cause back or flank pain. An extra long appendix, with an inflamed tip, may produce pain in the left lower quadrant or the right upper quadrant. A retroileal appendix may cause testicular pain (from irritation of the ureter and spermatic artery). A pelvic appendix may cause suprapubic pain. In pregnancy, the appendix migrates to the right upper quadrant as the uterus enlarges.

7. What percentage of the population has a retrocecal appendix?

Approximately 15%.

8. Describe some of the signs found in appendicitis.

Psoas sign: The patient lies on the left side while the examiner extends the right thigh, stretching the iliopsoas muscle. A positive test results if this maneuver causes pain.

Obturator sign: With the patient supine, the examiner flexes the right thigh and performs passive internal rotation. A positive test results in pain with stretching of the obturator internus muscle.

Rovsing's sign: A positive test results when pressure exerted in the left lower quadrant produces pain in the right lower quadrant.

Involuntary guarding: The patient has localized tenderness to palpation with involuntary (reflex) guarding of muscles.

Rebound tenderness: After applying pressure to the abdomen, the hand is removed quickly. If the patient reports pain, there is rebound tenderness.

Heel tap sign: With the patient supine and the straight, the examiner taps on the bottom of the patient's heel. This test is positive if the patient feels pain in the right lower quadrant (peritoneal sign).

9. Where is McBurney's point, and what does it signify?

McBurney's point is one third the distance from the anterior superior iliac spine to the umbilicus. It represents the point of maximum tenderness in patients with an anterior appendix. It also marks the point through which an appendectomy incision or laparoscopy is done.

10. What vital sign changes are observed in appendicitis?

In uncomplicated appendicitis, the vital signs are only minimally abnormal. If the patient's temperature is elevated, it is seldom more than 1°C above normal. The pulse rate may be normal or slightly elevated. If the vital signs are significantly abnormal, suspect either a complication (e.g., a perforation) or another diagnosis.

11. Which laboratory tests should I order?

White blood cell count: > 10,000 per mm^3 is seen in approximately 90% of cases (but may be normal).

Urinalysis: Use this to rule out renal calculus or pyelonephritis. Mild pyuria or hematuria may be present when an inflamed appendix lies near the bladder or ureter.

β-Human chorionic gonadotropin: Use this to rule out ectopic pregnancy as a cause of right upper quadrant pain.

12. What is the value of imaging studies?

Abdominal and chest radiographs can be of value if one suspects pneumonia or viscus perforation. An appendiceal fecalith is present in approximately 5% of abdominal films. Renal calculi, gallstones, and bowel obstruction also may be evident on plain films.

Abdominal CT is becoming a routine screening examination done with intravenous and oral or rectal contrast enhancement. It has been reported to have nearly 98% sensitivity and specificity. Helical CT has been proved to be cost-effective and reduces negative laparotomy rates. Findings include fecaliths, dilated appendiceal lumen, phlegmon, and abscess. CT scan may show other pathology responsible for the patient's symptoms.

Abdominal ultrasound may be better than CT to exclude other gynecologic pathology, including tuboovarian abscess, cysts, and ectopic pregnancy. It can be useful if experienced examiners can visualize an appendix. Its specificity and sensitivity can be good (approaching 90%), but there may be inadequate studies as a result of patient body habitus or with retrocecal appendices. Ultrasound should be considered if there is availability of an experienced sonographer and the patient is able to cooperate. Nonvisualization of the appendix does not rule out the diagnosis of appendicitis.

13. Name the clinical findings that have the highest predictive value for appendicitis.

Migration of pain to the right lower quadrant and rebound tenderness have a greater than 90% positive predictive value.

14. What are the MANTREL Scores?

This is a clinical assessment tool described by Alvarado that gives a numerical score to each of the following clinical findings: **m**igration, **a**norexia, **n**ausea and vomiting, **t**enderness, **r**ebound, **e**levation of temperature, **l**eukocytosis, shift to left. Tenderness and leukocytosis are given scores of 2, whereas the others are given a score of 1.

Patient score	Appendicitis
5–6	Likely
7–8	Probable
9–10	Very probable

15. Do all untreated episodes of appendicitis result in perforation?

No. Many patients with histologically proven appendicitis provide a history of previous similar episodes of right lower quadrant abdominal pain. Pathologic examination of appendices from these patients sometimes reveals thickening and scarring, suggestive of old, already healed acute inflammations.

16. What is the incidence of appendiceal perforation?

From the onset of symptoms, approximately 25% perforate by 24 hours; 50%, by 36 hours; and 75%, by 48 hours. Perforation rates are much higher in young, elderly, and gravid patients.

17. What is the differential diagnosis of patients with right lower quadrant abdominal pain?

Acute ileitis	Inflammatory bowel disease
Diverticulitis	Acute cholecystitis
Perforated gastric or duodenal ulcer	Volvulus
Intussusception	Early small bowel obstruction
Inflammation of Meckel's diverticulum	Uterine or tuboovarian pathology
Gonadal torsion	Acute epididymitis
Tubal pregnancy	Mittelschmerz
Mesenteric adenitis	Incarcerated inguinal hernia

18. Okay, I have made a diagnosis of appendicitis. What do I do next?

Prompt surgical consultation is mandatory. Intravenous fluids are started immediately, and the patient is given nothing by mouth. Intravenous antibiotics also are started and cover mixed colonic flora, including aerobic and anaerobic organisms, especially *Bacteroides fragilis*. Early administration of antibiotics has been shown to reduce morbidity.

19. List some of the pitfalls in caring for patients who may have appendicitis.

1. Relying on elevated white blood cell count to make the diagnosis.
2. Not considering the diagnosis in the very young, the elderly, and in pregnant women.
3. Performing only a single examination without subsequent examination or early follow-up in patients who may have early appendicitis.
4. Misinterpreting the ultrasound or CT scan.

20. When can I discharge the patient? What should be my follow-up instructions?

All patients should be informed that appendicitis can be a difficult diagnosis to make. Patients who have nonlocalized tenderness without vomiting and who are well hydrated can be reexamined in a few hours or followed as an outpatient with instructions to return immediately if pain increases, vomiting occurs, or pain or tenderness migrate to the lower abdomen.

BIBLIOGRAPHY

1. Alvarado A: A practical score for the early diagnosis of acute appendicitis. Ann Emerg Med 15:557–564, 1986.
2. Blackbourne LH: Surgical Recall. Baltimore, Williams & Wilkins, 1994.
3. Gwynn LK: The diagnosis of acute appendicitis: Clinical assessment versus computed tomography evaluation. J Emerg Med 21:119–123, 2001.
4. Harwood-Nuss AL, Linden C, Luten RC, et al (eds): The Clinical Practice of Emergency Medicine, 2nd ed. Philadelphia, Lippincott-Raven, 1996.
5. Paulman AA, Huebner DM, Forrest TS: Sonography in the diagnosis of acute appendicitis. Am Fam Physician 44:464–468, 1991.
6. Rao PM, Rhea JT, Novelline RA, et al: Effect of computed tomography of the appendix on treatment of patients and use of hospital resources. N Engl J Med 338:141–146, 1998.
7. Rosen P, Barkin RM (eds): Emergency Medicine: Concepts and Clinical Practice, 5th ed. St. Louis, Mosby, 2001.
8. Soda K, Nemoto K, Yoshizawa S, et al: Detection of pinpoint tenderness on the appendix under ultrasonography is useful to confirm acute appendicitis. Arch Surg 136:1136–1140, 2001.
9. Tintinalli JE, Kelen GD, Stapczynski JS: Emergency Medicine: A Comprehensive Study Guide. New York, McGraw-Hill, 2000.
10. Worrell JA, Drolshagen LF, Kelly TC, et al: Graded compression ultrasound in the diagnosis of appendicitis: A comparison of diagnostic criteria. J Ultrasound Med 9:145–150, 1990.

38. LIVER AND BILIARY TRACT DISEASE

Kaushal Shah, M.D., and Larry A. Nathanson, M.D.

1. What are the common manifestations of biliary disease?

Cholelithiasis is the presence of gallstones in the gallbladder without evidence of infection. Among adults, 8% of men and 17% of women have gallstones, and the incidence increases with age. **Biliary colic** is right upper quadrant or epigastric pain sometimes radiating to the right shoulder or scapula. It usually lasts less than 6 hours, occurs after a fatty meal, and is thought to be due to transient obstruction of the cystic duct by a gallstone. Of patients with colic, 30% progress to **cholecystitis**, a bacterial overgrowth and infection of the gallbladder caused by obstruction of the cystic duct. **Choledocholithiasis** occurs when the gallstone lodges in the common bile duct and can cause cholecystitis or pancreatitis (if the ampulla of Vater is obstructed) or both. **Cholangitis** is a severe infection of the biliary tract that presents as right upper quadrant pain, fever and chills, and jaundice (Charcot's triad) and may include shock and mental status changes (Reynold's pentad). **Emphysematous cholecystitis** is caused by gas-forming bacteria and is seen with vascular insufficiency. It is more frequent in men and diabetic patients and often is accompanied by sepsis.

2. Do all gallstones produce pain? Does a lack of stones preclude cholecystitis?

Of patients with gallstones, 80% are asymptomatic. Fifteen percent to 30% of asymptomatic patients develop symptoms within 15 years. Of cholecystitis, 10% is not secondary to cholelithiasis and is termed *acalculus*. This can be a challenging diagnosis because these patients often have concomitant medical conditions, such as diabetes, burns, multisystem trauma, AIDS, or sepsis.

3. What is Murphy's sign?

The sign is named after a prominent Chicago surgeon, John B. Murphy (1857–1916). The patient is asked to take a deep breath while the examiner applies pressure over the area of the gallbladder. If the gallbladder is inflamed, the descending diaphragm forces it against the examiner's fingertips, causing pain and often a sudden halt to the inspiration. A sonographic Murphy's sign uses the ultrasound probe instead of the examiner's fingers and is positive when the site of maximal tenderness localizes to the gallbladder.

4. Can a plain radiograph of the abdomen aid diagnosis?

Maybe. Only 10% to 15% of gallstones contain sufficient calcium to be radiopaque. Air can be seen in the biliary tree or the gallbladder wall when infection is due to gas-forming bacteria or there is a biliary-intestinal fistula. In cases in which the cause of upper abdominal pain is unclear, a flat plate may help by showing free air, pancreatic calcifications, ileus, obstruction, pneumatosis, or lower lobe lung consolidation.

5. What is the gold standard for diagnosing cholecystitis?

Although ultrasound is the test of choice in the ED, a **HIDA scan** is 95% accurate if the gallbladder does not fill with radioisotope in 4 hours after injection.

6. Is an elevated temperature or white blood cell count necessary for diagnosis?

No, they are not helpful for diagnosis, as is seen in one study in which 71% of patients with acute nongangrenous cholecystitis were afebrile, and 32% had normal white blood cell count.

7. Describe the ultrasound findings in cholecystitis.

Gallstones can be detected directly or sometimes their presence can be inferred by interference with transmission of ultrasound waves (*acoustic shadowing*). Other helpful findings include an enlarged gallbladder (> 5 cm), a thickened gallbladder wall (> 4 mm), fluid collections around the gallbladder (*pericholecystic fluid*), and intrahepatic or common ductal dilation.

8. When should elective surgery be considered in patients with asymptomatic cholelithiasis?

Cholecystectomy should be considered in diabetics, patients with a porcelain gallbladder, and patients with a history of biliary pancreatitis.
  • Diabetics have increased morbidity and mortality when urgent cholecystectomy is done in the setting of cholecystitis.
  • Calcified or porcelain gallbladders have a 22% association with carcinoma.
  • The risks of pancreatitis may outweigh the risks of elective cholecystectomy.

9. What are Courvoisier's law, Klatskin's tumor, and Fitz-Hugh–Curtis syndrome?

Courvoisier's law states that a palpable gallbladder in the setting of painless jaundice is likely to represent obstruction of the common bile duct by a malignancy, usually carcinoma of the pancreatic head.

Klatskin's tumor is a malignant tumor located where the hepatic ducts form the common duct.

Fitz-Hugh–Curtis syndrome is caused by pelvic inflammatory disease extending up the right paracolic gutter, causing inflammation of the capsule of the liver (perihepatitis), and can lead to adhesions between the liver and abdominal wall.

10. What is a porcelain gallbladder?

A gallbladder with calcified walls. This is an important finding because 22% are associated with carcinoma, and it is an indication for cholecystectomy in asymptomatic patients. There is a higher incidence in women and Native Americans, especially members of the Pima tribe.

11. Are all gallstones created equal?

No. Cholesterol stones usually are found in the stereotypical, **female, fat, 40, fertile** patient. Asian patients and patients with parasitic infections, chronic liver/biliary disease, or chronic hemolysis states (i.e., sickle cell, spherocytosis) are more likely to have pigment stones.

12. What are liver function tests?

Elevated blood levels of the intracellular enzymes aspartate aminotransferase (AST) and alanine aminotransferase (ALT), correlate with liver injury, not function. **Liver function** is analyzed best by measuring factors affected by hepatic protein synthesis. Acute liver failure results in a decrease in vitamin K–dependent coagulation factors (except VIII), leading to a prolonged prothrombin time. The liver also synthesizes albumin, although its longer half-life makes it a better marker of subacute or chronic liver disease.

13. What is the difference between conjugated and unconjugated bilirubinemia?

Bilirubin is a breakdown product of hemoglobin and related proteins. In its **unconjugated**, hydrophobic form, it is unable to be excreted into bile, although it can traverse the blood-brain barrier and placenta. Bilirubin is **conjugated** in the liver with glucuronic acid, making it more water soluble for excretion into the bile. A predominance of unconjugated bilirubin occurs when there is overproduction (due to hemolysis) or decreased conjugation (due to inborn metabolism syndromes of medications). A primarily conjugated bilirubinemia results from reflux into the plasma from impaired excretion, secondary to biliary obstruction from cholestasis, gallstones, tumors, or strictures.

14. State the major causes of acute hepatitis.

Viruses such as hepatitis A through E viruses, Epstein-Barr virus, and cytomegalovirus. It also can result from exposure to toxins such as ethanol, *Amanita phalloides* mushrooms, carbon tetrachloride, acetaminophen, halothane, and chlorpromazine.

15. What are the risk factors for viral hepatitis? Which can result in a carrier state?

Hepatitis B and C are transmitted via blood and body fluid exposures: sexual intercourse, intravenous drug abuse, blood transfusions, tattoos or body piercings, hemodialysis, and needle sticks. Hepatitis A and E are transmitted via fecal/oral exposure (i.e., foreign travel, raw seafood ingestion, poor hygiene or sewage management, and close contact with a person infected with hepatitis). Hepatitis A and E are often self-limited, whereas hepatitis B and C can result in a carrier state and progress to chronic hepatitis.

16. What is the most common form of liver disease in the United States?

Alcoholic hepatitis. It is most often diagnosed by history, but the following are highly suggestive associated findings: spider angiomas, gynecomastia, palmar erythema, ascites, and an elevated AST and ALT in a ratio of greater than 2:1.

17. Which patients with hepatitis should be admitted?

Patients who are coagulopathic (international normalized ratio > 3), actively bleeding, are encephalopathic, who are unable to tolerate oral fluids, and whose social situation (including drug and alcohol abuse) would make proper care and follow-up difficult or impossible.

18. What are complications of chronic liver disease to watch for in the ED?

The most common complication of cirrhotic ascites is **spontaneous bacterial peritonitis**, which can present with fever, abdominal pain, or mental status changes. Paracentesis is diagnostic if it shows white blood cell count greater than 1000, neutrophils greater than 250, or a positive Gram stain or cultre. Portal hypertension causes the development of **esophageal varices**, which can lead to massive gastrointestinal bleeding. Management should focus on resuscitation, local control (balloon tamponade or endoscopic ligation/sclerotherapy), and reduction of portal pressure (vasopressin plus nitroglycerin, somatostatin/octreotide, and, if necessary, emergent transjugular intrahepatic portosystemic shunt). Patients with chronic liver disease are at greatly **increased risk of bleeding** because of deficits of the coagulation cascade proteins, platelet abnormalities, and increased fibrinolysis. Renal failure in cirrhotic patients with structurally normal kidneys represents the **hepatorenal syndrome**. One study showed 38% 1-year survival in patients with the hepatorenal syndrome.

19. Are there any special issues to watch for in the post–liver transplant patient?
    Transplant rejection is common and manifests as fever, pain, and elevated transaminases and bilirubin. This can be treated with high-dose steroids and increased immunosuppressive medication. Other causes of transplant dysfunction include biliary strictures, recurrence of viral hepatitis, and vascular thrombosis. Immunosuppressive therapy can cause nephrotoxicity, neurotoxicity, and hypertension. As with other immunosuppressed patients, opportunistic infections, such as cytomegalovirus, Epstein-Barr virus, mycobacteria, and *Pneumocystis*, and fungal infection should be considered.

BIBLIOGRAPHY

1. Feldman M (ed): Sleisenger and Fordtran's Gastrointestinal and Liver Disease, 6th ed. Philadelphia, W.B. Saunders, 1998.
2. Gruber PJ, Silverman RA, Gottesfeld S, et al: Presence of fever and leukocytosis in acute cholecystis. Ann Emerg Med 28:273–277, 1996.
3. Rosen CL, Brown DFM, Chang Y, et al: Ultrasonography by emergency physicians in patients with suspected cholecystitis. Am J Emerg Med 19:32–36, 2001.
4. Sheth S, Bedford A, Chopra S: Primary gallbladder cancer: Recognition of risk factors and the role of prophylactic cholecystectomy. Am J Gastroenterol 95:1402–1410, 2000.

39. BOWEL DISORDERS

Vikhyat Bebarta, M.D.

1. What are the two categories of small intestinal obstruction?
    A small intestinal obstruction can be secondary to a **mechanical obstruction** or an **adynamic ileus**. An adynamic ileus, also known simply as *ileus*, is more common , is self-limiting, and usually does not require surgery. A mechanical obstruction may be caused by extrinsic and intrinsic factors that physically block the passage of material through the small bowel. When the term *small bowel obstruction* (SBO) is used, it usually means mechanical obstruction. An SBO can be *complete*, in which case no air (flatus) or stool is able to pass, or it may be *partial*.

2. What are the common causes of SBO?
    Overall, adhesions, hernias, cancer account for more than 90% of cases. **Postoperative adhesions** are the most common cause of SBO (56%), followed by **incarcerated hernia** (25%). Approximately 5% of all postoperative celiotomy patients develop adhesive obstruction, usually long after surgery. Inguinal is the most common hernia, and femoral is the second most common. Consider obturator hernias in elderly women without a history of surgery who present with knee or thigh pain. **Cancer** ranks third (10%). Other less common causes include inflammatory bowel disease, gallstones, volvulus, intussusception, radiation enteritis, abscesses, congenital lesions, and bezoars.

3. What are the clinical features of SBO?

Patients usually present with abdominal pain and distention. The pain is crampy with occasional spasms and usually is referred to the epigastrium or periumbilical area. Distal obstructions display more significant abdominal distention. Vomiting and obstipation (inability to pass feces or flatus) are frequent symptoms. Vomiting that is later in onset or more feculent signifies a more distal obstruction. Obstipation occurs only after all the feces distal to the obstruction is emptied. An early complete SBO may be difficult to diagnose. A patient with partial SBO often continues to have flatus and some passage of stool. A partial and complete SBO may look similar initially. The abdominal examination usually reveals diffuse tenderness. Look carefully for hernias or masses. Auscultation may reveal high-pitched, hyperactive *tinkling* or *rushing* sounds. Rectal examination may reveal a mass or impacted stool but more commonly, an empty vault.

4. Why is SBO life-threatening?

When the bowel is obstructed, fluid fills the lumen because of a combination of decreased intestinal absorption and increased secretion. Gastric, pancreatic, and biliary secretions also accumulate in the intestinal lumen. Fluid can seep into the bowel wall (causing wall edema) and eventually into the peritoneum. These various fluid shifts, along with frequent vomiting, produce profound intravascular fluid and electrolyte losses, leading to hypovolemic shock. As the process continues, the bowel dilates, and ultimately vascular compromise from rising intraluminal pressure or simple mechanical strangulation can lead to bowel necrosis and perforation. Intestinal flora penetrate the compromised bowel wall. They proliferate and spill into the peritoneum and bloodstream, causing bacterial peritonitis and sepsis. When this occurs, mortality reaches 70%.

5. Which clinical findings suggest bowel strangulation?

A complete SBO is often difficult to differentiate from a complete SBO with strangulated bowel early on by clinical examination, laboratory studies, or radiographically. Patients with bowel strangulation may present with fever, tachycardia, marked abdominal tenderness, peritoneal signs, diminished bowel sounds, or a persistent mass later in the course. Laboratory studies may reveal metabolic acidosis or elevations in white blood cell count, creatine phosphokinase, amylase, or lactate dehydrogenase. A complete SBO must be observed closely, and the surgical team usually has a low threshold for taking the patient to the operating room.

6. Describe the radiographic findings in SBO.

SBO causes air-fluid levels in the distended loops of small bowel. In a mechanical SBO, peristaltic activity causes the multiple air-fluid levels to layer in a stepladder-like pattern proximal to the obstruction (see Figure, top of next page). When the obstructed intestine contains more fluid than gas, small round pockets of air may line up to form the *string of pearls* sign. Distal to the obstruction, there is usually a paucity of stool and gas. Radiographic signs of a closed loop obstruction include the *coffee bean sign* of cecal volvulus (single gas distended loop with lumina separated by a broad, dense band of edematous bowel), the pseudotumor sign (loop of bowel filled with fluid that resembles a mass), and fixation of a single loop in three views. Plain films have sensitivity of 41% to 86% and a specificity of 25% to 88%; many early or radiographically subtle presentations may be missed. Abdominal CT scan has a sensitivity of 100% and a specificity of 83%, making it a very helpful study when the plain films are not diagnostic.

7. What is the treatment for SBO?

Initial emergency management includes cardiopulmonary support, electrolyte replacement, decompression with a nasogastric tube, intravenous fluids, and antibiotics. Because it is difficult to differentiate a strangulated SBO from a complete bowel obstruction, early surgical consultation is essential, especially if strangulated bowel or a complete SBO is suspected. Partial SBOs usually are managed nonoperatively for approximately 48 hours because most will resolve in that time period. If not, intervention is warranted.

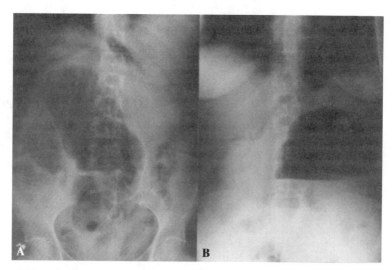

Small bowel obstruction. Note the dilated loops of small bowel on the supine film (*A*). The upright view reveals multiple air-fluid interfaces at different levels (***B***).

8. What are the characteristics of an ileus?

The terms *ileus* and *adynamic ileus* are used to describe a paralyzed intestine. The bowel is unable to perform peristalsis. This is the most common cause of an SBO. Causes include infections (e.g., peritonitis), drugs (e.g., narcotics, anticholinergics), electrolyte imbalances, spinal cord injuries, and postoperative states. Patients present with abdominal distention, mild nausea and vomiting, and obstipation. Abdominal pain is usually minimal or absent. Fever is usually absent, and the white blood cell count is often normal. Abdominal examination reveals decreased bowel sounds, relatively little or no tenderness, and absence of peritoneal signs, which all are uncommon in a complete mechanical SBO. Radiographs classically show minimally distended bowel throughout the entire gastrointestinal tract, with diffuse air-fluid levels, in small bowel.

9. How is an ileus treated?

Maintenance of intravascular volume; limiting oral intake; and correcting electrolytes, particularly hypokalemia. If abdominal distention is present and uncomfortable, placement of a nasogastric or orogastric tube is indicated for decompression. A review and discontinuence of medications, such as opiates, known to slow intestinal motility should be performed. If the ileus is prolonged (> 3 to 5 days), further imaging should be obtained to search for an underlying cause.

10. What are the causes of large bowel obstruction (LBO)?

LBO is caused most commonly by colon cancer (60%), volvulus (20%), and diverticular disease (10%). Primary adenocarcinoma accounts for most cancerous lesions. Other less likely causes include metastatic carcinoma, gynecologic tumors, inflammatory bowel disease (IBD), intussusception, and fecal impaction. In infants, consider congenital disorders, such as Hirschsprung's disease or an imperforate anus. Hernias and adhesions are uncommon causes of LBO.

11. What are the two main types of volvulus?

Volvulus is caused when a bowel segment rotates on its mesenteric axis. In colonic volvulus, 75% involve the sigmoid, and 25% involve the cecum. **Sigmoid volvulus** generally afflicts elderly and institutionalized individuals who suffer from chronic constipation and stretching of the sigmoid colon. Radiography shows a left-sided dilated bowel loop with both ends pointing toward the pelvis, the *bent inner tube* appearance (Figure). Barium enema reveals the characteristic *bird's beak* or *ace of spades* sign. Treatment is initial rectal tube decompression usually followed by elective resection because recurrence rates are almost 90%. **Cecal volvulus** can occur at any age but usually is seen in persons 25 to 35 years old. Radiography reveals a large oval dilated bowel loop somewhere in the midabdomen and signs of an SBO. Barium enema or colonoscopy is diagnostic, and treatment is surgical. Volvulus involving the transverse colon and splenic flexure is uncommon.

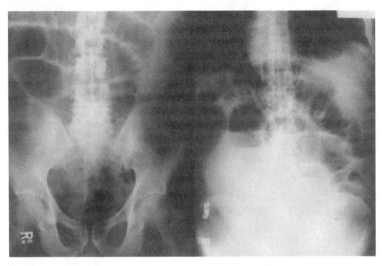

Dramatic dilation of a single loop of colon in the central abdomen should immediately suggest the diagnosis of sigmoid volvulus. Both ends of the loop are located in the pelvis with the bow oriented superiorly. Also note that there is no rectal bubble and very little if any small bowel gas.

12. What is Ogilvie's syndrome?

A pseudoobstruction of the colon with dilation that occasionally can involve the distal small bowel. The onset of symptoms is associated with recent surgery, sepsis, respiratory failure, or other medical or surgical stress. The patient presents with colicky abdominal pain and constipation. Examination reveals a distended tympanic abdomen, with absent bowel sounds. Radiography shows a dilated colon, predominately in the cecum. A cecum measuring greater than 11 to 12 cm is associated with a high risk of perforation. Treatment includes bowel rest, intravenous fluids, repletion of electrolytes, removal of contributing factors, and surgery if necessary. Neostigmine is effective in resolving Ogilvie's syndrome with limited side effects.

Ogilvie's syndrome is related to LBO in a manner similar to an ileus to a mechanical SBO.

13. How do I differentiate between large and small bowel radiographs?

The small intestine is centrally located and has circular folds that completely traverse the bowel called *plicae circulares*. The large intestine is located peripherally and has haustra that are short, blunt, and thick and indent the bowel but do not traverse the wall completely. Haustra are less numerous and are farther apart from each other than plicae circulares.

14. What are the major risk factors for mesenteric vascular occlusion?

Age greater than 50 years, valvular or atherosclerotic heart disease, peripheral vascular disease, congestive heart failure, recent myocardial infarction, arrhythemias (e.g., atrial fibrillation), critical illness with hypotension or sepsis, and the use of diuretics or vasoconstrictive drugs. The final common pathway is insufficient blood flow to the intestines caused by arterial emboli or thrombosis, venous thrombosis, or nonocclusive hypoperfusion (hypotensive states).

15. What are the causes of mesenteric ischemia?

Acute mesenteric ischemia is divided into occlusive (usually the superior mesenteric artery) and nonocclusive. Occlusive mesenteric ischemia is divided into arterial and venous (most commonly mesenteric vein thrombosis). Finally, arterial mesenteric ischemia is divided into embolic (the most common form of mesenteric ischemia) and thrombotic. Embolic mesenteric ischemia has the most abrupt onset. Mesenteric vein thrombosis has the most indolent course, and thrombotic mesenteric ischemia is in-between. Nonocclusive mesenteric ischemia usually is seen in seriously ill patients with low flow states resulting in reduced blood flow to the bowel. Chronic mesenteric ischemia also occurs.

16. What is intestinal angina?

Intestinal angina (chronic mesenteric ischemia) is caused by atherosclerosis of the visceral arteries. It is rare and occurs mostly in women. Patients have crampy abdominal pain that usually occurs 15 to 30 minutes after eating and lasts 1 to 4 hours.

17. How do patients with mesenteric ischemia present?

Most patients present with acute abdominal pain that is intially dull and diffuse. In this early state, patients frequently complain of severe pain but have minimal physical findings, the characteristic "pain out of proportion to the examination." This lack of physical findings explains why this disease is such a diagnostic challenge. As the infarction develops, peritoneal signs develop. Vomiting, hematochezia, hematemesis, abdominal distention, fever, and shock are late signs that often indicate dead bowel.

18. What tests should I order when I suspect mesenteric ischemia?

Laboratory findings include leukocytosis, hemoconcentration, metabolic acidosis, and elevated amylase, creatine phosphokinase, and lactate dehydrogenase. These findings may indicate ischemic bowel but lack sensitivity and specificity. Unfortunately, they are the least helpful in the early period of ischemia, which is the time when making the diagnosis can decrease morbidity and mortality significantly. Elevation of phosphate was thought to be a sensitive marker but later was confirmed to have a sensitivity of 25% to 33%. Serial lactate levels that are normal have been shown to be helpful, but an elevated lactate is nonspecific.

Abdominal plain films are usually normal early in the course but can be used to exclude other diagnoses. Late x-ray findings suggestive of advanced ischemia include gassless bowel, thumbprinting (caused by submucosal edema or hemorrhage), pneumatosis intestinalis (gas in the bowel wall), and portal venous gas. CT scan and ultrasound show vessel occlusion and are helpful in further delineating extraluminal air and bowel wall edema. Mesenteric angiography is the most useful tool for diagnosis and treatment, allowing for selective vasodilator infusion. It is the gold standard and should be done when a strong clinical suspicion of mesenteric ischemia exists.

19. How is mesenteric ischemia treated?

Initial treatment includes vigorous resuscitation, correction of predisposing factors, nasogastric tube suctioning, parenteral antibiotics, and surgical consultation. Digitalis and vasopressors should be avoided if possible. Definitive management involves selective vasodilator infusion, such as papaverine, an inhibitor of phophodiesterase, during angiography. Laparotomy may be necessary to undertake embolectomy or bowel resection.

20. What is ischemic colitis, and how is it different from mesenteric ischemia?

Ischemic colitis is ischemia of the large bowel and has little to do with mesenteric ischemia. It occurs predominantly in the elderly. Of patients, 60% present with diffuse or lower abdominal pain with diarrhea that often is mixed with blood. Often dysentery and a lower gastrointestinal bleed or in the differential diagnosis.

Ischemic colitis usually is due to small vessel disease, and an angiogram is not helpful diagnostically or therapeutically. In most cases, part of the mucosa or submucosa is sloughed. In a few serious cases, full-thickness infarctions can ensue, and bowel necrosis and peritonitis can develop. Sigmoidoscopy is the diagnostic procedure of choice with 100% sensitivity and 100% specificity.

21. What is intussusception?

Intussusception is caused when an intestinal segment invaginates and telescopes into an adjacent segment.

22. Is intussusception seen only in children?

No. Of intussusceptions, 5% occur in adults. In contrast to the idiopathic nature of childhood intussusceptions, a pathologic mechanical lesion, or *lead point*, is found in more than 90% of adult cases. Half of these cases originate in the small bowel, and half originate in the colon. Typical pathologic lesions include tumors, Meckel's diverticulum, and inflammatory lesions. The high frequency of mass lesions in adults mandates surgical exploration.

23. What are diverticula?

The word *diverticulum* is derived from the Latin, meaning a "wayside shelter or lodging." Diverticula are saclike outpouchings of the colonic mucosa that occur through weakened areas of the muscularis. In the strictest terms, purists regard these colonic diverticula as *pseudodiverticula* because they lack a muscularis layer.

24. In which part of the bowel are diverticula most likely to occur?

In Western societies, diverticula occur most commonly in the sigmoid colon, although they can be found in any area of the large bowel. Rectal diverticula are rare. Japanese, Chinese, and Hawaiians are more prone to right-sided colonic diverticula.

25. Which patients develop diverticular disease?

Diverticular disease is mostly isolated to Western societies, where the prevalence may be 20%. The incidence increases with age; 50% of persons in Western countries have diverticula by age 65 years, and 65% of persons have diverticula by age 85.

26. How does diverticular disease present, and what are the two major complications?

Most patients with **diverticular disease** remain asymptomatic; however, 10% to 20% eventually develop symptoms such as abdominal pain. Patients with diverticula may describe intermittent left lower quadrant abdominal pain that is exacerbated by eating and relieved by defecation. Patients may have flatulence, diarrhea, or constipation.

Diverticulitis is inflammation of the diverticula caused by fecal impaction that abrades the mucosal surface. These patients may describe persistent localized abdominal pain, low-grade fevers, malaise, vomiting, and rectal bleeding. Urinary symptoms may be present because of inflammation of the adjacent ureter or bladder. The diagnosis of uncomplicated diverticulitis usually can be made clinically. Patients younger than age 40 frequently have worse disease and often need to be treated aggressively with surgery.

Diverticular bleeding is another complication of diverticular disease. It is usually painless and results from erosion into the penetrating artery of the diverticulum. Bleeding subsides spontaneously in most patients.

27. What are other common causes of lower gastrointestinal bleeding?

Diverticulosis is the most common cause. Angiodysplasia is common and may be as common as diverticulosis. It most commonly causes venous bleeding located in the right colon. Other causes are neoplasms, IBD, upper gastrointestinal bleeding, anorectal disorders, ischemic colitis, and infectious diarrhea.

28. What are the complications of diverticulitis?

In uncomplicated diverticulitis, inflammation is confined to the bowel wall. Approximately 15% to 30% of patients with diverticulitis develop complications, including perforation, generalized peritonitis, abscess or fistula formation, or bowel obstruction. Patients with these complications manifest severe abdominal pain, fever, and peritoneal signs. Immunocomprosmised and elderly patients may not develop these signs. The most common fistula is the colovesical fistula. Patients with a colovesical fistula may report pneumaturia, fecaluria, urinary tract infection symptoms, or recurrent urinary tract infections. In the emergent setting, CT scan is the test of choice to investigate complications or to uncover alternative diagnoses. Abdominal radiographs may be helpful. Contrast enemas and colonscopy should be avoided in acute diverticulitis because of the risk of perforation.

29. How are diverticulosis and diverticulitis treated?

Diverticular disease rarely requires hospitalization. Local heat and anticholinergics may help to relieve bowel spasm. Bulk laxatives, a high-fiber diet, and stool softeners help decrease intraluminal pressure. Patients with **diverticulitis** and mild symptoms without acute complications can be treated as outpatients with a clear liquid diet, nonopioid analgesics, and oral antibiotics, such as levofloxacin and metronidazole. Any patient with complications, such as perforation or abscess formation, requires admission for surgical management and intravenous antibiotics. A **bleeding diverticulum** can cause significant blood loss, and some patients require admission and blood transfusion. Patients who continue to bleed despite conservative treatment (5% to 25% of patients) need definitive treatment with colonoscopy, selective arterial embolization, or potentially surgery to control the ongoing hemorrhage.

30. What is IBD?

An idiopathic, chronic inflammatory disease of the intestine. It encompasses two main groups: **Crohn's disease (CD)** and **ulcerative colitis (UC)**. CD is also known as *regional enteritis* or *granulomatous ileocolitis*. CD and UC are rising in incidence.

31. What are the differences between CD and UC?

CD causes inflammation through all layers of the bowel wall and can occur anywhere in the gastrointestinal tract. It is most common in Jews, whites, women, and those with a family history of CD. It does not cause continuous bowel involvement, forming *skip lesions* and a cobblestone-like appearance of the mucosa. Granulomas are found commonly in the mucosa. Although rectal involvement is uncommon, anorectal fistulas and abscesses are common complications. There is a peak incidence between 15 and 22 years and 55 and 60 years. Smoking has been associated with an increased recurrence rate of CD.

UC is confined to the large bowel and causes superficial mucosal and submucosal inflammation in a continuous fashion throughout the entire large colon (no skip lesions). It's peak incidence is in the 20 to 30 age group. UC more commonly involves the rectum. Because of its superficial inflammation, it is less likely to cause fistulas, abscesses, strictures, or obstruction. Crypt abscesses are common. UC is more likely to cause rectal bleeding and is associated more frequently with toxic megacolon and colon cancer. UC is also more prevalent in whites and those with a family history, and there is a slight male predominance.

32. How do CD and UC present?

Although they are pathologically distinct diseases, CD and UC can present in a similar fashion. They both affect all age groups. The incidence of CD and UC is approximately the same worldwide. Both diseases may present with diarrhea, abdominal pain, fevers, anorexia, weight loss, and bloody diarrhea. UC is more likely to have bloody diarrhea. In nonfulminating colitis, the diagnosis can be confirmed by endoscopy or barium enema.

33. What are the life-threatening complications of IBD?

Perforation, hemorrhage, intraabdominal abscess, bowel obstruction, and fulminant colitis leading to **toxic megacolon**. Fulminant colitis is a severe form of colitis seen more frequently in UC than in CD. It can lead to toxic megacolon and perforation. Patients with fulminant colitis are severely ill with abdominal tenderness, fever, tachycardia, bloody diarrhea, and more than six bowel movements per day. Laboratory workup may reveal anemia, elevated erythrocyte sedimentation rate, and hypoalbuminemia. Toxic megacolon is colonic dilation and dysmotility caused by fulminant colitis. The onset of toxic megacolon may be heralded by increased abdominal distention, peritoneal signs, or a sharp decrease in the number of daily stools. Radiographs confirm the diagnosis, showing a dilated segment of colon, loss of haustra, orr thumbprinting from bowel wall edema. Approximately one third of patients with toxic megacolon perforate the bowel wall. The mortality of toxic megacolon perforation is 50%.

34. What is the treatment for IBD?
Patients with mild disease who have no signs of life-threatening complications can be treated as outpatients with close follow-up. Treatment usually consists of sulfasalazine; steroids (oral or enema); steroid-sparing agents such as 6-mercaptopurine; and antidiarrheal agents such as loperamide, Lomotil, and cholestyramine. These antidiarrheal agents should be used with caution because they may predispose to toxic megacolon. Metronidazole may help treat the chronic perirectal complications of CD. Patients should be admitted if they have more severe disease or any life-threatening complications. Fulminant colitis is treated with bowel rest, vigorous fluid and electrolyte replacement, intravenous steroids, and broad-spectrum intravenous antibiotics. If patients do not improve or if they get worse, surgery is a final option. Toxic megacolon is treated similarly with bowel rest, antibiotics, and surgery if necessary. Treating toxic megacolon with steroids is controversial.

35. What are the extraintestinal complications of regional enteritis?
The incidence of systemic manifestations is 25% to 30% in patients with IBD. These symptoms may precede intestinal symptoms (especially in children) and so may be the initial presenting complaint. Extraintestinal manifestations are divided into arthritic (19%), dermatologic (4%), hepatobiliary (4%), and vascular (1.3%), and ocular (episcleritis and uveitis). Of IBD patients, 20% may have ankylosing spondylitis.

Extraintestinal Complications of Inflammatory Bowel Disease

HEPATOBILIARY DISEASE	OTHERS
Gallstones	Aphthous ulcers
Pericholangitis	Erythema nodosum
Chronic active hepatitis	Pyoderma gangrenosum
Primary sclerosing cholangitis	Nongranulomatous anterior uveitis
Cholangiocarcinoma	Polyarteritis
Cirrhosis	Nephrolithiasis
	Pneumaturia
	Thromboembolism

BIBLIOGRAPHY

1. Bitterman RA; Disorders of the large intestine. In Rosen P, Barkin RM (eds): Emergency Medicine: Concepts and Clinical Practice, 4th ed. St. Louis, Mosby, 1998, pp 2022–2037.
2. Brandt LJ, Smithline AE: Ischemic lesions of the bowel. In Feldman M, Sleisenger MH, Scharschmidt BF (eds): Sleisenger and Fordtran's Gastrointestinal and Liver Disease: Pathophysiology, Diagnosis, Management, 6th ed. Philadelphia, W.B. Saunders, 1998, pp 2009–2024.
3. Gallagher EJ: Acute abdominal pain. In Tintinalli JE, Kelen GA, Stapczynski JS (eds): Emergency Medicine: A Comprehensive Study Guide, 5th ed. New York, McGraw-Hill, 2000, pp 497–515.
4. Greenfield RH, Henneman PL: Disorders of the small intestine. In Rosen P, Barkin RM (eds): Emergency Medicine: Concepts and Clinical Practice, 4th ed. St. Louis, Mosby, 1998, pp 2005–2022.
5. Ponec RJ, Saunders MD, Kimmey MB: Neostigmine for the treatment of acute colonic pseudo-obstruction. N Engl J Med 341:137–141, 1999.
6. Schelble DT, Peter DJ: Lower gastrointestinal bleeding. In Harwood-Nuss A, Wolfson AB, Linden CH, et al (eds): The Clinical Practice of Emergency Medicine, 3rd ed. Philadelphia, Lippincott Williams & Wilkins, 2001, pp 809–812.

7. Silen W: Acute intestinal obstruction. In Braunwald E, Fauci AS, Kasper DL, et al (eds): Harrison's Principles of Internal Medicine, 15th ed. New York, McGraw-Hill, 2001, pp 1703–1705.
8. Turnage RH, Bergen PC: Intestinal obstruction and ileus. In Feldman M, Sleisenger MH, Scharschmidt BF (eds): Sleisenger and Fordtran's Gastrointestinal and Liver Disease: Pathophysiology, Diagnosis, Management, 6th ed. Philadelphia, W.B. Saunders, 1998, pp 1799–1810.
9. Vicario SJ, Price TG: Intestinal obstruction. In Tintinalli JE, Kelen GA, Stapczynski JS (eds): Emergency Medicine: A Comprehensive Study Guide, 5th ed. New York, McGraw-Hill, 2000, pp 539–543.
10. Werman HA, Mekhjian HS, Rund DA: Ileitis, colitis, and diverticulitis. In Tintinalli JE, Kelen GA, Stapczynski JS (eds): Emergency Medicine: A Comprehensive Study Guide, 5th ed. New York, McGraw-Hill, 2000, pp 547–556.

40. ANORECTAL DISORDERS

Gregory W. Burcham, M.D.

1. What anorectal problems will I see in the ED?

The most frequent anorectal complaints are pain and bleeding. Pruritus, masses or swelling, difficulty with bowel movements, and discharge are less common complaints. The most common problems are hemorrhoids, anal fissures, abscesses and fistula, and infections. Other problems include foreign bodies, trauma, tumors, strictures, and prolapse. Bleeding, infection, strictures, trauma, and prolapse can be life-threatening emergencies. Because of the sensitive nature of the area and the complaints, patients often wait until the symptoms become intolerable before seeking medical attention.

2. How do I evaluate these disorders?

A good **history** includes the duration and character of symptoms, character of bowel habits and stool, prior gastrointestinal (GI) or anorectal complaints, medications, recent procedures or instrumentation, and sexual history and practices. The **digital rectal examination** is vital to diagnosis of most anorectal disorders. The physician should explain the procedure thoroughly to help the patient relax and to enlist the patient's cooperation. Adequate analgesia should be provided to permit a thorough examination. The patient should be placed either in the lateral decubitus position with the hips and knees flexed or on the elbows and knees. After visual examination of the buttocks and anal orifice, the examiner should apply gentle pressure against the anal orifice until the external sphincter relaxes and allows insertion. Asking the patient to bear down may help the sphincter relax. The examiner should note sphincter tone and function. The entire circumference of the anus and distal rectum should be palpated, followed by the prostate or cervix. A bidigital examination can examine masses for fluctuance, induration, or tenderness. When the finger is removed, the material on the glove should be examined for feces, blood, mucus, and pus.

3. Is there a way to examine the rectum visually?

Anoscopy can provide a direct view of the anus and distal rectum and is done easily in the ED. A lubricated anoscope with the obturator in place is advanced gently through the anal orifice. The obturator is removed to view the distal rectal mucosa, and the anoscope is withdrawn slowly, revealing the hemorrhoidal cushions, anal crypts, dentate line, and anal canal.

4. What are hemorrhoids?

Hemorrhoids are displaced anal cushions; they are not prolapsed veins. They are well vascularized and often present with bleeding. Hemorrhoids are the most common cause of hematochezia. Development is exacerbated by a prolonged increase in resting pressure in the anal canal, as seen in pregnancy, excessive straining, and in certain occupations (e.g., truck driver).

Patients also may complain of swelling, burning, itching, or masses. Many patients who complain of hemorrhoids have other conditions.

5. How do internal and external hemorrhoids differ?

Internal hemorrhoids arise above the dentate line, are covered by mucosa, and are not usually palpable or painful. They are seen easily during anoscopy. They typically present as bright red blood in the toilet bowl or on toilet paper. **External hemorrhoids** are covered by skin and are easily visible and palpable at the anal orifice. They typically present with pain and thrombosis. Bleeding is infrequent.

6. How are internal hemorrhoids treated?

Treatment depends on the degree of the hemorrhoid and the patient's symptoms:
- **First-degree hemorrhoids** project into the anal canal but do not prolapse through the anal opening.
- **Second-degree hemorrhoids** prolapse with defecation or straining but reduce spontaneously.
- **Third-degree hemorrhoids** prolapse and require manual reduction.
- **Fourth-degree hemorrhoids** prolapse and are irreducible.

Severe bleeding should be treated as any other GI bleed, starting with the ABCs (airway, breathing, circulation), volume and blood replacement, and emergent control of the hemorrhage with direct pressure. Treatment for mildly symptomatic first-degree, second-degree, and third-degree hemorrhoids should begin with sitz baths, stool softeners, a high-fiber diet, proper anal hygiene, and topical steroids. Nonthrombosed prolapsed hemorrhoids should be reduced gently, and conservative therapy should be initiated. Patients with intractable symptoms or fourth-degree hemorrhoids need surgical referral.

7. How are external hemorrhoids treated?

The conservative measures used for internal hemorrhoids are appropriate for nonthrombosed external hemorrhoids as well. Thrombosed external hemorrhoids can be excised if they present within 72 hours of onset of symptoms. Excision is done by infiltrating the area with a local anesthetic, preferably 0.5% bupivacaine with epinephrine. An elliptical incision is made over the hemorrhoid, and the skin and underlying thrombus are removed. The wound is left open and dressed, and the patient is discharged with stool softeners, sitz baths, and analgesics. The patient should have a wound check in 2 days. Thrombosed external hemorrhoids that present more than 72 hours from the time of onset respond well to conservative therapy plus analgesics and often do not require excision.

8. What else can cause rectal bleeding?

The most common cause of a lower GI bleed is an **upper GI bleed**. Upper GI sources usually present with melena but can bleed briskly enough to cause hematochezia. Besides hemorrhoids, common causes of rectal bleeding are anal fissures, abscesses, proctitis, and infectious colitis. Colorectal conditions, such as neoplasms, inflammatory bowel disease, rectal ulcers, polyps, diverticulosis, aortoenteric fistula, and ischemia, also must be considered.

9. What is an anal fissure?

A linear crack or ulcer in the epithelium in the distal anal canal. Anal fissures are the most common cause of anorectal pain. They usually extend outside the anal orifice and are visible by spreading the buttocks and applying gentle traction on the skin around the anal opening. The presence of a skin tag at the anal verge suggests a chronic fissure. Most are idiopathic, but any trauma to the anal canal can cause a fissure. Most benign anal fissures occur in the posterior midline, followed by the anterior midline. Fissures in other locations are associated more frequently with Crohn's disease, infection, malignancy, or immunodeficiency.

10. How do I treat an anal fissure?

Most anal fissures can be managed with sitz baths, stool softeners, a high-fiber diet, bulk laxatives, and analgesics. For recurrent or intractable symptoms, topical nitroglycerin ointment and botulinum toxin can decrease anal sphincter tone and have been successful in healing fissures. Chronic fissures and fissures that do not respond to conservative therapy should be referred to a surgeon for lateral internal sphincterotomy.

11. What are anorectal abscesses, and where are they located?

Anorectal abscesses are infections in the deep tissues around the dentate line. The abscess probably begins with infection of an anal gland where it drains into the anal crypt. The infection spreads to one of four abscess sites (Figure). Mixed aerobic-anaerobic flora typically are present, including, *Escherichia coli*, *Proteus*, *Staphylococcus*, *Streptrococcus*, *Bacteroides*, and *Peptostreptococcus*.

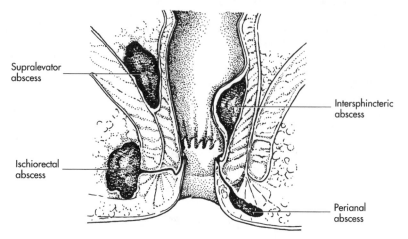

Location of common anorectal abscesses. (From Coates WC: Disorders of the anorectum. In Rosen P, Barkin RM (eds): Emergency Medicine: Concepts and Clinical Practice, 4th ed. St. Louis, Mosby, 1998, pp 2037–2052; with permission.)

Perianal abscesses are the most common (40% to 50%). These result from superficial extension and are located adjacent to the anal orifice, where they usually are obvious. They present as a visible, palpable, painful mass. Fever and leukocytosis are rare.

Ischiorectal abscesses result from lateral extension of the infection into the ischiorectal space. They are less obvious on external examination but may show induration, erythema, and tenderness in the buttock. Bidigitial rectal examination can help delineate these abscesses.

Intersphincteric abscesses, also called *submucosal abscesses*, result from local spread of infection in the anal gland. As the name indicates, the abscess is located between the internal and external sphincters. Abscesses present with rectal pain that is worsened during bowel movements. External examination is normal. A tender mass is palpable on digital examination at the dentate line.

Supralevator or **ischiorectal abscesses** are the least common (2% to 9%). They result from proximal spread of infection above the levator ani. Patients may complain of severe perirectal or deep buttock pain or low pelvic or abdominal pain. The external examination is normal, and the mass may be distal to the examiner's finger. These patients can appear toxic, and fever and an elevated white blood cell count are common. CT is often necessary to localize intersphincteric and supralevator abscesses.

12. Can any anorectal abscesses be treated in the ED?

Incisional drainage should be attempted only in small superficial abscesses. Most perianal and some ischiorectal abscesses are appropriate. The skin should be prepared with an iodine solution, and the roof and the periphery of the abscess should be well infiltrated with local anesthetic.

The acidic nature of the abscess and the well-innervated skin in the perianal area make good anesthesia difficult, and oral or parenteral narcotics and sedation may be necessary. The abscess should be incised as close to the anal verge as possible, pus drained, and loculations broken up using a finger for blunt dissection. The wound should be packed lightly with iodoform gauze, which the patient should remove in 24 hours. The patient should begin sitz baths and, if possible, daily irrigation and packing changes. A wound check should be done in 48 hours. The patient should be referred to a surgeon to be evaluated for the development of a fistula. Intersphincteric and supralevator abscesses and some deep or complicated ischiorectal abscesses require admission and surgical or CT-guided drainage.

13. Does a fistula always develop from an abscess?

Anorectal fistulas develop after ischiorectal abscesses in 50% to 66% of cases and less frequently after other anorectal abscesses. They also are seen with Crohn's disease, malignancy, trauma, and tuberculosis. The patient may complain of a chronic draining sinus on the buttock and give a history of prior anorectal complaints. Fistula should not be probed, and patients should be referred to a surgeon for fistulotomy or marsupialization of the fistula. If a fistula and abscess occur together, the abscess should be drained and the fistula left intact for delayed treatment.

14. What is Fournier's gangrene?

An acute life-threatening fasciitis in the perineal tissue planes. Mixed GI flora are usually the cause, often from a perirectal abscess or fistula, but any perineal or genital cellulitis or abscess can precipitate Fournier's gangrene. The infection is seen most commonly in diabetics and elderly men. Fournier's gangrene typically starts in the scrotum or perineum and progresses rapidly up the abdominal wall. Necrosis of the overlying skin and subcutaneous tissues occurs, leading to sepsis. Even with prompt surgical débridement and broad-spectrum antibiotics, mortality can be 50%.

15. Discuss other infections that occur in the anorectum.

Chlamydia and **gonorrhea** are common causes of proctitis. Chlamydia can cause lymphogranuloma venereum. Chlamydia and gonorrhea are transmitted via anorectal or oral-anal intercourse. Most patients infected with chlamydia are symptomatic, whereas only about 10% of patients infected with gonorrhea are symptomatic. Proctitis presents with rectal pain and tenesmus. Anoscopic examination reveals an erythematous, friable mucosa with a bloody or mucoid discharge and ulcerations. Untreated lymphogranuloma venereum can result in fistulas, abscesses, or rectal strictures. Strictures can be a surgical emergency requiring emergent dilation. Symptomatic patients should be treated for both organisms because of the high rate of coinfection. Doxycycline, 100 mg orally twice daily for 7 days, and azithromycin, 1 g orally once, plus ceftriaxone, 125 mg intramuscularly, are acceptable regimens. Sexual contacts also should be treated.

Herpes simplex virus is another common cause of proctitis. It is especially common in homosexual men. Rectal and anal ulceration is seen. Rectal pain, tenesmus, mucopurulent discharge, and pruritus are common. Strictures occur frequently with chronic disease. Treatment consists of oral acyclovir, 400 mg orally five times daily for 10 days. Analgesics and stool softeners also are necessary.

Anal condylomata are caused by **human papillomavirus**. Lesions appear as cauliflower-like or warty projections around the anal opening. Patients complain of pruritus, bleeding, and pain. Intraanal lesions are common. Serial treatments are necessary, and these patients should receive referral and prompt follow-up.

16. What is rectal prolapse?

The eversion and protrusion of the rectum through the anal opening during defecation, similar to a sock turning inside out as it is removed. It is most common in children younger than age 5 years and women older than 50 years. In children, this is a temporary condition relating to immaturity of the rectal floor in the face of constipation and straining. It can be associated with cystic fibrosis. Treatment consists of dietary advice and toilet retraining. In older women, the pelvic floor is fatigued and lax, nearly always due to chronic constipation and straining. Bulk laxatives can lessen constipation, and surgical procedures or sclerotherapy are options for recurrent cases. In most cases, applying gentle steady pressure to the rectal tissue easily reduces the prolapse.

17. How do I remove a foreign body from the rectum?

Foreign bodies in the rectum can be ingested orally or inserted through the anus. Patients often invent interesting stories to explain their condition, but an accurate history is necessary before attempting removal. Plain radiographs can be helpful to evaluate the object and can diagnose perforation if free air is noted. Ingested foreign bodies pass spontaneously. Most other foreign bodies can be retrieved manually with an adequately relaxed and sedated patient, allowing relaxation of the anal sphincters. Placing the patient in the lithotomy position allows the examiner to apply suprapubic pressure to assist in expulsion. For difficult objects, a Foley catheter can be advanced beyond the foreign body, the balloon inflated, and gentle traction applied. Plaster of Paris has been used in hollow foreign bodies to cement a handle or string in place to assist with retraction. General anesthesia sometimes is necessary. After removal, thorough examination of the rectum with an anoscope or sigmoidoscope is mandatory to rule out perforation.

BIBLIOGRAPHY

1. Andrews NJ, Jones DJ: Rectal prolapse and associated conditions. BMJ 305:243–246, 1992.
2. Brenner BE, Simon RR: Anorectal emergencies. Ann Emerg Med 12:367–376, 1983.
3. Coates WC: Anorectum. In Marx JA, et al (eds): Rosen's Emergency Medicine: Concepts and Clinical Practice, 4th ed. St. Louis, Mosby, 2002.
4. Fry RD: Anorectal trauma and foreign bodies. Surg Clin North Am 74:1491–1505, 1994.
5. Hancock BD: Haemorrhoids. BMJ 304:1042–1044, 1992.
6. Janicke DM, Pundt MR: Anorectal disorders. Emerg Med Clin North Am 14:757–788, 1996.
7. Jones DJ, Irving MH: Investigation of colorectal disorders. BMJ 304:974–977, 1992.
8. Loder PB, Kamm MA, Nicholls RJ, Phillips RKS: Haemorrhoids: Pathology, pathophysiology, and aetiology. Br J Surg 81:946–954, 1994.
9. Lund JN, Scholefield JH: Aetiology and treatment of anal fissure. Br J Surg 83:1335–1344, 1996.
10. Mazier WP: Hemorrhoids, fissures, and pruritus ani. Surg Clin North Am 74:1277–1292, 1994.
11. Nelson H, Dozois RR: Anus. In Townsend CM (ed): Sabiston's Textbook of Surgery: The Biological Basis of Modern Surgical Practice, 16th ed. Philadelphia, W.B. Saunders, 2001.

VIII. Genitourinary Tract

41. RENAL COLIC

Christopher M.B. Fernandes, M.D., and Grant D. Innes, M.D.

1. What are the most common forms of renal stones?

Calcium stones account for 80% of all renal stones: Two thirds are calcium oxalate, and the remainder are calcium phosphate. Struvite (magnesium ammonium phosphate), uric acid, and cystine account for 20% of renal stones.

2. List factors that predispose to stone formation.

Calcium stones:
   Chronic dehydration
   Antacid use
   Hypercalciuria
   Hyperoxaluria
   Acid urine
   Ingestion of vitamins A, C, and D

Struvite stones:
   Chronic infection by urea-splitting organisms

Cystine stones:
   Cystinuria

3. Name the lethal conditions that often are misdiagnosed as renal colic.

Aortic and iliac aneurysms. A careful search for bruits and pulsatile masses is mandatory when renal colic is suspected.

4. What clinical features help distinguish renal colic from other causes of abdominal pain?

Renal colic usually begins abruptly, causing terrible pain in the flank, costovertebral angle, lateral abdomen, and genitals. Patients often are profoundly distressed, more so than patients with other abdominal pathologies. Pallor, diaphoresis, restlessness, and nausea are prominent. Renal colic causes flank tenderness, but in contrast to other causes of lateralized abdominal pain (e.g., appendicitis, diverticulitis, cholelithiasis, and ectopic pregnancy), it produces little or no abdominal tenderness.

5. In which patients would imaging be absolutely indicated to confirm the diagnosis of renal colic?

 • Patients with a first episode of renal colic
 • Patients in whom the diagnosis is unclear
 • Patients in whom a proximal urinary tract infection, in addition to a calculus, is suspected

6. What is the role of the abdominal flat plate in diagnosing renal colic?

The abdominal flat plate, or *kidneys-ureter-bladder (KUB)*, is less sensitive and less specific than the clinical examination and, by itself, has no role in the workup of suspected renal colic. If a stone is diagnosed on ultrasound, it may be appropriate to view the stone on a plain film. Subsequent radiographs may be helpful to document stone progression.

7. Has helical CT supplanted the intravenous pyelogram (IVP) as the diagnostic test of choice? Why or why not?

Helical noncontrast CT has replaced IVP as the preferred diagnostic test. The IVP pinpoints stone size and location, clarifies the degree of obstruction, and shows ongoing renal function. Helical CT has been shown to be 97% sensitive and 96% specific in diagnosing renal stones. Used for this purpose, helical CT does not require intravenous contrast material and is faster than IVP—requiring only 1 to 2 minutes of scanner time to complete a study. Even though helical CT provides no information about renal function, this can be ascertained by a urinalysis and serum creatinine. The marginal cost is less, and it can identify other important causes of flank pain.

8. Name the two major contraindications to an IVP.

Allergy to contrast material and renal failure. Allergic reactions are uncommon. If a patient claims to be allergic to IVP dye, ask what his or her reaction was. Flushing and nausea often occur after injection and are not allergic reactions. Urticaria, stridor, wheezing, and syncope suggest a true allergy. If the patient has had a significant reaction in the past, there is a 15% chance of recurrence. Asthmatics are at higher risk of allergic reactions. In patients at risk of allergy or contrast-mediated nephrotoxicity, nonionic (low osmolar) contrast material is preferable.

9. In what other patients might intravenous contrast material be hazardous?

Patients older than 60 years and patients with underlying renal disease, diabetes, or myeloma all are at risk of contrast-mediated nephrotoxicity. Determine the blood urea nitrogen (BUN) and creatinine levels in all such patients, and reconsider the need for the IVP if serum creatinine is greater than 2.0. If the IVP is deemed necessary despite a risk factor, hydrate the patient adequately before contrast infusion or consider helical CT.

10. Is pregnancy a contraindication to IVP?

Ultrasound is the investigation of choice in pregnant patients, but if ultrasound is nondiagnostic, a limited IVP (scout film and 20 minutes postinjection film, preferably coned to the area of concern) is appropriate.

11. What IVP findings suggest a renal stone?

Typical findings include a delayed, intense, and often prolonged nephrogram on the involved side, delayed filling and dilation of the affected collecting system (hydroureter and hydronephrosis), and an uninterrupted column of dye extending from the kidney to the calculus. An unobstructed ureter, because it is peristaltic, does not normally appear opacified with contrast in its entirety.

12. Why is the postvoid film important, and what other special views are helpful?

Contrast in the bladder obscures the distal ureter. The postvoid film provides optimal visualization of the distal ureter and the ureterovesical junction. The postvoid film also shows whether the bladder is emptying completely. Oblique views help to confirm that a visualized stone is in, rather than overlying, the ureter. Prone films often provide a better view of the ureter than do standard supine films.

13. What if the ureter is not visualized on the standard IVP?

In high-grade ureteral obstruction, contrast material may not reach the distal ureter for many hours. If the ureter cannot be visualized at 1 hour, take a 2-hour film. If this fails, take a 4-hour film. The interval between films should be doubled until adequate visualization is achieved. It is important not to abandon the IVP until contrast material reaches the calculus.

14. Name the most common sites of stone impaction.

The ureteropelvic junction, the pelvic brim (where the ureter crosses the iliac vessels), and the ureterovesical junction (the most narrow point in the ureter).

15. Can the likelihood of spontaneous passage be predicted based on the size and location of the stone?

Stones reaching the distal ureter are more likely to pass than those impacting proximally. Stones smaller than 4 mm pass 90% of the time, stones 4 to 6 mm pass 50% of the time, and stones larger than 6 mm pass 10% of the time. When estimating stone size, remember that the x-ray image is magnified; the actual size is 80% of what is measured on the films.

16. What if the imaging study is normal, but the patient still appears to have renal colic?

Reexamine the patient carefully to ensure that you have not missed another cause of abdominal pain and that the patient is not developing a condition requiring surgery. If the physical examination is still compatible with renal colic, treat the patient, not the test result. Occasional false-negative results occur with all tests, and imaging modalities may miss small stones, but this may not be clinically relevant because small stones are unlikely to require specific therapy.

17. Isn't an ultrasound just as accurate as helical CT or an IVP?

Ultrasound is safe and noninvasive but is more prone to false-negative results than the other studies. Ultrasound is sensitive for stones in the bladder and renal pelvis but often fails to visualize those in the mid and distal ureter—the most common sites for stone impaction. When ultrasound fails to identify a stone, however, it may show dilation of the renal collecting system, providing evidence of ureteral obstruction.

18. List secondary signs of ureteral obstruction shown on helical CT.
* Unlateral obstruction
* Stranding of perinephric fat
* Hydronephrosis
* Nephromegaly

19. What is the soft tissue rim sign on helical CT, and how is it useful?

This sign shows soft tissue attentuation around a ureteral calculus and helps differentiate a calculus from a phlebolith.

20. What other tests are useful in the ED?

Urine dipsticks are sensitive for microscopic hematuria, which is present in 80% of patients with renal colic. Urinalysis is recommended to rule out pyuria and bacteriuria. Urine culture is indicated if symptoms, signs, or urinalysis findings suggest infection. Determination of BUN, creatinine, and electrolyte levels is helpful if the patient has been vomiting or if presence of an underlying renal disease is suspected. There is no need for a more extensive metabolic workup in the ED.

21. Why is coexistent infection a major problem?

Bacteria in an obstructed collecting system can cause abscess formation, renal destruction, and bacteremia quickly. The presence of infection in an obstructed ureter mandates immediate consultation with a urologist and high-dose intravenous antibiotics.

22. Has lithotripsy supplanted percutaneous and open surgical methods of stone removal?

Not always. Optimal therapy depends on the size, type, and location of the stone. Ureteroscopic techniques probably are still preferable for lower ureteral stones. Extracorporeal shock wave lithotripsy (ESWL) is optimal for stones 2 cm in size, particularly those in the renal pelvis. Percutaneous stone removal techniques are indicated for larger stones, when there is obstructive uropathy, and when less invasive techniques have failed. For some stones, a combination of ESWL followed by percutaneous instrumentation is optimal. Some large stones still require open surgery. The method of removal is best determined by a urologist.

23. What are the basics of ED treatment of renal colic?

Hydration, analgesia, and antiemetics. Unless the patient is elderly or has a history of renal or congestive heart failure, normal saline should be infused in volumes sufficient to produce a urine output of at least 100 mL/h. Various analgesics and antiemetics are available for rapid control of symptoms (see Table). Intravenous opioids, which provide the most rapid onset of effective analgesia, should be given immediately. Rectal or intravenous nonsteroidal antiinflammatory drugs (NSAIDs), which inhibit renal prostaglandin synthesis, are effective and may be given concurrently with opioids. Optimal ED pain control involves the combined administration of NSAIDs and opioids (balanced analgesia).

Analgesics and Antiemetics for Renal Colic

Opioid Analgesics			
Meperidine (Demerol)	IV 25–50 mg	q 5–10 min	prn
	IM 1–2 mg/kg	q 2 hr	prn[*]
Morphine sulphate	IV 3–5 mg	q 5–10 min	prn
	IM 0.1–0.2 mg/kg	q 3 hr	prn[*]
Oxycodone and acetylsalicylic acid (Percodan)	PO 2 tabs	q 4 hr	prn
Oxycodone and acetaminophen (Percocet)	PO 2 tabs	q 4 hr	prn
Anileridine (Leritine)	PO 50 mg	q 4 hr	prn
Antiemetics			
Metoclopramide (Reglan)	IV 10–20 mg	q 15 min	prn
Perphenazine (Trilafon)	IM 5 mg	q 6 hr	prn[*]
	PO 4 mg	q 6 hr	prn
Prochlorperazine (Compazine)	IV 5–10 mg	q 4 hr	prn
	IM 5–10 mg	q 6 hr	prn[*]
	PO 5–10 mg	q 4 hr	prn
Nonsteroidal Analgesics			
Ketorolac (Toradol)	IV 30 mg	q 6 hr[†]	
	IM 30 mg	q 6 hr[†]	
Indomethacin	50- or 100-mg suppositories, 200 mg/day		
Diclofenac (Voltaren)	50- or 100-mg suppositories, 150 mg/day		

[*] IM route not recommended for ED management of acute, severe pain
[†] Not to exceed 150 mg/day

24. Who requires hospitalization?

Patients with high-grade obstruction, intractable pain or vomiting, associated urinary tract infection, a solitary or transplanted kidney, and in whom the diagnosis is uncertain. Obtain urologic consultation for patients with stones larger than 6 mm in diameter, regardless of symptoms.

25. What advice should I give to patients being discharged from the ED?

Patients should be advised to drink plenty of fluids, strain their urine, follow-up with their family physician in 3 days, and return to the ED if they develop symptoms of infection or recurrent severe pain.

26. Which analgesics are recommended for outpatient pain control?

Gastrointestinal irritation limits the usefulness of oral NSAIDs in patients with renal colic; however, rectal NSAIDs (diclofenac, indomethacin) may provide adequate analgesia. If necessary, oral opioids can be combined with NSAIDs in patients with documented ureteral calculi.

27. What should I tell patients about long-term prevention of renal stones?

Patients prone to stone formation should hydrate themselves to the point that they are passing dilute urine. Elimination of rhubarb, beets, spinach, beer, cola, coffee, citrus fruit, and vitamin C from the diet may reduce the risk of calcium oxalate stones. A variety of specific treatment regimens exists, depending on the type of stone produced by the patient. Given the uncertainty of recurrence—only 50% to 70% of patients have recurrent stones—and the fact that lifetime compliance with dietary modification and drugs is poor, prophylactic measures for renal colic may not be reasonable.

28. When should patients return to the ED?

Patients should be instructed to seek medical care immediately if they have continued or increasing pain, nausea and vomiting, fever or chills, or any other new symptoms.

BIBLIOGRAPHY

1. Begun FP, Foley WD, Peterson A, White B: Patient evaluation: Laboratory and imaging studies. Urol Clin North Am 24:97–116, 1997.
2. Cordell WH, Larson TA, Lingeman JE, et al: Indomethacin suppositories vs. intravenous titrated morphine for the treatment of ureteral colic. Ann Emerg Med 23:262–269, 1994.
3. Escobar JI, Eastman ER, Harwood-Nuss AL: Selected urologic problems. In Marx JA, Hockberger RS, Walls RM (eds): Rosen's Emergency Medicine, 4th ed. St. Louis, Mosby, 2002, pp 1414–1421.
4. Fontanarosa PB: Radiologic contrast induced renal failure. Emerg Med Clin North Am 3:601–613, 1988.
5. Hendricks SK, Ross SO, Krieger JN: An algorithm for diagnosis and therapy of management and complications of urolithiasis during pregnancy. Surg Gynecol Obstet 172:49–54, 1991.
6. Hetherington JW, Philp NH: Diclofenac sodium versus pethidine in acute renal colic. BMJ 292:237–238, 1986.
7. Juul N, Burns J, Torp-Pedersen S, Fredfeldt KE: Ultrasound versus intravenous urography in the initial evaluation of patients with suspected obstructing urinary calculi. Scand J Urol Nephrol Suppl 137:45–47, 1991.
8. Manthey DE: Nephrolithiasis. Emerg Med Clin North Am 19:633–654, 2001.
9. Mutgi A, Williams JW, Nettleman M: Renal colic—utility of the plain abdominal roentgenogram. Arch Intern Med 151:1589–1592, 1991.
10. Segura JW: Current surgical approaches to nephrolithiasis. Endocrinol Metab Clin North Am 19:919–935, 1990.
11. Segura JW: Role of percutaneous procedures in the management of renal calculi. Urol Clin North Am 17:207–216, 1990.
12. Sheley RC: Helical CT in the evaluation of renal colic. Am J Emerg Med 17:279–282, 1999.
13. Sinclair D, Wilson S, Toi A, Greenspan L: The evaluation of suspected renal colic: Ultrasound scan versus excretory urography. Ann Emerg Med 18:556–559, 1989.
14. Spencer BA: Helical CT and ureteral colic. Urol Clin North Am 27:231–241, 2000.
15. Stewart C: Nephrolithiasis. Emerg Med Clin North Am 6:617–629, 1988.
16. Van Arsdalen KN, Banner MP, Pollack HM: Radiologic imaging and urologic decision making in the management of renal and ureteral calculi. Urol Clin North Am 17:171–190, 1990.

42. SCROTAL PAIN

Robert E. Schneider, M.D.

1. What is the differential diagnosis in a patient with acute scrotal pain?

Testicular torsion always must be considered in any patient with a history of acute scrotal pain. The differential diagnosis is age dependent. In patients 15 years old or younger, the differential diagnosis includes testicular torsion; torsion of a testicular or epididymal appendix; epididymitis; and, rarely, orchitis, acute hematocele, or idiopathic scrotal edema. In patients older than 15, the differential diagnosis includes testicular torsion, epididymitis, torsion of a testicular or epididymal appendix, and testicular tumor.

2. What is testicular torsion?

The result of a congenital developmental abnormality that involves the testicle and the tunica vaginalis. In the normal state, the visceral tunica vaginalis covers the anterolateral portion of the testis and the lateral portion of the epididymis, whereas the parietal tunica vaginalis acts as an envelope and fixes the testis and epididymis to the posterior scrotal wall. This fixation eliminates the freedom for rotation and subsequent torsion. In the abnormal state, both layers of the tunica vaginalis totally encircle the testis and epididymis (similar to a clapper in a bell, hence bell-clapper deformity) so that these structures are free to rotate on their cord secondary to any stimulus that may promote cremaster muscle contraction. This can lead to varying degrees of testicular torsion.

3. When is testicular torsion most likely to occur?

The first year of life and puberty are the ages of peak occurrence. It is 10 times more likely to occur in a patient with an undescended testis.

4. How is testicular torsion diagnosed?

Surgical exploration is the only definitive diagnostic method. For complete torsion, the window of warm ischemia is 4 to 6 hours. No clinical findings, laboratory tests, or radiographic studies can approach the sensitivity of surgical exploration. Adjunctive studies used in the diagnosis include

1. Physical examination to document the presence or absence of the cremasteric reflex.
2. Attempted manual detorsion with or without the aid of a Doppler stethoscope.
3. Radionuclide testicular scan.
4. Duplex color Doppler ultrasonography.
5. MRI.

5. What is the significance of cremasteric reflex?

The cremasteric reflex is a spinal cord reflex encompassing T12–L2 nerve roots and is elicited by stroking the inner aspect of the involved thigh. In a normal state, the ipsilateral testis retracts in a superior fashion as the cremaster muscle contracts. Any inflammatory process that fixes the testis to the surrounding scrotal wall or inhibits contraction of the cremaster muscle prevents elicitation of this reflex. A torsed testis may lose its cremasteric reflex as a result of twisting of the spermatic cord.

6. What is manual detorsion, and how do I perform it?

A maneuver used to untwist the spermatic cord to reestablish blood flow to the testis. This procedure should be done in any patient with suspected testicular torsion while the patient is being readied for the operating room. Because most testes torse lateral to medial, the procedure is as follows. If you were to stand at the foot of the patient's bed, you would perform the detorsion maneuver for either testis just as you would open a book, rotating each testicle in a medial to lateral direction. If testicular torsion has progressed to the point where there is fixation of the scrotal contents to the overlying scrotal skin, testicular detorsion is not possible. Successful detorsion results in immediate reduction of pain or complete pain relief and allows an emergent operative procedure to be done electively within 24 to 48 hours. In many cases, detorsion is not successful or the testis twists again; surgical fixation is still indicated.

7. What is Doppler evaluation of the spermatic cord?

Doppler evaluation is done by placing a Doppler stethoscope over the superior portion of the at-risk spermatic cord and attempting to measure arterial flow to the involved testis. The interpretation of this examination is subjective and by itself is not diagnostic. Absent or diminished arterial flow strongly supports the diagnosis of torsion. The presence of flow does *not* exclude this diagnosis. The use of this technique in conjunction with manual detorsion to confirm an increase in blood flow after the detorsion maneuver has some merit.

8. What is the utility of radionuclide scans and Doppler ultrasound?

After injection of a radionuclide substance into a peripheral vein, a scanner is used to document the presence of the radionuclide substance in the testis, showing arterial inflow. This examination is invasive, time-consuming, and reader dependent and has no place in the time-sensitive diagnostic armamentarium of testicular torsion. Duplex color Doppler ultrasonography is noninvasive, can be done much faster, and has a specificity of 100%. It also is reader dependent, however, and should not delay surgical exploration.

9. How are these tests helpful in the management of testicular torsion?
These studies are truly adjunctive and in no way should preclude or delay surgical exploration when the diagnosis of testicular torsion is suspected.

10. What is the treatment of choice for testicular torsion?
Surgical exploration. The involved testis must be detorsed surgically, then evaluated for viability. If the testis is deemed to be salvageable, it is fixed (pexed) to the medial and lateral scrotal wall with nonabsorbable suture material. If it is deemed unsalvageable, the testis is removed. Because testicular torsion is a bilateral phenomenon, the uninvolved testis should be pexed prophylactically to prevent subsequent development of torsion.

11. What is torsion of the appendix testis and appendix epididymis?
The testicular and epididymal appendices are müllerian and wolffian duct remnants that have no physiologic function. They are subject to torsion because of their anatomic stalk. In contrast to torsion of the testis, physical examination of a torsed appendix early in its course discloses point tenderness over the involved appendix. Late in its course, generalized scrotal tenderness may be encountered, making differentiation from testicular torsion impossible and necessitating scrotal exploration. In an unequivocal case of appendiceal torsion, ice, bed rest, nonsteroidal antiinflammatory drugs, and pain medication are the treatment modalities. The affected appendix subsequently necroses over 10 to 14 days and becomes asymptomatic.

12. What is orchitis, and how common is it?
Inflammation of the testis. It usually is unilateral, and it occurs most commonly in association with mumps. Its relatively infrequent occurrence should prompt reconsideration of the history and physical findings to be certain not to miss a more serious diagnosis, such as testicular torsion, epididymitis, or testicular tumor.

13. What is epididymitis? What are the physical findings?
Inflammation of the epididymis, the tubular structure that lies on the posterolateral portion of the testis. Epididymitis begins in the area of the ejaculatory ducts found in the prostatic urethra. Infected and occasionally sterile urine refluxes in a retrograde fashion down the vas deferens to the globus minor or tail of the epididymis, initiating the inflammatory response. The history is usually that of a gradual onset of unilateral scrotal pain reaching a peak over several days and associated with fever. When evaluated at this stage, the examiner feels an isolated mass at the inferiormost portion of the epididymis adjacent to the testis. The remainder of the testis and scrotal contents are normal. With inflammation confined solely to the epididymis, the sulcus or groove that separates the epididymis from the testis is uninvolved and easily identifiable during examination. If the process is allowed to progress, inflammation spreads to the body of the epididymis and subsequently to the superiormost portion of the epididymis known as the *globus major* or *head of the epididymis*.

14. What is epididymoorchitis?
Severe inflammation of the epididymis that has progressed onto the contiguous testis. The normally palpable sulcus between the epididymis and testis is obliterated, and a large tender scrotal mass results. This severe form of epididymitis must be treated aggressively.

15. List the most common causes of epididymitis in a 20-year-old man. What about a 50-year-old man?
In a **20-year-old man**, the most common cause of epididymitis is related to sexually transmitted diseases. The most common organisms are *Chlamydia trachomatis*, followed by *Neisseria*

gonorrhoeae and *Ureaplasma urealyticum.* In contrast, the most common cause of epididymitis in a **50-year-old man** is gram-negative rods, such as *Escherichia coli* and *Klebsiella,* and, rarely, *Pseudomonas* species. The older patient with epididymitis presents an additional diagnostic challenge because the physician must discover why the patient's urine is infected (e.g., is it outlet obstruction or a urethral stricture?).

16. What is the treatment for epididymitis or epididymoorchitis?

A patient who is febrile and toxic should be admitted to the hospital for intravenous antibiotics and possible diagnostic studies to exclude a scrotal or testicular abscess (testicular ultrasound). Otherwise, outpatient therapy includes bed rest with placement of a folded towel between the legs to elevate the affected hemiscrotum. Ice is placed on the affected testis or epididymis for 10 minutes at a time, three or four times a day. The patient may get up to eat or to go to the bathroom. When he is pain-free at rest, he may begin to ambulate with some type of scrotal supporter. If pain recurs, the patient should resume absolute bed rest and begin the process again.

When sexually transmitted disease is suspected to be the cause of the epididymitis, the patient should be cultured for chlamydia and gonorrhea, then treated empirically with ceftriaxone, 125 mg intramuscularly; cefixime, 400 mg orally; ciprofloxacin, 500 mg orally; or ofloxacin, 400 mg orally, and doxycycline, 100 mg twice a day for 7 to 10 days, or azithromycin (Zithromax), 1 g orally, in the ED before discharge. The patient's sexual partner should be referred for evaluation and treatment. When gram-negative organisms are thought to be the cause of the epididymitis, treatment is based on the suspected organism. For patients who have not been sexually active, a 14-day treatment with trimethoprim-sulfamethoxazole or ciprofloxacin is appropriate.

All patients should be treated with antiinflammatory agents. If it becomes necessary to prescribe narcotics, it is prudent to place the patient on stool softeners to avoid straining to have a bowel movement because this may exacerbate the inflammatory process. All patients should be referred to a urologist within 1 week of initiation of outpatient therapy. If a large inflammatory mass is present, the urologist will need to proceed with testicular ultrasound to ensure the patient does not have a testicular abscess or testicular tumor.

BIBLIOGRAPHY

1. Cattolica EV: Preoperative manual detorsion of the torsed spermatic cord. J Urol 133:803–805, 1985.
2. Chen DC, Holder LE, Melloul M: Radionuclide scrotal imaging: Further experience with 210 patients: Part II. Results and discussion. J Nucl Med 24:841–853, 1983.
3. Edelsberg JS, Surh YS: The acute scrotum. Emerg Med Clin North Am 6:521–546, 1988.
4. Escobar JI, Eastman ER, Harwood-Nuss AL: Selected urologic problems. In Marx JA, Hockberger RS, Walls RM (eds): Rosen's Emergency Medicine, 4th ed. St. Louis, Mosby, 2002, pp 1414–1421.
5. Kaver I, Matzkin H, Braf ZF: Epididymo-orchitis: A retrospective study of 122 patients. J Fam Pract 30:548–552, 1990.
6. Lindsey D, Stanisic TH: Diagnosis and management of testicular torsion: Pitfalls and perils. Am J Emerg Med 6:42–46, 1988.
7. Melekos MD, Asbach HW, Markou SA: Etiology of acute scrotum in 100 boys with regard to age distribution. J Urol 139:1023–1025, 1988.
8. Middleton WD, Siegel BA, Melson GL, et al: Acute scrotal disorders: Prospective comparison of color Doppler US and testicular scintigraphy. Radiology 177:177–181, 1990.
9. Rabinowitz RL: The importance of the cremasteric reflex in acute scrotal swelling in children. J Urol 132:89–90, 1984.
10. Smith GI: Cellular changes for graded testicular ischemia. J Urol 73:355, 1955.

43. ACUTE URINARY RETENTION

Samuel J. Killian, M.D., and John P. Marshall, M.D.

1. What is acute urinary retention (AUR)?

A painful inability to urinate. AUR is most commonly the result of bladder outlet obstruction, but it also may result from neurogenic, pharmacologic, or other causes of detrusor muscle dysfunction. Urine is produced normally but is retained in the bladder, which then becomes distended and uncomfortable.

2. Is there chronic urinary retention?

Yes. It generally represents prolonged retention. The hallmarks of chronic urinary retention are the absence of pain and common association with overflow incontinence. It most frequently occurs in mentally debilitated or neurologically compromised patients.

3. What is the most common cause of AUR? Who gets it?

Obstruction of the lower urinary tract (bladder and urethra) is the most common cause encountered in the ED. The usual site of obstruction is the prostate gland, but lesions of the urethra or penis also may cause retention. In general, AUR is a disease of older men, although it occasionally is encountered in women. Patients with indwelling catheters (suprapubic or Foley) are at risk for episodes of retention because of obstruction or dysfunction of these drainage systems.

4. How does benign prostatic hypertrophy (BPH) cause AUR?

BPH with bladder neck obstruction is the most common cause of AUR. Of men older than age 60, 50% have histologic evidence of BPH. As the prostate hypertrophies, urine outflow is obstructed by enlargement of the median lobe of the gland impinging on the internal urethral lumen. The typical patient with BPH gives a progressive history suggestive of urinary outlet obstruction. Symptoms such as hesitancy, diminished stream quality, dribbling, nocturia, and the sensation of incomplete bladder emptying may precede the episode of acute retention. New medications or increased fluid loads may precipitate an acute episode of retention in these patients.

5. List the other causes of AUR.

- **Obstructive**: BPH, prostate carcinoma, prostatitis, urethral stricture, posterior urethral valves, phimosis, paraphimosis, meatal stenosis, calculi, blood clots, clogged or crimped Foley catheter.
- **Neurogenic**: Spinal cord injuries, herniated lumbosacral discs (cauda equina syndrome), tumors, diabetes, multiple sclerosis, tabes dorsalis, syringomyelia, herpes.
- **Pharmacologic**: Anticholinergics, antihistamines, tricyclic antidepressants, antispasmodics, narcotics, amphetamines, sympathomimetics, antipsychotics, antiparkinsonian agents (see question 14).
- **Psychogenic**: Diagnosis of exclusion.

6. What are the important features in the history and physical examination?

When taking the history, any previous prostate or urethral conditions should be elicited. Patients often have a history of chronic voiding hesitancy, a decreased force to the urinary stream, a feeling of incomplete bladder emptying, or nocturia. Information about neurologic symptoms, trauma, previous instrumentation, back pain, and current medication is essential. On physical examination, the distended bladder often is palpable above the pubic rim. The genitalia are usually normal. The penis and particularly the urethra should be examined carefully for any signs of stricture, which may be evident on palpation. A rectal examination is essential and often provides clues to the diagnosis of BPH, prostate carcinoma, or prostatitis. A careful neurologic examination, including rectal tone and perineal sensation, is vital in any patient suspected of having a neurologic lesion.

7. Are there any red flags in the history and physical examination that might indicate a more serious, potentially surgical, cause?

Yes. New urinary symptoms, particularly obstruction, in patients with a history of trauma or back pain should alert the examiner to the possibility of **spinal cord compression** resulting from disc herniation, fracture, epidural hematoma, epidural abscess, or tumor. Be especially suspicious if there is no prior history of bladder, prostate, or urethral conditions.

8. How do I treat AUR?

Catheterization and bladder decompression using a Foley catheter.

9. What if I can't pass a Foley catheter?

Occasionally, simple passage of a 16F or 18F Foley catheter cannot be accomplished. One trick that often helps is to fill a 30-mL syringe with lidocaine (Xylocaine) jelly and inject it into the urethral meatus. Still no luck? Try a 20F coudé catheter. The coudé-tipped catheter has a gentle upward curve in the distal 3 cm that may be helpful in pointing the catheter up and over the enlarged prostatic lobe. Never force a catheter through an area of significant resistance because this can cause urethral perforation, false lumens, and subsequent stricture formation.

10. Is bigger better?

A loaded question. If you are unable to pass a 16F (standard adult) catheter, it is generally recommended to move up in size to a 18F or 20F Foley catheter. Usually the stiffness and larger bulk of the bigger catheter is more successful in passing through the bladder neck than a smaller, more flexible catheter. Remember, never force a catheter through significant resistance.

11. What if nothing is working?

If you still cannot pass a catheter, the obstruction may be more severe than anticipated, or a stricture may be present. One clue to the presence of a stricture is that the obstruction occurs less than 16 cm from the external meatus. If this is the case, more sophisticated instrumentation may be required, such as filiforms and followers or catheter guides. These techniques should be done only by a urologist or practitioner with extensive training in their use. If AUR cannot be relieved by transurethral bladder catheterization, placement of a suprapubic catheter may be necessary.

12. What is suprapubic catheterization? How is it done?

A procedure used to pass a urinary catheter directly into the bladder through the lower anterior abdominal wall. It is indicated when bladder drainage is necessary and other methods have failed or when urethral damage from trauma is suspected. The procedure is done under sterile conditions with local anesthesia. The bladder is percussed or visualized by ultrasound, and a small incision is made 2 cm above the symphysis pubis midline. Depending on the technique, either a needle or a trocar is used to penetrate the bladder through the incision. When urine is aspirated, a catheter is advanced over the cannula.

13. What diagnostic studies are useful in the evaluation of AUR?

Bedside ultrasonography can be helpful during the initial evaluation, and if needed, suprapubic aspiration can be done. Always check a urinalysis with microscopic examination and urine culture. It is generally recommended to check blood urea nitrogen and creatinine levels to evaluate renal function, especially in cases of suspected chronic retention.

14. Which medications may cause AUR?

Sympathomimetics (α-adrenergic)
Ephedrine
Phenylephrine hydrochloride (Neo-Synephrine)
Phenylpropanolamine hydrochloride (Contac)
Pseudoephedrine (Sudafed, Actifed)
Cocaine
Sympathomimetics (β-adrenergic)
Isoproterenol
Terbutaline
Antidepressants
Tricyclics
Antiarrhythmics
Quinidine
Procainamide
Anticholinergics
Antihistamines
Antiparkinsonian Agents
Trihexyphenidyl (Artane)
Benztropine (Cogentin)
Amantadine (Symmetrel)
Levodopa (Sinemet)
Hormonal agents
Progesterone
Estrogen
Testosterone

Antipsychotics
Haloperidol
Chlorpromazine (Thorazine)
Prochlorperazine (Compazine)
Antihypertensives
Hydralazine
Muscle Relaxants
Diazepam (Valium)
Cyclobenzaprine (Flexeril)
Narcotics
Morphine sulfate
Codeine
Meperidine
Hydromorphone hydrochloride (Dilaudid)
Miscellaneous
Nifedipine (Procardia)
Indomethacin
Carbamazepine (Tegretol)
Amphetamines
Mercurial diuretics
Dopamine
Vincristine
MDMA

15. Summarize the different neurogenic causes of AUR.

1. **Upper motor neuron lesions**: Lesions located in the spinal cord above the sacral mic-turition center (L2 vertebral level, S2–4 spinal segments) result in a spastic or reflex bladder. Common causes are spinal cord trauma, tumor, and multiple sclerosis. Lesions of the cerebral cortex (e.g., acute stroke, bleed) usually cause chronic loss of bladder control and incontinence except in the acute phase, when the lesions typically produce AUR.

2. **Lower motor neuron lesions**: Lesions at the micturition center in the cauda equina interrupt the sacral reflex arc and produce vesical dysfunction. There is loss of sensation of bladder fullness leading to overstretch, muscle atony, and poor contraction. Large residuals are common. The most common causes include spinal trauma, tumor, herniated intervertebral discs, and multiple sclerosis.

3. **Bladder afferent and efferent nerve dysfunction**: Dysfunction in this pathway disrupts the micturition reflex arc that is necessary for proper urination, causing AUR. Common causes include diabetes mellitus, herpes simplex infection, and the postoperative state.

16. Name the most common complications of AUR.

Infection, hemorrhage, and postobstruction diuresis. All three are more common in patients with chronic urinary retention.

17. What is autonomic dysreflexia/hyperreflexia, and what does it have to due with AUR?

An abnormality of the autonomic nervous system seen in patients with long-standing cervi-cal or high thoracic spinal cord lesions (i.e., quadriplegics and high paraplegics). It is caused pri-marily by unchecked reflex sympathetic discharge secondary to some visceral or somatic stimuli below the level of the spinal injury. This potentially life-threatening syndrome includes severe paroxysmal hypertension, diaphoresis, tachycardia or bradycardia, anxiety, headache, flushing, seizures, and coma. Morbidity has resulted in cerebrovascular accident, subarachnoid hemorrhage, and respiratory arrest. One of the most common precipitating stimuli is overdistention of the bladder (AUR) owing to a plugged or kinked catheter. It is always important to evaluate these types of patients for potential Foley catheter problems.

18. What is postobstruction diuresis, and how is it managed?
The inappropriate excretion of salt and water after relief of urinary obstruction. Patients with abnormal renal function or chronic urinary retention are most susceptible. A physiologic diuresis is normal because the kidneys excrete the overload of solute and volume retained while obstructed. If urine output persists at high levels, significant fluid and electrolyte abnormalities may develop. Any patient who exhibits a continuous diuresis after clinical euvolia is reached requires hospitalization for hemodynamic monitoring and fluid and electrolyte repletion.

19. Who can I send home? Who needs admission? Can I remove that catheter?
Most patients with AUR caused by an obstruction require Foley catheterization with continuous drainage. Reliable patients in good health and without signs of serious systemic infection are candidates for careful outpatient management with a leg bag and timely urologic follow-up. The use of prophylactic antibiotics in these patients is controversial. Patients with new neurogenic causes, severe infection, systemic toxicity, or any lesion that may need surgical intervention require hospital admission. Some younger patients with pharmacologic urinary retention may have the catheter removed after decompression. The causative medication should be discontinued, and the patient should be discharged with instructions to return if symptoms recur. It is prudent to have patients void on their own while they are still in the ED.

CONTROVERSY

20. I have heard that gradual emptying of the distended bladder best helps to prevent complications. Is this true?
Traditionally the medical literature has recommended gradual emptying of the obstructed, distended bladder to decrease the risk of hematuria, hypotension, and postobstructive diuresis. The validity of this practice has long been questioned and, until more recently, inadequately studied. A group of physicians from the Mayo Clinic reviewed all of the literature and all of the available studies for each of these complications and compared quick, complete decompression with gradual emptying. Their review revealed that although hematuria, transient hypotension, and postobstructive diuresis occasionally do occur after rapid emptying of the bladder, they are rarely of any clinical significance and do not require any treatment. The recommendation is that gradual, incremental bladder decompression is unnecessary.

BIBLIOGRAPHY

1. Dawson C, Whitfield H: ABC of urology: Urologic emergencies in general practice (education and debate). BMJ 312:838–840, 1996.
2. Fontanarosa PB, Roush WR: Acute urinary retention. Emerg Med Clin North Am 6:419–437, 1988.
3. Givre S, Freed HA: Autonomic dysreflexia: A potentially fatal complication of somatic stress in quadraplegics. J Emerg Med 7:461–463, 1989.
4. Harwood-Nuss AL, Etheredge W, McKenna I: Urologic emergencies. In Rosen P, Barkin RM (eds): Emergency Medicine: Concepts and Clinical Practice, 4th ed. St. Louis, Mosby, 1998, pp 2227–2260.
5. Hastie KJ, Dickinson AJ, Ahmad R, Maoisey CU: Acute retention of urine: Is trial without catheter justified? J R Coll Edinb 35:225–227, 1990.
6. Higgins PM, French ME, Chadalavada VS: Management of acute retention of urine: A reappraisal. Br J Urol 67:365–368, 1991.
7. Jones DA, George NJR: Interactive obstructive uropathy in man. Br J Urol 69:337–345, 1992.
8. Nyman MA, Schwenk NM, Silverstein MD: Management of urinary retention: Rapid vs. gradual decompression and risk of complications. Mayo Clin Proc 72:951–956, 1997.
9. Peterson NE: Urinary incontinence and retention. In Harwood-Nuss AL, Linden C, Luten RC, et al (eds): The Clinical Practice of Emergency Medicine, 2nd ed. Philadelphia, Lippincott-Raven, 1996, pp 258–263.
10. Samm BJ, Domchowski RR: Urologic emergencies: Conditions affecting the kidney, bladder, prostate, and ureters. Postgrad Med 100:177–180, 183–184, 1996.

44. URINARY TRACT INFECTION: CYSTITIS, PYELONEPHRITIS, AND PROSTATITIS

Nicola E. E. Schiebel, M.D.

1. Define the terms relevant to the spectrum of urinary tract infection (UTI).

Bacteriuria: The presence of bacteria anywhere in the urinary tract.

Cystitis: Significant bacteriuria with bladder mucosal invasion. Clinically, cystitis is characterized by dysuria, urgency, frequency, and sometimes suprapubic discomfort.

Pyelonephritis: An infection of the renal parenchyma and collecting system. It is characterized by flank pain, fever, costovertebral angle tenderness, and significant bacteriuria.

Urethritis or **acute urethral syndrome**: The clinical syndrome of dysuria, frequency, and urgency in the absence of significant bacteriuria.

Prostatitis: A chronic or acute syndrome of prostatic inflammation that presents with a wide range of symptoms.

2. Define *significant bacteriuria.*

The traditional gold standard of greater than or equal to 10^5 colony-forming units (CFU)/mL of a single uropathogen on voided midstream urine was based on studies done 40 years ago of women with acute pyelonephritis and asymptomatic bacteriuria. More recent studies suggested that this cutoff results in poor sensitivity for acute cystitis when suprapubic aspiration is used as the reference standard. Of cases with acute cystitis, 30% to 50% grow less than 10^5 uropathogens per mL on voided midstream urine specimens. A definition of greater than or equal to 100 CFU/mL has been reported to provide the best combination of sensitivity (95%) and specificity (85%) for diagnosing acute cystitis in women. Many clinical laboratories cannot detect bacteria at this level. The Infectious Diseases Society of America (IDSA) consensus definition of significant bacteriuria for use in antimicrobial treatment studies is greater than or equal to 10^3 CFU/mL for cystitis in women, greater than or equal to 10^4 CFU/mL for pyelonephritis (sensitivity 90% to 95%), and greater than or equal to 10^4 CFU/mL in acute uncomplicated UTI in men. Any growth of bacteria (except skin contaminants) on suprapubic aspiration should be considered significant. A reasonable cutoff for catheter specimens is greater than or equal to 100 CFU/mL.

3. What are the most common causes of UTI?

Escherichia coli is the most common pathogen. In immunocompromised or chronically ill patients and in complicated UTI, *Pseudomonas* and many members of the Enterobacteriaceae family, such as *Klebsiella*, *Proteus*, and *Enterobacter*, are commonly involved. *Proteus* and *Klebsiella* predispose to stone formation and grow more frequently in patients with calculi.

4. What is asymptomatic bacteriuria?

The presence of greater than or equal to 10^5 uropathogens/mL on voided midstream urine from an asymptomatic patient. When two consecutive specimens contain the same organism at this concentration, the probability of true bacteriuria rises from 80% to 95%.

5. When should asymptomatic bacteriuria be treated?

During pregnancy because it is associated with a 20% to 40% risk of developing symptomatic UTI, including pyelonephritis. Pyelonephritis during pregnancy is associated with increased risk of prematurity and low birth weight. Treating asymptomatic bacteriuria before urologic surgery decreases the risk of postoperative complications, including bacteremia. There is no evidence to support the treatment of asymptomatic bacteriuria in catheterized patients or in the elderly.

6. List the differential diagnoses of dysuria.
- **Infectious**: Cystitis, urethritis, pyelonephritis, epididymitis, prostatitis, vulvovaginitis.
- **Structural**: Calculi, occasionally neoplastic lesions.
- **Traumatic**: Blunt trauma, sexual intercourse, sexual assault, chemical irritants, allergy.

7. When should a pelvic examination be done in a female patient with dysuria?

Whenever there is a suspicion that the cause is not a classic UTI. Clinical situations include external dysuria suggestive of vulvovaginitis, low abdominal pain or bilateral flank pain to rule out pelvic inflammatory disease, any history of trauma or chemical irritant, and any patient at high risk for a sexually transmitted disease or sexual abuse. Any patient who fails to respond to empirical antibiotic therapy for cystitis or who has a negative urinalysis or cultures with a suspected UTI should have a pelvic examination.

8. What is a routine urinalysis?

There is no standardization of what constitutes a *routine urinalysis* in the literature. The definition of *significant bacteriuria* depends on the relatively costly and slow results of urine culture. Many screening tests have been evaluated to try to detect UTI earlier and to predict negative cultures, reducing the number of full urine cultures ordered. These screening tests include:

Pyuria: This involves the measurement of white blood cells (WBCs) in the urine. The most commonly used technique is to examine microscopically centrifuged urine sediment and to quantitate the number of WBCs per high-power field (HPF) (> 5 WBCs/HPF is abnormal). The accuracy and reproducibility of this technique are hampered severely by a lack of standardization. Variations in speed, volume, and duration of centrifuge; volume resuspended; volume under coverslip; degree of magnification; and observer bias all contribute to variability of test results. The most accurate method to measure pyuria is with a hemocytometer on unspun urine (≥ 10 leukocytes/mm^3 is considered abnormal). This test is not widely available.

Microscopic evaluation for bacteria: Variable techniques include examination of unstained and Gram-stained specimens of centrifuged and uncentrifuged urine. Standardization of this technique is poor, and it is an insensitive test because pathogens in quantities less than 10^4 CFU/mL are difficult to find by this technique.

Epithelial cells: Estimates of epithelial cells/HPF are used mainly to estimate perineal contamination of midstream specimens. Although epithelial cells can be derived from anywhere in the urinary tract, their presence on urinalysis is usually from vaginal epithelial cells and suggests contamination.

Leukocyte esterase: This test depends on the ability of any leukocytes present to convert indoxyl carboxylic acid to an indoxyl moiety. When positive, it is suggestive of but not confirmatory for pyuria.

Nitrite: This test depends on the ability of most urinary pathogens to reduce urine nitrates to nitrite. To be positive, the bacteria must act on the urine for 6 hours, making a first-voided morning specimen necessary for optimal testing. Methods used to detect leukocyte esterase and nitrite include urine dipsticks and automated urine analyzers in the laboratory.

9. What is the role of urinalysis and urine dipsticks in the diagnosis of UTI?

The reported sensitivities, specificities, and likelihood ratios for the above-mentioned screening tests vary widely in the literature. Given that the clinical presentation of most UTIs is classic, the utility of any of the screening tests becomes questionable. The pretest probability of cystitis in a population of patients presenting with any symptoms of dysuria, frequency, or urgency has been estimated to be approximately 70%. Estimates of screening test sensitivities and specificities vary so much that the predictive value of a positive test ranges from 75% to 99%, and the predictive value of a negative test ranges from 40% to 99%. Evidence suggests that urinalysis and dipstick testing done under practice conditions are not as reliable as when done under research protocol conditions. The role of urine screening tests is unclear. As a result, it may be sensible to continue to develop clinical guidelines involving the empirical treatment of uncomplicated

UTI, limiting the use of screening tests to only patients with low-to-moderate pretest probability estimates.

10. When should I order a urine culture?

A urine culture generally is not required to treat presumptively uncomplicated cystitis in women. Most clinicians recommend a culture with sensitivities in suspected pyelonephritis because of the potential for serious sequelae if an inappropriate antibiotic is used. All cases of potentially complicated UTI should have a urine culture done.

11. What is the difference between complicated and uncomplicated UTI?

A complicated infection is associated with a clinical condition that increases the risk for acquiring infection, patients who have failed initial therapy, and patients who have increased morbidity. This definition does not depend on anatomic localization of infection to the lower urinary tract. Acute pyelonephritis can be uncomplicated in an otherwise healthy host infected with a virulent uropathogen. Factors that predispose to a complicated UTI include structural abnormalities (e.g., calculi, urinary catheters, stents, prostatic infection, and urinary diversion procedures), metabolic or hormonal abnormalities (e.g., diabetes or pregnancy), immunocompromise, recent urinary tract instrumentation, male gender, the elderly, young children, unusual pathogens, recent antibiotic use or failed treatment for UTI, and presence of symptoms for longer than 7 days. It can be argued that true uncomplicated UTIs occur only in nonpregnant, heathly women with no neurologic or structural dysfunction; 80% of UTIs fall into this group.

12. How should acute, uncomplicated cystitis be treated?

The causative agents are quite predictable. The IDSA has recommended that a 3-day regimen of trimethoprim-sulfamethoxazole (TMP-SMX) be standard therapy for acute uncomplicated cystitis. There is also reasonable evidence that trimethoprim alone is equivalent to TMP-SMX. Fluoroquinalones, such as ofloxacin, norfloxacin or ciprofloxacin, for 3 days are considered to have similar effectiveness as TMP-SMX, but are considerably more expensive. Also, in an effort to postpone emergence of resistance to these drugs the IDSA dose not recommend them as initial empirical therapy except in regions with known resistance to TMP-SMX of greater than 10–20% among uropathogens. Nitrofuratoin for 7 days or a single dose of fosfomycin may become more useful as resistance to TMP-SMX increases.

13. How should acute, uncomplicated pyelonephritis be treated?

There are few properly designed trials for management of acute pyelonephritis, and those that exist are several years old. This, therefore, makes recommendations firmly based on recent evidence impossible. The IDSA recommends 14 days of antimicrobial therapy for young, nonpregnant women with normal urinary tracts. In mild cases, oral fluoroquinolones are considered the first choice for outpatient treatment of pyelonephritis (e.g., ciprofloxacin, 500 mg every 12 hours; levofloxacin, 250 mg daily; or ofloxacin, 200 to 300 mg every 12 hours). Trimethoprim-sulfamethoxazole for 14 days is an inexpensive option, but because of increasing antibiotic resistance to this agent in pyelonephritic strains, the IDSA recommends it be used only if the organism is known to be susceptible. In patients with a contraindication to fluoroquinolones, alternatives include cefixime, 400 mg daily, and cefpodoxime proxetil, 200 mg every 12 hours, for 14 days. A single-dose parenteral antibiotic (gentamicin or ceftriaxone) followed by any of the aforementioned regimens is an acceptable alternative.

14. Which patients with pyelonephritis should be admitted?

Admission should be strongly considered for patients who are unable to maintain oral hydration or to take oral medications and patients with uncertain social support or concern about compliance. Other indications include uncertain diagnosis or severe illness with extreme pain or marked debility. Any patients with evidence of complicated UTI also should be considered for admission. There is increasing evidence that some subsets of complicated pyelonephritis can be treated successfully on an outpatient basis. Pregnant patients at less than 24 weeks' gestation who are hemodynamically stable have been treated safely as outpatients if they can be reached easily by phone and are likely to be compliant with medication and follow-up. Further study is needed to define what other subsets of complicated pyelonephritis may be managed safely outside of the hospital.

15. When should emergency imaging of the urinary tract be obtained in acute pyelonephritis?
If the patient remains febrile for more than 72 hours on appropriate antibiotic therapy, CT or ultrasound should be considered to rule out obstruction and renal or perinephric abscess.

16. What are the signs and symptoms of acute bacterial prostatitis?
The presentation can be dramatic and usually includes frequency, urgency, dysuria, and some obstructive voiding symptoms in greater than 80% of patients. Other common complaints include fever (60%), rigors, myalgias, and perineal discomfort (38%). Some patients also complain of low back pain or rectal pain. The prostate is warm, swollen, and extremely tender.

17. How is acute prostatitis managed?
The pathogen usually can be isolated from voided urine. Prostatic massage and urethral catheterization should be avoided because they are painful and may precipitate bacteremia. Severely ill patients should be admitted and treated with intravenous antibiotics. An aminoglycoside-penicillin derivative combination is often used. Less severely ill patients respond well to oral fluoroquinolones or trimethoprim-sulfamethoxazole. In one study, more than 95% of cultured organisms were sensitive to aminoglycosides, cephalosporins, ciprofloxacin, and imipenem as opposed to 83% sensitivity to trimethoprim-sulfamethoxazole. The duration of therapy should be at least 30 days to prevent chronic bacterial prostatitis. Supportive measures include hydration, nonsteroidal antiinflammatory drugs, sitz baths, and stool softeners. If urinary retention is a problem, suprapubic aspiration or suprapubic catheter placement is recommended.

18. Name the most common cause of recurrent UTI in men?
Chronic bacterial prostatitis.

19. What are the signs and symptoms of chronic bacterial prostatitis?
This is a syndrome of relapsing subacute illness characterized by mild symptoms of frequency, urgency, and dysuria. Other symptoms may include back pain, scrotal or perineal pain, voiding dysfunction, hematospermia, and painful ejaculation. Fever and rigors should not occur. Symptoms must be present for more than 3 months. Examination is highly variable and may be normal. A premassage and postmassage of the prostate urinalysis generally should be done and show repeated postmassage bacteriuria with the same organism.

20. How is chronic bacterial prostatitis treated?
Treatment is difficult with poor cure rates and frequent relapse. Prolonged treatment (2 to 3 months) with fluoroquinolones is the mainstay of therapy. Recalcitrant infection may require long-term, low-dose therapy or resection of the prostate. Referral to a urologist generally is recommended, if possible, before treatment with antibiotics. α_1-Blocking agents show some promise for relief of symptoms and prevention of recurrence.

BIBLIOGRAPHY

1. Gupta K, Scholes D, Stamm WE: Increasing prevalence of antimicrobial resistance among uropathogens causing acute uncomplicated cystitis in women. JAMA 281:736–738, 1999.
2. Hooton TM, Stamm WE: Diagnosis and treatment of uncomplicated urinary tract infection. Infect Dis Clin North Am 11:551–581, 1997.
3. Lummus WE, Thompson I: Prostatitis. Emerg Med Clin North Am 19:691–707, 2001.
4. Patterson TF, Andriole VT: Detection, significance, and therapy of bacteriuria in pregnancy. Infect Dis Clin North Am 11:593–608, 1997.

5. Sheets C, Lyman JL: Urinalysis. Emerg Med Clin North Am 4:263–280, 1986.
6. Stamm WE: Measurement of pyuria and its relation to bacteriuria. Am J Med 75:53–58, 1983.
7. Sultana RV, Zalstein S, Cameron P, Campbell D: Dipstick urinalysis and the accuracy of the clinical diagnosis of urinary tract infection. J Emerg Med 1:13–19, 2001.
8. Warren JW, Abrutyn E, Hebel JR, et al: Guidelines for antimicrobial treatment of uncomplicated acute bacterial cystitis and acute pyelonephritis in women. Clin Infect Dis 29:745–758, 1999.
9. Winkens RAG, Leffers P, Trienekens TAM: The validity of urinary examination for urinary tract infections in daily practice. Fam Pract 12:290–293, 1995.

45. CHRONIC RENAL FAILURE AND DIALYSIS

Allan B. Wolfson, M.D.

1. Isn't renal failure just another genitourinary disorder?

No. **End-stage renal disease (ESRD)** is a complex multisystem disorder. The absence of renal function has obvious consequences for the regulation of total body fluid and electrolyte balance, limiting the ability of dialysis patients to handle fluid and electrolyte loads. Chronic renal failure results in subtle metabolic abnormalities, such as glucose intolerance and lipid disturbances. Renal failure is associated with numerous end-organ effects, ranging from pericarditis to renal osteodystrophy, that compromise comfort and normal function.

2. What are the special concerns in patients with renal failure?

Iatrogenic illness is one important consideration, whether through overadministration of fluids or drug toxicity. Because the effects of renal failure on drug metabolism and disposition are often complex, it is always advisable to check recommended dosage adjustments for patients with ESRD before administering or prescribing medications. Even apparently innocuous drugs, such as antacids and cathartics, may cause morbidity and mortality if used improperly. Patients with ESRD also have complications from underlying disease that may have caused renal failure and complications from dialysis therapy. They have a limited capacity to respond to infection, trauma, or other intercurrent illnesses.

3. How is hemodialysis performed?

In hemodialysis, the patient's blood is brought into contact with a semipermeable artificial membrane, on the other side of which is a chemically balanced aqueous dialysis solution. Metabolic waste and electrolytes flow from the patient's blood into the dialysate, and other substances (e.g., calcium) may flow from the dialysate into the blood, acting to normalize blood chemistries. To achieve adequate total body clearances over the time available for hemodialysis, a high blood flow rate is necessary. This requires the cannulation of large vessels or, for long-term dialysis, the creation of an artificial vascular access that can be used repeatedly. Hemodialysis typically is performed for 4 to 5 hours, three times per week.

4. How is peritoneal dialysis performed?

The patient's peritoneal membrane serves as the semipermeable barrier between the blood (in the peritoneal capillaries) and a balanced dialysate solution, which is introduced into the patient's peritoneal cavity and allowed to dwell for a period of hours before being drained and replaced. An osmotic gradient is created by using a dialysate with high concentrations of glucose that, through osmosis, pulls water from the intravascular space into the dialysate, acting to correct volume overload. For patients with ESRD on **chronic ambulatory peritoneal dialysis (CAPD)**, about 2 L of dialysate dwell continuously within the peritoneal cavity. It is exchanged for fresh dialysate in a sterile fashion by the patient four times a day. Special peritoneal access is required in the form of a surgically implanted Teflon catheter (Tenckhoff catheter), through which dialysate is infused and drained.

5. What is the most common problem relating to the vascular access device in the ED?

Thrombosis should be suspected when patients report loss of thrill in the vascular device. More often, they present to the ED when there has been a problem establishing adequate flow during a hemodialysis session. The only intervention necessary is a prompt call to a vascular surgeon. An angiogram defines the nature and extent of the obstruction and delineates anatomic lesions, allowing the surgeon to revise or replace the access.

6. How do I diagnose and treat a vascular access infection?

Infection is obvious when the patient presents with signs of inflammation localized to the access area. The difficulty is that many patients present only with fever and without specific localizing signs. A useful rule of thumb in such instances is to assume that an endovascular access infection is present and to treat accordingly. Patients typically can be sent home after one dose of an appropriate antibiotic, provided that they look well and are reliable for follow-up. Vancomycin, 1 g intravenously, is the treatment of choice because most infections are staphylococcal, and the drug's duration of action is 5 to 7 days in ESRD. Vancomycin is not hemodialyzable, and its major toxicity is to the kidneys. If gram-negative infection is suspected, a third-generation cephalosporin, aztreonam, or an aminoglycoside should be added to the regimen. Careful follow-up should be arranged with the patient's dialysis nurse or physician. Blood cultures should be obtained before treatment is initiated.

7. When can the vascular access device be used for giving intravenous infusions or for drawing blood?

Hemodialysis patients are instructed never to allow their blood pressure to be taken in the arm with the vascular access or to allow their blood to be drawn or intravenous fluids to be infused through the vascular access. This is to protect the access device, which is truly the patient's lifeline. Occasionally, there is no reasonable alternative but to use the access device for blood drawing or intravenous lines. In these situations, cautious use of the vascular access device is permissible, provided that certain guidelines are followed.

When using the access to draw blood, a tourniquet should not be used. At most, one finger can be used to tourniquet the vein lightly. The presence of a thrill should be documented before and after the procedure. The area should be cleaned thoroughly with povidone-iodine or another antiseptic, and sterile technique should be observed. Care should be taken not to puncture the back wall of the vessel, and after the puncture, firm but nonocclusive pressure should be applied to the site for several minutes to ensure that extravasation does not occur. Obvious aneurysms should not be punctured.

When using the vascular access for an intravenous line, similar precautions should be observed. Because the vessel is under arterial pressure, a pressure bag or, preferably, an automated infusion device is an absolute requirement (certainly when infusing medications).

8. How is CAPD-associated peritonitis diagnosed?

Peritonitis associated with CAPD occurs about once per year in even the most fastidious and well-motivated patients. In contrast to other types of peritonitis, it tends to be mild clinically, and most patients can be managed without hospital admission. CAPD-associated peritonitis is caused most commonly by gram-positive organisms, which are thought to be introduced during the exchange procedure. The diagnosis is suspected by the patient on the basis of the new appearance of cloudiness of the dialysis effluent. Patients are instructed to seek medical attention promptly when this occurs, and for this reason most episodes of peritonitis are relatively mild. If the patient delays seeking attention, however, the symptoms tend to become progressively more severe. Most patients have abdominal pain and tenderness, but only a few have fever, nausea, vomiting, or even (at least early on) an elevated peripheral white blood cell count. Localized peritoneal findings are suggestive of an acute surgical abdomen rather than CAPD-induced peritonitis.

9. How is CAPD-associated peritonitis treated?

When fluid has been obtained through the effluent bag and laboratory studies have confirmed the presence of a significant number of white cells (> $100/mm^3$ with > 50% polymorphonuclear leukocytes) or a positive Gram stain, antibiotic treatment is initiated. Commonly, vancomycin (30 mg/kg) is given intraperitoneally and may be repeated weekly. Gram-negative coverage, with a third-generation cephalosporin, azotreonam, or an aminoglycoside, can be added if thought appropriate. These may be given intraperitoneally as well and should be followed by daily intraperitoneal maintenance doses as an outpatient. One commonly recommended initial regimen consists of cefazolin and ceftazidime given intraperitoneally in each bag of dialysate. Usually, each center has its own protocols for treatment, so the patient's nephrologist or dialysis nurse should be consulted. Follow-up should be in 48 hours, at which time cultures and clinical findings are rechecked and therapy adjusted as necessary. Admission criteria include severe pain, nausea and vomiting, a toxic appearance, or the inability of the patient to comply with outpatient therapy and follow-up.

10. Name the indications for emergency dialysis.

Acute pulmonary edema, life-threatening hyperkalemia, or life-threatening intoxication or overdose secondary to dialyzable toxins that ordinarily are excreted by the kidneys.

11. What is unique about a dialysis patient with cardiac arrest?

Two potentially reversible entities always should be considered in an ESRD patient with cardiac arrest:

1. Severe hyperkalemia may cause severe rhythm disturbances and ultimately cardiac arrest without any other warning or clinical signs. When a patient suffers an arrest from whatever cause, respiratory and metabolic acidosis and the efflux of potassium from cells can be expected to produce hyperkalemia secondarily. In the patient who already may have a tendency toward hyperkalemia, this further increase could cause the patient to be refractory to standard advanced cardiac life support (ACLS) interventions. ESRD patients in cardiac arrest always should be given intravenous calcium if they do not respond immediately to the first round of ACLS measures.

2. Acute pericardial tamponade may result from accumulation of pericardial fluid or spontaneous bleeding into the pericardial sac. Patients with tamponade tend to display refractory hypotension or pulseless electrical activity or both. Although less likely than other entities to be the cause of refractoriness to resuscitation measures, the possibility of pericardial tamponade always should be considered in patients in whom other measures have failed. Emergency pericardiocentesis may be life-saving.

12. What are the treatment options for acute pulmonary edema in patients with ESRD?

ESRD patients with pulmonary edema do not have the ability to rid themselves of excess fluids through the kidneys and ultimately require dialysis to correct volume overload. Interventions that are useful in patients with functioning kidneys also are useful in patients with ESRD before dialysis can be initiated. The patient should be given oxygen and placed in a sitting position. Nitrates administered sublingually or intravenously are the mainstay of temporizing therapy. Sublingual nitroglycerin can be given every 3 minutes to decrease preload and afterload as blood pressure permits. Intravenous nitroglycerin is a useful alternative. Intravenous morphine, although less popular, also may be helpful in decreasing pulmonary venous hypertension, although patients may be more likely to require intubation and mechanical ventilation because of its sedative action. Intravenous furosemide, although it cannot act as a diuretic, has some action in decreasing pulmonary venous pressure.

Dialysis is the definitive therapy and should be instituted as early as possible. The CAPD patient with acute pulmonary edema presents a slightly different problem because intensified dialysis, even with 4.25% glucose solution, is a slow means of removing fluid and because the presence of 2 L of dialysate in the peritoneal cavity tends to have an adverse effect on diaphragmatic excursion and pulmonary mechanics. Intubation and mechanical ventilation may be necessary while continuing hourly exchanges of high-concentration dialysate.

13. What about air embolism?

Air embolism is an uncommon but well-reported complication of hemodialysis. Although air embolism has become rare with the advent of sophisticated monitoring and alarm systems on hemodialysis machines, when it does occur it is often a devastating event and one for which the patient almost surely will be brought to the nearest ED.

Air embolism should be suspected when a patient experiences a sudden acute decompensation during the course of hemodialysis treatment. Several immediate measures are thought to be helpful. Any intravenous lines should be clamped. The patient should be given 100% oxygen and laid on the left side with the head down, in an attempt to cause the air to collect at the apex of the right ventricle. At this point, if the patient is reasonably stable, an interventional radiologist or cardiologist can be consulted for consideration of passage of a central venous catheter into the right ventricular apex, through which the air can be aspirated directly out of the heart. For patients who are in close proximity to a hyperbaric chamber, treatment with 100% oxygen at several atmospheres can shrink directly the size of the bubbles and enhance resorption of the gas. One should be certain before embarking on this course, however, that the patient's symptoms are due to air embolism rather than, for example, a sudden spontaneous pneumothorax.

14. How should a patient with acute shortness of breath be evaluated?

The rule of thumb: If they are short of breath, dialyze them because volume overload is the most common cause. It is sometimes difficult to make the diagnosis of volume overload. The patient's weight may be the best guide. Physical examination is not always helpful, and chest radiographs may be misleading.

15. What are the main differential diagnostic elements of chest pain in ESRD?

Always think first of either **angina** or **pericarditis**. Some patients with ESRD, particularly those who are anemic, may have angina and cardiac ischemia even if a previous cardiac catheterization has shown a *noncritical* coronary obstruction. This is due to increased cardiac oxygen demands and decreased oxygen delivery to the heart. Although cardiac enzyme levels may be altered in ESRD, renal failure does not obscure the usual ECG and enzyme changes of acute myocardial infarction.

16. What is the differential diagnosis of hypotension in a patient with ESRD?

Hypovolemia after dialysis, hemorrhage, acute pericardial tamponade, and sepsis.

17. What are the major causes of altered mental status in patients with ESRD?

Dysequilibrium syndrome, caused by rapid solute shifts during hemodialysis, is a common consideration, but a major pitfall is to attribute every change in mental status to this entity. Drug effects are a major cause, as is spontaneous intracranial hemorrhage. Any patient with localizing signs should have a CT scan of the head; patients without localizing signs probably should as well because subdural hematoma may not cause focal findings.

BIBLIOGRAPHY

1. Aronoff GR, Perns JS, Frier ME, et al: Drug Prescribing in Renal Failure: Dosing Guidelines for Adults, 4th ed. Philadelphia, American College of Physicians, 1999.
2. Keane WF, Bailie GR, Boeschoten E, et al: Adult peritoneal dialysis-related peritonitis treatment recommendations: 2000 update. Perit Dial Int 20:396–411, 2000.
3. Wolfson AB, Maenza RL: Renal failure. In Marx J, Hockberger R, Walls R (eds): Rosen's Emergency Medicine: Concepts and Clinical Practice, 5th ed. St. Louis, Mosby, 2002, pp 1360–1390.
4. Wolfson AB: Chronic renal failure and dialysis-related emergencies. In Harwood-Nuss A, Wolfson AB (eds): The Clinical Practice of Emergency Medicine, 3rd ed. Philadelphia, Lippincott Williams & Wilkins, 2001, pp 867–872.
5. Wolfson AB: End-stage renal disease: Emergencies related to dialysis and transplantation. In Wolfson AB, Harwood-Nuss A (eds): Renal and Urologic Emergencies. New York, Churchill Livingstone, 1986, pp 23–50.
6. Wolfson AB, Singer I: Hemodialysis-related emergencies (part I). J Emerg Med 5:543–553, 1987.
7. Wolfson AB, Singer I: Hemodialysis-related emergencies (part II). J Emerg Med 6:61–70, 1988.

IX. Hematology/Oncology

46. HEMOSTASIS AND COAGULOPATHIES

Stephen C. Altmin, M.D., M.P.H.

1. I memorized the clotting cascade in medical school. Do I need to memorize it again?

No. But a basic knowledge of hemostasis is important in the management of patients with bleeding in the ED.

2. What do I need to know about hemostasis?

Hemostasis can be divided into three phases.

Primary hemostasis after tissue injury is achieved through vasoconstriction, platelet adhesion, and platelet aggregation. Disorders of primary hemostasis include vascular abnormalities (e.g., hereditary hemorrhagic telangiectasia) and disorders of platelet function or quantity (e.g., thrombocytopenia, von Willebrand's disease [vWD]). Disorders in primary hemostasis may be assessed by the platelet count or bleeding time.

Secondary hemostasis describes the reinforcement of the platelet plug by cross-linked fibrin from the coagulation cascade. Coagulation factor deficiencies (e.g., hemophilia A and B) or production of inactive factors (e.g., warfarin use) can disrupt the coagulation cascade leading to bleeding. Disorders in secondary hemostasis can be assessed by the partial thromboplastin time (PTT) and prothrombin time (PT). The PTT measures defects in the intrinsic and common pathways of the coagulation cascade, whereas the PT measures defects in the extrinsic and common pathways.

Tertiary hemostasis or the fibrinolytic system involves the breakdown of fibrin clot via the proteolytic enzyme plasmin. Plasmin is activated by tissue plasminogen activator, which is released from endothelial cells and converts plasminogen to plasmin. Plasmin breaks down fibrinogen and fibrin into fibrin split products and D-dimers. Increased release of fibrinolytic activators or deficiencies of fibrinolytic inhibitors (e.g., protein C, protein S, antithrombin III) can cause an increase in bleeding.

3. What questions should I ask in the history if I suspect a bleeding abnormality?

In patients with known bleeding disorders, ask the patient about the management of their disease. They will frequently know more than you. In patients with suspected bleeding disorders, it is useful to ask about a family history of bleeding disorders, medications, past medical history (e.g., liver or kidney disease, malignancy), and previous challenges to hemostasis, such as tooth extraction or operative procedures.

4. How can the physical examination help me determine the type of bleeding disorder?

Patients with platelet defects or deficiencies cannot initiate primary hemostasis. They present with prolonged superficial bleeding, epistaxis, gingival and mucosal bleeding, purpura, and petechiae. When bleeding stops, fibrin clot formation usually prevents recurrence. Patients with coagulation factor defects (e.g., hemophiliacs) cannot effectively reinforce platelet-initiated hemostasis. They present with recurrent bleeding into deep structures, such as the subcutaneous tissues, muscles, joints, and retroperitoneum. Ecchymosis, gastrointestinal bleeding, and menorrhagia can occur with almost any bleeding disorder.

5. List the causes of thrombocytopenia.

1. Pseudothrombocytopenia (laboratory error)
2. Platelet dilution or loss (e.g., massive transfusion)
3. Platelet sequestration (e.g., hypersplenism)
4. Decreased platelet production, acquired or congenital
5. Immune-mediated destruction (e.g., infection, idiopathic thrombocytopenic purpura [ITP])
6. Mechanical or toxic destruction (e.g., disseminated intravascular coagulation [DIC], thrombotic thrombocytopenic purpura [TTP])

6. What is ITP?

ITP is thought to be an autoimmune phenomenon whereby IgG antibodies are produced that target platelets and facilitate their destruction. ITP is a diagnosis of exclusion after other causes of thrombocytopenia have been ruled out. It can be either acute or chronic. **Acute ITP** is most common in children 2 to 6 years old, typically occurring several weeks after a viral infection. **Chronic ITP** typically is seen in women (similar to most autoimmune disorders). There is an association between ITP and *Helicobacter pylori*, HIV, and hepatitis C infections. These infections should be treated.

7. How is ITP treated?

Acute ITP is typically self-limited and marked by spontaneous remission in 90% of patients within several weeks to months. The platelet count generally decreases to less than 20,000/mm^3. Treatment is supportive, and steroid therapy does not alter the disease.

Chronic ITP has a more insidious onset and typically presents with ecchymosis, mucosal bleeding, prolonged menses, petechiae, or purpura. Platelet counts generally range from 30,000 to 100,000/mm^3. Spontaneous remission is rare. Treatment options include:
- Corticosteroids
- Intravenous immunoglobulin, intravenous anti-D antibodies
- Plasmapheresis
- Immunosuppressive (e.g., cyclophosphamide, azathioprine, vincristine)
- Danazol
- Splenectomy
- Newer experimental therapies: thrombopoietin, anti-CD40 ligand, rituximab, and autologous bone marrow transplantation

Platelet transfusions are used only for severe, life-threatening bleeding.

8. What is TTP, and how is it treated?

TTP is caused by injured microvascular endothelial cells, leading to microangiopathic hemolytic anemia and thrombocytopenia. Patients present with a classic pentad of clinical findings: (1) altered mental status, (2) thrombocytopenia, (3) fever, (4) microangiopathic hemolytic anemia, and (5) renal impairment. TTP usually occurs in young adults with a peak incidence at age 25 (age range, 10 to 40 years). Recognized triggers to TTP include pregnancy, cancer, drugs, and infections; however, frequently no trigger is identified. Laboratory workup may show anemia, thrombocytopenia, hematuria, proteinuria, elevated blood urea nitrogen, elevated creatinine, and elevated lactate dehydrogenase. Peripheral blood smear reveals fragmented red blood cells. Untreated, the disease progresses to death in 80% of patients within 1 to 3 months. Aggressive use of plasmapheresis has reduced mortality from 90% to 17%. Additional therapeutic options include steroids, splenectomy, and antiplatelet agents (e.g., aspirin). Platelet transfusions should be reserved for life-threatening bleeding because platelets may worsen microvascular thrombi.

9. What is the difference between TTP and hemolytic-uremic syndrome (HUS)?

HUS and TTP are part of the same disease spectrum. HUS tends to cause more kidney damage and fewer central nervous system effects. Patients with HUS are usually younger and often have a preceding bacterial gastroenteritis (e.g., *Escherichia coli* 0157).

10. What is the HELLP syndrome?

The **HELLP** syndrome (**h**emolysis, **e**levated **l**iver function tests, and **l**ow **p**latelets) is a preeclampsia variant that occurs most commonly in white, multiparous women older than age 25. Criteria for diagnosis include (1) microangiopathic hemolytic anemia, (2) serum aspartate aminotransferase levels greater than 70 U/L, and (3) thrombocytopenia less than 100,000 platelets/mL. HELLP is associated with higher maternal and fetal morbidity and mortality than preeclampsia. Treatment is generally supportive, but platelet transfusion may be needed before cesarean section. DIC may complicate HELLP and can be managed with fresh-frozen plasma. A small subset of patients may develop prolonged thrombocytopenia (> 4 to 5 days) and multiorgan failure after delivery. In these patients, plasmapharesis or corticosteroids may be indicated.

11. What is HIT, and why do I have to worry about it?

Heparin-induced thrombocytopenia (HIT) was seen previously in inpatients receiving heparin therapy. As heparin is used more frequently in the outpatient setting (e.g., deep venous thrombosis), emergency physicians are likely to diagnose HIT and be responsible for the initial management. The diagnosis must be considered in any patient presenting with an unexplained fall in platelet count of at least 30% to 40% or the development a new thromboembolic complication 5 to 10 days after the initiation of heparin therapy. Although low-molecular-weight heparins are less likely to cause HIT than unfractionated heparin, HIT can occur with both.

The most dreaded complication of HIT is the development of paradoxical arterial or venous thrombosis, termed *heparin-induced thrombocytopenia with thrombosis (HITT)*. Also called *white clot syndrome*, HITT has been associated with 20% mortality rates and 10% limb amputation rates. Without therapy, approximately 30% of patients with HIT develop HITT.

Treatment of HIT and HITT involves immediate discontinuation of heparin therapy and any contact with heparin, such as heparin-coated intravenous lines. Two new drugs have become available to treat HIT and HITT:

- **Lepirudin** is an anticoagulant that acts directly on circulating and clot-bound thrombin. Lepirudin has been shown to reduce death, amputations, and thromboembolic complications.
- **Argatroban** is a direct thrombin inhibitor that inhibits soluble and clot-bound thrombin.

12. When does a patient with thrombocytopenia need platelet transfusions?

Normal platelet counts range from 140,000 to 400,000/μL. Patients are typically asymptomatic at levels between 75,000 and 140,000/μL. Increased bruising, increased menstrual blood loss, and epistaxis may occur at platelet levels between 20,000 and 75,000/μL. At platelet levels less than 20,000/μL, petechiae, spontaneous purpura, dental bleeding, and spontaneous renal hemorrhage may occur. At platelet levels less than 10,000/μL, spontaneous cerebral hemorrhage may occur and severe gastrointestinal bleeding in the presence of infections, such as gastritis, colitis, or proctitis.

In the nonbleeding patient with thrombocytopenia, the decision concerning when to transfuse is controversial and depends on the type of thrombocytopenia, coexisting disease, other bleeding risk factors, and the rate of platelet decline. In the past, a platelet count of less than 20,000/μL was considered the threshold at which to transfuse a nonbleeding patient. More recent studies showed that prophylactic platelet transfusion can be withheld safely until platelet counts decrease to less than 10,000/μL. As mentioned previously, platelet transfusions in patients with ITP or TTP should be avoided except in severe life-threatening bleeding. In surgical patients, a platelet count of 50,000/μL is the standard preoperative platelet target.

In thrombocytopenic patients with life-threatening bleeding, platelet transfusion should be initiated regardless of the cause of the thrombocytopenia or the platelet count.

13. How much can I expect the platelet count to rise with a platelet transfusion?

A typical platelet transfusion consists of 6 to 10 bags of random donor platelets (RDP) or 1 U of single donor apheresis platelets (SDP). A SDP unit is usually equivalent to about 6 to 8 RDP. A single RDP unit generally can be expected to increase the adult platelet count by

5000/µL, assuming no peripheral destruction or hypersplenism. A multitude of variables may affect platelet recovery, however, including (1) factors inherent in the platelet concentrates, such as age of the concentrate and ABO compatibility; (2) clinical settings, such as DIC, infection, and hypersplenism; and (3) immune causes, such as ITP. A 1-hour posttransfusion platelet count should be obtained to assess rapid destruction or consumption.

14. What is vWD?

vWD is the most common (0.1% of population) inherited bleeding disorde, and is a result of a deficiency or dysfunction of von Willebrand factor (vWF). vWF plays a role in primary and secondary hemostasis by mediating the adhesion of platelets at the site of vascular injury and stabilizing factor VIII. Consequently, patients with vWD have an elevated bleeding time and PTT. In contrast to the common hemophilias, vWD is autosomal dominant and affects men and women. There are 3 types of vWD that are characterized by the amount, nature, and inheritance pattern of the protein deficiency. Type I disease is the most common.

15. How do I treat vWD?

There are two main therapeutic agents used to treat vWD: (1) desmopressin (DDAVP) and (2) blood products that contain factor VIII and vWF such as cryoprecipitate and factor VIII concentrates rich in bound vWF. However, different vWD subtypes respond differently to treatment. Treatment regimens include:

- DDAVP (0.3 ug/kg IV) increases the release of vWF from endothelial cells and is most useful in patients with type 1 vWD. Also available in subcutaneous and intranasal preparations.
- Cryoprecipitate contains 5 to 10 times more VIII and vWF than fresh frozen plasma (FFP). Standard dose is 1 bag/10 kg for minor bleeding or 2 bags/10 kg for major bleeding. Cryoprecipitate carries a small risk of blood borne infection transmission because common laboratory virucidal techniques cannot be applied to cryoprecipitate. Therefore, virus-inactivated factor VIII-vWF (e.g., Humate-P) concentrates are often preferred over cryoprecipitate in patients not responsive to DDAVP.
- Factor VIII-vWF concentrates (e.g., Humate-P; dose 30-50 U/kg).

16. What is classic hemophilia?

Classic hemophilia or **hemophilia A** is the second most common inherited coagulopathy, after vWD, occurring in 1 in 5000 males. Patients with hemophilia A produce a defective factor VIII secondary to a mutation on the X chromosome. The affected male usually inherits the defective gene from his carrier mother, but approximately 30% of cases arise from spontaneous mutation. Hemophilia occurs in mild (6% to 30% factor activity), moderate (2% to 5%), and severe (< 1%) forms. Patients with mild hemophilia usually bleed only after trauma or surgery, whereas patients with severe hemophilia can bleed spontaneously. Patients with severe hemophilia typically have 20 to 30 episodes/year of spontaneous or excessive bleeding after minor trauma. Screening tests reveal a prolonged PTT with a normal platelet count and PT.

17. How do I treat hemophilia A?

Plasma concentrates of coagulation factors became available for the treatment of hemophilia in the 1970s, revolutionizing hemophilia treatment. The success of early factor therapy was tampered, however, by the transmission of hepatitis B and C in nearly all recipients and later by HIV. Since then, donor factor therapy has become safer, and recombinant factor therapy has become more widely available. Currently, genetically engineered recombinant factor therapy is 2 to 3 times more expensive than donor factor therapy. In the United States, about 60% of patients with severe hemophilia use recombinant factor.

The treatment of hemophilia A is based on the location and severity of bleeding. Minimal bleeding (scrape) does not require treatment. Minor bleeding (mild laceration, early hemarthrosis, mild epistaxis, mild hematuria) requires 12.5 U/kg factor VIII concentrate. Moderate bleeding requires 25 U/kg of factor VIII. Major or life-threatening bleeds need 50 U/kg, which brings the factor VIII level to 100%. Desmopressin (0.3 µg/kg) has been shown to increase factor VIII levels and can be tried for mild hemophiliacs with mild bleeding. Cryoprecipitate (100 U of factor VIII/10 mL bag) can supply factor VIII if purified concentrate is not available.

18. What is Christmas disease?

Christmas disease or **hemophilia B** is an X-linked recessive disorder leading to a defective factor IX. The name of the disease originates from its first description in the *British Medical Journal's* 1952 Christmas issue. The disease occurs in 1 in 30,000 males. Similar to hemophilia A, patients have an elevated PTT and a normal PT and platelet count.

19. How do I treat hemophilia B?

The indications and dosage of factor IX replacement are generally the same as for factor VIII replacement in hemophilia A. Life-threatening bleeds require 50 U/kg of factor IX. Cryoprecipitate is not used because it does not contain any factor IX. When factor IX concentrate is unavailable, large doses of fresh-frozen plasma can be used.

20. What characterizes a *life-threatening* bleed?

Bleeding in the central nervous system, retroperitoneum, neck, and oropharynx. Bleeding in the neck or mouth may obstruct the airway.

21. What about gene therapy in hemophilia?

Three clinical trials of gene therapy in patients with hemophilia A or B are currently under way with encouraging results. Although much work needs to be done, experts predict that hemophilia is likely to be the first common severe genetic disease that is cured by gene therapy.

22. How do I treat patients with factor inhibitor?

Antibodies to factor VIII or IX occur in 30% of patients with severe hemophilia A and less commonly (1% to 4%) in patients with hemophilia B. These antibodies are called *inhibitors* because they inhibit or neutralize factor coagulant activity. Although inhibitors may be detected during routine comprehensive hemophiliac screening, they also may be detected by the clinical unresponsiveness to clotting factor during a bleeding episode.

The treatment of bleeding in patients with factor inhibitor can be challenging and should be coordinated with a hematologist. The inhibitor antibody concentration is measured in Bethesda units (BU). One way to treat patients with inhibitor antibody is to provide additional or more frequent factor to overwhelm the antibodies. In patients with a Bethesda titer of 10 BU or greater, even high-dose factor therapy is ineffective. In this case, other measures are necessary, such as plasmapheresis or the use of porcine factor. Other treatments include bypass therapy, which involves concentrates of activated prothrombin complex concentrates or prothrombin complex concentrates that bypass the requirement for factor VIII or IX to develop clot. Desmopressin, intravenous immunoglobulin, and immunosuppression with cyclophosphamide or prednisone also have been used to treat patients with high titer inhibitors.

23. Why do patients with liver disease have hemostasis problems?

The liver is the site of production of nearly all coagulation factors. Patients with cirrhosis may have thrombocytopenia as a result of hypersplenism and poor platelet function.

24. Why do patients with renal failure have hemostasis problems?

Bleeding disorders in patients with uremia are usually multifactorial in nature involving primary and secondary hemostasis; however, platelet abnormalities seem to predominate. Mild thrombocytopenia and uremic toxin–mediated platelet function defects occur. Platelet transfusions in patients with uremia are often of little value because the uremic toxin persists. Dialysis is the treatment of choice. Desmopressin, conjugated estrogens, and cryoprecipitate also have been used successfully in managing bleeding. Heparin administration during hemodialysis may play a role in bleeding disorders.

25. Why do alcoholics have hemostasis problems?

Alcoholics with liver disease have decreased hepatic synthesis of clotting factors and decreased marrow production of platelets. Splenic sequestration reduces the number of circulating platelets. Alcohol also has a toxic effect on platelet function.

26. How is heparin-induced bleeding managed?

Heparin works by potentiating antithrombin III activity, which inactivates multiple coagulation factors, including heparin. Because the half-life of heparin is only about 1 hour, minor bleeding can be treated by stopping the heparin. Major bleeding may require treatment with protamine sulfate, at a dose of 1 mg for every 100 U of heparin in circulation. Protamine works by binding to and inactivating heparin.

27. How do I treat bleeding in patients who are on warfarin?

Warfarin inhibits the vitamin K–dependent clotting factors II, VII, IX, and X. Prolongation of the PT or elevation of the international normalized ratio without bleeding and without planned surgical procedures may be treated by simply withholding the warfarin. If the patient has additional risk factors for bleeding or minor bleeding, vitamin K should be given. Correction of the PT with vitamin K is not immediate and requires at least 4 to 6 hours. Doses of vitamin K range from 0.5 to 5 mg depending on the degree of anticoagulation. With significant bleeding that requires immediate reversal of anticoagulation, fresh-frozen plasma is required because it contains all the vitamin K–dependent coagulation factors.

28. How is DIC diagnosed and treated?

DIC is a hemostatic disorder marked by microthrombosis and diffuse microvascular bleeding, which occurs in a variety of clinical settings (e.g., retained fetal products, shock, sepsis, cancer, major trauma, burns). Laboratory analysis shows a prolonged PT and PTT, decreased platelets and fibrinogen, and elevated fibrin degradation products. The definitive treatment of DIC is correction of the underlying disease process. While the underlying disorder is being corrected, patients may need transfusions of red blood cells, platelets, cryoprecipitate, and fresh-frozen plasma. In patients who do not show improvement with blood products, low-dose heparin and antithrombin III concentrates have been used. Both treatments are controversial and should be used only in consultation with a hematologist.

29. Will there ever be an artificial blood substitute?

Yes. There already is. Because of the frequent red blood cell donor shortages and the risk of transmission of infections, the search for a pharmacologic product that can carry and deliver oxygen has made significant progress. Multiple agents have undergone clinical trials and now are awaiting Food and Drug Administration (FDA) approval. The two major groups of blood substitutes in development include the perfluorocarbons and the hemoglobin-based solutions. Currently, most of the agents in phase III clinical trials or awaiting FDA approval are based on human or bovine hemoglobin solutions. Of particular interest to emergency medicine physicians, PolyHeme, a polymerized human hemoglobin concentration, has finished phase III clinical trials for use in trauma patients requiring large-volume transfusions and is awaiting FDA approval.

BIBLIOGRAPHY

1. DiMichele D, Neufeld EJ: Hemophilia: A new approach to an old disease. Hematol Oncol Clin North Am 12:1315–1344, 1998.
2. George JN, Rizvi MA: Thrombocytopenia. In Beutler E (ed): Williams Hematology, 6th ed. New York, McGraw-Hill, 2001, pp 1495–1539.
3. Hamilton GG, Janz TG: Disorders of hemostasis. In Rosen P, Barkin RM (eds): Emergency Medicine: Concepts and Clinical Practice, 5th ed. St. Louis, Mosby, 2002, pp 1688–1700.

4. Humphries JE: Transfusion therapies in acquired coagulopathies. Hematol Oncol Clin North Am 8:1181–1201, 1994.
5. Lusher JM: Transfusion therapy in congenital coagulopathies. Hematol Oncol Clin North Am 8:1167–1180, 1994.
6. Mannucci PM: How I treat patients with von Willebrand disease. Blood 97:1915–1919, 2001.
7. Roberts HD, Hoffman M: Hemophilia A and hemophilia B. In Beutler E (ed): Williams Hematology, 6th ed. New York, McGraw-Hill, 2001, pp 1639–1655.
8. Stowell CP, Levin J, Winslow RM: Progress in the development of RBC substitutes. Transfusion 41:287–299, 2001.

47. SICKLE CELL ANEMIA

Linda L. Hanson, M.D.

1. What is sickle cell anemia?

An autosomal dominant disease that results from substitution of valine for glutamine at the sixth position on both chains of the β-globulin chain in a hemoglobin molecule. When conditions are right, this chemical change can cause the hemoglobin molecule to assume an abnormal shape that is reflected in the red blood cell, which appears sickle-shaped instead of round.

2. What factors promote sickling?

Low pH independent of oxygen tension by shifting the oxygen dissociation curve to the right. Low oxygen tension from any cause induces sickling. Causes include cardiovascular disease, circulatory stasis that results in local tissue hypoxia, high altitude, and breathing through special devices as when scuba diving or during anesthesia. A high intracellular concentration of sickle hemoglobin from dehydration promotes sickling. Low temperature promotes sickling through vasoconstriction.

3. Why do patients with sickle cell anemia develop clinical problems?

Sickled cells produce sludging in the microcirculation and chronic hemolysis, with obstruction of flow causing regional hypoxia and acidosis, further increasing sickling and obstruction of flow. Ischemic injury and infarcts occur, resulting in a propensity for infection and chronic organ damage.

4. Describe the various types of sickle cell crises.

Vasoocclusive (painful) crisis is caused by ischemic tissue injury, which can lead to infarction. The presenting complaint is usually pain, which may affect any organ, but common sites include bone, abdomen, and chest. **Hemolytic crisis** usually occurs in response to infection, resulting in a more rapid rate of hemolysis. A rapidly falling hematocrit, an elevated reticulocyte count, pallor, and jaundice are observed. **Aplastic crisis** often is induced by infection and, rarely, folic acid deficiency. Patients present with a decreased hematocrit, depressed reticulocyte count, fatigue, dyspnea, or pallor. **Sequestration crisis** occurs when large numbers of red blood cells pool in the spleen. The inciting event is thought to be infection. Patients present with splenic enlargement, abdominal pain, a falling hematocrit, pallor, tachycardia, and dyspnea. Pooling can be so massive that hypovolemic shock and death can ensue. It usually occurs between the ages of 5 months and 2 years and is the most dangerous crisis for young children.

5. Why is sequestration crisis more common in very young children?

Fetal hemoglobin inhibits sickling and has a protective effect until about 4 months of age, when it declines. Splenic sequestration is unusual until after 4 months of age, when the spleen may undergo repeated infarcts that result in autosplenectomy (usually before the age of 2).

6. Why do patients with sickle cell anemia have an increased risk of infection?

Patients with sickle cell anemia experience repeated splenic infarctions that lead to functional asplenia. Ischemic tissue produced by sludging in the microcirculation by sickled cells serves as a site for infection. Phagocytic activity is depressed because of blockage of sinusoids in the liver and spleen. Decreased nonantibody opsonic activity and decreased IgM antibody production also contribute to infection.

7. Why should I worry about a child with sickle cell anemia who presents with fever?

Fever in children, especially children younger than age 5 years, may indicate life-threatening infection. Severe overwhelming sepsis secondary to *Streptococcus pneumoniae* is the most common cause of death during early childhood. Patients with sickle cell anemia should receive the pneumococcal vaccine. A twofold increase in the incidence of *Haemophilus influenzae* in nonimmunized patients is seen. Appropriate cultures should be done, and antibiotics should be used liberally.

8. What is the *acute chest syndrome*?

An acute pulmonary process that occurs in patients with sickle cell anemia. Typical findings include fever, pleuritic chest pain, and radiographic evidence of an acute pulmonary process. Hypoxemia and leukocytosis may be present. The differential diagnosis includes viral, bacterial, or mycoplasmal infections or pulmonary infarcts resulting from pulmonary emboli. It may be difficult to determine whether infection or infarction is responsible for the condition.

9. Which diagnostic studies are indicated in acute chest syndrome?

In general, diagnostic studies are indicated only when deep venous thrombosis is suspected, in which case a venous Doppler study should be done. Because the hypertonicity of contrast agents may produce cellular dehydration (resulting in more sickling), pulmonary angiograms and venograms are contraindicated. Ventilation-perfusion scans can be done safely in patients with sickle cell anemia; however, interpretation is often difficult, owing to previous repeated pulmonary insults, unless baseline ventilation-perfusion scans are available.

10. How is acute chest syndrome treated?

Patients should be admitted to the hospital. Analgesics, intravenous hydration, and oxygen for hypoxemia are the basic treatment strategies. Early treatment with broad-spectrum antibiotics and oral erythromycin is instituted until culture results are available. In severe, rapidly progressive cases with marked hypoxemia, exchange transfusion is indicated to lower the concentration of hemoglobin S (HgS) acutely.

11. Is heparin beneficial in the treatment of acute chest syndrome?

No. It is dangerous. Patients with sickle cell anemia and acute chest pain syndrome have not been shown to benefit from heparin, and it imposes the risk of bleeding. Severe cases should be treated with exchange transfusion to lower the concentration of HgS acutely, which retards sickling. Heparin should be reserved for cases with unequivocal proof of pulmonary emboli or deep venous thrombosis.

12. Are neurologic complications a predominant feature in patients with sickle cell disease?

Yes. They occur in 26% of all patients with sickle cell anemia. Most such complications result from vascular occlusion and embolic events. Possible complications include transient ischemic attacks, cerebrovascular accidents (CVAs), meningitis, seizures, coma, and subarachnoid and intracerebral hemorrhage.

13. Which neurologic complications occur more frequently in young patients?

CVAs. Children and young adults are more likely to have recurrent CVAs. CVAs occur in 10% to 20% of sickle cell anemia patients by age 20. The mean age of onset of CVA is 10. The youngest patient reported to have a CVA was 6 years old. CVAs account for 16% of deaths in children. Of patients who have one stroke, 67% will suffer another, usually within 36 months, presumably secondary to stasis.

14. What steady-state laboratory abnormalities are present in sickle cell anemia?

Patients with sickle cell anemia at steady-state have underlying hemolytic anemia. Hemoglobin levels are generally between 5 and 10 g/dL. Reticulocyte counts are in the range of 5% to 30%. Polymorphonuclear leukocytosis is common from demargination. Increased indirect bilirubin and lactate dehydrogenase result from hemolysis. Increased alkaline phosphatase results from increased bone metabolism.

15. Which screening tests are helpful?

The diagnostic workup is guided by the presentation of the patient. Minimum screening tests are complete blood count, reticulocyte count, and oxygen saturation, which are compared with the patient's baseline values to determine severity and type of crisis. Severely ill patients with toxemia or hypoxemia require screening of all systems and panculture because of the potential for multiple organ failure and sepsis.

16. How do I treat a patient with a painful sickle cell crisis?

The mainstays of treatment are supplemental oxygen, hydration, and adequate analgesia. Parenteral and oral narcotics are often necessary to attain optimal analgesia. Agents such as morphine, meperidine (Demerol), and codeine often are indicated. Patients with frequent painful crises may develop a tolerance to narcotics and require higher doses.

17. What is the fluid of choice and rate for intravenous hydration?

Aggressive rehydration is one of the mainstays of therapy. The fluid of choice is 5% dextrose in half-normal saline because it is relatively hypotonic and restores intracellular volume. This reduces the intracellular concentration of sickle hemoglobin and retards sickling. Severely ill patients with hypovolemia should be given normal saline, then switched to 5% dextrose in half-normal saline as intravascular volume is repleted. Adults should be given 200 to 300 mL/h; children should be given 100 mL/kg/d.

18. What is the rationale for the use of rapid partial exchange transfusion?

Rapid partial exchange transfusion is used to decrease rapidly the sickle hemoglobin concentration to less than 30%, which decreases sludging in the microcirculation and increases tissue perfusion and limits infarct size.

19. What are some indications for rapid partial exchange transfusion?

Life-threatening events, including acute impending or suspected CVA or transient ischemic attack, acute hepatic or splenic sequestration in the face of a falling hematocrit, acute priapism unresponsive to medical management after 6 hours, acute progressive lung disease, fat embolization, before surgery, and before administration of intravenous contrast material or other hypertonic fluids.

20. Name the new treatment modalities that are being researched or are currently in use to increase the percentage of fetal hemoglobin in the erythrocyte, protecting the sickle cell anemia patient against crises.

Hydroxyurea has been used for many years with some success. Five azacytidine has been used along with other antineoplastic agents with a rise in the concentration of fetal hemoglobin and increased hemoglobin. Bone marrow transplantation is curative when it works.

BIBLIOGRAPHY

1. Buetler E: The sickle cell diseases and related disorders. In Buetler E (ed): Williams Hematology, 6th ed. New York, McGraw-Hill, 2001, pp 581–605.
2. Charache, S, Dover JG, Moore RD, et al: Hydoxyurea: Effects on hemoglobin F production in patients with sickle cell anemia. Blood 79:2555, 1992.

3. Charache S, Lubin B, Reid C: Management and therapy for sickle cell disease. National Institutes of Health Publication No. 85-2117. Bethesda, MD, U.S. Department of Health and Human Services, 1985, p 485.
4. Charache S, Scott J, Charache P: Acute chest syndrome in adults with sickle cell anemia. Arch Intern Med 139:67–69, 1979.
5. Galloway S, Harwood-Nuss A: Sickle cell anemia: A review. J Emerg Med 6:213–226, 1988.
6. Golden C, Styles L, Vichinsky E: Acute chest syndrome and sickle cell disease. Curr Opin Hematol 5:89, 1998.
7. Hargis C, Claster S: Acute chest syndrome in sickle cell disease. Crit Dec Emerg Med 11:11, 1997.
8. Mirchev R, Ferrone FA: The structural link between polymerization and sickle cell disease. J Mol Biol 265:475, 1997.
9. Shapiro BS: The management of pain in sickle cell disease. Pediatr Clin North Am 36:1029–1045, 1989.
10. Walters MC, Patience M, Leienring W, et al: Bone marrow transplantation for sickle cell disease. N Engl J Med 335:369, 1996.

48. ONCOLOGIC EMERGENCIES

Nicholas J. Jouriles, M.D.

1. What is an oncologic emergency?

A life-threatening or limb-threatening problem in a patient with an underlying neoplastic disease. These problems may be caused by the cancer or its systemic effects or by therapeutic maneuvers used in treatment.

2. Is an oncologic emergency important?

Yes. Cancer is the second leading cause of death in the United States. It is second only to trauma in years of potential life loss.

3. List several oncologic emergencies.

Airway compromise
  Head and neck mass
  Tracheal compression
Adrenal crisis
  Primary tumor
  Metastatic lesion
Anemia
  Bone marrow replacement
    with tumor
  Chemotherapy effects
Bleeding
  Primary mass
  Low platelet count
  Abnormal clotting factors
    secondary to liver metastases
Carcinoid syndrome
Complications of chemotherapy
  Bone marrow suppression
  Cardiac toxicity
  Gastrointestinal toxicity
  Pulmonary toxicity
  Renal toxicity

Graft-versus-host disease
Hemorrhagic cystitis
  Chemotherapy induced
  Radiotherapy induced
Hyperviscosity syndrome
Infection
  With neutropenia
  Postobstructive pneumonia
Intestinal obstruction
Intestinal perforation
Malignant pericardial effusion with tamponade
Metabolic abnormalities
  Hypercalcemia
  Acute tumor lysis syndrome
  Hyponatremia/syndrome of inappropriate
    secretion of antidiuretic hormone
  Hyperuricemia
  Hypoglycemia
Obstructive jaundice
Obstructive uropathy
Pain
Peptic ulcer disease

Complications of radiotherapy
  Dermatitis
  Gastrointestinal toxicity
Emotional stress
  Death and dying
  Do not resuscitate orders
  Family issues

Priapism
Seizures
Spinal cord compression
  Motor/sensory loss
  Incontinence
  Back pain
Superior vena cava syndrome
Tinnitus

4. Which on this list are life-threatening or limb-threatening?

The life-threatening diseases are those that can lead to shock or death. They can be divided into the standard categories of shock: volume loss (bleeding) or impaired vascular return (superior vena cava syndrome), pump impairment (cardiac tamponade), and derangement of systemic vascular resistance or afterload (infection or sepsis). In addition to life-threatening problems, there are diseases that can cause serious metabolic derangements (hypercalcemia) and diseases that can lead to neurologic impairment (spinal cord compression).

5. Discuss diseases that can cause serious metabolic derangements and that can lead to neurologic impairment.

Superior vena cava syndrome is caused by obstruction of the superior vena cava. Although it may be caused by such relatively benign processes as mediastinitis or aortic aneurysms, it most often is caused by a neoplastic process. Lung cancer is the most common cause, usually the small cell or squamous types. Adenocarcinoma of the breast, lymphoma, and thymus neoplasms are common. Superior vena cava syndrome also may occur secondary to metastatic lesions from distant primary sites. Treatment usually involves radiation therapy.

Pericardial tamponade occurs secondary to metastatic disease to the pericardium and has been found in 2% to 21% of patients dying of cancer. Patients with pericardial tamponade usually have a large tumor burden and poor 6-month survival. The diagnosis of a malignant pericardial tamponade is suspected clinically in the hypotensive patient with muffled heart sounds, elevated neck veins, and an enlarged cardiac silhouette on chest radiograph. It is seen most commonly in lung and breast carcinomas and lymphoma. Treatment involves pericardial drainage. Emergency physician bedside ultrasound is the best way to make the diagnosis and to guide drainage.

Infections. Because all patients with tumors are by definition immunocompromised, the variety of infections is unlimited. Immune status may be compromised further by chemotherapeutic agents. When patients become neutropenic secondary to treatment, any type of infection may occur (bacterial, viral, or fungal), potentially leading to septic shock, adult respiratory distress syndrome, and death. The neutropenic febrile patient should be treated immediately with prophylactic broad-spectrum antibiotics.

Hypercalcemia occurs in approximately 5% of patients followed in a hospital-based oncology practice. Neoplasms that lead to metastatic involvement of the skeletal system commonly are associated with hypercalcemia. Common presenting signs are lethargy, constipation, and altered mental status. Treatment involves hydration with normal saline followed by forced calcium excretion and agents, such as pamidronate or mithromycin, that act against calcium.

Spinal cord compression occurs in 5% of all patients with metastatic disease. The spinal cord or nerve root is directly compromised by an extradural mass, causing secondary neurologic dysfunction. The most common causes of spinal cord compression are lung, breast, and prostate cancer and multiple myeloma. The most common presenting symptom is back pain. Any patient with an underlying malignancy who presents with back pain, motor or sensory loss, or incontinence should be considered to have spinal cord compression until proved otherwise. Prompt diagnosis and treatment can save neurologic function. All patients who fit the clinical criteria should undergo MRI, including those with negative plain radiographs. Of patients with spinal cord compression, 40% may have normal plain radiographs. Treatment is emergent surgical decompression or radiation therapy. Steroids can be used in the ED.

6. Are these common problems?

Of the life-threatening problems, **spinal cord compression, infection**, and **hypercalcemia** are relatively common.

7. Which problems are common in patients with an underlying malignancy?

The most common problems are complications of cancer treatment. Each chemotherapeutic agent has side effects, including nausea and vomiting, renal involvement (e.g., cisplatin), pulmonary toxicity (e.g., bleomycin), cardiac toxicity (e.g., doxorubicin), and diarrhea or enteritis secondary to radiation. These problems usually are treated by the oncologist before the patient leaves the clinic or office. Onset of symptoms may be delayed, however, and the patient may present to the ED for treatment. Other problems include pain and death.

8. How is a patient with a terminal neoplastic disease treated?

Often the best treatment for a patient with a terminal malignancy is adequate analgesia, comfort measures, and supportive care. The emergency physician must deal with problems related to do not resuscitate orders in the ED and the out-of-hospital arena.

9. How is an oncologic emergency diagnosed?

The most important element is clinical suspicion. In any patient with an underlying neoplastic process (not only patients with an ongoing process, but also patients who had a cure in the remote past), a complication related to that process should be suspected. After concentrating on the ABCs (airway, breathing, and circulation) and vital signs, an extensive history should be taken, followed by a complete physical examination. A presumptive diagnosis should be made and appropriate data obtained (Table).

Management of Selected Oncologic Emergencies

CLINICAL PROBLEM	PRESENTING SYMPTOMS	ED DATA BASE	ED PRIORITIES
Superior vena cava syndrome	Plethora Cyanosis Dyspnea Dilated head/arm veins Jugular venous distention Cough Chest pain	Mediastinal mass on chest film	Emergency radiotherapy Consider tissue biopsy Consider chemotherapy Consider surgical debulking
Infection	Fever Varies with source	CBC with differential Urinalysis Chest film Blood cultures Wound culture Catheter culture Lumbar puncture if not contraindicated	Complete physical exam to locate source Culture all possible sources Protective isolation if neutropenic Begin broad-spectrum antibiotics (varies with known community antibiotic resistance patterns)
Malignant pericardial effusion	Chest pain Cardiac rub Jugular venous distention Distant heart sounds Hypotension	Elevated CVP Low-voltage ECG Cardiomegaly on chest film Pericardial fluid on echocardiogram CVP/PCWP pressure equalization	IV fluid challenge (NS or LR) Drainage Pericardial window (preferred) Pericardiocentesis (ultrasound guided)

(*Table continued on next page.*)

Management of Selected Oncologic Emergencies (cont.)

CLINICAL PROBLEM	PRESENTING SYMPTOMS	ED DATA BASE	ED PRIORITIES
Hypercalcemia	Dehydration Constipation Lethargy Altered mental status	Elevated free calcium Abnormal ECG	IV fluid rehydration (NS) Furosemide Consider calcitonin Consider prednisone, pamidronate
Spinal cord compression	Back pain Motor/sensory deficits Incontinence	Spinal x-ray abnormality Image spinal cord (MRI preferred)	Initiate high-dose steroids Analgesics Emergent surgical decompression Emergent radiotherapy

CBC, complete blood count; CVP, central venous pressure; IV, intravenous; NS, normal saline; LR, lactated Ringer's; PCWP, pulmonary capillary wedge pressure.

10. What symptoms can be related to an underlying neoplastic emergency?

Any presenting symptom can be caused by a neoplastic process. A neoplastic process should be considered in any patient who presents with pain, weakness, dizziness, altered mental status, headache, or seizure. The common symptoms of back pain and abdominal pain can be the initial presentation for an oncologic process that has led to spinal cord compression (back pain) or intestinal obstruction or perforation (abdominal pain).

11. What treatment is used for patients with oncologic emergencies?

Treatment is identical to that for patients without an underlying neoplastic process and should be initiated early. Treatment of selected life-threatening problems is provided in the table in question 9.

12. When should the patient be admitted?

All patients with life-threatening or limb-threatening disease must be admitted. Patients in whom the diagnosis of an oncologic process is made first in the ED usually are admitted. Patients who need to be admitted are those who lack the resources at home to care for themselves. It is common for families to give so much of themselves that they need a break, and an admission for respite care is indicated.

For all other patients, it probably is best to discuss the matter with the patient and the primary physician. Most patients with neoplastic processes have a primary oncologist who knows the patient and his or her situation in detail. One needs to balance the medical risks of the current problem with the patient's psychological needs. Many patients already have spent much time at the hospital and want to spend as much time at home as possible.

13. Can cancer be cured?

Modern therapies offer excellent success with medical (testicular, lymphoma, leukemia), surgical (lung, colon, breast), and combination (radiotherapy and chemotherapy for head and neck, anal) treatments. Many patients today survive long-term, and today's research will find new treatment methods and more success.

BIBLIOGRAPHY

1. Bodey GP, Rolston KV: Management of fever in neutropenic patients. J Infect Chemother 7:1–9, 2001.
2. Coleman RE: Metastatic bone disease: Clinical features, pathophysiology and treatment strategies. Cancer Treat Rev 27:165–176, 2001.
3. DeVita VT, Hellman S, Rosenberg SA (eds): Cancer: Principles and Practice of Oncology, 5th ed. Philadelphia, Lippincott-Raven, 1997.

4. Grant R, Papadopoulos SM, Sandler HM, Greenberg HS: Metastatic epidural spinal cord compression: Current concepts and treatment. J Neurooncol 19:79–92, 1994.
5. Lamy O, Jenzer-Closuit A, Burckhardt P: Hypercalcaemia of malignancy: An undiagnosed and undertreated disease. J Intern Med 250:73–79, 2001.
6. Markman MA: Diagnosis and management of SVC syndrome. Cleve Clin J Med 66:59–61, 1999.
7. Santolaya ME, Alvarez AM, Becker A, et al: Prospective, multicenter evaluation of risk factors associated with invasive bacterial infection in children with cancer, neutropenia, and fever. J Clin Oncol 19:3415–3421, 2001.
8. Shepherd FA: Malignant pericardial effusion. Curr Opin Oncol 9:170–174, 1997.

X. Metabolism and Endocrinology

49. FLUIDS AND ELECTROLYTES

Corey M. Slovis, M.D.

1. Why is the study of fluid and electrolytes so difficult?

Most people who teach fluid and electrolytes are very educated and talk about things like "the negative log of the hydrogen ion concentration," "idiogenic osmols," and "pseudo-pseudo triple acid-base disturbances." Luckily, this chapter is not written by a person who believes in, or understands, negative logarithms.

2. What is the anion gap?

The anion gap (AG) measures the amount of negatively charged ions in the serum (unmeasured anions) that are not bicarbonate (HCO_3^-) or chloride (Cl^-). The AG is calculated by subtracting the sum of HCO_3^- and Cl^- values from the sodium (Na^+) value, the major positive charge in the serum. Potassium (K^+) values are not generally used in the calculation because of the huge amount of intracellular potassium (155 mEq) and the relatively low amount of potassium in the serum (only about 4 mEq). The formula for determining AG is as follows:

$$AG = Na^+ - (Cl^- + HCO_3^-)$$

The normal upper limit for the AG is generally accepted at 8 to 12, although some centers use 10 to 14.

3. Why must AG be calculated each time an electrolyte panel is evaluated?

An elevated AG means there is some unmeasured anion, toxin, or organic acid in the blood. If you do not calculate the gap, you could miss one of the only clues to a potentially life-ending disease or overdose. The AG also allows acidosis to be divided into two types: wide gap (anion gap > 12 to 14) and normal gap (anion gap < 12 to 14).

4. There are two types of acidosis: wide gap and normal gap. What is a hyperchloremic metabolic acidosis?

A hyperchloremic acidosis is just another name for a normal gap acidosis. Just think: If the AG is going to be normal, and the formula for AG = $Na^+ - (Cl^- + HCO_3^-)$, if HCO_3^- goes down, Cl^- has to rise, or, more simply, you become hyperchloremic—hence the name *hyperchloremic metabolic acidosis*.

5. Is there an easy way to remember the differential diagnosis for wide gap metabolic acidosis?

My favorite is taken from Goldfrank and is called **MUDPILES**.

M	=	Methanol	**P**	=	Paraldehyde
U	=	Uremia	**I**	=	INH (Isoniazid) and Iron
D	=	DKA and AKA	**L**	=	Lactic acidosis
			E	=	Ethylene glycol
			S	=	Salicylates

221

6. What are the clues to each of the entities in MUDPILES?

DISEASE	CLUES
Methanol	Alcoholism, blindness or papilledema, profound acidosis
Uremia	Chronically ill-appearing, history of chronic renal failure, BUN > 100 mg/dL, and creatinine > 5 mg/dL
DKA	History of diabetes mellitus, polyuria, and polydipsia, glucose > 500 mg/dL
AKA	Ethyl alcohol, glucose < 250 mg/dL, nausea and vomiting
Paraldehyde	Alcoholism, distinctive breath, access to this now-hard-to-find drug
INH	Tuberculosis, suicide-prone, refractory status seizures
Iron	Pregnant or postpartum, hematemesis, radiopaque tablets on abdominal film (unreliable finding)
Lactic acidosis	Hypoxia, hypotension, sepsis
Ethylene glycol	Alcoholism, oxalate crystals in urine with or without renal failure, fluorescent mouth or urine (from drinking antifreeze—unreliable finding))
Salicylates	History of chronic disease requiring aspirin use (i.e., rheumatoid arthritis); mixed acid-base disturbance (primary metabolic acidosis plus primary respiratory alkalosis); aspirin level > 20 to 40 mg/dL

7. What are the causes of narrow gap acidosis?

Memorize the mnemonic **HARDUPS**.

H = **H**yperventilation (chronic)
A = **A**cetazolamide; **A**cids (e.g., hydrochloric); **A**ddison's disease
R = **R**enal tubular acidosis
D = **D**iarrhea
U = **U**terosigmoidostomy
P = **P**ancreatic fistulas and drainage
S = **S**aline (in large amounts)

If you do not want to memorize anything, it is important to know that diarrhea, especially in children, and renal tubular acidosis, especially in adults, are the two most common causes of a narrow gap acidosis.

8. Why should normal saline (NS) or lactated Ringer's (LR) solution rather than 0.5 NS or dextrose in 5% water (D_5W) be given to someone who needs volume replacement?

Fluid goes into three different body compartments: (1) inside blood vessels (intravascular), (2) into cells (intracellular), and (3) in-between the two (interstitial). NS and LR solution go into all three compartments, and only 25% to 33% stays in the intravascular compartment. A person who lost 2 U of blood (1000 mL) would need 3 to 4 L of crystalloid for volume resuscitation. One-half NS (0.45 NS) provides only half of what NS or LR provide; each liter of 0.45 NS provides 125 to 175 mL to blood vessels (versus 250 to 333 mL for NS and LR). D_5W is the worst for trying to give intravascular volume; it puts only about 80 mL per 1000 mL of D_5W into the vasculature. The rest goes into cells and the interstitium.

9. Which solution is better, NS or LR?

Both fluids are excellent for early volume replacement. **NS** has a pH of 4.5 to 5.5 and has a sodium *and* chloride content of 155 mEq/L each. It is acidotic, has an osmolarity of 310, and has a little more sodium than serum and a lot more chloride than serum (155 mEq/L of Cl⁻ in NS vs. about 100 mEq/L of Cl⁻ in serum). Too much NS too quickly may cause hyperchloremic metabolic acidosis.

LR is considered more physiologic in that it is much closer to serum in its content. Its sodium content is lower than NS at 130 mEq/L, and its chloride is only 109 mEq/L (vs. 155

mEq/L of NS). The solution is called lactated because it has 28 mEq/L of bicarbonate in the form of lactate, which becomes bicarbonate when it is in the body. LR has 4 mEq of potassium (none in NS) and has 3 mEq/L of calcium. Critics of LR do not like all the bicarbonate in it and believe that potassium therapy should be individualized. The bottom line is that neither NS nor LR is better; both are equal in quantities of 2 to 3 L over 24 hours. Patients with protracted vomiting should be given NS, which is higher in chloride. Patients with severe dehydration and the resultant hyperchloremic metabolic acidosis should be given LR, which has the equivalent of 0.5 ampule of bicarbonate per liter.

10. What is the most dangerous electrolyte abnormality? What are its five most common causes?

Hyperkalemia. It may result in sudden arrhythmogenic death because of its effect on the cells' resting membrane potential. The most common cause of hyperkalemia is often referred to as "laboratory error." Actually the laboratory does a perfect analysis, but the serum sample has hemolyzed after, or while, it is being drawn.

1. The number one cause of hyperkalemia is *spurious*.

Other common causes are

2. *Chronic renal failure* (the true number one cause of hyperkalemia)
3. *Acidosis* (potassium moves out of the cell as the pH falls)
4. *Drug induced* (including nonsteroidal antiinflammatory drugs, potassium-sparing diuretics, digoxin, angiotensin-converting enzyme inhibitors, and administration of intravenous potassium chloride)
5. *Cell death* (when potassium comes out of injured muscle or red cells). This category includes burns, crush injuries, rhabdomyolysis, tumor lysis syndrome and intravascular hemolysis.

Much less common causes of hyperkalemia include adrenal insufficiency, hyperkalemic periodic paralysis, and hematologic malignancies.

11. What ECG changes are associated with hyperkalemia?

The first ECG change seen in hyperkalemia is usually a tall, peaked T wave that may occur as potassium values rise to 5.5 to 6.5 mEq/dL. Loss of the P wave may follow as potassium levels rise to 6.5 to 7.5 mEq/dL. The most dangerous ECG finding (generally associated with levels of ≥ 8.0 mEq/dL) is widening of the QRS, which may merge with the abnormal T wave and create a sine wave-appearing ventricular tachycardia.

12. Summarize the best treatment for hyperkalemia.

Treatment is based on (1) serum levels, (2) the presence or absence of ECG changes, and (3) underlying renal function. If the patient has life-threatening ECG changes of hyperkalemia (widening QRS or a sine wave-like rhythm), 10% calcium chloride should be given in an initial dose of 5 to 10 mL to reverse temporarily potassium's deleterious electrical effects. Most patients with hyperkalemia usually require moving potassium intracellularly, then removing potassium from the body, rather than receiving a potentially dangerous calcium infusion.

13. How can potassium be moved intracellularly?

The most effective way is by giving glucose and insulin. Glucose and insulin work by activating the glucose transport system into the cell. As glucose is carried intracellularly, potassium is carried along. The usual dose of glucose is 2 ampules of $D_{50\%}$ (100 mL) and 10 U of insulin. Bicarbonate may be used to drive potassium into the cell, but it is effective *only* in acidotic patients. Usually 1 to 2 ampules of bicarbonate (44.6 to 50 mEq of bicarbonate per ampule) is given over 1 to 20 minutes, depending on how sick or acidotic the patient is. Another method of driving potassium into the cell is use of inhaled β-agonist bronchodilators. β-Agonists may be helpful in a renal failure patient with fluid overload because it may help treat the bronchospasm of pulmonary edema. Intravenous magnesium also drives potassium into the cell, which is advantageous if the patient is having ventricular ectopy but is potentially dangerous if the patient has hypermagnesemia in association with chronic renal failure. Magnesium, in a dose of 1 to 2 g over 10 to 20 minutes may, similar to β-agonists, lower serum potassium by 0.5 mEq.

14. After potassium's electrical effects have been counteracted (if indicated) and potassium has been driven intracellularly, how do you remove it from the body?

Potassium can be removed from the body by (1) diuresis, (2) potassium-binding resins, and (3) hemodialysis. Diuresis with saline, supplemented by furosemide, is an excellent way to lower total body potassium. Most patients have renal failure, however, and cannot make much urine, which is how they became hyperkalemic in the first place. Sodium polystyrene sulfonate (Kayexalate) is a sodium-containing resin that exchanges its sodium content for the patient's potassium. Each 1 g of Kayexalate can remove about 1 mEq of potassium from the patient's body. The best method of lowering potassium is by hemodialysis, and it is the method of choice for any severely ill, acidotic, or profoundly hyperkalemic patient.

15. Discuss the most common causes of hyponatremia.

Hyponatremia is a serum sodium of less than 135 mEq/dL. Most patients with mild hyponatremia (levels > 125 to 130 mEq/dL) are on diuretics or have some degree of fluid overload as a result of congestive heart failure (renal failure or liver disease). Diuretic-induced hyponatremia is most common in the elderly. Patients with congestive heart failure, liver failure, and renal failure develop hyponatremia as a result of secondary hyperaldosteronism. Aldosterone is released because of renal hypoperfusion resulting in volume overload and dilutional hyponatremia (even in the face of total body sodium excess). Moderate-to-severe hyponatremia (levels < 125 mEq/dL) are most commonly due to the syndrome of inappropriate secretion of antidiuretic hormone (SIADH) and psychogenic polydipsia (compulsive water drinking).

16. What is SIADH?

Abnormally high levels of hormone from the posterior pituitary gland, which blocks free water excretion. Normally, when sodium levels fall, levels of this hormone also decrease, resulting in urinary losses of water (diuresis). In this syndrome, antidiuretic hormone (ADH) is released inappropriately, and serum sodium levels fall as more excess free water is retained (antidiuresis). The hallmark of this syndrome is relatively concentrated urine, rather than the maximally dilute urine one sees in a water-overloaded patient. Patients cannot be given this diagnosis if they are taking diuretics or have a reason to be water overloaded (i.e., congestive heart failure, chronic renal failure, or liver failure).

17. What are the classic neurologic signs of hyperkalemia? What are the classic ECG signs of hyponatremia?

No, not a misprint, just a trick to wake you up after antidiuresing. Potassium causes cardiovascular symptoms via its effects on the ECG (see question 11). Sodium causes no ECG changes but does affect the brain because of its effects on osmolality; symptoms include dizziness, confusion, coma, and seizures.

18. How fast should hyponatremia be corrected?

There has been much debate over how rapidly (about 2 mEq/h) or how slowly (about 0.5 mEq/h) sodium should be corrected. Patients should be corrected slowly over 1 to 2 days, and serum sodium should be allowed to rise by no more than 0.5 mEq/h. This approach avoids the possible development of central pontine myelinosis (which is now called the *osmotic demyelinating syndrome* by some purists), a catastrophic neurologic illness of coma and paralysis, seen with too-rapid correction.

19. Should sodium levels *ever* be treated quickly?

There are some specific indications for raising a patient's sodium rapidly by infusing 3% saline at 100 mL/h for a maximum of 2 to 3 hours. Patients who have serum sodium levels of less than 120 mEq/L *and* who have acute alterations in mental status, seizures, or focal findings should have their levels raised about 4 to 6 mEq/dL over a few hours. Other than these rare patients with severe, symptomatic hyponatremia, slow correction by water restriction, slow infusion of saline, and judicious use of furosemide should be employed.

20. What is osmolality? What is the osmolal gap?

Osmolality is calculated by multiplying the serum sodium by 2 and adding the glucose (GLU) divided by 18, plus the blood urea nitrogen (BUN) divided by 2.8. Normal is approximately 280 to 290 mOsm.

$$Osmolarity = 2 \times Na + GLU/18 + BUN/2.8$$

The osmolal gap is determined by using this formula, then asking the laboratory to determine the osmolality by the molal freezing point depression. The difference should be only about 10; if it is more, something else is in the serum (e.g., an alcohol, intravenous contrast media, or mannitol).

$$Osmolal\ gap = laboratory\text{-}determined\ osmolarity - calculated\ osmolarity$$

21. How do you use the osmolal gap in figuring out if someone has ingested methanol or ethylene glycol?

If osmolal gap is elevated, you should measure the patient's serum ethanol level immediately. Because of ethanol's molecular weight, every 4.2 mg/dL of alcohol "weighs" 1 mOsm. If the alcohol level is 100 mg/dL, the patient's osmolal gap should be about 30 to 35 (about 25 from alcohol, added to the normal osmolal gap, which is about 5 to 10).

If there is a higher gap, these unaccounted osmols may represent methanol, ethylene glycol, or isopropyl alcohol. Because isopropyl alcohol causes ketosis without acidosis, acidosis plus an unexplained osmolal gap may mean a life-threatening overdose. Hints to methanol and ethylene glycol overdose appear in answer 6.

22. What are the most common causes of hypercalcemia, and how do they present?

Mild hypercalcemia is usually due to dehydration, thiazide diuretics, or hyperparathyroidism. It is often asymptomatic, but mild fatigue, renal stones, or nonspecific gastrointestinal symptoms may be present. Severe hypercalcemia, with levels greater than 2 to 3 mg/dL above normal, presents as alteration in mental status with the signs and symptoms of profound dehydration.

23. Describe the emergency treatment of hypercalcemia.

Hypercalcemia is treated symptomatically by aggressive volume resuscitation with saline supplemented by furosemide when intravascular volume has been normalized. Hypercalcemia is one of the only true indications left for forced diuresis (rhabdomyolysis may be the only other). Patients should receive 200 to 400 mL of NS plus enough furosemide to keep urine flow high. Saline blocks the proximal tubules from absorbing calcium, and furosemide blocks distal tubular absorption. Older patients and patients with impaired cardiac function should not receive more than about 200 mL of saline per hour when they are volume repleted—otherwise turn to the chapter on congestive heart failure.

BIBLIOGRAPHY

1. Adrogué HJ, Madias NE: Hyponatremia. N Engl J Med 342:1581–1589, 2000.
2. Adrogué HJ, Madias NE: Hypernatremia. N Engl J Med 342:1493–1499, 2000.
3. Edelson GW, Kleerekoper M: Hypercalcemic crisis. Med Clin North Am 79:79–92, 1995.
4. Halperin ML, Kamel KS: Potassium. Lancet 352:135–140, 1998.
5. Hoffman RS: Fluid, electrolyte, and acid-base principles. In Goldfrank LR, Flomenbaum NE, Lewin NA, et al (eds): Goldfrank's Toxicologic Emergencies, 7th ed. New York, McGraw-Hill, 2002, pp 364–380.
6. Narins RG, Emmett M: Simple and mixed acid-base disorders—a practical approach. Medicine 59:161–187, 1980.

7. Narins RG, Jones ER, Stom MC, et al: Diagnostic strategies in disorders of fluid, electrolyte and acid-base homeostasis. Am J Med 77:496–519, 1982.
8. Slovis C, Jenkins R: ABC of clinical electrocardiography: Conditions not primarily affecting the heart. BMJ 324:1320–1323, 2002.

50. ACID-BASE DISORDERS

Stephen L. Adams, M.D.

1. Name the four types of acid-base disorders seen in the ED, and give a common example of each.

Actually, there are five:

1. Metabolic acidosis (e.g., cardiac arrest)
2. Respiratory acidosis (e.g., chronic obstructive pulmonary disease with carbon dioxide [CO_2] retention)
3. Metabolic alkalosis (e.g., protracted vomiting)
4. Respiratory alkalosis (e.g., hyperventilation syndrome)
5. Mixed acid-base disorder (e.g., respiratory alkalosis and metabolic acidosis, as seen in an adult with salicylate intoxication; metabolic acidosis with respiratory compensation)

2. What does pulse oximetry contribute to the understanding of the patient's acid-base status?

Nothing. Pulse oximetry measures oxygen saturation and does not provide a measurement of acid-base or ventilatory status. Arterial blood gas analysis is necessary to determine acid-base status.

3. What are the most commonly cited causes of an elevated anion gap?

An elevated anion gap, usually indicating a low bicarbonate level, should give the clinician cause to consider the presence of a metabolic acidosis. The differential diagnoses may be remembered by the mnemonic **DR. MAPLES**:

D = Diabetic ketoacidosis
R = Renal failure

M = Methanol
A = Alcoholic ketoacidosis
P = Paraldehyde
L = Lactic acidosis
E = Ethylene glycol
S = Salicylate intoxication

These are only some of the causes of a metabolic acidosis.

4. Name some obscure causes of an elevated anion gap metabolic acidosis.

Sulfuric acidosis, short bowel syndrome (D-lactic acidosis), nalidixic acid, methenamine, mandelate, hippuric acid salt, rhubarb (oxalic acid) ingestion, and inborn errors of metabolism, such as the methylmalonic acidemias and isovaleric acidemia. Toluene intoxication can cause either an elevated anion gap metabolic acidosis or a hyperchloremic metabolic acidosis (no anion gap).

5. Is the size of the anion gap clinically useful?

In one study, an anion gap of greater than 30 mEq/L was usually the result of an identifiable organic acidosis (i.e., lactic acidosis or ketoacidosis). Almost 30% of patients with an anion gap of 20 to 29 mEq/L had neither a lactic acidosis nor a ketoacidosis.

6. What are some causes of lactic acidosis?
Shock, seizure, hypoxemia, isoniazid (INH) toxicity, metformin, cyanide poisoning, ritodrine, inhaled industrial acetylene, phenformin ingestion, iron intoxication, ethanol abuse, and carbon monoxide poisoning. Sodium nitroprusside, povidone-iodine ointment, sorbitol, xylitol, and streptozocin are other drugs that have been listed as causing increased lactic acid formation.

7. How severe is the acid-base disturbance that results from a grand mal seizure? How long does it take to resolve the acidosis?
A grand mal seizure can result in a profound lactic acidosis. The pH levels may plummet to 6.9 or lower. The acidosis in an uncomplicated seizure usually resolves spontaneously within 1 hour.

8. Can a patient have a metabolic acidosis without evidence of an elevated anion gap?
Yes. A patient with a hyperchloremic metabolic acidosis may have no evidence of an elevated anion gap. This condition is caused, in effect, by adding hydrogen chloride to the serum. The fall in serum bicarbonate is offset by the addition of Cl^-; consequently, there is no increased anion gap.

9. How can I remember some of the causes of a normal anion gap metabolic acidosis?
Use the mnemonic **USED CARP**:

U	=	Ureteroenterostomy	C	= Carbonic anhydrase inhibitors
S	=	Small bowel fistula	A	= Adrenal insufficiency
E	=	Extra chloride	R	= Renal tubular acidosis
D	=	Diarrhea	P	= Pancreatic fistula

10. In a patient with DKA who is improving with appropriate therapy, why might the measurement of serum ketones show an increase?
There are three ketone bodies: β-hydroxybutyrate (BHB), acetoacetate (AcAc), and acetone. BHB and AcAc are acids; acetone is not. The proportion of BHB to AcAc depends on the oxidation-reduction status of the patient. A patient who is in DKA on presentation often is severely dehydrated, and the preponderance of ketone bodies may be in the form of BHB. The test by which ketones are noted is the nitroprusside reaction test (Acetest, Ketostix), which measures AcAc and acetone but is not sensitive to BHB. In the patient with DKA, as fluids and insulin therapy are instituted, the amount of BHB converted to AcAc increases, and the nitroprusside reaction, which initially may have been weakly positive or even negative, becomes increasingly positive.

11. List nine disorders that can cause a hyperketonemic state.

Isopropyl alcohol intoxication	Cyanide intoxication
DKA	Industrial acetylene inhalation
Alcoholic ketoacidosis	Hyperemesis gravidarum
Starvation	Bovine ketosis
Paraldehyde intoxication (pseudoketosis)	Stress hormone excess

12. What may contribute to metabolic acidosis in an abuser of alcohol?
Ketoacidosis has been well documented in the chronic alcoholic who binges, then presents with nausea, vomiting, abdominal pain, and poor caloric intake. Lactic acid, acetic acid, and indirect loss of bicarbonate in the urine (nonanion gap metabolic acidosis) also may contribute to an alcoholic acidosis.

13. Which electrolyte is affected most commonly by a change in acid-base status?
Serum potassium. Patients with severe acidosis tend to have elevated serum K^+ levels, whereas patients with severe alkalosis tend to have low serum K^+ levels. A change of pH of 0.10 is consistent with a corresponding change in serum K^+ of about 0.5 mEq/L (range, 0.3 to 0.8 mEq/L). If the pH is elevated by 0.10, the serum K^+ falls by about 0.5 mEq/L. If the pH is diminished

by 0.10, the serum K^+ rises by about 0.5 mEq/L. This concept is well known to clinicians who treat patients who present in DKA. Although the patient's total body K^+ may be severely depleted, initial serum K^+ levels may be elevated in the severely acidotic patient. As the patient is treated appropriately and acidosis resolves, K^+ supplementation is indicated because serum levels may fall precipitously.

14. What is a pseudometabolic acidosis?

Underfilling of Vacutainer tubes can cause a significant decline in bicarbonate and an increase in anion gap that may be mistaken for metabolic acidosis. It is theorized that because atmospheric pressure contains less than 5% CO_2, the lower partial pressure of CO_2 over the blood in an underfilled tube causes CO_2 to diffuse out of the venous solution, decreasing the bicarbonate with which it is in equilibrium. Tubes should be filled completely to prevent creating a pseudometabolic acidosis.

15. Are there any potential ill effects of using paper bag rebreathing in the treatment of hyperventilation syndrome?

Yes. When normal volunteers hyperventilated into a brown paper bag, inspired oxygen was decreased sufficiently so as to endanger hypoxic patients. Paper bag rebreathing therapy probably should not be used unless myocardial ischemia can be ruled out and arterial blood gas analysis or pulse oximetry excludes hypoxia.

16. How does core temperature affect arterial blood gases?

Uncorrected arterial blood gases yield a falsely elevated pH and a falsely decreased PO_2 and PCO_2 in hypothermia. For every $1°C$ decrease in body temperature, the pH is elevated 0.015, PCO_2 (mm Hg) decreases 4.4%, and PO_2 decreases 7.2% ($37°C$ reference). Hyperthermia decreases the pH and increases the PCO_2 and PO_2 by an equivalent amount. The clinical use of corrected versus uncorrected pH determinations in hypothermia is controversial.

17. What acid-base alterations are seen commonly in heatstroke?

Metabolic acidosis (81% of patients in one study) and respiratory alkalosis (55% of patients). The prevalence of metabolic acidosis was associated significantly with the degree of hyperthermia. Of patients, 63% with a rectal temperature of $41°C$, 95% with a temperature of $42°C$, and 100% with a temperature of $43°C$ had a metabolic acidosis. This association was not true for respiratory alkalosis. Patients who had a metabolic acidosis had a large anion gap (24 ± 5).

18. What disease process can present with an anion gap *higher* than the serum glucose?

Alcoholic ketoacidosis, a well-known cause of an elevated anion gap metabolic acidosis, may present with hypoglycemia. One case report presented a patient with alcoholic ketoacidosis and a concomitant illness, pneumonia, with an anion gap of 36 and a serum glucose of less than 20 mg/dL. Severe hypoglycemia may cause a lactic acidosis and usually occurs in the setting of a defect in gluconeogenesis, which may be seen in a patient with chronic alcohol ingestion. A concomitant illness commonly is seen in the patient with alcoholic ketoacidosis.

19. How may patients with HIV have an abnormality in the anion gap?

A patient with HIV may have a low anion gap. Hypergammaglobulinemia, resulting from an increased number of immunoglobulin-secreting B cells because of failure in immunoregulation, has been reported in patients with HIV. Consequently an elevation of IgG and IgA may occur. The anion gap may be low because of the cationic charge of IgG. One case report described a patient with HIV with lactic acidosis, which should elevate the anion gap, who had a "deceptively" normal anion gap. A patient with hyperlactacidemia and a normal anion gap acidosis should prompt an evaluation of coexisting illnesses that may be responsible for the low anion gap.

20. Besides the toxic alcohols, name two entities causing a metabolic acidosis with an elevated anion gap that have been associated with an elevated osmolal gap.

Alcoholic ketoacidosis and lactic acidosis. It has been speculated that in patients with lactic acidosis, organic substances of low molecular weight are released from ischemic tissues, accounting for unmeasured osmols. In alcoholic ketoacidosis, it has been speculated that an increased osmolal gap could be attributed to acetone, an uncharged ketone of low molecular weight that may be elevated if the ketoacidosis is severe and prolonged. The exact pathogenesis of the gap in these two entities is not certain, however. As can be seen, the elevated osmolal gap is not specific for a toxic alcohol ingestion.

21. Is there a mathematical model of the outer medullary collecting duct of the rat? Will you ever find an ED attending physician who can cite the article?

Yes. No.

BIBLIOGRAPHY

1. Adams SL: Alcoholic ketoacidosis. Emerg Med Clin North Am 8:749–760, 1990.
2. Bouchama A, De Vol EB: Acid-base alterations in heatstroke. Intensive Care Med 27:680–685, 2001.
3. Callaham M: Hypoxic hazards of traditional paper bag rebreathing in hyperventilating patients. Ann Emerg Med 18:622–628, 1989.
4. Gabow PA, Kaehny WD, Fennessey PV, et al: Diagnostic importance of an increased serum anion gap. N Engl J Med 303:854–858, 1980.
5. Herr RD, Swanson T: Pseudometabolic acidosis caused by underfill of Vacutainer tubes. Ann Emerg Med 21:177–180, 1992.
6. Marinella MA: Alcoholic ketoacidosis presenting with extreme hypoglycemia. Am J Emerg Med 15:280–281, 1997.
7. Orringer CE, Eustace JC, Wunsch CD, Gardner LB: Natural history of lactic acidosis after grand mal seizures. N Engl J Med 297:796–799, 1977.
8. Reuler JB: Hypothermia: Pathophysiology, clinical settings, and management. Ann Intern Med 89:519–527, 1978.
9. Schelling JR, Howard RL, Winter SD, Linas SL: Increased osmolal gap in alcoholic ketoacidosis and lactic acidosis. Ann Intern Med 113:580–582, 1990.
10. Schwartz-Goldstein BH, Malik AR, Sarwar A, Brandstetter RD: Lactic acidosis associated with a deceptively normal anion gap. Heart Lung 25:79–80, 1996.
11. Slucher B, Levinson SS: Human immunodeficiency virus infection and anion gap. Ann Clin Lab Sci 23:249–255, 1993.
12. Weinstein AM: A mathematical model of the outer medullary collecting duct of the rat. Am J Physiol Ren Physiol 279:F24–45, 2000.

51. DIABETES MELLITUS

Christina Johnson, M.D.

1. Describe the physiologic and clinical differences between type 1 diabetes mellitus (DM) and type 2 DM.

Type 1 DM is also known as *juvenile-onset diabetes* or *insulin-dependent DM*. It is thought to be initiated by an immunologic stimulus that destroys pancreatic islet cells, which produce insulin. Patients with type 1 DM have little or no endogenous insulin production. Without adequate insulin, these patients are prone to developing diabetic ketoacidosis. Dietary modifications and oral hypoglycemic agents are inadequate therapy. In contrast, patients with type 2 DM generally develop the disease after age 40. Obesity is a contributing factor in the development of the disease. These patients produce insulin, but their insulin response to glucose is diminished, and there is resistance to the insulin. Type 2 diabetics are non–insulin dependent, although they may be taking insulin to control their glucose levels further. Their glucose levels generally respond to dietary modification and oral hypoglycemic agents.

2. List the physiologic complications of hyperglycemia.
Complications of type 1 or type 2 DM:
  Osmotic diuresis
  Electrolyte abnormalities
  Impaired leukocyte function with predisposition to infection
  Retinopathy
  Nephropathy
  Neuropathy
  Coronary artery and cerebrovascular disease
  Peripheral vascular disease
Only type 1 diabetics develop diabetic ketoacidosis.

3. What types of infections are seen more commonly in diabetics than in other patients?
Malignant otitis externa, caused by *Pseudomonas aeruginosa*, is unique to diabetics. Starting in the external auditory canal, this infection can spread rapidly to the nearby skin, cartilage, and bone without appropriate antibiotics. The diagnosis can be made on clinical grounds, but CT scan is useful to delineate the extent of disease. Invasive disease requires admission of the patient and IV antipseudomonal antibiotic administration. Outpatient therapy for noninvasive disease consists of topical antibiotic drops and oral ciprofloxacin. Diabetics also may develop invasive **mucormycosis**. This infection originates in the nasal or paranasal sinuses and invades locally. Complications include orbital spread, necrosis of the sinuses, and cerebral abscesses. CT scan is indicated, and treatment includes administration of amphotericin B. **Emphysematous pyelonephritis** and **emphysematous cholecystitis** are more common in diabetics and present similar to typical pyelonephritis and cholecystitis, with the additional finding of gas on plain films; IV antibiotics and surgical therapy are required for treatment. **Cellulitis** progresses more quickly in diabetics and leads more frequently to complications, such as necrotizing fasciitis, osteomyelitis, and sepsis.

4. What are the common manifestations of diabetic neuropathy?
Typically the neuropathy is a peripheral *stocking-glove* polyneuropathy. Sensory loss in the feet predisposes diabetics to foot ulceration and risk of amputation. Diabetic patients may present with acute mononeuropathy multiplex, cranial mononeuropathy, and autonomic insufficiency such as gastroparesis or urinary retention. They tend to have a higher incidence of silent ischemia.

5. Describe the pertinent clinical and laboratory findings of diabetic ketoacidosis (DKA).
A patient with DKA presents with hyperglycemia; osmotic diuresis with resultant dehydration; polyuria, polydipsia, and polyphagia; weight loss; metabolic acidosis secondary to lipolysis with production of acetoacetate and β-hydroxybutyrate; tachypnea; Kussmaul breathing; fruity breath odor (similar to nail polish remover); and potassium, sodium, chloride, calcium, magnesium, and phosphorus depletion. Some patients with DKA also complain of nausea, vomiting, or abdominal pain secondary to gastric distention or stretching of the liver capsule. Others may have some degree of altered mentation.

6. What causes DKA?
DKA occurs only in patients with insulin deficiency. When there is deficient insulin, glucose transfer into the cells is prohibited, and the resultant cellular deprivation leads to increased stress hormone levels. The body's stress hormones are glucagon, catecholamines, cortisol, and growth hormone. These hormones increase glycogenolysis and gluconeogenesis, increasing the blood glucose level. Glucagon and catecholamines also stimulate lipolysis, which leads to the breakdown

of triglycerides into fatty acids. The fatty acids are oxidized to form ketone bodies called *acetoacetate* and β-*hydroxybutyrate*. Accumulation of these ketone bodies leads to metabolic acidosis.

Acute precipitants of DKA include insufficient or absent insulin administration and stressors such as infection, stroke, myocardial infarction, pancreatitis, trauma, or pregnancy. Pneumonia or urinary tract infections are found in 30% to 50% of cases of DKA. Patients with new-onset type 1 DM frequently present in DKA.

7. How does one make the diagnosis of DKA?

The diagnosis is made when a patient presents with the following laboratory parameters:
- Hyperglycemia (glucose > 250 mg/dL)
- Low bicarbonate (< 15 mEq/L)
- Low pH (pH < 7.3) with ketonemia and moderate ketonuria

8. How should DKA be treated in the ED?

- **Fluid resuscitation**. Estimated volume deficit approaches 5 L in most patients. Normal saline should be administered at a rate of 500 mL/h for several hours in the otherwise healthy adult. In children, give 10 to 20 mL/kg/h of fluid for the first hour. This bolus may be repeated, but do not give more than 50 mL/kg of IV fluid in the first 4 hours. After this time, IV fluids can be given at 1.5 times the 24-hour maintenance rate.
- **Insulin therapy**. Initial insulin dosage should be 0.1 to 0.4 U/kg followed by 0.1 U/kg/h via IV infusion. Serum glucose levels should be checked frequently, with the goal being a decrease in glucose level by 50 to 75 mg/dL/h.
- **Potassium replacement**. In most patients, the serum potassium drops quickly with administration of fluid and insulin. When insulin has been given, the addition of 20 to 40 mEq of potassium to each 1 L of fluid should correct the deficit slowly. The potassium level should be maintained between 4 and 5 mEq/L.
- **Phosphorus and bicarbonate**. Therapy with these agents is controversial and should be reserved for patients with severe deficits (phosphorus < 1, pH < 6.9).
- **Glucose**. When the serum glucose level decreases to less than 250 mg/dL, IV fluids should be switched to half-normal saline with the addition of 5% dextrose. Generally the insulin requirement decreases at this point.

9. Do all patients with DKA need to be admitted to the hospital?

Not anymore. Traditionally, all patients with DKA have been admitted to the hospital. Patients with mild DKA may respond rapidly to therapy. Patients who do not have underlying illnesses that mandate admission, have normal vital signs and mentation, have corrected laboratory abnormalities, are taking oral fluids and food, and can comply with instructions regarding treatment and follow-up of their diabetes may be able to be treated and discharged from the ED.

10. List the potential complications of therapy for DKA in the ED.

Cerebral edema (with overly aggressive correction of fluid or sodium and glucose abnormalities)
Adult respiratory distress syndrome (particularly in patients with pneumonia or cardiac disease)
Hyperchloremic acidosis
Hypoglycemia
Hypokalemia
A common mistake in managing patients with DKA in the ED is failure to identify and treat the underlying precipitants of DKA.

11. What is hyperosmolar hyperglycemic nonketotic coma?

This is defined by a plasma osmolarity greater than 350 mOsm/kg water, a serum glucose concentration greater than 600 mg/dL, and absence of ketoacidosis in a patient with altered mentation. The patient may be lethargic or confused rather than comatose.

12. How is plasma osmolarity determined?

Osmolarity (mOsm/kg water) = 2 × (serum sodium) + (serum glucose)/18 + blood urea nitrogen)/2.8. The degree of hyperosmolarity and the rate with which it develops predict the extent of alteration in patient mental status.

13. What occurs pathophysiologically to cause hyperosmolar hyperglycemic nonketotic coma (HHNC)?

In the absence of insulin, glucose remains extracellular and creates an osmotic gradient. Extracellular volume expands at the expense of intracellular dehydration. Elevated glucose levels overcome renal filtration, and glucosuria results. Osmotic diuresis occurs as a result of the glucosuria. Along with loss of free water, there is loss of potassium, often to a profound degree. Why these patients are not ketotic remains controversial. Some authors report that there is inhibition of lipolysis with higher insulin levels than are seen in DKA, whereas others report that free fatty acids are metabolized differently in patients with HHNC.

14. What are the precipitants of HHNC?

HHNC may be the initial presentation of previously unrecognized diabetes in an adult with type 2 DM. Elderly diabetic patients seem to be at greater risk for this illness. Other precipitants include corticosteroids, propranolol, calcium channel blockers, cimetidine, mannitol, phenytoin, and thiazide diuretics. Concomitant renal disease, gastrointestinal bleeding, hypertension, and congestive heart failure are common in patients with HHNC. As with DKA, the presence of infection, myocardial infarction, stroke, pancreatitis, or trauma may precipitate HHNC.

15. What are the four key points in ED management of patients with HHNC?

1. **Fluid administration**. Initially, 1 to 2 L of normal saline should be given. Subsequent liters may be half-normal saline. Usual fluid deficits are on the order of 10 L. Care should be taken not to administer IV fluids too rapidly to patients with renal, pulmonary, or cardiac disease.

2. **Potassium**. Assuming normal renal function, potassium should be repleted at a rate of 10 to 20 mEq/h.

3. **Insulin**. Although most patients with HHNC do not receive insulin therapy, patients with acidosis, hyperkalemia, or renal failure need insulin to lower glucose and resolve metabolic derangements. A starting dose of 0.15 U/kg of insulin given intravenously, with an infusion rate of 0.1 U/kg/h, is reasonable in these patients.

4. **Glucose**. Glucose should be added to the IV fluids when the serum level decreases to less than 250 mg/dL.

16. Which patients with HHNC should be admitted to the hospital?

All patients with HHNC should be admitted. Most require at least 24 hours of monitoring for treatment of electrolyte abnormalities, fluid administration, and evaluation of precipitating causes.

17. Define hypoglycemia.

A serum glucose level less than 50 mg/dL.

18. Who develops hypoglycemia?

Patients with DM are at greatest risk. Excessive insulin or oral hypoglycemic agent dosing for the patient's activity or oral intake results in hypoglycemia. Other patients at risk include those taking pentamidine, aspirin, or haloperidol; very young or very old patients; and patients with insulinomas or renal failure, adrenal insufficiency, sepsis, alcoholism, or heart failure.

19. Overdoses of which oral hypoglycemic agents do not cause hypoglycemia?

Metformin reduces hepatic glucose release and enhances insulin sensitivity. Metformin overdose leads to nausea, vomiting, abdominal pain, and lactic acidosis. Treatment of the lactic acidosis may require intubation or dialysis or both. Acarbose and miglitol act in the small intestine to inhibit breakdown of carbohydrates into glucose and absorption of glucose. Symptoms of overdose with one of these agents include bloating, abdominal pain, and diarrhea.

20. What are the presenting signs and symptoms of a patient with hypoglycemia?

Sweating, trembling, light-headedness, palpitations, irritability, inability to concentrate, confusion, focal neurologic deficits, and seizures. If due to hypoglycemia, these signs and symptoms should resolve quickly with administration of glucose to the patient.

21. Which patients with hypoglycemia require admission to the hospital?

Patients with persistent alterations in mental status after glucose administration

Patients who have taken excessive oral hypoglycemic agents or long-acting insulin preparations

Patients who are unable to tolerate oral fluids and food

Patients who are suicidal

Patients who have other underlying illnesses that require hospitalization

Out-of-hospital paramedic administration of glucose and evaluation for medical clearance is safe and cost-effective in selected populations.

BIBLIOGRAPHY

1. Atkinson MA, Maclaren NK: The pathogenesis of insulin-dependent diabetes mellitus. N Engl J Med 321:1428–1436, 1994.
2. Braaten JT: Hyperosmolar nonketotic diabetic coma: Diagnosis and management. Geriatrics 42:83–92, 1987.
3. Carlton FB: Recent advances in the pharmacologic management of diabetes mellitus. Emerg Med Clin North Am 18:745–753, 2000.
4. Kitabchi AE, Umpierrez GE, Murphy MB, et al: Management of hyperglycemic crises in patients with diabetes. Diabetes Care 24:131–148, 2001.
5. Kitabchi AE, Wall BM: Diabetic ketoacidosis. Med Clin North Am 79:9–37, 1995.
6. Rutledge J, Couch R: Initial fluid management of diabetic ketoacidosis in children. Am J Emerg Med 18:658–660, 2000.
7. Service FJ: Hypoglycemias. West J Med 154:442–454, 1991.
8. Socransky SJ, Pirrallo RG, Rubin JM: Out-of-hospital treatment of hypoglycemia: Refusal of transport and patient outcome. Acad Emerg Med 5:1080–1085, 1998.

52. THYROID DISORDERS

W. Jared Scott, M.D.

1. Which thyroid-related conditions are considered true emergencies?

True emergencies are represented by the life-threatening extremes of myxedema coma and thyroid storm. Thyroid disease is common. The frequency of hypothyroidism in adults in the United States is 1 in 20. Myxedema coma is rare, however, accounting for significantly less than 1% of hypothyroid cases. Thyroid storm occurs in 1% to 2% of thyrotoxic patients. The mortality of thyroid storm and myxedema coma without treatment is 80% to 100%, and with treatment, it is 15% to 50%. Rarely, ophthalmologic complications of Graves' disease may require emergent treatment.

2. When should thyroid function tests be sent from the ED?

The results of thyroid function tests are rarely available in a timely fashion to aid in ED diagnosis and management of thyroid disease. At best, most initial thyroid function tests take several hours to complete and, with a few exceptions, need not be sent from the ED. For patients with appropriate outpatient follow-up, thyroid tests may be sent to help guide long-term management by other providers (i.e., patients with unexplained weight loss, constitutional symptoms, or persistent tachycardia). Thyroid function tests also are mandatory for patients being admitted with new-onset atrial fibrillation or suspicion of thyroid storm or myxedema coma.

3. What is the difference between thyrotoxicosis and hyperthyroidism?

Thyrotoxicosis refers to the condition of excess circulating thyroid hormone originating from multiple causes (e.g., thyroid hormone overdose, thyroid inflammation, or thyroid hyperfunction). **Hyperthyroidism** refers to excess circulating hormone resulting only from thyroid *gland* hyperfunction.

4. What are the most common causes of thyrotoxicosis, and how do they present?

- **Excess thyroid hormone production**: (1) Graves' disease accounts for 85% of all cases of thyrotoxicosis. Most commonly, patients are women 20 to 40 years old who have a goiter and exophthalmos. (2) Toxic multinodular goiter is the second most common cause of thyrotoxicosis. The usual patient is elderly and has cardiovascular abnormalities, with congestive heart failure and tachyarrhythmias predominating. (3) Exposure to iodine can precipitate thyrotoxicosis in patients with toxic multinodular goiter or Graves' disease. Sources of exposure may include radiographic contrast material, potassium iodine solution, amiodarone, and large doses of topical povidone-iodine.
- **Leakage of thyroid hormone**: (1) Subacute thyroiditis is an inflammatory condition commonly seen in young women. This common cause of postpartum thyrotoxicosis typically presents with a goiter. (2) Radiation-induced inflammation is another cause.
- **Exogenous thyroid hormone administration**: (1) Thyrotoxicosis factitia is a Munchausen-type syndrome in which thyroid hormone is taken to cause illness. (2) Thyroid hormone overdose or ingestion of meat containing beef thyroid tissue also can cause thyrotoxicosis.

5. List the common clinical manifestations of thyrotoxicosis.

Constitutional: fatigue, weakness, heat intolerance, diaphoresis, fever, weight loss
Neuropsychiatric: tremor, hyperreflexia, apathy, anxiety, emotional lability, psychosis
Ophthalmologic: exophthalmos, lid lag, eye dryness
Cardiovascular: tachycardia, palpitations, congestive heart failure
Hematologic: anemia, leukocytosis
Gastrointestinal: diarrhea
Dermatologic: hair loss, onycholysis

6. Is goiter always found in thyrotoxicosis?

No. A goiter is often not present in a patient with thyrotoxicosis. Two thyrotoxic states without goiter are exogenous administration of thyroid hormone and apathetic thyrotoxicosis. A goiter may be present in hypothyroidism. The latter case is seen in goiterous forms of thyroiditis, in which, in advanced stages, the gland is "burned out," and scar tissue causes gland enlargement.

7. What is apathetic thyrotoxicosis?

An atypical and frequently missed presentation of hyperthyroidism seen commonly in the elderly but noted at any age, even in children. The typical patient is 70 to 80 years old with a small or no palpable thyroid gland. Few patients exhibit ophthalmologic findings characteristic of hyperthyroidism. The diagnosis should be considered in elderly with chronic weight loss, proximal muscle weakness, depressed affect, new-onset atrial fibrillation, or congestive heart failure.

8. What differentiates thyroid storm from thyrotoxicosis?

Most thyrotoxic states may be managed as an outpatient, whereas thyroid storm is a medical emergency. No absolute diagnostic criteria exist for thyroid storm, but the clinical picture usually includes (1) exaggerated manifestations of thyrotoxicosis; (2) temperature greater than 100°F

(37.7°C); (3) tachycardia out of proportion to fever; and (4) dysfunction of the central nervous system, cardiovascular system, or gastrointestinal system.

9. What conditions are included in the differential diagnosis of thyroid storm?
Thyroid storm may mimic the symptoms of toxicity caused by cocaine, amphetamines, other sympathomimetics, and anticholinergics and alcohol withdrawal syndromes or infections such as encephalitis, meningitis, and sepsis. A history of thyroid disease or previous thyroid treatment or surgery is helpful in distinguishing thyroid storm from these other conditions.

10. What role do thyroid function tests have in making the diagnosis of thyroid storm?
Although thyroid function tests in the patient with thyroid storm are abnormal, they may not be appreciably different from those with thyrotoxicosis and do not differentiate between the two. The diagnosis is a clinical one.

11. List conditions that precipitate thyroid storm.
Emotional stress
Infection or serious illness
Surgery
Trauma
Childbirth
Withdrawal of antithyroid therapy
Recent thyroid ablation therapy

12. How is thyroid storm treated?
ED management of thyroid storm is essentially the same as for thyrotoxicosis, only more urgent.

Step Therapy of Decompensated Thyrotoxicosis

A. Supportive Care
General: Oxygen, cardiac monitor
Fever: External cooling, acetaminophen (aspirin is contraindicated because it may increase free T_4)
Dehydration: Intravenous fluids
Nutrition: Glucose, multivitamins, including folate (deficient secondary to hypermetabolism)
Adrenal replacement (depletion secondary to hypermetabolism): Hydrocortisone, 200 mg IV initially, then 100 mg three times a day until stable
Cardiac decompensation (atrial fibrillation, congestive heart failure): digoxin (increased requirements), diuretics, sympatholytics as required
Treat precipitating event: Therapy as indicated

B. Inhibition of hormone biosynthesis—thionamides:
Propylthiouracil (PTU),* 1200 to 1500 mg/day given as a loading dose of 600 to 1000 mg followed by 200 to 250 mg q 4 hr PO, by nasogastric tube, or rectally (also blocks peripheral conversion of T_4 to T_3)
or
Methimazole, 120 mg/day given as 20 mg PO q 4 hr (or 40 mg crushed in an aqueous solution rectally) with or without a loading dose of 60 to 100 mg

C. Blockade of hormone release—iodides* (at least 1 hour after step B):
Lugol's solution, 30–60 drops/day orally divided three or four times a day
or
Ipodate (Orografin) 0.5 to 3 g/day (especially useful with thyroiditis or thyroid hormone overdose)
or
Lithium carbonate (if allergic to iodine or agranulocytosis occurs with thionamides), 300 mg PO q 6 hr and subsequently to maintain serum lithium at 1 mEq/L

(Table continued on next page.)

Step Therapy of Decompensated Thyrotoxicosis (cont.)

D. Antagonism of peripheral hormone effects—sympatholytics:

Propranolol,* 2 to 5 mg IV q 4 hr or IV infusion at 5 to 10 mg/hr. For less toxic patients use PO at 20 to 200 mg q 4 hr (contraindicated in bronchospastic disease† and congestive heart failure; digitalize patients with congestive heart failure before starting propranolol)

or

Reserpine, 2.5 to 5 mg IM q 4 hr, preceded by 1-mg test dose while monitoring blood pressure (use if β-blocker contraindicated and congestive heart failure and hypotension and cardiac shock not present)

or

Guanethidine, 30 to 40 mg PO q 6 hr

* Preferred medication.
† Consider esmolol if history of pulmonary disease. Effective dose may be higher than recommended. Begin with 500 mg/kg load over one minute, followed by 50 mg/kg/min IV. Repeat load and double infusion as necessary.

13. How is thyroid hormone overdose treated?

Thyroid hormone overdose presents as thyrotoxicosis and is most common after chronic ingestions. Fatalities are rare with acute ingestion. Toxicity after massive acute overdose may occur within 4 to 12 hours or may be delayed for 5 to 11 days, particularly with T_4 (levothyroxine) ingestion. Acute overdose management is as usual, including charcoal and workup for possible coingestants. Gastric lavage may be considered for patients who present within 1 hour of ingestion. If the chronic overdose is iatrogenic, the patient's dose of levothyroxine is held for 1 week and restarted at a reduced dose.

14. Describe Graves' ophthalmopathy.

Graves' ophthalmopathy is usually a self-limited process associated with a history of current or previous Graves' hyperthyroidism. Clinical features variably present include eyelid retraction, proptosis, chemosis, periorbital edema, and diplopia with poor eye movement. Clinically evident ophthalmopathy occurs in about half of Graves' patients.

15. When is treatment of Graves' ophthalmopathy an emergent condition?

With severe ophthalmopathy, the patient may complain of days or weeks of visual blurring persisting with eye closure and diminished color brightness. These symptoms may signal compression of the optic nerve. Chronic corneal exposure can cause keratitis or corneal ulceration presenting as eye pain, photophobia, conjunctival injection, visual loss, and a flare of cells in the anterior chamber. Immediate consultation with an ophthalmologist is required for either of these conditions. Optic neuropathy initially is treated with high-dose steroids (e.g., prednisone, 1 to 2 mg/kg PO). Corneal ulcers, with or without keratitis, require culture and topical antibiotics. The use of cycloplegics should be discussed with the consulting ophthalmologist.

16. What are the causes of hypothyroidism?

Hypothyroidism is simply a deficiency of thyroid hormone. The major mechanisms include (1) **primary**—dysfunction of the gland; (2) **secondary**—deficiency of thyroid-stimulating hormone (TSH) from the pituitary; and (3) **tertiary**—deficiency of thyrotropin-releasing hormone (TRH) from the hypothalamus. Primary hypothyroidism is the most common, and causes include autoimmune and subacute thyroiditis, end-stage Graves' disease, postthyroidectomy or postirradiation, drug induced (iodides, lithium, thionamides, amiodarone), congenital, and tumor.

17. What are the common clinical manifestations of hypothyroidism?

Constitutional: cold intolerance, weight gain, hypothermia, weakness, lethargy, hoarse or deep voice, slow speech, drowsiness

Neuropsychiatric: delayed deep tendon reflexes, dementia, psychosis, paresthesia

Cardiovascular: angina, bradycardia
Respiratory: pleural effusion, dyspnea, hypoventilation
Musculoskeletal: joint pains, muscle cramps
Dermatologic: cool, dry skin; hair loss; nonpitting edema
Gynecologic: menorrhagia

18. How is myxedema coma diagnosed?

The hallmark clinical features of myxedema coma are hypothermia (75%) and coma. A history of thyroid disease, thyroid replacement therapy, or previous thyroid surgery is helpful. Classic physical findings of hypothyroidism may be present. Laboratory evaluation may reveal anemia, electrolyte abnormalities, hypercarbia, respiratory acidosis, or respiratory failure. ECG and chest radiograph may show bradycardia and pleural effusion or frank congestive heart failure.

19. What precipitates myxedema coma in the hypothyroid patient?

Triggers include pulmonary infection, sedatives and anesthetic agents (owing to decreased drug metabolism), cold exposure, trauma, myocardial infarction or congestive heart failure, cerebrovascular accident, and gastrointestinal hemorrhage. Contributing metabolic conditions include hypoxia, hypercapnia, hyponatremia, and hypoglycemia.

20. What is the treatment for myxedema coma?

(1) **Supportive care**: Immediate life threats are assessed and treated, beginning with airway control, oxygen, IV access, and cardiac monitor. Patients should be intubated and hyperventilated for respiratory failure. Hypotension is treated with crystalloids. Patients may be refractory to vasopressors without thyroid hormone replacement. Baseline thyroid function studies should be sent. Hypothermia is treated with passive rewarming. Hydrocortisone, 100 to 200 mg IV, is indicated because of the metabolic stress associated with hypothyroidism. (2) **Thyroid replacement therapy**: A dose of 4 μg/kg lean body weight of IV T_4 (levothyroxine or thyroxine) is given as a bolus, followed in 24 hours by 100 μg IV, then 50 μg IV until oral medication is tolerated. Because of the risk of decreased T_3 generation from T_4 in severely hypothyroid patients, a simultaneous bolus of T_3 (liothyronine), at 20 μg IV followed by 10 μg IV every 8 hours until the patient is conscious, should be given. (3) **Identify and treat precipitating factors**. (4) **Treat metabolic abnormalities**: Hyponatremia is managed by free water restriction or infusion of saline and furosemide. Hypertonic saline is rarely indicated. Hypoglycemia and hypercalcemia are seen occasionally.

21. What is the significance of a palpable thyroid nodule in an asymptomatic patient?

Solitary thyroid nodules are a common physical finding in the general population. Most are benign colloid nodules that may change in size or disappear over time. Because a small percentage of solitary nodules are thyroid carcinomas, referral for fine-needle aspiration biopsy is indicated for all patients with palpable nodules. Biopsy results identify 70% of nodules to be benign, 5% to be malignant, and the remainder to be cytologically indeterminate with surgical follow-up required.

22. What is the significance of a nonpalpable thyroid nodule incidentally found on a radiologic study (incidentaloma)? When does it require further workup?

Thyroid nodules less than 1 cm are usually not detected on physical examination but may be identified incidentally on magnetic resonance imaging, computed tomography, or ultrasound. Nonpalpable thyroid nodules are common and detectable by ultrasound in 30% to 50% of the general population. Patients do not need to be referred for biopsy unless a nonpalpable nodule is greater than 1.5 cm or a personal history of neck irradiation or family history of thyroid cancer is present. Radiologic findings suggestive of malignancy, such as calcifications, also may warrant referral. Nodules larger than 1.5 cm should be referred for fine-needle aspiration biopsy on an outpatient basis.

23. How does amiodarone affect thyroid function?

Amiodarone is 37% organic iodine by weight and as such can have many effects on thyroid function. Normal maintenance doses result in iodine loads of 10 to 20 times the normal dietary requirement of iodine. Greater than 50% of patients on long-term amiodarone have abnormalities of thyroid function tests, including increased levels of T_4 and rT_3, decreased T_3, and increased TSH. Chronic amiodarone use may cause either a hypothyroid or a thyrotoxic state in 20% to 30% of patients. Amiodarone administration also has been cited in the literature as a precipitant of thyroid storm, although not in the setting of acute cardiac resuscitation in the ED.

BIBLIOGRAPHY

1. Bravermann LE, Utigar RD (eds): Werner and Ingbar's The Thyroid: A Fundamental and Clinical Text, 8th ed. Philadelphia, Lippincott Williams & Wilkins, 2000.
2. Burch HB, Wartofsky L: Life-threatening thyrotoxicosis-thyroid storm. Endocrinol Metab Clin North Am 22:263–277, 1993.
3. Harjai KJ, Licata AA: Effects of amiodarone on thyroid function. Ann Intern Med 126:63–73, 1997.
4. Hermus AR, Huysmans DA: Treatment of benign nodular thyroid disease. N Engl J Med 338:1438–1446, 1998.
5. Jordan RM; Myxedema coma: Pathophysiology, therapy, and factors affecting prognosis. Med Clin North Am 79:185–194, 1995.
6. Klein I, Ojamaa K: Thyroid hormone and the cardiovascular system. N Engl J Med 344:501–509, 2001.
7. Nicoloff JT, LoPresti JS: Myxedema coma: A form of decompensated hypothyroidism. Endocrinol Metab Clin North Am 22:279–290, 1993.
8. Tan GH, Gharib H: Thyroid incidentalomas: Management approaches to nonpalpable nodules discovered incidentally on thyroid imaging. Ann Intern Med 126:226–231, 1997.
9. Tietgens ST, Leinung MC: Thyroid storm. Med Clin North Am 79:169–184, 1995.
10. Weetman AP: Medical progress: Grave's disease. N Engl J Med 343:1236–1248, 2001.

53. ADRENAL DISORDERS

Michael W. Brunko, M.D.

1. Since adrenal emergencies are rare, why should I spend time learning about them?

Adrenal emergencies are rare, but if you are confronted with one and do not recognize it, the results can be devastating. Untreated adrenal insufficiency has a mortality rate approaching 100%. Overall, the treatment is simple, but you must understand some adrenal physiology to recognize a problem and know how to treat it.

2. What are the adrenal emergencies that I need to worry about?

The most serious adrenal emergency is acute adrenal insufficiency. Hypercortisolemia, or Cushing's disease, is rare, and it is unlikely you will make that diagnosis in the ED.

3. Will I ever need to worry about hypercortisolemia in the ED?

Cortisol excess can lead to psychoemotional disturbances, such as insomnia, mood disorders, mania, depression, and psychosis. If a woman presents with signs of masculinization or a man presents with signs of feminization and the above-mentioned symptoms, think of hypercortisolemia.

4. What adrenal physiology do I need to know?

The primary functions of the glucocorticoid cortisol and the mineralocorticoid aldosterone.

5. Describe the primary effects of cortisol.

Cortisol has essential effects on all organ systems. It influences fat, protein, and carbohydrate metabolism. It affects immunologic and inflammatory responses, bone and calcium metabolism, growth and development, the gastrointestinal tract, and the central nervous system. It is a major mediator of the stress response—affecting the heart, the vascular bed, water excretion, and electrolyte balance.

6. What are the primary effects of aldosterone?
To maintain sodium and potassium concentrations and to regulate extracellular volume.

7. How is normal secretion of cortisol controlled?
Cortisol is secreted from the cortex of the adrenal gland in response to direct stimulation by adrenocorticotropic hormone (ACTH). ACTH secretion is stimulated by the hormone corticotropin-releasing factor (CRF) from the hypothalamus. This occurs in a diurnal rhythm, with higher levels secreted in the morning and lower levels in the evening. By negative feedback inhibition, plasma cortisol levels act to suppress release of ACTH.

8. How is secretion of aldosterone controlled?
Primarily by the renin-angiotensin system and the serum potassium concentration. The renin-angiotensin system controls aldosterone levels in response to changes in volume, posture, and sodium intake. Potassium influences the adrenal cortex directly to increase secretion of aldosterone.

9. What causes acute adrenal insufficiency?
Adrenal insufficiency may be due to either destruction of adrenal gland (primary adrenal insufficiency) or inadequate production of ACTH (secondary adrenal insufficiency). Adrenal crisis often presents in a patient with chronic adrenal insufficiency who undergoes some form of stress, such as an acute myocardial infarction, surgery, or trauma, and is unable to mount a stress response by increasing circulating cortisol levels.

10. List the causes of adrenal insufficiency.

Primary adrenal insufficiency
   Idiopathic (autoimmune)
   Tuberculosis
   Miscellaneous
      Bilateral adrenal hemorrhage or infarction
      Acquired immunodeficiency syndrome (AIDS)
      Drugs: adrenolytic agents (metyrapone, aminoglutethimide, mitotane), ketoconazole
      Infections: fungal, bacterial sepsis
      Infiltrative disorders: sarcoidosis, hemochromatosis, amyloidosis, lymphoma, metastatic cancer
      Bilateral surgical adrenalectomy
      Hereditary: adrenal hypoplasia, congenital adrenal hyperplasia, adrenoleukodystrophy, familial
         glucocorticoid deficiency
Secondary adrenal insufficiency
   Exogenous glucocorticoid administration
   Pituitary or suprasellar tumor
   Pituitary irradiation or surgery
   Head trauma
   Infiltrative disorders of the pituitary or hypothalamus: sarcoidosis, hemochromatosis, histiocytosis
      X, metastatic cancer, or lymphoma
   Infectious diseases: tuberculosis, meningitis, fungal
   Isolated ACTH deficiency

---

11. What are the most common causes of primary adrenal insufficiency?
Tuberculosis and autoimmune destruction account for 90% of the cases of primary adrenal insufficiency.

12. Has primary adrenal insufficiency increased since there has been an increased incidence of tuberculosis?

This has yet to be shown in the literature, but with the increasing spread of tuberculosis associated with AIDS, more cases of primary adrenal insufficiency are being reported.

13. How can AIDS cause primary adrenal insufficiency?

Human immunodeficiency virus (HIV) has been found in the adrenal gland, where it may cause impaired function of the gland. Opportunistic infections may cause adrenal insufficiency; cytomegalovirus, *Cryptococcus* and *Mycobacterium* species, and Kaposi's sarcoma have been found in the glands of patients with AIDS. Some drugs used to treat AIDS can cause adrenal insufficiency. Ketoconazole is an inhibitor of steroid hormone synthesis, and rifampin alters cortisol metabolism and decreases cortisol bioavailability.

14. What is the most common cause of secondary adrenal insufficiency?

Long-term therapy with pharmacologic doses of glucocorticoid is the most common cause of secondary adrenal insufficiency. These drugs are used to treat a wide variety of medical problems, and if they are used for any significant time, some degree of suppression of the hypothalamic-pituitary-adrenal (HPA) axis occurs.

Diseases in Which Glucocorticoids Are Therapeutically Effective

1. Rheumatoid arthritis	21. Idiopathic thrombocytopenic purpura
2. Psoriatic arthritis	22. Autoimmune hemolytic anemia
3. Gouty arthritis	23. Lymphomas
4. Bursitis and tenosynovitis	24. Immune nephritis
5. Systemic lupus erythematosus	25. Tuberculous meningitis
6. Acute rheumatic carditis	26. Urticaria
7. Pemphigus	27. Chronic active hepatitis
8. Erythema multiforme	28. Ulcerative hepatitis
9. Exfoliative dermatitis	29. Regional enteritis
10. Mycosis fungoides	30. Nontropical sprue
11. Allergic rhinitis	31. Dental postoperative inflammation
12. Bronchial asthma	32. Cerebral edema
13. Atopic dermatitis	33. Subacute nonsuppurative
14. Serum sickness	thyroiditis
15. Allergic conjunctivitis	34. Malignant exophthalmos
16. Uveitis	35. Hypercalcemia
17. Retrobulbar neuritis	36. Trichinosis
18. Sarcoidosis	37. Myasthenia gravis
19. Löffler's syndrome	38. Organ transplantation
20. Berylliosis	39. Alopecia areata

15. What period of time is required to cause suppression of the HPA axis?

Any patient who is on larger doses of steroids (e.g., > 20 mg/day of prednisone) for 2 weeks or more has the potential for long-term suppression of the HPA axis. It depends on the dose and potency of the glucocorticoid, the time of day the drug was taken (suppression is greater when taken in the evening), and the potency of the drug. Recovery of the HPA axis may take a few months to a year.

16. I understand that adrenal insufficiency is difficult to diagnose and treat. Why is that?

The clinical features of adrenal insufficiency are nonspecific and usually masked by coexisting illnesses or therapies. Currently used diagnostic criteria may not be valid or practical to use in the critically ill patient because time and access to the tests usually prevents emergent use, such as in the ED.

17. List some signs and symptoms of primary adrenal insufficiency.
Fatigue
Weakness
Weight loss
Anorexia
Hyperpigmentation
Gastrointestinal symptoms (nausea, vomiting, abdominal pain, and diarrhea)
Hypotension (usually with orthostatic changes)

18. What are the characteristic laboratory findings?
Hyperkalemia, hyponatremia, and hypoglycemia are usually present with primary adrenal insufficiency. If the patient is dehydrated, volume depletion may lead to azotemia. A mild metabolic acidosis is often present.

19. How is the presentation of secondary adrenal insufficiency different from that of primary adrenal insufficiency?
In secondary adrenal insufficiency, there is no deficiency of aldosterone secretion. The volume depletion and hypotension are not as severe (unless crisis is present), hyperkalemia is absent, and hyponatremia, if present, is due to water retention and not salt wasting, as in primary adrenal insufficiency. Patients usually have a cushingoid appearance because of long-term glucocorticoid use. If the patient has a pituitary or hypothalamic cause for the adrenal insufficiency, findings may include symptoms of other pituitary hormone deficiencies, such as hypothyroidism and amenorrhea.

20. When does acute adrenal crisis usually occur?
It usually occurs in response to a major stress, such as acute myocardial infarction, sepsis, surgery, major injury, or other illness in any patient with primary or secondary adrenal insufficiency.

21. What is the most frequent iatrogenic cause of acute adrenal crisis?
Rapid withdrawal of steroids in patients with adrenal atrophy secondary to long-term steroid administration.

22. Describe the most common clinical features of acute adrenal insufficiency.
Patients appear to be profoundly ill. They are significantly volume-depleted with hypotension and shock. Nausea, vomiting, and severe abdominal pain, many times mimicking an acute abdomen, are present. Fever may occur as a result of infection or the adrenal insufficiency itself. Central nervous system symptoms of confusion, disorientation, and lethargy may be present.

23. Will these patients always be hyponatremic and hyperkalemic?
No. If a patient has been taking mineralocorticoid replacement, such as fludrocortisone, these laboratory findings may be near-normal.

24. Why do these patients have a metabolic acidosis?
There are multiple reasons. Volume depletion and shock lead to increased lactate production. If aldosterone deficiency is present, decreased renal acid secretion is also present, contributing to a metabolic acidosis.

25. How is adrenal crisis diagnosed in the ED?
First, you must suspect adrenal crisis if a patient has been taking high-dose steroids and presents with the symptoms mentioned. The most useful and practical laboratory test in the ED is the **rapid ACTH stimulation test**.

26. How is the rapid ACTH stimulation test performed?

A baseline sample of blood is drawn at time 0 for a cortisol level. Then, 0.25 mg of cosyntropin (synthetic ACTH) is given intravenously. Cortisol levels are checked at 30 minutes, 1 hour, and 6 hours.

27. Does performance of the rapid ACTH stimulation test delay treatment of the patient with glucocorticoids?

No. You can begin treatment using a glucocorticoid that will not cause an increase in measurable cortisol levels. Dexamethasone (6–10 mg) is generally recommended.

28. Are there any imaging studies that may be useful in the ED in determining the cause of primary adrenal insufficiency?

Computed tomography (CT) scans may be useful. Enlargement of the adrenal glands on CT scan may be a sign of active tuberculosis, fungal infections, metastatic disease, or lymphoma. Calcifications of the adrenal glands also may indicate tuberculosis infection. A rounded enlargement of the adrenal gland on CT scan may be the result of blunt trauma. Atrophic adrenal glands on CT scan may be a finding of autoimmune adrenalitis. Imaging studies, including CT scan, should be held until the patient is hemodynamically stable.

29. How is acute adrenal insufficiency treated?

Intravenous hydrocortisone (100 mg minimum) and crystalloid IV fluids containing dextrose must be initiated early. A detailed history and examination should be done to attempt to elicit what may have instigated the stress that caused the acute adrenal insufficiency. If a cause is found, supportive and definitive measures need to be instituted in the ED. Mineralocorticoid replacement is usually unnecessary if salt and water replacement is adequate and if the patient receives hydrocortisone—100 mg of hydrocortisone has the salt-retaining effect of 0.1 mg of fludrocortisone.

30. What about the patient with chronic adrenal insufficiency who presents to the ED with a minor illness or injury? Should I treat this patient any differently?

Yes. These patients usually require 20 to 30 mg/day of hydrocortisone. Some also require mineralocorticoid replacement. If these patients experience a minor illness or injury, they should be told to double their daily cortisol dose for 24 to 48 hours until symptoms improve. Increasing the mineralocorticoid dose is usually not necessary. Follow-up care should be coordinated closely with the primary care physician or endocrinologist. Patients should be told that if nausea or vomiting develops and they are unable to keep down the medication, they should seek immediate medical care.

BIBLIOGRAPHY

1. Aron DC: Endocrine complications of the acquired immunodeficiency syndrome. Arch Intern Med 149:330–333, 1989.
2. Beale MB, Belzberg H: Adrenal insufficiency. In Grenvik A (ed): Textbook of Critical Care, 4th ed. Philadelphia, W.B. Saunders, 2000, pp 806–816.
3. Brunko MW, Wolfe R: An unusual cause of an acute surgical abdomen. J Emerg Med 6:411–416, 1988.
4. Loriaux DL, McDonald WJ: Adrenal insufficiency. In DeGroot LJ (ed): Endocrinology, 4th ed. Vol. 2. Philadelphia, W.B. Saunders, 2001, pp 1683–1690.
5. Nelson DH: Diagnosis and treatment of Addison's disease. In DeGroot LJ (ed): Endocrinology. Vol. 2. New York, Grune & Stratton, 1985, pp 1193–1201.
6. Orth DN: Adrenal insufficiency. In Bardin CW (ed): Current Therapy in Endocrinology and Metabolism, 6th ed. St. Louis, Mosby, 1997.
7. Orth DN, Kovacs WJ, DeBold CR: The adrenal cortex. In Wilson JD, Foster DW (eds): Williams' Textbook of Endocrinology, 8th ed. Philadelphia, W.B. Saunders, 1992, pp 489–619.
8. Wogan JM: Selected endocrine disorders. In Marx JA, et al (eds): Rosen's Emergency Medicine: Concepts and Clinical Practice, 5th ed. St. Louis, Mosby, 2002, pp 1770–1785.

XI. Infectious Disease

54. SOFT-TISSUE INFECTIONS

Harvey W. Meislin, M.D., and K. Alexander Malone, M.D.

1. How do I differentiate cellulitis from an abscess?

Cellulitis is a soft tissue infection of the skin and subcutaneous tissue usually characterized by blanching erythema, swelling, tenderness, and local warmth. A cutaneous abscess is a localized collection of pus that results in a painful soft tissue mass that is often fluctuant but surrounded by firm granulation tissue and erythema.

2. What are the causes of cellulitis? How does it progress?

Although most often acute, cellulitis may be subacute or chronic. Minor trauma is often the predisposing cause, but hematogenous and lymphatic dissemination may account for its appearance in previously normal skin. Cellulitis caused by bacterial infection tends to spread radially proximately and distally with associated swelling. Nonbacterial or inflammatory cellulitis tends to stay localized. Cellulitis may progress to ascending lymphangitis and septicemia.

3. What are the causes of abscesses? How do they progress?

Abscesses occur on all areas of the body, although they have a predominance for the head and neck, upper extremities, and torso. Abscesses usually are caused by interruptions of the integrity of the protective epithelium, but they may be associated with obstruction of apocrine glands or spread via mucosal involvement in the oral and anorectal areas. Superficial abscesses tend to remain localized and often rupture through the skin if not incised and drained.

4. What is the significance of the presence of pus?

Abscesses contain pus; cellulitis does not. Although soft tissue infections tend to spread, and abscess and cellulitis may be present in the same anatomic area, the presence of pus defines the presence of the abscess and the need for incision and drainage. Pus itself is a heterogeneous mix of cellular material in various stages of digestion by polymorphonuclear neutrophil leukocytes (PMNs). These PMNs are drawn to sites of inflammation, infection, or trauma by various chemotactic factors to defend the host against potential pathogens.

5. How do I know if pus is present?

In cutaneous abscesses, a raised painful mass with a fluctuant center surrounded by erythematous tissue signifies the presence of pus. Adjunctive techniques, such as ultrasound or CT scanning, may be useful for deeper soft tissue infections but are indicated rarely in superficial abscesses. The use of a localizer needle is often helpful, especially in wounds in which the purulence is loculated. Needle aspiration of the involved area with a needle large enough to withdraw thick pus often helps to define the location of purulence for incision and drainage and makes the process more comfortable by decreasing the pressure and pain in the area.

6. What is the differential diagnosis of cellulitis and abscess?

The differential is one of **bacterial versus nonbacterial infection**. Nonbacterial cellulitis includes arthropod envenomation, chemical or thermal burns, arthritis, and healing wounds. Nonbacterial cellulitis usually is localized and often does not have the presence of lymphangitic streaking. The differential diagnosis of abscesses includes sterile abscesses, cutaneously borne bacterial abscesses, and mucous membrane abscesses. Abscesses of the oral and anorectal area usually originate from flora of the oral or rectal cavity. Sterile abscesses, which occur approximately 5% of the time, tend to be associated with drug abuse and subcutaneous injections.

7. Is it useful to culture cellulitis or abscesses?

Culturing cellulitis is often futile, with only 10% to 50% of such efforts yielding successful results. Often there is secondary skin contamination. Culturing can be useful, however, in patients who do not respond to initial management, in patients with recurrent disease, or in patients with sepsis. Culturing the portal of entry may be useful, even if distal to the site of the cellulitis. Culturing of cutaneous abscesses seldom is clinically indicated because normal host defenses tend to contain and localize the process. In recurrent abscess or failure of initial therapy, Gram stain and culture may be indicated.

8. Is there any role for routine laboratory studies?

Laboratory studies are generally not helpful in the treatment of superficial soft tissue infections, unless signs or symptoms of systemic illness are present. These patients are often not systemically ill, and even an elevated white blood cell (WBC) count does not differentiate bacterial from nonbacterial infection, identify the presence of abscess or cellulitis, or show systemic involvement. An exception may be *Haemophilus influenzae* cellulitis, in which WBC counts often exceed 15,000 with a left shift; this usually occurs in children. Laboratory analysis may be useful in the immunocompromised host or in patients who appear to be septic or systemically ill.

9. Summarize appropriate treatment of soft tissue infections.

The time-honored treatment for cellulitis is immobilization, elevation, heat or warm moist packs, analgesics, and antibiotics directed toward suspected pathogens. The treatment for cutaneous abscesses is a properly performed incision and drainage, done most commonly with local anesthesia and a No. 11 blade scalpel.

Oral Therapy of Superficial Soft Tissue Infections

Group A Streptococcus	
Penicillin V (phenoxymethylpenicillin)	250–500 mg q.i.d.
First-generation cephalosporin	250–500 mg q.i.d.
Erythromycin	250 mg-1 g q 6 h
Azithromycin	500 mg × 1 dose, then 250 mg qd × 4
Clarithromycin	500 mg b.i.d.
Staphylococcus aureus **(not methicillin-resistant *S. aureus*)**	
Dicloxacillin	125–500 mg q.i.d.
Cloxacillin	250–500 mg q.i.d.
First-generation cephalosporin	250–500 mg q.i.d.
Erythromycin (variable effectiveness)	250–500 mg q.i.d.
Azithromycin	500 mg × 1 dose, then 250 mg qd × 4
Clarithromycin	500 mg b.i.d.
Clindamycin	150–450 mg q.i.d.
Amoxicillin-clavulanate	250–500 mg t.i.d.
Ciprofloxacin	500 mg b.i.d.
Haemophilus influenzae	
Amoxicillin-clavulanate	250–500 mg t.i.d.
Cefaclor	250–500 mg t.i.d.
Trimethoprim (TMP)-sulfamethoxazole (SMX)	160 mg TMP/800 mg SMX b.i.d.
Azithromycin	500 mg × 1 dose, then 250 mg q.d. × 4
Clarithromycin	500 mg b.i.d.

10. Should I routinely prescribe antibiotics for patients with an abscess?

No. Antibiotics are not indicated in patients with a cutaneous abscess and with normal host defenses. In patients with complications of diabetes, AIDS, leukemia, neoplasms, significant vascular insufficiency, trauma, or thermal burns, antibiotics should be considered as prophylaxis to prevent spread into local tissues or the bloodstream. Prophylactic antibiotics, although not necessary, could be considered for abscesses of the face, groin, and hand. The selection of antimicrobial agents can be facilitated by knowing the flora associated with the anatomic area involved and if the abscess is from a cutaneous or mucosal process.

11. Are there anatomic areas of significance in a patient with an abscess or cellulitis?

Cellulitis of the midface, especially in the area of the orbits, must be treated aggressively. The venous drainage of these infections is through the cavernous sinus of the brain, with the potential for causing cavernous sinus thrombosis. In true orbital cellulitis, there must be aggressive intravenous antibiotic therapy. Often a CT scan is performed to detect abscess formation. *H. influenzae* cellulitis usually occurs in children, resulting in high fevers, high WBC counts, and bacteremia. Perirectal or perianal abscesses that are large or extend into the supralevator or ischiorectal space often need surgical management, removing not only the abscess, but also the fistulas that are often associated with it. Deep space abscesses of the groin and head and neck region often must be drained in the operating room because of their proximity to major neurovascular structures.

12. When are antibiotics always indicated for cellulitis or abscesses?

Antibiotics are indicated for cellulitis along with other supportive therapies, such as immobilization, elevation, and heat. Cutaneous cellulitis occurs most often in the upper or lower extremities; initial therapy to cover common skin organisms such as *S. aureus* and streptococcus can be oral cephalosporins, erythromycin, or dicloxacillin. If there is no response to such therapy, one must search aggressively for a causative factor and attempt to culture the cellulitis. A broader spectrum antibiotic or multiple antibiotics may be indicated. The treatment for most abscesses is incision and drainage, and neither antibiotics nor cultures are indicated in patients with normal host defenses as long as the abscess is localized. For abscesses associated with immunocompromised or progressing cellulitis and for abscesses that may be penetrating into deeper soft tissues, incision and drainage, antibiotic therapy, culture, and Gram stain constitute a reasonable initial approach. The choice of antibiotics depends on the location and the most likely cause of the infection.

13. Describe appropriate follow-up care.

Most patients with simple cellulitis and localized abscesses need to be seen only once or twice in the ED. The packing usually can be removed after 48 to 72 hours, and the patient can irrigate the abscess cavity by bathing or showering at home. It is important to ensure that the cellulitis is responding to therapy and, with abscesses, that all pus has been drained and evacuated. Further follow-up is indicated only when the processes are recurrent, when there is no response to therapy, or when the patient is immunocompromised.

14. Who should be admitted to the hospital?

Patients who appear septic, are immunocompromised, or are not responding to treatment; patients with soft tissue infections in certain anatomic sites, such as the central area of the face, and patients with infections that potentially may cause airway closure. Examples are sublingual and retropharyngeal abscesses and Ludwig's angina. Close attention must be paid to immunosuppressed patients, who may develop abscesses or cellulitis as secondary infections from gram-negative or anaerobic gas-forming organisms. Abscesses in the perineal area may spread quickly through the fascial planes, resulting in Fournier's gangrene.

15. Is there an association between abscesses or cellulitis and systemic disease?

Patients who are immunocompromised or have peripheral vascular disease have a tendency to develop superficial soft tissue infections. Recurrent abscesses in the head and neck or groin regions may be associated with hidradenitis suppurativa, which is a disease of chronic suppurative abscesses of the apocrine sweat glands. Inflammatory bowel disease, diabetes, malignancies, and pregnancy have been associated with a higher incidence of perirectal abscesses. Recurrent abscesses in the perineal and lower abdominal area may signify the presence of associated inflammatory bowel disease. All patients with recurrent soft tissue infections, whether superficial or deep, should be evaluated for underlying systemic disease such as diabetes.

16. What is the best advice overall for treating cellulitis and abscesses?

Cellulitis usually responds to antibiotic therapy and immobilization. Cutaneous abscesses respond to adequate incision and drainage; antibiotics are not indicated. All soft tissue infections should be observed to ascertain that healing is occurring. Selection of antibiotics, when indicated, is guided by the location and cause of the infection.

17. What is necrotizing fasciitis?

A life-threatening and limb-threatening bacterial infection of the fascia often extending to the skin and subcutaneous tissue. Multiple bacteria usually are involved. The most common are gram-positive cocci (*Streptococcus* and *Staphylococcus*), gram-negative organisms (*Enterococcus, Proteus,* and *Pseudomonas*), and anaerobes (*Clostridium, Escherichia coli, Bacteroides fragilis*). Bacteria usually enter the subcutaneous tissue through a break in the skin, often caused by minor or trivial trauma. Blood-borne and postoperative infection may lead to necrotizing fasciitis.

18. How is necrotizing fasciitis diagnosed?

The diagnosis should be considered in any patient who has pain and tenderness out of proportion to the visible degree of cellulitis. It also should be considered in patients without any skin changes who have exquisite muscle tenderness with no obvious reason, such as a history of musculoskeletal trauma. Some patients may have subcutaneous emphysema. Most develop sepsis late in the course, and in severe cases disseminated intravascular coagulopathy develops. Any patient experiencing exquisite tenderness over or adjacent to an area of cellulitis should have a surgical consultation. A soft tissue radiograph may be helpful to visualize subcutaneous emphysema. CT and MRI are helpful when this diagnosis is suspected.

19. Why should I get a surgical consultation?

Necrotizing fasciitis is a surgical disease and must be treated with extensive incision, drainage, and débridement of necrotic tissue. Additional therapy includes antibiotics and in-hospital supportive care.

20. What is Fournier's gangrene?

A necrotizing subcutaneous infection of the perineum occurring primarily in men, usually involving the penis, scrotum, or rectum. It most commonly affects individuals who are immunologically compromised or diabetic. Typically, it begins as a benign infection or small abscess that quickly progresses and leads to end-artery thrombosis in subcutaneous tissues. Ultimately, it leads to widespread necrosis of adjacent areas. Any patient complaining of lesions or pain in the aforementioned areas should be approached with this diagnosis in the differential.

21. How can the risk of developing necrotizing fasciitis be minimized?

Always meticulously scrub and irrigate all wounds, particularly those of the extremities and perineum. Consider delayed primary closure of contaminated wounds (see Chapter 120, Wound Management). Take special care with immunocompromised patients, such as diabetics, and follow such patients closely so that the diagnosis can be made early in the course of this disease, improving the prognosis.

22. List the most common (and concerning) organisms found in the following wounds and their accompanying cellulitis.

Cat bites?

Pasteurella multocida (80%), *Staphylococcus, Streptococcus.*

Dog bites?
Pasteurella, Enterobacter, Pseudomonas, Capnocytophaga canimorsus (rare, but 25% fatality in immunocompromised).
Human bites?
Streptococcus, Staphylococcus, H. influenzae, Eikenella corrodens, Enterobacter, Proteus.
Open water wounds?
Aeromonas hydrophila, Bacteroides fragilis, Chromobacterium, Mycobacterium marinum, Vibrio.

23. What question must be asked of all patients presenting with cellulitis or abscesses?
When was your last tetanus booster? Current recommendations suggest tetanus-diphtheria toxoid (Td), 0.5 mL IM × 1 if it has been more than 5 years since the previous booster.

24. What is the most important word to remember when describing how much pus is in a wound?
Purulent. Many a medical student and intern has been shamed when trying to spell the word for "that which contains pus." Although a wound with significant blood is bloody, and a wound that is malodorous is smelly, a wound with pus should *never* be spelled with "sy" at the end.

BIBLIOGRAPHY

1. Brandt MM, Corpron CA, Wahl WL: Necrotizing soft tissue infections: A surgical disease. Am Surg 66:967–971, 2000.
2. Dong SL, Kelly KD, Oland RC, et al: ED management of cellulitis: A review of five urban centers. Am J Emerg Med 19:535–540, 2001.
3. Kilic A, Aksoy Y, Kilic L: Fournier's gangrene: Etiology, treatment, and complications. Ann Plast Surg 47:523–527, 2001.
4. Llera JL, Levy RC: Treatment of cutaneous abscess: A double-blind clinical study. Ann Emerg Med 14:15–19, 1985.
5. Meislin HW, Guisto JA: Soft-tissue infections. In Rosen P, Barkin RM (eds): Emergency Medicine: Concepts and Clinical Practice, 5th ed. St. Louis, Mosby, 2002, pp 1944–1957.
6. Meislin HW, Lerner SA, Graves MH, et al: Cutaneous abscesses: Anaerobic and aerobic bacteriology and outpatient management. Ann Intern Med 87:145–149, 1977.
7. Meislin HW, McGehee MD, Rosen P: Management and microbiology of cutaneous abscesses. J Am Coll Emerg Physicians 7:186–191, 1978.
8. Stevens DL: The flesh eating bacterium: What's next? J Infect Dis. 179(suppl 2):S366–374, 1999.
9. Stone DR, Gorbach SL: Necrotizing fasciitis: The changing spectrum. Dermatol Clin 15:213–220, 1997.
10. Struk DW, Munk PL, Lee MJ, et al: Imaging of soft tissue infections. Radiol Clin North Am 39:277–303, 2001.

55. HIV INFECTION AND AIDS

Catherine A. Marco, M.D.

1. What is the significance of AIDS in the ED?
Disease caused by human immunodeficiency virus (HIV) infection, ranging from asymptomatic infection to acquired immunodeficiency syndrome (AIDS), with serious, possibly life-threatening complications, is encountered commonly in the ED. As of 2001, more than 790,000 cases of AIDS had been reported in the United States. It is estimated that more than 440,000 persons are living with HIV infection and AIDS currently in the United States. Seroprevalence among ED patients varies greatly depending on the location and type of hospital. Among inner-city ED patients, seroprevalence ranges from 4.2% to 8.9%. Knowledge of HIV infection and related

disease is essential to diagnose and treat disease and to ensure adequate protection of health care workers.

2. How is the diagnosis of AIDS made?

AIDS is diagnosed by laboratory evidence of HIV infection and the presence of one of the indicator diseases, some of which are listed in the following table. HIV infection should be suspected in all patients with known risk factors or with presenting symptoms suggestive of opportunistic infection. Questioning the patient directly about risk factors may be crucial to diagnosing HIV-related disease. Risk factors that are commonly associated with HIV infection include men who have sex with men, injecting drug use, heterosexual exposure, blood recipients before 1985, and maternal-neonatal transmission.

Testing for HIV rarely is indicated in the ED because of difficulty in maintaining confidentiality and ensuring appropriate reporting and counseling. Referral for testing and counseling can be initiated in the ED, however.

AIDS-Defining Conditions

Laboratory evidence of HIV infection plus any of the following:

Esophageal candidiasis	Brain lymphoma	HIV wasting syndrome
Cryptococcosis	*Mycobacterium avium* complex	Disseminated histoplasmosis
Cryptosporidiosis	*Pneumocystis carinii* pneumonia	Isosporiasis
Cytomegalovirus retinitis	Progressive multifocal leukoencephalopathy	Disseminated *Mycobacterium tuberculosis* disease
Herpes simplex virus	Brain toxoplasmosis	Recurrent *Salmonella* septicemia
Kaposi's sarcoma	HIV encephalopathy	CD4 lymphocyte count < 200/μL
Pulmonary tuberculosis	Invasive cervical cancer	

3. How do patients with HIV infection present to the ED?

Patients may present with involvement of virtually any organ system. HIV infection should be suspected in any patient who presents with abnormally severe symptoms of a common disease or with symptoms of opportunistic infection or other debilitating HIV-related disease, such as AIDS wasting syndrome or AIDS dementia. Among AIDS patients, systemic infection or malignancy always must be considered and may present with malaise, anorexia, fever, weight loss, gastrointestinal complaints, or other symptoms. Because of the wide spectrum of disease related to HIV infection, many specific diagnoses cannot be made definitively in the ED; treatment focuses on recognition of disease, institution of initial therapy, and admission or outpatient follow-up.

4. How is the HIV-positive patient with systemic symptoms evaluated in the ED?

In addition to a complete history and physical examination, appropriate laboratory investigations may include electrolytes, complete blood count, blood cultures (aerobic, anaerobic, and fungal), urinalysis and culture, liver function tests, chest radiography, serologic testing for syphilis, blood tests for cryptococcal antigen, and *Toxoplasma* and *Coccidioides* serologies. Lumbar puncture also may be appropriate if no other source of fever is identified.

5. Explain the significance of fever in these patients.

Fever may indicate bacterial, fungal, viral, or protozoal infection. The most common causes of fever include HIV-related fever, systemic infections such as *Mycobacterium avium* complex, cytomegalovirus, Hodgkin's disease, and non-Hodgkin's lymphoma.

Many HIV-infected patients with fever may be managed as outpatients. Outpatient management may be attempted if the source of the fever does not dictate admission, if appropriate laboratory studies have been initiated, if the patient is able to function adequately at home (able to ambulate and tolerate oral intake), and if appropriate medical follow-up can be arranged.

6. **What are the common neurologic complications of AIDS?**

The most common acute symptoms are altered mental status, seizures, headache, and meningismus. ED evaluation should include a complete neurologic examination and, when appropriate, CT or MRI and lumbar puncture. Specific cerebrospinal fluid studies that may be of value include cell count, glucose, protein, Gram stain, India ink capsule stain, bacterial culture, viral culture, fungal culture, *Toxoplasma* and cryptococcal antigen, and coccidioidomycosis titer. The most common causes of neurologic symptoms include *Toxoplasma gondii*, AIDS dementia, *Cryptococcus neoformans*, *Mycobacterium tuberculosis*, and herpes simplex virus.

7. **What is AIDS dementia?**

An organic brain syndrome manifested by decline in attention, cognitive reasoning, speech, motor function, and motivation. AIDS dementia is the most common neurologic problem and affects 33% to 60% of patients. It may be the presenting sign of overt AIDS in 25% of patients. Other causes of dementia must be ruled out.

8. **What are the pulmonary complications of HIV infection, and how are they managed?**

Common presenting pulmonary complaints are cough, hemoptysis, shortness of breath, and chest pain. After history and lung examination, arterial blood gases, chest radiography, sputum culture, Gram stain, acid-fast stain, and blood cultures should be obtained if clinically indicated. The most common pulmonary complication is *Pneumocystis carinii* pneumonia, which occurs in 70% to 80% of seropositive patients and typically presents with dyspnea, nonproductive cough, fever, and weight loss. Rapid institution of therapy with trimethoprim-sulfamethoxazole (weight-based dosing), steroids, dapsone, or pentamidine may prevent excessive morbidity and mortality. Other causes include *M. tuberculosis* pneumonia, *Histoplasma capsulatum*, and neoplasm.

ED management includes supplemental oxygen, volume repletion if indicated, and, when appropriate, antibiotic therapy. Admission should be considered for patients with new-onset pulmonary symptoms or patients with a significant deterioration in respiratory status.

9. **How should gastrointestinal complaints be managed?**

Approximately 50% of AIDS patients present with gastrointestinal complaints at some time during their illness. The most common presenting symptoms are abdominal pain, bleeding, and diarrhea. Diarrhea is the most common gastrointestinal complaint and is estimated to occur in 50% to 90% of AIDS patients. Helpful laboratory studies include microscopic examination of stool for leukocytes, acid-fast stain, examination for ova and parasites, and bacterial culture of stool and blood. *Cryptosporidium* and *Isospora* infections in particular are common causes and are associated with prolonged watery diarrhea. Other common infectious agents include *Candida*, Kaposi's sarcoma, *M. avium* complex, herpes simplex virus, cytomegalovirus, *Campylobacter jejuni*, *Entamoeba histolytica*, *Shigella*, *Salmonella*, *Giardia*, *Cryptosporidium*, and *Isospora*. Management should be directed at repletion of fluid and electrolytes and appropriate antibiotic coverage.

10. **What are the common cutaneous presentations of AIDS, and how are they treated?**

Kaposi's sarcoma is the most common unique cutaneous manifestation of AIDS. It usually is widely disseminated and may involve mucous membranes. Exacerbation of any underlying dermatologic condition in an HIV-infected patient is common. Complaints such as xerosis (dry skin) and pruritus are common and may be manifested before development of opportunistic infections. Traditional therapy is employed. Xerosis may be treated with emollients and, if necessary, with mild topical steroids. Pruritus may respond to oatmeal baths and, if necessary, antihistamines. Infections, including *Staphylococcus aureus* (presenting as bullous impetigo, ecthyma, or folliculitis), *Pseudomonas aeruginosa* (which may present with chronic ulcerations and macerations), herpes simplex, herpes zoster, syphilis, and scabies, are common and should be treated with standard therapies.

Other dermatologic conditions that occur with increased frequency in HIV-infected patients include seborrheic dermatitis, psoriasis, atopic dermatitis, and alopecia. Dermatologic consultation generally is indicated. Admission may be indicated for patients with any disseminated cutaneous infection requiring intravenous antibiotics or antiviral agents.

11. Describe ophthalmologic emergencies that occur in AIDS patients.

Eye complaints such as change in visual acuity, photophobia, redness, and pain are common and may represent retinitis or invasion of eye or periorbital tissues with a malignant or infectious process. Cytomegalovirus retinitis occurs in 30% of AIDS patients and accounts for most retinitis among AIDS patients. It has a characteristic appearance of fluffy white retinal lesions, often perivascular (sometimes referred to as "tomato and cheese pizza" appearance). Ophthalmology consultation is indicated followed by treatment with foscarnet or ganciclovir for 2 weeks and long-term maintenance therapy.

12. Should HIV-infected patients receive tetanus immunization?

According to the U.S. Public Health Service Immunizations Practices Advisory Committee, routine immunization recommendations for diphtheria (DPT); tetanus (Td); and measles, mumps, and rubella (MMR) are unchanged for HIV-infected patients.

13. How should symptoms of side effects from drugs be managed?

Reactions to pharmacologic therapy are common in HIV-infected patients and always must be considered as the cause of new symptoms. In one series, 5% of ED visits by symptomatic HIV-positive patients were related to complications of pharmacologic therapy. Certain commonly used pharmaceutical agents cause a particularly high incidence of adverse drug reactions, including trimethoprim-sulfamethoxazole (TMP-SMZ), which has a 65% incidence of adverse drug reactions in AIDS patients, and pentamidine, which has a 50% incidence of adverse reactions. A decision about discontinuing therapy depends on balance between the benefit of the drug and the severity of side effects.

Common Drug Reactions Seen in HIV-Infected Persons

	FEVER	RASH	NAUSEA/ VOMITING	DIAR- RHEA	HEAD- ACHE	Δ MENTAL STATUS	NEUR- OPATHY	OTHER
Antiretroviral								
Zidovudine	X	X	X	X	X	X		
Didanosine		X	X	X	X	X	X	Pancreatitis
Zalcitabine	X	X	X	X	X		X	
Saquinavir		X	X	X				
Ritonavir			X	X	X			Paresthesias
Indinavir		X	X		X			Nephrolithiasis
Lamivudine	X		X	X	X		X	Cough
Antibiotics								
TMP-SMZ	X	X	X					
Pentamidine		X						
Isoniazid	X	X	X					Hepatitis
Azithromycin		X	X	X	X			
Antifungals								
Amphotericin	X		X		X			Nephrotoxicity
Ganciclovir			X	X				
Ketoconazole			X	X				
Fluconazole		X	X	X	X			
Itraconazole		X	X	X	X			
Antiviral								
Foscarnet	X		X	X				Nephrotoxicity, seizures

Note. This table shows only a representative sample of drug reactions that may occur in HIV-infected persons. Note in particular the frequency of gastrointestinal effects of many medications. Additional references should be consulted for complete information.

Laboratory Abnormalities in HIV-Infected Persons

	↑LFT	↑GLUC	↓GLUC	↓MG	↓K	↓WBC	↓HCT	↓PLT
Antiretroviral								
Zidovudine	X					X	X	
Didanosine	X							
Zalcitabine								
Saquinavir								
Ritonavir	X							
Indinavir	X							
Lamivudine								
Antibiotics								
TMP-SMZ	X					X		X
Pentamidine		X	X			X	X	
Isoniazid	X					X	X	X
Azithromycin								
Antifungals								
Amphotericin				X	X	X	X	X
Ganciclovir						X		
Ketoconazole	X							
Fluconazole	X							
Itraconazole	X							
Antiviral								
Foscarnet				X	X		X	

LFT, liver function test; GLUC, glucose; Mg, magnesium; K, potassium; WBC, white blood cell count; HCT, hematocrit; PLT, platelets.

14. Discuss common ethical problems.

Several important ethical considerations are HIV testing in patients and physicians, confidentiality, and resuscitation efforts. Routine testing for HIV is generally not indicated in the ED, and many EDs have adopted strict policies against HIV testing because of difficulties in ensuring adequate confidentiality and availability of counseling. One important exception to this general guideline may include source patients of needlestick injuries. This policy may change as the need for early identification and treatment of patients is shown. Initiation of counseling and referral for testing are recommended for patients at high risk.

Confidentiality regarding HIV-related diagnoses is paramount to providing appropriate patient care. Discretion when discussing the patient's diagnosis and condition with staff members and with the patient's family and friends helps to maintain confidentiality.

Resuscitation of patients with advanced AIDS is controversial. Decisions about life-support measures are best made before the need for their institution. Discussions with the family and the primary care physician may aid in making appropriate decisions. Because ED physicians may not have sufficient information about individual patients, their wishes, and the state of their disease, it is recommended that appropriate therapy and resuscitative measures be undertaken unless specifically otherwise stated.

15. How can physicians protect themselves from acquiring HIV?

Health care workers often are exposed to HIV-infected patients and their body fluids. Precautions in handling potentially infectious fluids are crucial. Because HIV infection is often undiagnosed at the time of the ED encounter, the use of universal precautions is strongly recommended, including the appropriate use of gown, gloves, mask, and goggles for procedures in all patients. The Needlestick Safety and Prevention Act of 2000 mandates that safety-engineered devices be used whenever possible and that institutions maintain exposure control plans. With the use of universal precautions, the risk of acquiring HIV infection by occupational exposure is extremely low.

16. Should postexposure prophylaxis (PEP) be administered after exposure to blood and body fluids?

PEP should be considered in all occupational and nonoccupational exposures. Decisions to treat should be based on the type of exposure, the risk of HIV in the source patient, and careful consideration of the risks and benefits of therapy. PEP is most effective if administered within 30 minutes of the exposure. PEP may consist of a basic regimen (zidovudine plus lamivudine) or an expanded regimen for high-risk exposures (zidovudine, lamivudine plus either indinavir or nelfinavir). Ideally, each health care institution should have written protocols that are formulated in consultation with occupational medicine and infectious disease specialists for health care workers who have had an exposure.

17. Should health care workers be tested for HIV?

Routine testing for HIV in health care workers is not currently recommended. To date, there have been no documented cases of direct physician-to-patient transmission of HIV among 22,000 patients being studied by the Centers for Disease Control. Current recommendations state that mandatory disclosure of HIV status by health care workers is unnecessary for low-risk procedures, but that practice restrictions may be appropriate if patients are at risk.

BIBLIOGRAPHY

1. Carpenter CC, Cooper DA, Fischl MA, et al: Antiretroviral therapy in adults. JAMA 283:381, 2000.
2. Centers for Disease Control: Case-control study of HIV seroconversion in health-care workers after percutaneous exposure to HIV-infected blood—France, United Kingdom, and United States. January 1988–August 1994. MMWR Morb Mortal Wkly Rep 44:929–933, 1995.
3. Centers for Disease Control and Prevention: HIV/AIDS Surveillance Report. Atlanta, CDC, 12(No. 2):5–7, 2000.
4. Centers for Disease Control and Prevention: Public Health Service guidelines for the management of health-care worker exposures to HIV and recommendations for postexposure prophylaxis. MMWR Morb Mortal Wkly Rep 47:1–19, 1998.
5. Deeks SG, Smith M, Holodniy M, Kahn JO: HIV-1 protease inhibitors: A review for clinicians. JAMA 277:145–154, 1997.
6. Enger C, Graham N, Peng Y, et al: Survival from early, intermediate, and late stages of HIV infection. JAMA 275:1329–1334, 1996.
7. Hawkins CC, Gold JW, Whimbey E, et al: *Mycobacterium avium* complex infections in patients with the acquired immunodeficiency syndrome. Ann Intern Med 105:184–188, 1986.
8. Hu DJ, Dondero TJ, Rayfield MA, et al: The emerging genetic diversity of HIV. JAMA 275:210–216, 1996.
9. Kinloch-de Loes S, Hirschel BJ, Hoen B, et al: A controlled trial of zidovudine in primary human immunodeficiency virus infection. N Engl J Med 333:408–413, 1995.
10. Marco CA: HIV infection and AIDS. In Tintinalli JE (ed): Emergency Medicine: A Comprehensive Study Guide, 4th ed. New York, McGraw-Hill, 1996, pp 701–707.
11. Musher DM, Hamill RJ, Baughn RE: Effect of human immunodeficiency virus (HIV) infection on the course of syphilis and on the response to treatment. Ann Intern Med 113:872–881, 1990.

56. TOXIC SHOCK SYNDROME

Scott Miner, M.D., and Bruce Evans, M.D.

1. What is toxic shock syndrome (TSS)?

TSS describes the constellation of symptoms associated with an exotoxin-mediated immune response to infection. In 1978, Todd et al. reported seven pediatric cases (ages 8 to 17) in which high fever, headache, confusion, conjunctival hyperemia, and gastrointestinal symptoms were accompanied by a scarlatiniform rash and severe shock. *Staphylococcus aureus* related to phage group 1 was isolated from infected or mucosal sites in these cases, prompting fears that the bacterium was expressing a newly discovered toxin.

2. Why did a bacterium begin to express a new and deadly exotoxin in the late 1970s?

Todd's report led to additional associations between TSS and *S. aureus*. In retrospect, the syndrome may had been described as early as 1927. Some researchers believe that the syndrome may have been responsible for the plague that ended the Golden Age of Athens.

3. Who gets TSS?

Menses were associated with 91% of cases reported by 1980, which quickly pointed to the use of new high-absorbency tampons as a risk factor. Such tampons, made with cross-linked carboxymethylcellulose and polyester foam, were thought to provide an ideal environment for the expression of TSS toxin and subsequently were removed from the market.

4. Is tampon use required for the patient to develop TSS?

No. Three of the patients identified in the 1978 report were male. Although the media focused on the association with high-absorbency tampons, clinical interest in the syndrome identified a wide variety of causes in the early 1980s. TSS has been reported in all age groups, in burn and postsurgical patients, after childbirth, and in association with the nasal packing commonly used to control epistaxis.

5. Describe the pathophysiology of TSS.

Three stages have been identified in the progression of the syndrome: (1) the local proliferation of toxin-producing bacteria, such as the site of a foreign body; (2) the toxin production, which is thought to require an aerobic environment; (3) the immune response to the toxin, which sets off the inflammatory cascade and leads to multisystem organ involvement. Air-containing foreign bodies seem to be a common risk factor.

6. There was heavy media coverage of TSS in the early 1980s because of the high case fatality rate. Has mortality been reduced?

The initial fatality rate was 13% for the first 55 cases, with white females in the 15- to 19-year old range thought to be at greatest risk. By 1984, 27% of reported cases were not associated with menses. Nonmenstrual TSS now accounts for about half of all cases. Reanalysis of early cases suggests that significant reporting bias was a factor in the high fatality rate, which is now stable at less than 3%. Also, TSS now may be recognized and treated before the patient becomes ill enough to meet the criteria that define the syndrome.

7. List the criteria for defining a case of TSS.

In 1980, the CDC defined six criteria:
1. Fever ≥ 38.9° C
2. Diffuse macular erythematous rash
3. Desquamation, usually of the palms or soles, after 1 to 2 weeks
4. Orthostasis or hypotension (with systolic blood pressure < 90 mm Hg in adults or less than the 6th percentile in children)
5. Involvement of three or more of the following organ systems:
   - Gastrointestinal: vomiting or diarrhea
   - Muscular: myalgias or elevated creatine phosphokinase (twice normal)
   - Renal: elevated blood urea nitrogen or creatinine (twice normal) or pyuria in the absence of urinary tract infection
   - Hepatic: total bilirubin, alanine aminotransferase, aspartate aminotransferase at least twice the upper limit of normal
   - Hematologic: platelets < 100,000/mm^3
   - Central nervous system: disorientation or alteration in consciousness without focal neurologic signs (when fever and hypotension are absent)

6. Negative results of the following, if obtained:
- Blood, throat, or cerebrospinal fluid cultures (blood cultures may be positive for *S. aureus*)
- Rise in titer to Rocky Mountain spotted fever, leptospirosis, or rubeola

8. Describe the rash associated with TSS.

The rash is a macular erythroderma that blanches and is not pruritic. It may be diffuse or localized and often is described as sunburn-like. It appears early in the illness and fades in about 3 days. It may be subtle and can be missed in dark-skinned patients.

9. When is desquamation likely to occur?

Loss of skin, usually of the distal extremities, invariably occurs in survivors 5 to 12 days after the illness starts. Delayed alopecia and fingernail loss may occur later and seem to depend on the level of hypotension during the acute illness.

10. Given the above-mentioned criteria, list the differential diagnosis.

Kawasaki disease

Staphylococcal scalded skin syndrome

Streptococcal scarlet fever

Rocky Mountain spotted fever

Leptospirosis

Stevens-Johnson syndrome

Erythema multiforme

Toxic epidermal necrolysis

Sepsis

Colorado tick fever

11. What is streptococcal TSS?

Group A streptococcus (*Streptococcus pyogenes*) can cause a severe systemic reaction similar to TSS. The toxin is similar to that of TSS. Diagnosis requires the isolation of group A streptococci from a sterile or nonsterile site, hypotension, and multisystem organ involvement (at least two or more of the following: renal impairment, coagulopathy causing disseminated intravascular coagulopathy or thrombocytopenia, hepatitis, adult respiratory distress syndrome, necrotizing soft tissue infections, or skin changes similar to those seen in TSS).

12. Summarize the treatment for TSS.

1. Supportive care including intravenous fluids for hypotension, with supplemental pressor support as needed.
2. Identification and removal of the source of infection (tampon, abscess, nasal packing).
3. Antibiotics.

13. Do antibiotics help?

No prospective studies show that antibiotics alter the severity of the course of TSS. Antibiotics reduce the recurrence rate (which can be 28%), however, and are considered standard of care.

14. What antibiotics should I use?

Pencillinase-resistant penicillins and **first-generation cephalosporins** are considered the antibiotics of choice. Vancomycin or clindamycin may be used in penicillin-allergic patients. Clindamycin has the added advantage of a direct antitoxin effect. High-dose penicillin is the treatment of choice for streptococcal TSS.

15. Do steroids help control the immune response to the toxin?

Theoretically, steroids should help attenuate the systemic response to the toxin, but there are no prospective data to show they are effective. Steroid use in sepsis still is debated, and steroids are not routinely used in the management of TSS.

16. Do all patients with TSS need admission?

Patients in whom TSS is suspected should be admitted because this toxin-mediated disease can progress rapidly. In most patients, the systemic signs of illness (hypotension, fever, and multisystem organ involvement) are present in the ED, clearly indicating the need for inpatient supportive care.

BIBLIOGRAPHY

1. Davis D, Gash-Kim TL, Heffernan EJ: Toxic shock syndrome: Case report of a post-partum female and a literature review. J Emerg Med 16:607–614, 1998.
2. Davis JP, Chesney PJ, Wand PJ, et al: Toxic-shock syndrome. N Engl J Med 303:1429–1435, 1980.
3. Hoge CW, Schwartz B, Talkington DF, et al: The changing epidemiology of invasive group A streptococcal infections and the emergence of streptococcal toxic shock-like syndrome. JAMA 269:384–389, 1993.
4. Russell NE, Pachorek RE: Clindamycin in the treatment of streptococcal and staphylococcal toxic shock syndromes. Ann Pharmacother 34:936–939, 2000.
5. Spijkstra JJ, Girbes ARJ: The continuing story of corticosteroids in the treatment of septic shock. Intensive Care Med 26:496–500, 2000.
6. Todd J, Fishaut M, Kapral F, et al; Toxic-shock syndrome associated with phage-group-1 staphylococci. Lancet 2:1116–1118, 1978.
7. Working Group on Severe Streptococcal Infections: Defining the group A streptococcal toxic shock syndrome: Rationale and consensus definition. JAMA 269:390–391, 1993.
8. Wright SW, Trott AT: Toxic shock syndrome: A review. Ann Emerg Med 17:268–273, 1988.

57. FOOD POISONING

Jeff S. Beckman, M.D.

1. Name the causes of food poisoning.
- Exotoxins produced by microorganisms
- Microorganisms (e.g., bacteria, fungi, viruses, parasites [these may be classified further as invasive, noninvasive, or toxin-producing organisms])
- Toxic substances present in the food naturally (e.g., amatoxins [mushrooms], dinoflagellates, or thallophytes)

2. List the common symptoms of food poisoning.
Nausea
Vomiting
Diarrhea
Low-grade fever
Crampy abdominal pain

3. What history is suggestive of food poisoning?
Presence of similar symptoms in other family members or others who ingested the same food or water, presence of blood in stools, and recent travel to underdeveloped countries or to mountainous regions. Other historical points include course of disease (acute versus subacute versus chronic), recent food ingested, other medical problems (HIV status, hypertension), previous abdominal surgeries, sexual history, and pets at home.

4. What are the usual physical findings?
Generally the abdomen is soft and minimally tender without peritoneal signs. Bowel sounds can be hyperactive or normal, and blood may be present in the stool.

5. Which physical findings are atypical in food poisoning?
Discrete areas of abdominal tenderness, peritoneal signs, and grossly bloody stools or melena should be warning signs that further investigations, including surgical consultation or

gastroenterology consultation, may be warranted. High fever is not a common feature of bacterial diarrhea with the exception of shigellosis.

6. Differentiate diarrhea caused by invasive versus noninvasive organisms.

Organisms that invade the mucosa (*Escherichia coli, Salmonella, Shigella, Campylobacter,* and *Yersinia*) cause bloody mucoid stools. Enterotoxins produced by other organisms (viruses, *Vibrio cholerae, E. coli, Staphylococcus aureus, Clostridium perfringens, Clostridium difficile,* and *Bacillus cereus*) affect the cyclic adenosine monophosphate pump on the gut mucosa and produce watery diarrhea.

7. Describe the initial ED treatment of food poisoning.

When a history and physical examination have been obtained and the working diagnosis is that of gastroenteritis (regardless of the cause), the degree of dehydration must be assessed and treated. Be especially diligent in infants and children; diarrheal disease continues to be a leading cause of infant death throughout the world, including the United States. Intravenous hydration with crystalloids may be required. Oral rehydration is accomplished with isotonic glucose-containing fluids (which help to facilitate sodium and water absorption). Antiemetics may be administered. The patient should be able to tolerate fluids in the ED before being discharged.

8. What is the best test for diagnosing invasive diarrhea?

The presence of fecal leukocytes and occult blood is a sensitive and specific predictor for an invasive bacterial cause of diarrhea and the likelihood of a positive bacterial stool culture.

9. What is *Montezuma's revenge*?

Most cases of traveler's diarrhea (also known as *turista* or *Montezuma's revenge*) come from Mexico, South America, or Africa. Watery diarrhea typically begins after a few days of travel and most often is caused by enterotoxigenic *E. coli. E. coli* can produce diarrhea by three mechanisms: (1) Enterotoxigenic strains produce a toxin that causes watery diarrhea similar to that which occurs in cholera. (2) Enteropathogenic strains colonize the bowel, causing outbreaks of diarrhea in hospital nurseries. (3) Enteroinvasive strains (*E. coli* 0157:H7) may cause a shigella-like illness with bloody mucoid stools.

10. Describe the treatment for traveler's diarrhea.

Fluids and electrolytes, along with agents to decrease stool volume, are the mainstay of treatment for traveler's diarrhea. Bismuth subsalicylate (Pepto-Bismol) reduces the number of unformed stools by approximately 50%; loperamide (Imodium) reduces diarrhea by 80%. For patients who do not respond to these measures, consider antibiotic therapy. Double-strength trimethoprim-sulfamethoxazole (160 mg of trimethoprim and 800 mg of sulfamethoxazole), one tablet twice daily, is recommended for travelers to noncoastal areas of Mexico during the summer. For other areas and other seasons, fluoroquinolone antibiotics are the drugs of choice. Ciprofloxacin (750 mg), levofloxacin (500 mg), norfloxacin (800 mg), or azithromycin (1,000 mg) may be used as single-dose therapy in the ED or given as a 3-day regimen for more seriously ill patients.

11. Is there any role for prophylaxis against traveler's diarrhea?

Prophylactic antibiotics may be appropriate for patients with significant underlying health impairments who are traveling to high-risk areas. Patients with inflammatory bowel disease, insulin-dependent diabetes, heart disease (in elderly patients), or AIDS may consider prophylaxis using trimethoprim-sulfamethoxazole or a fluoroquinolone antibiotic, depending on the area to which they are traveling (see question 10). Travelers without underlying illness who wish to take some type of chemoprophylaxis are advised to use bismuth subsalicylate at a dose of two tablets, four times daily. This product should not be used by patients on anticoagulants or salicylates or by people who are allergic to salicylates.

12. Which diarrhea-producing agent is associated with febrile seizures in children?

Shigella infections in young children often cause high fevers with febrile seizures before the onset of diarrheal illness. The disease can be quite severe, and death has been known to occur within 8 hours of the onset of diarrhea secondary to dehydration. Abdominal pain and fever usually precede the diarrhea. Stools are typically bloody, mucoid, and explosive. Elevated white blood cell counts may be seen, and a marked leftward shift is typical.

13. Describe a patient with *Salmonella* food poisoning.

Typically, patients have watery diarrhea and abdominal cramping usually without vomiting about 12 to 36 hours after ingestion of contaminated food. Food sources include eggs, poultry, meat, turkey, and unpasteurized milk or juice. Pet turtles are common reservoirs. If septicemia is present, systemic symptoms of fever, cough, headache, and meningismus occur. Enteric fever should be treated with hospitalization and antibiotics.

14. Which bacterial organism proliferates in precooked or poorly reheated meat and typically causes abdominal cramps and diarrhea 12 hours after eating contaminated food?

C. perfringens frequently is associated with food-service establishments where food is prepared in advance. Usual symptoms include diarrhea, abdominal pain, and occasionally nausea. Fever and vomiting are unlikely.

15. What food-borne diseases cause symptoms within 1 to 6 hours?

S. aureus enterotoxin is heat stable; causes vomiting, cramping, and mild diarrhea; and is produced in cooled meats, produce, dairy, and bakery goods left at room temperatures for prolonged periods. *B. cereus* enterotoxin typically is found in cooked rice and results in profuse vomiting.

16. What is the most common bacterial food-borne infection in the United States?

Campylobacter jejuni infection causes abdominal pain with diarrhea and in one third of cases has a prodromal influenza-like illness before the onset of gastrointestinal symptoms. Mostly found in raw or undercooked poultry, *C. jejuni* may induce a Guillain-Barré syndrome or reactive arthritis within 12 weeks of infection.

17. What food-borne disease can mimic acute appendicitis in older children and adults?

Yersinia enterocolitica infection may result in acute symptoms of right lower abdominal pain, high fevers, vomiting, and leukocytosis with mild diarrhea. This syndrome, referred to as *pseudoappendicitis* or *mesenteric adenitis*, has resulted in many unnecessary appendectomies.

18. What is scombroid?

Histamine fish poisoning (or scombroid) is caused by histamine or biogenic amine buildup in poorly refrigerated tuna, bluefish, mackerel, marlin, or mahi-mahi. Symptoms of flushing, urticaria, dizziness, and paresthesias present minutes to hours after ingestion of contaminated food. Most cases are self-limited, and diphenhydramine and cimetidine may be used for symptomatic relief. Selected patients may experience toxicity equivalent to acute anaphylaxis and require more aggressive management.

19. Which parasite should be highly suspected in a camper with chronic abdominal bloating and intermittent diarrhea with constipation?

Giardia lamblia is endemic to many areas of the United States and is the most common parasite in the country. Infection is acquired through drinking contaminated water or person-to-person contact. Of the population, 7% harbors the parasite in the cyst stage. Treatment with metronidazole frequently has been used effectively, although its use for this infection is not approved.

20. Should antibiotics be used for bacterial diarrhea?

The use of antibiotics in diarrhea is controversial and is not indicated for noninvasive causes. Any antibiotic has the potential to result in an overgrowth of *C. difficile* with resulting pseudomembranous colitis. Antibiotic treatment of bloody diarrhea in children generally is not recommended because of the association of hemolytic-uremic syndrome with *E. coli* 0157:H7 infections. Adults with a diarrheal illness of less than 2 weeks' duration, fever, and fecal leuko-cyte or Hemoccult-positive stools may be treated with empirical therapy; reasonable choices include 3- to 5-day courses of trimethoprim-sulfamethoxazole (1 DS tablet b.i.d.), ciprofloxacin (500 mg b.i.d.), norfloxacin (400 mg b.i.d.), levofloxacin (500 mg q.d.), or azithromycin (500 mg q.d.).

21. Should symptomatic relief be offered to patients?

Historically, symptomatic relief was offered only to patients with noninvasive diarrhea (no fecal leukocytes in stool smears). Patients with invasive diarrhea can develop toxic megacolon and have continued shedding of the organism if they are placed on antimotility drugs. More re-cently, however, loperamide has been used safely for all forms of gastroenteritis, but diphenoxy-late (Lomotil) should be avoided in invasive diarrhea.

22. What is an appropriate disposition for a patient with food poisoning?

Most patients can be discharged to home with instructions to avoid lactose-containing foods until the diarrhea stops. They should receive instructions on proper use of clear liquids and how to advance their diet. Follow-up should be arranged if the symptoms persist for 1 week. Be sure to rule out other causes of vomiting and diarrhea in the elderly. Close follow-up to assess for de-hydration is crucial in young infants.

BIBLIOGRAPHY

1. Adachi JA, Ostrosky-Zeichner L, DuPont HL: Empirical antimicrobial therapy for traveler's diarrhea. Clin Infect Dis 31:1079–1083, 2000.
2. Becker K, Southwick K, Reardon J: Histamine poisoning associated with eating tuna burgers. JAMA 285:1327–1330, 2001.
3. Bitterman RA: Acute gastroenteritis. In Marx JA, et al (eds): Rosen's Emergency Medicine: Concepts and Clinical Practice, 5th ed. St. Louis, Mosby, 2002, pp 1301–1326.
4. DuPont HL, Ericsson CD: Prevention and treatment of traveler's diarrhea. N Engl J Med 328:1821–1827, 1993.
5. Hogan DE: The emergency department approach to diarrhea. Emerg Med Clin North Am 14:673–694, 1996.
6. Karras DJ: Incidence of foodborne illnesses: Preliminary data from the foodborne diseases active sur-veillance network (FoodNet). Ann Emerg Med 35:92–93, 2000.
7. Larson SC: Traveler's diarrhea. Emerg Med Clin North Am 15:179–189, 1997.
8. Mead PS, Slutsker L, Dietz V: Food-related illness and death in the United States. Emerg Infect Dis 5:607–625, 1999.
9. Restuccia MC: Food poisoning. In Harwood-Nuss AL, Linden C, Luten RC, et al (eds): The Clinical Practice of Emergency Medicine, 2nd ed. Philadelphia, Lippincott-Raven, 1996, pp 1331–1334.
10. Wong CS, Jelacie S, Habeeb RL: The risk of the hemolytic-uremic syndrome after antibiotic treatment of *E. coli* 0157:H7 infections. N Engl J Med 342:1930–1936, 2000.

58. BOTULISM

Scott E. Rudkin, M.D., and Mark I. Langdorf, M.D., M.H.P.E.

1. What is the causative agent of botulism, and how does it cause disease?

Botulism is caused by the toxin produced by *Clostridium botulinum*. This toxin binds to pe-ripheral presynaptic cholinergic membranes, preventing the release of acetylcholine and produc-ing a life-threatening, paralytic illness. Adrenergic synapses are unaffected. By weight, botulism toxin is the most potent toxin known.

2. State the three most common ways that a patient can contract botulism.

1. Botulism most commonly is contracted by ingesting food that contains the toxin. Most cases are caused by home-canned or home-prepared foods and occur in isolation or in small clusters.

2. Wound botulism occurs when *C. botulinum* organisms contaminate traumatic wounds, most often in wounds in intravenous drug users and in wounds grossly contaminated by soil. Children are at greater risk because they often sustain extremity injuries while playing in the dirt. The incubation period for the development of wound botulism is 4 to 14 days, and the wound may appear clean at the time of initial medical evaluation.

3. Infant botulism occurs when *C. botulinum* spores are ingested and proliferate in the infant's gastrointestinal tract, most commonly from contaminated raw honey. This is the most common form of botulism in the United States, usually occurring in infants 3 to 20 weeks of age.

3. How does infant botulism present?

Often the first sign is constipation. This is followed by a feeble cry, floppy or weak neck, pooling of oral secretions or food in the oropharynx, decreased gag reflex, hypotonia, and areflexia. Cranial nerve deficits also occur, including flaccid facial expression, ptosis, and ophthalmoplegia. Respiratory arrest occurs in 50% of infants affected. Infants with botulism are afebrile and have normal cerebrospinal fluid. *C. botulinum* toxin does not cross the blood-brain barrier.

4. Describe the treatment for infant botulism.

Supportive care, including respiratory support, is the mainstay of treatment. Antitoxin is not recommended because infants recover without it, and there is high risk for anaphylaxis, caused by the horse serum in the antitoxin. The organism and toxin may remain in the bowel for 8 weeks after recovery. It has been suggested that infant botulism accounts for some cases of sudden infant death syndrome (SIDS). Reports have identified botulism organism or toxin in 5% to 10% of SIDS cases.

5. How can food-borne botulism be prevented?

Foods contaminated with botulism may have a normal appearance and taste, and only a small amount of toxin is necessary to cause disease. Appropriate processing of foods is vital to preventing illness. Botulism spores are heat resistant. Even when home-prepared food is cooked before canning, the spores still can produce toxin. Proper methods of cooking canned foods before eating, either by boiling for 10 minutes or heating at 80°C (176°F) for 30 minutes, destroy botulism toxin.

6. How does a patient with adult botulism present?

Early symptoms are nonspecific and usually begin 12 to 36 hours (range, 6 hours to 8 days) after ingestion. These symptoms include nausea, vomiting, weakness, lassitude, and dizziness. The patient then develops anticholinergic symptoms, including extreme dry mouth unrelieved by fluids, decreased lacrimation, constipation, and urinary retention. Neurologic symptoms, which may be delayed 3 days after the appearance of anticholinergic symptoms, most often involve cranial nerves first. The patient develops diplopia, blurred vision, photophobia, dysphonia, and dysphagia—all ocular and bulbar symptoms. The patient also develops symmetric descending weakness of the extremities. The weakness may progress to involve respiratory muscles.

7. What are the characteristic physical findings?

Postural hypotension, ptosis, extraocular palsies, and dilated, fixed pupils. Deep tendon reflexes may be normal, increased, or absent. Sensory examination is normal, as is body temperature in the absence of wound infection. The patient may have decreased bowel sounds and abdominal distention from an ileus. Pulmonary function tests may reveal decreased vital capacity. The constellation of postural hypotension, dilated and unreactive pupils, dry mucous membranes, descending paralysis with progressive respiratory weakness, and absence of fever strongly suggests the diagnosis of botulism.

8. What is the differential diagnosis of botulism?

There are many causes of acute weakness, such as disorders of nerves, muscles, or the neuromuscular junction: myasthenia gravis, Guillain-Barré syndrome, multiple sclerosis, tick paralysis, Eaton-Lambert syndrome, periodic paralysis (hyperkalemic and hypokalemic), diphtheria, polio, paralytic shellfish poisoning, and coral snake envenomation. Drug-induced disorders of neuromuscular transmission caused by aminoglycosides, phenytoin, lithium, organophosphates, and carbamate insecticides also can mimic botulism.

9. How can the diagnosis be confirmed?

Diagnosis is made by isolating the organism or the toxin from the patient or from the contaminated food that has been eaten. Laboratory examination of the patient's stool, blood, wound, and, in the case of infant botulism, gastric contents should be performed. Consider consultation with a poison control center, the Centers for Disease Control, or the local health department because this is a reportable condition.

10. How is adult botulism treated, and which organ system requires the most intensive monitoring?

Treatment is largely supportive. The most life-threatening effect of botulism is respiratory failure. Intensive monitoring of vital capacity and negative inspiratory force, preferably in an ICU, is mandatory. Early and controlled intubation is preferable to crash intubation because patients can deteriorate within minutes. Nasogastric suction, total parenteral nutrition, and bladder catheterization are necessary for profound ileus and urinary retention. Penicillin may eradicate colonization of the intestine but is of unproven value. Aminoglycosides should be avoided because of their potential for aminoglycoside-induced neuromuscular blockade. Botulism antitoxin, available through state health departments, should be given as soon as possible. Even if diagnosis is delayed, antitoxin still should be administered because toxin has been shown in the blood for 30 days. It is an equine antitoxin, effective against types A, B, and E. Patients must be tested for hypersensitivity to horse serum before administration, as described on the antitoxin package insert. Equine antitoxin should be avoided in infants because of an increased risk for anaphylaxis. Human botulism immune globulin is under investigation. Tetanus prophylaxis should be administered.

11. How could botulism be used as a bioterrorism weapon, and how would it present?

Botulism can be spread by either food-borne or aerosolized mechanisms. The clinician must be concerned about unsual clusters of cases. After a 12- to 72-hour latency period, the botulism toxin would cause acute symmetric, descending flaccid paralysis with bulbar palsies (diplopia, dysarthria, dysphonia, and dysphagia).

12. What is the prognosis of a patient with botulism?

With the use of antitoxin and respiratory support, adult mortality has decreased from 60% to 25%. Recovery is gradual over weeks to months.

BIBLIOGRAPHY

1. Arnon SS: Botulinum toxin as a biological weapon: Medical and public health management. JAMA 285:1059–1070, 2001.
2. Case records of the Massachusetts General Hospital: Weekly clinicopathological exercises. Case 22—1997: A 58-year-old woman with multiple cranial neuropathies. N Engl J Med 337:184–190, 1997.
3. Cox N, Hinkle R: Infant botulism. Am Fam Physician 65:1388–1392, 2002.
4. Diagnosis and management of foodborne illnesses, 2001. MMWR Morb Mortal Wkly Rep 50(RR-2):1–69, 2001.
5. Goetz CG, Meisel E: Biological neurotoxins. Neurol Clin 18:719–740, 2000.
6. Long SS: Infant botulism. Pediatr Infect Dis 20:707–709, 2001.
7. Masselli RA, Ellis W, Mandler RN, et al: Cluster of wound botulism in California: Clinical, electrophysiologic, and pathologic study. Muscle Nerve 20:1284–1295, 1997.
8. McGarrity L: Wound botulism in injecting drug users. Anaesthesia 57:301–302, 2002.

9. Microbiological investigation into wound botulism. Commun Dis Rep CDR Wkly 10:185, 188, 2000.
10. Mitchell PA, Pons PT: Wound botulism associated with black tar heroin and lower extremity cellulitis. J Emerg Med 20:371–375, 2001.
11. Muensterer OJ: Infant botulism. Pediatr Rev 21:427, 2000.

59. TETANUS

James Mathews, M.D.

1. No one I know has seen a clinical case of tetanus. Why should I worry about it?

Because of mandated immunization in the United States, the incidence of tetanus is less than 1 case per 1 million per year. Many people are at risk, however, including immigrants from countries in which tetanus prophylaxis is not mandated and elderly people who have lost their immunity.

2. Worldwide, what is the most common cause of death from tetanus?

The neonatal form, arising from poor hygiene of the umbilical stump or from circumcision practices.

3. What are *tetanus-prone* wounds?

Wounds that produce anaerobic conditions, including puncture wounds, crush injuries, and burns (even superficial ones). Any wound heavily contaminated with debris, such as soil or feces, is at high risk.

4. Name other problems that may lead to tetanus.

Otitis media, tonsillar crypt infection, septic abortion, and problems with the lower gastrointestinal tract.

5. What bacterium causes tetanus?

Clostridium tetani, which is an obligate anaerobe. It is shaped like a drumstick and produces spores. This organism is ubiquitous in soil and feces and occurs worldwide. The organism itself is killed easily by heat and antiseptics, but the spores are extremely tough. Disease occurs when the spores germinate, multiply in tissue under anaerobic conditions, and produce the toxin.

6. How can I diagnose tetanus?

The most common presenting symptom is **trismus**, possibly associated with dysphagia, excessive pain in the area of injury, and a painful stiff neck. This usually begins within 10 to 15 days of injury, and onset is over a 2- to 5-day period. Onset is the period between earliest symptoms and the first generalized spasm. Onset over less than 48 hours is associated with severe disease. Progression of the disease involves increasing numbers of spastic muscle groups and increasing pain during spasm.

7. Which muscle group is often profoundly affected?

The muscles of the neck and back. Severe spasm of these muscles may produce opisthotonos to the extent that only the heels and the back of the head are touching the bed. In the worst cases, these spasms have caused rupture of the rectus abdominis muscles and fractured vertebrae.

8. Are there systemic symptoms?

Yes, but these may be minimal. In severe cases, high fever and wide swings in blood pressure and heart rate may be seen. These signs seem to be due to excessive catecholamines.

9. What usually causes death?

In modern developed countries, the most common causes of death are the autonomic problems, especially fatal arrhythmias and hyperpyrexia. In the past and in underdeveloped countries, the most common cause of death was and is respiratory failure secondary to spasm of the muscles of respiration.

10. What diseases may mimic tetanus?

In the established case, tetanus can be confused only with strychnine poisoning. In strychnine poisoning, the jaw muscles usually are involved late or not at all, and between spasms there is no rigidity. Early tetanus may be confused with dental infections that produce trismus and dystonic reactions. Observation reveals that trismus secondary to dental infection does not progress, and the patient with a dystonic reaction can open the mouth, which does not occur with true trismus.

11. Which laboratory studies are helpful?

There are no diagnostic laboratory studies. Routine testing includes ECG, arterial blood gases, and vital capacity. These last two should be followed closely to recognize early respiratory failure. The site of infection should be identified.

12. What do I do in the ED?

An intravenous line should be started and human tetanus immunoglobulin given, 1,000 U intravenously and 2,000 U intramuscularly. Immunoglobulin must be given before surgical wound débridement to bind any released toxin. Penicillin is the drug of choice in a dose of 1 million U intravenously every 6 hours. Penicillin-allergic patients are treated with erythromycin, 500 mg intravenously every 6 hours (see Figure).

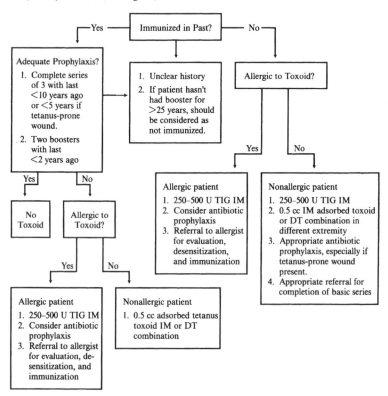

Guidelines for tetanus immunization.

13. What about supportive measures?

If vital capacity is less than 50% predicted, the patient must be paralyzed with long-acting agents, such as curare or pancuronium, and placed on a ventilator. If vital capacity is greater than 50% but trismus is severe with compromise of the airway, either an endotracheal tube or tracheostomy is indicated. Mild disease may be controlled with sedatives such as diazepam. A nasogastric tube should be placed.

14. How can tetanus be prevented?

Mandatory **immunization**. Proper wound care and good hygiene are important components of prevention. Proper cleansing irrigation and débridement must be done on all wounds, and appropriate immunization is mandatory (see question 12). Tetanus immunization always must be confirmed and documented. If there is any doubt regarding earlier immunizations, toxoid and tetanus immunoglobulin should be given.

15. What are the pitfalls?

The early symptoms of tetanus are easy to ascribe to psychoneurotic disorders. A dystonic reaction should respond immediately to 50 mg of intravenous diphrenhydramine. The careful observer should not make this error.

BIBLIOGRAPHY

1. Adams EB, Laurence DR, Smith DWG: Tetanus. Oxford, Blackwell Scientific Publications, 1969.
2. Alagappan K, Rennie W, Narang V, Auerbach C: Immunologic response to tetanus toxoid in geriatric patients. Ann Emerg Med 30:459–462, 1997.
3. Bovier PA, Chamot E, Bouvier Gallacchi M, Loutan L: Importance of patients' perceptions and general practitioners' recommendations in understanding missed opportunities for immunizations in Swiss adults. Vaccine 19:4760–4767, 2001.
4. Cook TM, Protheroe RT, Handel JM: Tetanus: A review of the literature. Br J Anaesth 87:477–487, 2001.
5. Davies-Adetugbo AA, Torimiro SE, Ako-Nei KA: Prognostic factors in neonatal tetanus. Trop Med Int Health 3:9–13, 1998.
6. Dowell VR Jr: Botulism and tetanus: Selected epidemiologic and microbiologic aspects. Rev Infect Dis 6(suppl 1):S202–S207, 1984.
7. Ernst ME, Klepser ME, Fouts M, Marangos MN: Tetanus: Pathophysiology and management. Ann Pharmacother 31:1507–1513, 1997.
8. Furste W: Tetanus: a new threat. J Trauma 51(2):416–417, 2001.
9. Marak I, Baykan Z, Aksakal FN, et al: Tetanus immunization in pregnant women. Public Health 115:359–364, 2001.
10. Patel JC, Mehta BC: Tetanus: Study of 8,697 cases. In Proceedings of the Fourth International Conference on Tetanus, April 6-12, 1975, Dakar, Senegal. Lyon, France, Foundation Merieux, 1975.
11. Tetanus among injecting-drug users-California, 1997. MMWR Morb Mortal Wkly Rep 47:149–151, 1998.

60. SEXUALLY TRANSMITTED DISEASES

Kerry B. Broderick, M.D.

1. What are the most common sexually transmitted diseases (STDs)?

The true incidence of most STDs is unknown because not all cases are reported. Overall, it is estimated that STDs affect about 12 million people in the United States each year. **Chlamydia** is estimated to infect 4 million people annually and is a major health problem for young women because of the sequelae of infertility and ectopic pregnancy. In 1996, 498,884 cases were reported. The incidence of **gonorrhea** peaked at more than 1 million cases per year in the late 1970s but declined steadily in the 1980s and 1990s. There are an estimated 600,000 new cases reported per year. The rate of gonococcal infections is highest among adolescent girls. Approximately 5.5 million annual cases of genital **human papillomavirus** (HPV) are found. More than 30 types of HPV can cause genital tract infection. Genital warts usually are caused by HPV type 6 or 11. Several types are associated with cervical dysplasia. Each year, 500,000 new cases of **genital herpes** are diagnosed. **Syphilis** is on the decline after an epidemic from 1986–1990. In 1996, 52,976 cases were reported. Syphilis is substantially more common in non-Hispanic blacks than in other ethnic groups. It is also endemic in the South. Cases of **HIV**—the deadly STD—continue to accumulate. In 1996, 66,885 new cases were reported.

2. How should I evaluate abnormal vaginal discharge?

The first thing to do is to take a complete **sexual history**:

1. How many partners has she had in the last several months (men or women)?
2. Has she used protective barriers such as condoms and dental dams with each episode?
3. Ask about previous STDs.
4. Establish when the last menstrual period was because pregnancy would affect any decision about antimicrobial therapy (although it is prudent to trust no one and to obtain a pregnancy test).

The appearance of the discharge on **pelvic examination** is important. Always take a sample for wet preparation and potassium hydroxide. **Vulvovaginal candidiasis** (not an STD) causes a white, curdlike discharge that clings to vaginal walls. Hyphae are present on potassium hydroxide preparation. Recent antibiotic usage is a risk factor for this, as are diabetes and HIV. Treatment is single-dose oral fluconazole or any of the topical imidazoles. Patients frequently treat themselves with an over-the-counter antiyeast product before their ED visit, unaware that the cause of the discharge is an infection other than a yeast infection. **Bacterial vaginosis** is not an STD but an alteration of the microbial ecosystem with overgrowth of *Gardnerella vaginalis* and other species. Diagnosis is made by noting clue cells on the wet preparation, and treatment is with metronidazole. *Trichomonas* vaginitis, the third common cause, is a true STD. It causes a green, frothy discharge, and the cervix may be erythematous and friable (strawberry cervix). Diagnosis is based on finding the motile trichomonads on wet preparation or in urine. Treatment is with metronidazole. A discharge with significant leukocytes that does not include yeast, clue cells, or *Trichomonas* may be due to **mucopurulent cervicitis** (MPC).

3. A sexually active young man presents with dysuria. How likely is it that it resulted from a urinary tract infection?

About as likely as getting gonorrhea from sitting on a toilet seat. Dysuria in young men almost always is due to urethritis from an STD. The likely pathogens include gonorrhea, *Chlamydia, Ureaplasma, Trichomonas*, and herpes simplex virus. A purulent discharge most likely is caused by gonorrhea, whereas a mucoid discharge most likely is caused by infection with *Chlamydia*. The patient should be tested for both of these pathogens. *Chlamydia* also can infect the urethra of women, and they may present only with dysuria. Consider this diagnosis in a woman with dysuria and no bacteria on urinalysis, and do a pelvic examination.

4. Are there any single-dose treatment regimens for uncomplicated chlamydial infections?

Yes, a single 1-g dose of **azithromycin** is an effective treatment for lower tract chlamydial infections, including urethritis and cervicitis. Single-dose therapy is *not* appropriate for upper tract disease, such as epididymitis and pelvic inflammatory disease (PID). This simplified therapy should lead to more effective treatment in noncompliant patients.

5. Are there suitable oral alternatives to parenteral therapy for gonorrhea?

Uncomplicated urethral, endocervical, or rectal gonorrheal infections can be treated adequately with a single intramuscular injection of ceftriaxone (125 mg) or an equivalent third-generation cephalosporin antibiotic. Alternative oral regimens include cefixime (400 mg), ciprofloxacin

(500 mg), ofloxacin (400 mg), and levofloxacin (500 mg). Cases of quinolone-resistant *Neisseria gonorrhoeae* have been reported from many parts of the world and are becoming widespread in parts of Asia. Currently, quinolones can be used with confidence to treat these infections, but quinolone-resistant *N. gonorrhoeae* could increase in the future, forcing changes in recommended regimens. Because of possible concomitant chlamydial infections, these patients should be treated with an additional agent to address the *Chlamydia*.

6. What is the significance of finding MPC in a woman with lower abdominal pain?

The normal endometrial secretion, as noted on exit from the endocervical canal, should be transparent. The presence of a mucopurulent secretion from the os, which may appear yellow when viewed on a white cotton-tipped swab (positive *Q-tip sign*), suggests MPC. MPC, most commonly caused by gonorrhea or *Chlamydia*, is a precursor to upper tract infection (e.g., PID). PID is a diagnosis based on clinical criteria including cervical motion tenderness, adnexal tenderness, and lower abdominal tenderness. Patients who are severely ill with PID require hospitalization and intravenous antibiotics. Many patients with PID can be treated as outpatients with a single dose of intramuscular ceftriaxone and 2 weeks of doxycycline.

7. How do I evaluate a sexually active young woman who presents with an acutely swollen, warm, painful right ankle?

This patient, with acute monarticular arthritis, should be presumed to have a **disseminated gonococcal infection**. This is a syndrome of gonococcal bacteremia that leads to peripheral manifestations of disease, including dermatitis, tenosynovitis, and septic arthritis. Arthrocentesis should be done on the involved joint, and the fluid should be sent for Gram stain, culture for gonococcus (GC) and regular aerobic cultures, and cell count. GC is cultured from less than 50% of joints. A pelvic examination must be done to culture the cervix for GC. Consider culturing the rectum and urethra. A patient suspected of having disseminated gonococcal infection should be admitted and treated with parenteral antibiotics (ceftriaxone, 1 g intravenously q 12 h).

8. Discuss the most common causes of genital ulcers.

Genital ulcers can represent infection with herpes simplex virus (HSV), chancroid, or syphilis. It is difficult to make a diagnosis based solely on history and physical examination. Always ask these patients about their travel history and about exposure to prostitutes in other regions. Genital ulcers are an important risk cofactor for HIV transmission.

- **Herpes simplex virus (HSV)**: In most areas of the United States, genital herpes caused by HSV is the most common cause of genital ulcers. Primary HSV infection results in severely ill patients who are toxic with fever, malaise, and inguinal adenopathy. Diagnosis is made by viral culture or antigen testing. HSV is a recurrent disease, and patients may shed the virus while they are asymptomatic. It cannot be cured, but treatment with antiviral agents, such as acyclovir, can shorten the duration of symptoms. Long-term suppressive therapy can prevent outbreaks of ulcers.
- **Chancroid**: Also called *soft sore*, this disease is caused by *Haemophilus ducreyi*, a bacterium that is difficult to culture. Incidence in the United States had decreased until the late 1980s, when outbreaks were noted in several inner cities. It is now endemic in some areas of the United States. Clinically, this syndrome causes a painful nonindurated papule that erodes into an ulcer. Painful inguinal adenopathy is found in more than 50% of cases. Treatment options include single-dose azithromycin or ceftriaxone or 1 week of erythromycin or ciprofloxacin.
- **Syphilis**: Primary syphilis presents with a painless indurated ulcer called a *chancre*. Diagnosis is best made by dark-field examination for spirochetes, although this is usually available only in public health laboratories. A Venereal Disease Research Laboratory (VDRL) test should be done on anyone with possible syphilis. Treatment for primary syphilis is penicillin G benzathine, 2.4 million U intramuscularly.

9. What is the Jarisch-Herxheimer reaction?

After initiation of treatment for syphilis, onset of fever, chills, myalgias, headache, tachycardia, increased respirations, increased neutrophil count, and mild hypotension. This occurs approximately 2 hours after initiation of treatment with peak temperatures at approximately 7 hours, with defervescence at 12 to 24 hours. This reaction occurs in 50% of primary syphilis, 90% of secondary syphilis, and 25% of early latent syphilis patients. In secondary syphilis patients, the mucocutaneous lesions may become more edematous and erythematous.

10. Proctitis is a problem primarily seen in men who have sex with men. Discuss the approach and treatment.

Any individual, male or female, with the onset of acute proctitis symptoms (rectal pain, discharge, tenesmus), who recently has had unprotected, receptive anal intercourse, is at risk for an STD-related problem. These patients should be examined by anoscopy and should be tested for gonorrhea, *Chlamydia*, and HSV. All patients should have serologic testing for syphilis. These patients should have empirical treatment for gonorrhea and *Chlamydia*. If ulcers are apparent on anoscopy, consider empirical antiviral therapy with acyclovir.

11. Do I need to report STD cases to the health department?

Yes. Accurate reporting of STDs is essential to national and local STD control efforts. HIV, gonorrhea, and syphilis are reportable infections in every state. Chlamydial infection is reportable in most states. It is the responsibility of each clinician to know his or her local reporting requirements. If you are unsure of what to report about a specific patient, contact your local health department.

12. What are the important points to address in the discharge instructions for STD patients?

1. Instruct patients to refer *all* their sexual partners for evaluation and treatment. Some physicians in the United States routinely provide additional antibiotic prescriptions for sexual partners. Although it is well intentioned, it is controversial to provide a prescription for a person you have not interviewed or examined. That person may be allergic to the medication or may have additional infections that you are not treating.

2. All patients should be instructed to avoid sexual contact with their partners until all parties have finished treatment. Because it is unrealistic to expect all patients to follow this advice, explain the importance of using condoms with every sexual contact to avoid further infections and to prevent infection with HIV.

3. Education about STDs is the responsibility of every ED physician because you may be the only contact the patient has with the medical system.

BIBLIOGRAPHY

1. Centers for Disease Control: 1998 guidelines for treatment of sexually transmitted diseases. MMWR Morb Mortal Wkly Rep 47:1–111, 1998.
2. Erbelding E, Quinn TC: The impact of antimicrobial resistance on the treatment of sexually transmitted diseases. Infect Dis Clin North Am 11:889–903, 1997.
3. Handsfield HH, McCormack WM, Hook EW 3d, et al: A comparison of single-dose cefixime with ceftriaxone as treatment for uncomplicated gonorrhea. N Engl J Med 325:1337–1341, 1991.
4. Holmes KK, Sparling PF, Mardh P-A, et al: Sexually Transmitted Diseases, 3rd ed. New York, McGraw-Hill, 1998.
5. Knapp JS: Fluoroquinolone resistance in *Neisseria gonorrhoeae*. Emerg Infect Dis 3:33–39, 1997.
6. Stamm WE: Azithromycin in the treatment of uncomplicated genital chlamydia infections. Am J Med 91:195–225, 1991.

61. TICK-BORNE ILLNESSES OF NORTH AMERICA

Gayle E. Long, M.D., and Cheryl Melick-Casanova, M.D.

1. Are tick-related illnesses of medical importance?

Yes. They transmit a greater variety of infectious agents than any other arthropod. They are the most important vector for human illness in North America and second only to mosquitoes worldwide. Lyme disease is the most common vector-borne illness in the United States, affecting more than 15,000 people a year.

2. Classify ticks.

Ticks are from the class Arachnida, which includes spiders, mites, and scorpions. There are two major families of ticks: the Ixodidae, or hard tick, and the Argasidae, or soft tick. All major tick-borne illnesses are transmitted by hard ticks except for relapsing fever.

3. What time of year do tick-related illnesses occur?

They can occur throughout the year, but most present in **May through September**. This is due partly to humans being outside during this time, allowing ticks to jump on them, and to the life cycle of ticks.

4. Name the vector and infectious agent for each North American tick-borne illness.

Tick-Borne Illnesses

DISEASE	VECTOR	AGENT	ORGANISM
Lyme disease	*Ixodes scapularis* (black legged tick or deer tick)	Spirochetal	*Borrelia burgdorferi*
	Ixodes pacificus	Spirochetal	*B. burgdorferi*
Relapsing fever	Various species in the genus *Ornithodoros*	Spirochetal	At least 13 *Borrelia* species worldwide
Rocky Mountain spotted fever	*Dermacentor andersoni*	Rickettsial	*Rickettsia rickettsii*
	Dermacentor variabilis	Rickettsial	*R. rickettsii*
Human monocytic ehrlichiosis	*Amblyomma americanum* (Lone Star tick)	Bacterial	*Ehrlichia chaffeensis*
Human granulocytic ehrlichiosis (HGE)	*Ixodes scapularis*	Bacterial	HGE agent
	Ixodes pacificus	Bacterial	HGE agent
Human ehrlichiosis	*A. americanum*	Bacterial	*Ehrlichia ewingii*
Q fever	Unknown	Rickettsial	*Coxiella burnetii*
Colorado tick fever	*D. andersoni*	RNA virus	Orbivirus
Encephalitis	Multiple	Viral	Arbovirus
Babesiosis	*I. scapularis*	Protozoan	*Babesia microti*
	I. pacificus	Protozoan	*Babesia equi* and others
Tularemia	*D. andersoni*	Bacterial	*Francisella tularensis*
	D. variabilis	Bacterial	*F. tularensis*
	Amblyomma americanum and others	Bacterial	*F. tularensis*
Tick paralysis	Multiple	Toxin	None

5. How does the life cycle of the *Ixodes scapularis* tick relate to its transmission of Lyme disease?

The *I. scapularis* tick goes through three stages in its 2-year life span: larva, nymph, and adult. In each stage, the ticks have one blood meal (usually lasting 2 to 15 days) from a vertebrate (often mice or deer and occasionally humans), and if they obtain the spirochete from one meal, it stays with them until their next stage. Nymphs and adults can infect humans, but most infections are caused by nymphs. This is due to various factors, including their small size (about that of a poppy seed), which allows them to avoid detection and removal, and their predominance during the spring and summer, when humans are more likely to be outside.

6. Describe the three clinical stages of Lyme disease.

1. **Early acute**. The hallmark of this stage is erythema migrans (EM), previously known as erythema chronicum migrans. EM is a painless erythematous macular skin lesion that appears in approximately 80% of infected individuals. It occurs 1 to 36 days after infection (average 7 to 10 days) at the site of the bite. The lesion expands centrifugally over days to weeks, attaining a size of at least 5 cm. A central papule, consisting of several millimeters of erythema, scale, or hyperpigmentation, is often present at the site of the tick bite (punctum). Initial reports indicated central clearing of the lesion, but less than 50% of individuals show this clearing 1 to 2 weeks into the development of the lesion. Approximately 20% of cases develop multiple lesions. Although some individuals with the expanding EM rash are asymptomatic, most have associated viral-like symptoms, including fatigue, myalgias, arthralgias, headache, stiff neck, fever, and chills.

2. **Early disseminated disease**. This may occur in untreated individuals in the weeks to months after the tick bite. Nervous system involvement occurs in 10% to 15% of individuals. Most common are a lymphocytic meningitis or cranial neuritis, particularly Bell's palsy, which may be bilateral. Radiculoneuritis consisting of burning, numbness, or tingling in the extremities also may be seen. Optic nerve problems or arthritis sometimes can occur in this time frame. Carditis may result from disseminated disease in about 5% of untreated patients. Symptoms include palpitations, light-headedness, chest pain, dyspnea, or syncope. Most commonly the sudden onset of second-degree or third-degree atrioventricular conduction defects, possibly requiring temporary pacing, is noted. Less common are tachyarrhythmias, myopericarditis, and, rarely, cardiomyopathy. In this stage and later, diagnosis is supported by serologic tests: an enzyme-linked immunosorbent assay followed by a confirmatory Western blot.

3. **Late or chronic**. Late or chronic manifestations may occur months to years after the onset of the illness. Lyme arthritis is the most common of these manifestations. This generally presents with brief recurrent attacks of a single or a few painful swollen joints, usually the knee. Associated significant systemic symptoms are rare. Syndromes including polyneuritis, encephalomyelitis (0.1%), encephalopathy, cranial neuropathies, chronic radiculopathies, and chronic meningitis have been identified. Less common are skin changes, such as acrodermatitis chronicum atrophicans, and *Borrelia* lymphocytoma. Ocular keratitis has been described.

7. What is the geographic distribution of Lyme disease?

The coastal regions of the Northeast, upper Midwest, and Pacific regions.

8. Who should get the vaccine for Lyme disease, and can people still contract Lyme disease after being vaccinated?

The vaccine series, which involves three injections over 1 year, is recommended for people 15 to 70 years old who live in or visit high-risk areas and have frequent or prolonged exposure to tick habitats. People who have received vaccine can still become infected because the full series is only 76% effective.

9. A patient comes to the ED having removed a tick that day. Should you treat the patient prophylactically for Lyme disease or other tick-borne illness?

In general, the incidence of disease from one bite is so low (about 3% in hyperendemic Lyme disease areas) that it is best not to treat presumptively. Recommend that the patient return immediately if he or she develops a rash in the area of the bite, a fever (>38°C, which may suggest ehrlichiosis or babesiosis), or other illness within 30 days. Some evidence suggests that in select cases, one dose of 200 mg of doxycycline may help to prevent Lyme disease. The criteria for use of this drug should include definitive recognition of an *I. scapularis* tick in a high-risk area, treatment within 72 hours of tick removal, and known tick attachment for at least 48 to 72 hours (infection rarely occurs before the tick has been attached for 48 hours). Engorgement of the tick suggests longer attachment.

10. What is relapsing fever?
Relapsing fever is caused by a spirochete and is the only tick-borne illness transmitted by the Argasidae, or soft-bodied tick. Outbreaks usually occur in backpackers from the Western mountains who stay in old cabins infested by rodents. The tick is harbored in the rodent's nest and feeds on the unwary for brief periods at night. The 4- to 18-day incubation period is followed by the abrupt onset of a high fever associated with chills, severe headache, myalgia, weakness, and occasional gastrointestinal complaints. Symptoms last 3 days, then resolve. If the condition is not treated, multiple relapses ensue at weekly intervals. In 25% of patients, an erythematous macular rash may develop. Diagnosis is made by identifying spirochetes on a peripheral blood smear using Giemsa or Wright stain, dark-field microscopy, or a quantitative buffy coat analysis.

11. What is Rocky Mountain spotted fever?
Infection by this rickettsial organism causes a disseminated vasculitis. Organisms multiply within the vascular endothelium with development of increased vascular permeability and microinfarction of organs. Onset is abrupt, with initial complaints of high fever, headache, and myalgia. The classic rash, which is initially macular, becomes petechial over several days. It begins on the palms and soles, then spreads centripetally to involve the trunk. It does not appear until the third or fourth day of illness but is absent in 10% to 15% of patients. The classic triad of fever, rash, and tick exposure is present in less than 20% of patients. Meningismus, focal neurologic signs, myocarditis, pneumonitis, and gastrointestinal symptoms may occur. Death is the result of multisystem organ failure with intracerebral hemorrhage, disseminated intravascular coagulation, and vascular collapse. Early treatment is based on clinical diagnosis; confirmatory laboratory tests include serology and identification of the organism in blood and tissues.

12. What is the mortality rate for Rocky Mountain spotted fever?
The case fatality rate has remained constant at 4%, with mortality the highest in the elderly (> 8%) and in patients whose treatment is begun after the third day of symptoms. In regions with endemic Rocky Mountain spotted fever, a trial of doxycycline is recommended for anyone who presents with fever, headache, and myalgia from May through September.

13. What is the geographic distribution of Rocky Mountain spotted fever?
Initially the condition was isolated and diagnosed in the Rocky Mountains, but a change in the epidemiology of the illness occurred around 1931. The illness now is seen almost exclusively in the southern Atlantic and western south-central parts of the United States. The states with the highest incidence are Oklahoma, Kansas, and the Carolinas.

14. What is human ehrlichiosis?
The causative agents are obligate intracellular gram-negative cocci, similar to true rickettsial organisms. Human monocytic ehrlichia first was described in humans in 1987. It is transmitted by the Lone Star tick and is seen primarily in the south-central and southeastern United States. Human granulocytic ehrlichia first was discovered in 1994. It is transmitted by the *I. scapularis* tick, the same tick responsible for Lyme disease, and its geographic distribution is also the upper midwestern and northeastern United States. Coinfection with human granulocytic ehrlichia and Lyme disease can occur. In 1999, it was found that *Ehrlichia ewingii*, the agent of canine granulocytic ehrlichiosis, also could cause disease in humans. Following an incubation period of 1 to

30 days after a tick bite (average 8 to 14 days), an acute flulike febrile illness associated with malaise, myalgias, headache, arthralgias, nausea, and occasionally some gastrointestinal and neurologic symptoms develops. A rash, if present, is fleeting and rare. Significant laboratory results include leukopenia, thrombocytopenia, and a mild elevation of liver function enzymes. A Wright stain smear of peripheral blood cells may show characteristic morulae—membrane-bound intracellular clusters of bacteria in white blood cells. Diagnosis ultimately is made by serologic confirmation comparing acute and convalescent titers or by cell culture or molecular methods. With a fatality rate estimated at 5%, it is recommended that anyone who presents with a flulike illness, associated laboratory findings, and a history of tick exposure promptly be treated empirically with a tetracycline agent.

15. What is Q fever?

Query (Q) fever is a highly infectious rickettsial infection in which a single inhaled organism is sufficient to initiate infection. The infection, although carried by and transmitted to animals by ticks, is rarely if ever transmitted to humans by this route. Most human infection follows exposure during parturition of livestock, especially sheep. After an incubation period of 14 to 39 days, an acute febrile illness associated with rigors, severe headache, malaise, myalgia, and chest pain develops. Pneumonia and hepatitis may be the primary manifestations. The most serious and often fatal complication of unrecognized and untreated Q fever is the development of endocarditis 1 to 20 years later. Diagnosis is by serology. Most patients recover without treatment; antibiotics are used for severe or prolonged disease.

16. What is Colorado tick fever?

After infection with this RNA virus, the incubation period averages 4 days (range, 1 to 14 days). Onset is sudden with high fever, chills, headache, myalgia, fatigue, retroorbital pain, and gastrointestinal symptoms. Meningeal or encephalitic symptoms are common in children. Rash is fleeting if present. The characteristic biphasic or *saddleback* fever lasts 2 to 3 days and abates for 1 to 2 days before returning. A marked leukopenia (1,000 to 3,000 range) develops, reaching its lowest point during the second fever spike. The diagnosis is made by identifying the virus in blood specimens. An erythrocyte viremia persists for 120 days, so blood donations should be avoided in this period. Recovery is complete after 3 weeks, with only supportive care required. Lifelong immunity develops. As the name implies, this illness is found in the Rocky Mountain states.

17. What is babesiosis?

A protozoan parasite of red blood cells whose incidence is increasing. The illness is characterized by a mild febrile illness with headache, fatigue, weakness, and anemia. The illness is most severe in elderly, immunocompromised, or asplenic patients. Diagnosis is by identifying parasitized red blood cells on peripheral blood smears or by serologic or polymerase chain reaction tests. It is endemic to areas in the northeastern United States. The major concern is that the same tick that transmits this illness also transmits Lyme disease, and coinfection with both organisms, causing a more severe illness, occurs in 10% to 23% of patients.

18. What is tularemia?

An illness caused by *F. tularensis*, a small, pleomorphic, gram-negative, intracellular and extracellular coccobacillus. Exposure occurs by multiple routes of transmission, including exposure to animal products and through tick bites. The ulceroglandular variety accounts for 85% of cases. About 48 hours after skin exposure, a firm erythematous papule develops. Ulceration develops within 2 days; regional lymph nodes enlarge and form suppurating buboes. Constitutional symptoms of fever, myalgia, headache, and cough are present. Mortality from untreated ulceroglandular tularemia is 5% to 7%. The disseminated typhoidal variety develops in 10% of cases and is characterized by severe disabling fatigue, weight loss, and pulmonary involvement. The pneumonic variety is associated with nonproductive cough, diffuse patchy infiltrates on chest radiograph, and a mortality approaching 30%. Serologic and other laboratory tests are used in diagnosis.

19. What is tick paralysis?

A rare toxin-mediated illness seen after prolonged attachment (4 to 7 days) and feeding of a female tick. The toxin is secreted in the saliva and affects central and peripheral nerves. Victims are usually children. Initially the victim is irritable, is restless, and may complain of paresthesia of extremities but has a normal neurosensory examination. Over the subsequent 24 to 48 hours, an ascending symmetric flaccid paralysis develops. Eventually, respiratory paralysis, stupor, myocarditis, and death may result, with mortality rates of 10%. Recovery is usually rapid when the tick is removed.

20. What is the proper method for tick removal?

Extensive folklore and home remedies exist. Most are ineffective or dangerous to the victim and increase the risk of transmission of infectious agents to the person involved in the removal. The best method for removal is to use a gloved hand to grasp the tick as close to the head or mouth as possible with forceps and to pull upward with steady traction. If any tick parts remain embedded, complete removal is not necessary to prevent infection. Cleanse the area and treat it with topical antibiotics.

21. Describe the best methods for prevention of tick-borne disease.

The best methods of prevention are appropriate awareness and use of precautions while outdoors. Long-sleeved shirts should be worn, and pants should be tucked into socks or boots. Light clothing allows identification of crawling ticks. Twice-daily tick checks aid early removal and prevention of transmission of illness. DEET repellents applied to skin repel ticks but in toxic amounts may cause seizures in children. Permethrin that is made for clothing kills ticks only on contact but is not readily available. Using DEET repellents and permethrin in combination is most effective.

Awareness of the seasonality of ticks is useful. The nymph stage, which is responsible for 90% of illness transmission, occurs in May and early summer. Being more vigilant for these small ticks or avoiding tick-infested regions at this time is helpful. On a more global scale, knowing the animals necessary for completion of the tick life cycle is beneficial. The number of *I. scapularis* ticks is significantly lower in areas with no white-tailed deer. Control of the deer population and avoiding forested landscapes where deer reside can diminish the risk of contact with the infected ticks. Treating an area with insecticides during May for 2 consecutive years kills the nymph stage, significantly decreasing the tick population.

22. Summarize the treatment for each tick-borne illness.

Treatment of Tick-Borne Illnesses

	DRUG	ADULT DOSAGE
SPIROCHETES		
Lyme disease (*B. burgdorferi*)		
Acute phase		
Drug of choice:	Doxycycline*	100 mg PO b.i.d. 14–21 d
Alternate:	Amoxicillin	500 mg PO t.i.d. 14–21 d
	Cefuroxime axetil	500 mg PO b.i.d. 14–21 d
Acute disseminated		
Neurologic disease with meningits or radiculopathy	Ceftriaxone	2 g IV qd 2-4 wk
Alternate:	Penicillin G	18–24 million U daily divided q 4 h
	Cefotaxime	2 g IV q 8 h
	Doxycycline	200–400 mg/d PO or IV divided b.i.d. 2–4 wk
Carditis, mild (first- or second-degree atrioventricular block)	Same as acute phase	

(*Table continued on next page.*)

Treatment of Tick-Borne Illnesses (cont.)

	DRUG	ADULT DOSAGE
Carditis, severe (third-degreee atrioventricular block)	Same as neurologic disease	
Chronic/late phase		
Lyme arthritis (without neuologic disease)	Doxycycline[*]	100 mg PO b.i.d. 4 wk
	Amoxicillin	500 mg PO t.i.d. 4 wk
Joint swelling months after initial antibiotics	Repeat 4 wk PO antibiotic	
	Or ceftriaxone	2–4 wk
Joint swelling persistent after second course antibiotics: NSAIDs/intraarticular steroids		
Joint and nervous system symptoms *or*		
Neuroborreliosis	Ceftriaxone	2 g IV qd 2–4 wk
Alternate:	Penicillin	18–24 million U IV q 4 h
	Cefotaxime	2 g IV q 8 h
Relapsing fever (*Borrelia*)		
Drug of choice:	Doxycycline[*]	200 mg PO single dose
More severe disease:	Penicillin, erythromycin, or ceftriaxone	
RICKETTSIAE		
Rocky Mountain Spotted Fever (*R. rickettsii*)		
Drug of choice:	Doxycycline[*]	100 mg PO b.i.d. 1–7 d
Alternate:	Chloramphenicol[†]	
Q fever (*C. burnetii*)		
Drug of choice:	Doxycycline[*]	100 mg PO b.i.d. 14–21 d
Alternate:	Fluoroquinolone[‡]	
Q fever meningoencephalitis	Flouroquinolone	
Q fever endocarditis		
Drug of choice:	Doxycycline[*]	100 mg PO b.i.d.
	plus choloroquine	200 mg PO t.i.d. for at least 18 mo
	Or doxycyline	100 mg PO b.i.d.
	Plus ofloxacin	200 mg PO t.i.d. for at least 3 y
PROTOZOA		
Babesiosis (*Babesia microti*)		
Drug of choice:	Clindamycin	1.2 g IV b.i.d. or 600 mg PO t.i.d. for 7 d
Plus:	Quinine	650 mg PO t.i.d. for 7 d
BACTERIA		
Ehrlichiosis		
Drug of choice:	Doxycycline[*]	100 mg PO b.i.d. for at least 7 d or for 3–5 days after defervescence
Tularemia (*Francisella tularensis*)		
Drug of choice:	Streptomycin	30–40 mg/kg/d IM divided b.i.d. for 3 d, then give half this does PO for 4–11 d
	Gentamicin	1–1.5 mg/kg/dose IM for 7–14 d
Alternate:	Doxycycline[§]	
	Chloramphenicol[§]	
TOXIN		
Tick paralysis		
Drug of choice:	None	

(*Table continued on next page.*)

Treatment of Tick-Borne Illnesses (cont.)

DRUG	ADULT DOSAGE
VIRUS	
Colorado tick fever and arbovirus encephalitides	
Drug of choice:	None: supportive care

* Tetracyclines generally are not recommended for pregnant women or children younger than 8 years.

† This is the drug of choice in pregnant women and children younger than 8 years. The penicillins, cephalosporins, aminoglycosides, sulfonamides, and erythromycins are not effective against rickettsial infections.

‡ Ciprofloxacin or ofloxacin. Neither of these agents is recommended for children.

§ Doxycycline and chloramphenicol control the acute phase but their bacteriostatic nature prevents eradication, and relapses may occur.

BIBLIOGRAPHY

1. Bakken JS, Dumler JS: Clinical and laboratory characteristics of human granulocytic ehrlichiosis (HGE). JAMA 275:199–205, 1996.
2. Centers for Disease Control: Babesiosis—Connecticut. MMWR Morb Mortal Wkly Rep 38:649–650, 1989.
3. Centers for Disease Control: Human ehrlichiosis—Maryland, 1994. JAMA 276:1212–1213, 1996.
4. Centers for Disease Control: Outbreak of Powassan encephalitis—Maine and Vermont, 1999–2001 MMWR Morb Mortal Wkly Rep 50:761–764, 2001.
5. Centers for Disease Control: Outbreak of relapsing fever—Grand Canyon National Park, Arizona, 1990. MMWR Morb Mortal Wkly Rep 40:296–297, 1991.
6. Edlow JA: Lyme disease and related tick-borne illnesses. Ann Emerg Med 33:680–693, 1999.
7. Goodpasture HC, Poland JD, Francy DB, et al: Colorado tick fever: Clinical, epidemiologic and laboratory aspects of 228 cases in Colorado in 1973–1974. Ann Intern Med 88:303–310, 1978.
8. Kamper CA, Chessman KH, Phelps SJ: Therapy reviews: Rocky Mountain spotted fever. Clin Pharmacol 7:109–116, 1988.
9. Maurin M, Raoult D: Q fever. Clin Micr Rev 12:518–553, 1999.
10. Nadelman RB, Nowakowski J, Fish D, et al: Prophylaxis with single-dose doxycycline for the prevention of Lyme disease after an *Ixodes scapularis* tick bite. N Engl J Med 345:79–84, 2001.
11. Orloski KA, Hayes EB, Campbell GL, Dennis DT: Surveillance for Lyme disease—United States, 1992–1998. MMWR Morb Mortal Wkly Rep 49:1–11, 2001.
12. Parola P, Raoult D: Ticks and tickborne bacterial diseases in humans: An emerging infectious threat. Clin Infect Dis 32:897–928, 2001.
13. Steere AC: Lyme disease. N Engl J Med 345:115–125, 2001.
14. Wormser GP, Nadelman RB, Dattwyler RJ, et al: Practice guidelines for the treatment of Lyme disease. Clin Infect Dis 31(suppl 1):S1–14, 2000.

62. ARTHRITIS

Catherine B. Custalow, M.D., Ph.D.

1. What is arthritis, and what are the signs and symptoms?

Arthritis is the inflammation of a joint, which may be characterized as monarticular (involving a single joint) or polyarticular (involving multiple joints). Patients typically report pain, swelling, redness, and limitation of motion about the involved joint. On examination, there may be tenderness, swelling, effusion, erythema, and painful decreased range of motion. Children may present with a limp or may avoid using an extremity.

2. List the common causes of acute arthritis.

Infection (bacterial, granulomatous, fungal, or viral)

Trauma (fracture, overuse)

Hemorrhage (traumatic hemarthrosis, inherited coagulopathy, or anticoagulant-induced)
Crystal deposition disease (gout or pseudogout)
Neoplasm (metastasis)
Inflammatory conditions (rheumatoid arthritis, rheumatic fever, lupus)
Degenerative conditions (osteoarthritis)

3. How do I differentiate between an intraarticular and a periarticular inflammation?

True **intraarticular** processes typically cause generalized joint pain, joint effusion, tenderness, warmth, swelling, and an increase in pain with active and passive range of motion. **Periarticular** processes, such as bursitis, tendinitis, or cellulitis, tend to have more localized areas of tenderness; there is no joint effusion or swelling; and the pain may not be reproduced by range of motion in certain directions.

4. What other physical findings may be helpful in a patient with arthritis?

A thorough physical examination may provide clinical clues to certain rheumatologic diseases, such as the finding of Heberden's nodes in osteoarthritis, skin lesions in psoriatic arthritis, urethral or cervical discharge in gonococcal arthritis, conjunctivitis in Reiter's syndrome, tophi in gout, and erythema chronicum migrans in Lyme disease.

5. Are radiographs helpful in the diagnosis of arthritis?

Often the only radiographic evidence of inflammation is soft tissue swelling; however, plain radiographs may reveal foreign bodies, calcifications, fractures, effusions, osteoporosis, or osteomyelitis. The radiographic changes of degenerative arthritis include asymmetric joint space narrowing, marginal osteophytes, ligamentous calcifications, and subchondral sclerosis. In advanced gout, there may be *punched-out* subchondral and marginal erosions, joint space narrowing, and periarticular calcified tophi.

6. What is the most important diagnostic test for determining the cause of acute arthritis?

Arthrocentesis. Synovial fluid analysis provides rapid, crucial diagnostic information and should be done on all patients with an acute joint effusion who have no contraindications. The procedure is simple and safe, and complications are rare when done under sterile conditions and with proper technique. The procedure may be therapeutic for a patient with an acutely swollen, painful joint. The fluid should be analyzed for cell count, differential, Gram stain, culture, and crystal analysis. Contraindications to arthrocentesis are overlying cellulitis and severe coagulopathy. If infection is suspected in a prosthetic joint, it is recommended that joint aspiration be done by an orthopedist.

7. Is the erythrocyte sedimentation rate (ESR) useful for the evaluation of acute arthritis?

No. The ESR has been used over the years to indicate the body's acute-phase response to inflammation and infection. A normal or elevated ESR is neither sensitive nor specific enough to confirm or rule out any particular disease. Septic arthritis cannot be excluded based on a normal ESR because false-negative rates may be 20% to 30%. When clinical suspicion is high, a joint should be aspirated regardless of the ESR.

8. Besides synovial fluid analysis, are there any other laboratory tests that are useful in the evaluation of arthritis?

The peripheral white blood cell count (WBC) is of limited value in diagnosing the cause of acute arthritis in the ED. Only 50% of patients with nongonococcal bacterial arthritis have an elevated WBC count. Blood cultures are positive in only 5% of patients with nongonococcal bacterial arthritis and only 20% of patients with gonococcal arthritis. In suspected disseminated gonococcal infection, cultures from the urethra and cervix should be obtained because the organism is recovered in less than 50% of purulent joints caused by disseminated gonococcal infection and is isolated more frequently from genital sources.

9. How do I interpret the results of the arthrocentesis?

Normal findings and those of various rheumatic disease states are shown in the Table. There is significant overlap among the various conditions, and many patients with septic arthritis have WBC counts less than 50,000/μL. Gram stain is also crucial for the evaluation of synovial fluid and may be positive in 75% of nongonococcal septic arthritis and 25% of gonococcal arthritis cases. Polarized light microscopy is helpful to identify crystals.

Synovial Fluid Analysis

DIAGNOSIS	APPEARANCE	TOTAL WBC COUNT (per mm³)	PMN (%)	MUCIN CLOT TEST	FLUID/BLOOD GLUCOSE (DIFF.) (mm/dL)	MISCELLANEOUS (CRYSTALS/ ORGANISMS)
Normal	Clear, pale	0–200 (200)	< 10	Good	NS	—
Group I (noninflammatory; degenerative joint disease, traumatic arthritis)	Clear to slightly turbid	50–4000 (600)	< 30	Good	NS	—
Group II (noninfectious, mildly inflammatory; SLE scleroderma)	Clear to slightly turbid	0–9000 (3000)	< 20	Good (occ. fair)	NS	Occ. LE cell, decreased complement
Group III (noninfectious, severely inflammatory)						
Gout	Turbid	100–160,000 (21,000)	70	Poor	10	Uric acid crystals
Pseudogout	Turbid	50–75,000 (14,000)	70	Fair-poor	Insuff. data	Calcium pyro-phosphate
Rheumatoid arthritis	Turbid	250–80,000	70	Poor	30	Decreased
Group IV (infectious, inflammatory)						
Acute bacterial	Very turbid	150–250,000 (80,000)	90	Poor	90	Positive cul-ture for bacteria
Tuberculosis	Turbid	2,500–100,000 (20,000)	60	Poor	70	Positive cul-ture for *M. tuberculosis*

PMN, polymorphonuclear cells; NS, not significant; SLE, systemic lupus erythematosus; LE, lupus erythematosus. (From Wyngaarden JB, Smith LH [eds]: Cecil Textbook of Medicine, 18th ed. Philadelphia, W.B. Saunders, 1988, p 1994, with permission.)

10. Discuss the most serious cause of arthritis.

Acute infectious arthritis is the most critical cause of acute monarticular arthritis. It can be due to bacteria, mycobacteria, fungi, and viruses, although a bacterial cause is the most common and the most serious. These infections carry a risk of permanent joint damage that may occur in 7 days and result in chronic disability. In children, septic arthritis can cause epiphyseal damage, resulting in growth impairment and limb-length discrepancy. Untreated septic arthritis carries a risk of sepsis and death.

11. How is acute bacterial arthritis diagnosed and treated?

It is diagnosed in most cases by a synovial fluid count with typical synovial fluid counts greater than 50,000 WBC/mm³, predominantly polymorphonuclear neutrophilic white blood cells, and a Gram stain positive for bacteria. Treatment is admission to the hospital; administration of intravenous antibiotics; and immediate orthopedic consultation for arthroscopic joint drainage, open joint drainage, or daily joint aspirations.

12. What is the difference between gout and pseudogout?

Gout develops when sodium urate crystals precipitate in a joint and initiate an inflammatory reaction. **Pseudogout** is caused by the deposition of calcium pyrophosphate crystals. When viewed with polarized light microscopy, gout crystals appear needle-shaped and negatively birefringent, whereas pseudogout crystals appear rhomboid in shape and positively birefringent.

13. Which joint most commonly is affected in gout?

The metatarsophalangeal joint of the great toe (75%). This type of gout is known as *podagra*. Other commonly involved joints are the tarsal joints, the ankle, and the knee. Gout is polyarticular in 40% of patients.

14. What are the treatment options for gout?

Nonsteroidal antiinflammatory drugs (NSAIDs), particularly indomethacin, are the primary agents used to treat gout. A newer, expensive class of drugs, the cyclooxygenase-2 (COX-2) inhibitors, act by inhibiting prostaglandin synthesis through inhibition of COX-2. Although COX-2 inhibitors, similar to nonselective NSAIDs, are contraindicated in advanced renal disease, they seem to be associated with less gastrointestinal ulceration. Colchicine is effective in treating acute attacks. It may be administered orally, 0.5 to 0.6 mg every hour until symptoms improve, until diarrhea or vomiting develops, or until the maximum dose of 4 mg has been reached. A single intravenous dose of 1 to 2 mg of colchicine administered over 10 minutes also may be effective. Corticosteroids may be administered orally, intravenously, or by intraarticular injection but only after bacterial infection has been ruled out. Drugs that decrease serum uric acid levels either by decreasing production (allopurinol) or by increasing excretion (probenecid) should not be given in the acute phase because they can exacerbate the condition. In patients with hyperuricemia and frequent exacerbations of gouty arthritis, the primary care physician may wish to prescribe these medications, but only after the gouty attack has subsided.

15. Which tick-borne infection causes arthritis?

Lyme disease, a tick-borne illness caused by the spirochete *Borrelia burgdorferi*, is known to cause arthritis in 60% of untreated patients. In certain endemic areas (> 15 states in the United States), the history of a tick bite and the characteristic annular rash of erythema chronicum migrans and constitutional symptoms are highly suggestive of Lyme disease. The arthritis is usually a manifestation of late disseminated disease. Although this arthritis usually responds to a course of doxycycline or amoxicillin, some patients develop chronic joint inflammation that does not respond to antibiotics.

BIBLIOGRAPHY

1. Goldenberg DL, Reed JI: Bacterial arthritis. N Engl J Med 312:764–771, 1985.
2. Heffner AC, Colluciello SA: Monoarticular arthritis. In Harwood-Nuss AL, Wolfson AB (eds): The Clinical Practice of Emergency Medicine, 3rd ed. Philadelphia, Lippincott Williams & Wilkins, 2001, pp 1063–1071.
3. Olshaker JS, Jerrard DA: The erythrocyte sedimentation rate. J Emerg Med 15:869–874, 1997.
4. Schwartz DT, Reisdorff EJ: Fundamentals of skeletal radiology. In Schwartz DT, Reisdorff EJ (eds): Emergency Radiology. New York, McGraw-Hill, 2000, pp 22–24.
5. Shell D, Perkins R, Cosgarea A: Septic olecranon bursitis: Recognition and treatment. J Am Board Fam Pract 8:217–220, 1995.

6. Steere AC: Lyme disease. N Engl J Med 345:115–125, 2001.
7. Talbot-Stern JK: Arthritis, tendinitis, and bursitis. In Rosen P, Barkin RM (eds): Emergency Medicine: Concepts and Clinical Practice, 4th ed. St. Louis, Mosby, 1998, pp 2729–2747.
8. Zink BJ: Bone and joint infections. In Rosen P, Barkin RM (eds): Emergency Medicine: Concepts and Clinical Practice, 4th ed. St. Louis, Mosby, 1998, pp 2662–2669.

63. SKIN DISEASES

Lela A. Lee, M.D., and Joanna M. Burch, M.D.

1. How are skin lesions best described?

It is helpful to remember dermatologic terms (see Table). Describing in plain terms how the lesions appear is acceptable, however. If you do not remember that a macule is a flat lesion and papules and plaques are raised, you may describe the lesions as either flat or raised. Communication with other care providers may be improved by the use of plain but accurately descriptive terms.

PRIMARY SKIN LESION	DESCRIPTION	EXAMPLE
Macule	Flat, circumscribed color change (nonpalpable) < 1 cm	Café-au-lait spot
Patch	Flat color change > 1 cm	Vitiligo
Papule	Raised lesion < 1 cm	Molluscum contagiosum
Plaque	Elevated, flat-topped lesion > 1 cm. Lesions with epidermal changes (e.g., scale) would be considered plaques	Psoriasis
Nodule	Raised lesion with a deeper palpable portion	Erythema nodosum
Vesicle	Raised, usually dome-shaped lesion filled with fluid and < 1 cm	Varicella
Bulla	Fluid-filled lesion > 1 cm	Bullous pemphigoid
Pustule	Raised lesion filled with exudative fluid, giving it a yellow appearance	Folliculitis
Cyst	Nodule filled with semisolid-to-solid material	Epidermoid cyst
Wheal	Flat-topped, firm, raised, edematous lesion; a hive	Urticaria

Characteristics helpful in establishing a diagnosis include the following:
Location and distribution
Color
Size
Presence of absence of scale
Contour change (e.g., raised, depressed, pitted)
Tactile characteristics (e.g., firm, spongy, fluctuant, blanchable or nonblanchable)
Apparent depth (e.g., superficial, dermal, subcutaneous)

2. Is photography useful?

Photography of lesions may be the most effective way to convey their appearance. The tactile characteristics are lost with photography, but most other relevant characteristics are retained.

3. What categories of skin conditions are life-threatening or associated with life-threatening disease?

Skin diseases resulting in extensive compromise to the cutaneous barrier

Skin signs of systemic infection

Skin cancers

Urticaria or angioedema with airway compromise

Skin signs of vascular compromise (including hemorrhage, emboli, thrombi, and vasculitis)

Skin findings of an introduced toxin (e.g., venomous snake bite)

Skin signs of physical abuse

4. List some cutaneous *red flags* (i.e., skin signs indicating an increased likelihood of disease requiring emergency attention).

- Extensive blisters or denuded areas of skin
- Acute total-body erythema, particularly in the elderly or frail
- Extensive erythematous eruption in a person who is febrile and systemically ill
- Petechiae, purpura, and ecchymoses
- Necrosis
- Urticaria
- Isolated, abnormal-appearing mole

5. What types of skin diseases result in potentially life-threatening compromise to the skin barrier?

Most of these are blistering diseases. When the blister breaks, the barrier is removed, and the individual is at risk for infection, fluid and electrolyte imbalance, and difficulties with heat regulation. Skin conditions that can be associated with an extensively compromised barrier include toxic epidermal necrolysis, Stevens-Johnson syndrome (also called *erythema multiforme major*), pemphigus and pemphigus-like chronic blistering diseases, and burns. Patients with erythroderma (total or near-total body erythema) also may have problems with infection, fluid and electrolyte balance, and heat regulation, particularly patients who have significant chronic health problems, such as congestive heart failure. Lesions of the oral cavity may compromise life if they are severe enough to prevent food or fluid intake.

6. Describe the skin findings in meningococcemia, Rocky Mountain spotted fever, toxic shock syndrome, and necrotizing fasciitis.

In **meningococcemia**, lesions may be irregularly shaped petechiae or purpura with dusky centers, located most commonly on the trunk and extremities. The lesions may involve the palms and soles.

In **Rocky Mountain spotted fever**, skin lesions appear at about day 4 of the acute febrile illness. Lesions begin on distal extremities, may involve palms and soles, and spread centripetally. After a few days, the lesions become petechial or purpuric. In practice, this eruption may be difficult to distinguish from that of meningococcemia.

Patients with **toxic shock syndrome** may have a scarlatiniform eruption, edema of the face and extremities, conjunctival erythema, and erythema of the oral or genital mucosa. There is desquamation of the hands and feet 1 to 2 weeks later.

Necrotizing fasciitis is characterized by a rapidly progressive erythema with development of duskiness and frank necrosis. There may be blisters. The overlying skin change is often mild compared with the necrosis occurring underneath.

7. Describe the skin findings of common or distinctive childhood exanthems.

Scarlet fever occurs in children between the ages of 2 and 10 years. Red macules and papules start on the neck and usually spread to the trunk and extremities. The skin may have a rough *sandpaper* feel on palpation and sometimes can be petechial. Erythema is usually most intense in the axillae, groin, and abdomen. Patients may exhibit Pastia's lines, which are petechiae in a linear pattern along the major skin folds. Palms and soles characteristically are spared. The face appears flushed with a circumoral pallor. Desquamation usually occurs as the eruption resolves in 1 to 3 weeks.

Staphylococcal scalded skin syndrome begins as faint erythema on the face, neck, axilla, and groin in a child younger than 5 years old, usually following upper respiratory symptoms. The skin is tender, and crusting may occur around the mouth, eyes, and neck. The skin separates through the epidermis with even slight rubbing, leaving a red, moist surface underneath (Nikolsky's sign). Mucous membranes are not involved. In neonates, the entire body is involved, whereas in infants and children the upper body is affected preferentially.

Varicella presents with abrupt onset of crops of faint macules that progress through several stages. The macules become edematous papules, then vesicles over 24 to 48 hours. Often there is a small vesicle on a larger erythematous macule, described as a "dew drop on a rose petal." The vesicles develop moist crusts and leave shallow erosions. Lesions tend to begin centrally and spread to the extremities. The palms, soles, and mucous membranes frequently are involved. Characteristically, lesions in multiple stages of development (macules, papules, vesicles, crusts, erosions) are present in the same patient. The number of lesions ranges from 10 to 1,500 (average 300). The lesions are usually pruritic. They do not scar. Scars from varicella are the result of patient scratching.

Erythema infectiosum (fifth disease) is a parvovirus B19 infection that results in intense erythema on the bilateral cheeks ("slapped cheeks"). After the facial erythema, a pink-to-red macular eruption develops with a reticular or *lacy* appearance. Although most children have the facial eruption with the slapped cheeks appearance, a few exhibit only the pink, lacy eruption on the body. The macular eruption tends to *reappear* with stimulation of cutaneous vasodilation, such as warm baths, exercise, or sun exposure. This can last for 4 months. Some patients develop a petechial eruption of the distal hands and feet with parvovirus B19 infection. This is the "purpuric gloves and socks syndrome."

Roseola (exanthem subitum) is a disease of infants and toddlers caused by infection with human herpesvirus 6. After 2 to 3 days of sustained fever, abrupt defervescence is followed by a pink maculopapular eruption. Periorbital edema sometimes is seen.

Hand-foot-and-mouth disease exhibits an abrupt onset of a few scattered papules that progress to oval or linear vesicles with an erythematous rim. As the name suggests, most lesions occur on the oral mucosa, palms, and soles. The oral lesions appear as small, discrete, whitish gray erosions. Coxsackieviruses cause this eruption.

Kawasaki disease is typified by an irritable child with conjunctival injection and slightly swollen, distinctly red lips. The hands may be edematous or desquamating. The skin findings ar nonspecific and variable, ranging from macules, maculopapules, to vesicles. The child must meet the clinical criteria of fever for 5 or more days plus four of five of the following: (1) nonpurulent conjunctivitis, (2) mucosal changes, (3) edema or desquamation of the distal extremities, (4) exanthem, and (5) cervical lymphadenopathy.

8. What is erythema multiforme (EM)?

A reaction pattern in the skin, characterized histologically by necrosis or apoptosis of individual keratinocytes. The lesions may not appear grossly necrotic, but the characteristic lesion has a dusky center with an erythematous periphery, the so-called target lesion. It is typical for most lesions of EM to be erythematous, whereas only a few lesions are truly target-like.

There are two major forms: EM minor and EM major (Stevens-Johnson syndrome). **EM minor** frequently follows herpes simplex infection. Mucous membranes usually are spared or affected mildly. Lesions are found on the dorsal hands and extensor extremities, and palms and soles frequently are involved. Although there may be some systemic symptoms, EM minor is not usually debilitating and generally is managed on an outpatient basis. EM minor may recur after subsequent episodes of herpes simplex. Antiviral therapy is useful only as suppressive therapy to prevent herpes simplex recurrences.

EM major is a serious, potentially life-threatening disease with prominent mucous membrane involvement. EM major usually is caused by a drug, in particular, sulfonamides, anticonvulsants, allopurinol, and certain nonsteroidal antiinflammatory drugs. Some authorities believe that EM major and toxic epidermal necrolysis are so similar in appearance and cause that they are, in essence, the same disease.

9. Which disease is most often mistaken for EM minor?

Acute urticaria. Urticarial lesions may be annular with concentric color changes and may occur on the palms and soles. Usually, urticarial lesions have a pale edematous center with an erythematous border, whereas EM lesions tend to have dusky centers. Lesions in urticaria are transient (< 24 hours), whereas the target-like lesions of EM are fixed and can be present 1 week or more. Urticarial lesions clear with subcutaneous epinephrine, whereas EM lesions do not.

10. Which skin cancers require urgent attention?

In general, **melanoma** requires the most urgent diagnosis and treatment. Surgical removal of melanoma before it has metastasized can be life-saving.

11. How do I recognize a melanoma?

Some characteristics that help identify lesions at higher risk to be melanoma are irregularity of pigmentation; irregular shape of the border; and presence of red, white, or blue-black color. An underemphasized finding that can be extremely helpful is a difference in appearance between the lesion in question and the patient's other moles. A brown macule on a fair-skinned person should be viewed with suspicion if the person does not have other similarly pigmented lesions, even if the brown macule is regularly pigmented, small, and perfectly round. A history of change in a mole is a risk factor, as is personal or family history of melanoma.

12. Which spider bites can cause a necrotic reaction?

Only a few species of spiders in North America produce bites that lead potentially to skin necrosis. Of these, bites of the brown recluse (*Loxosceles reclusa*) and the hobo spider (*Tegenaria agrestis*) are important because they may be fatal. The range of the brown recluse is limited, with the center of the endemic area being around eastern Arkansas, western Tennessee, and southern Missouri and the radius being several hundred miles in every direction. Outside the endemic area, brown recluse bites are uncommon, although they may occur because the spider may be transported on clothing or in boxes. The range of the hobo spider is the Northwest United States and western Canada. Other *Loxosceles* species may cause necrotic reactions, and many of these spiders live in the deserts of the Southwest United States. If one is outside an endemic area, the diagnosis of necrotic reaction to spider bite should be made with caution.

13. What skin lesions may be confused with a necrotic reaction to a spider bite?

Necrotizing fasciitis, ecthyma, pyoderma gangrenosum, vasculitis, and clotting disorders. Erythematous reactions to stings or bites, such as beestings or tick bites, occasionally may be confused with early reactions to spider bites.

14. Describe common benign skin conditions that mimic melanoma.

Seborrheic keratoses are extremely common benign lesions that usually first appear in middle age. They are growths of keratinocytes rather than pigment cells, but the keratinocytes may take up pigment and look alarmingly dark or irregularly pigmented. The scaling produced by the seborrheic keratosis may be so compact that it is difficult to discern, but detection of this rough scaling helps considerably in distinguishing this lesion from melanoma.

Venous lakes are vascular growths that often appear on the helix of the ears and on the lips of older persons with sun damage. The purple color may mimic that of a melanoma. Pressing firmly on the lesion drains much of the blood from the lesion and reveals it as a vascular growth.

15. Describe common benign skin conditions that mimic purpura resulting from systemic disease.

Solar purpura is common on the forearms and backs of hands of persons who have crhonic sun damage. Large areas of purpura may be evident and may have occurred with minimal, sometimes unnoticeable trauma. Solar purpura is restricted to chronically sun-damaged skin and is particularly common in patients on long-term systemic steroid therapy.

Schamberg's purpura is a benign condition characterized by petechiae primarily on the lower legs. The lesions tend to be pinpoint, nonpalpable, and extremely numerous. By contrast, purpuric lesions of leukocytoclastic (*hypersensitivity*) vasculitis tend to be slightly larger in diameter (often 2 to 4 mm), and frequently some of the lesions are palpable. (Although leukocytoclastic vasculitis sometimes is referred to as *palpable purpura*, it is common to find that most lesions are flat and only a few are palpable.)

16. Describe common skin conditions that mimic cellulitis.

A **kerion** caused by fungal infection in the scalp (tinea capitis) may be so intensely inflamed that it is mistaken for cellulitis. Because a kerion may produce permanent, scarring alopecia, it is important to recognize and institute therapy early. Kerions occur almost exclusively in children.

Stasis dermatitis sometimes may be confused with cellulitis. Stasis dermatitis is usually bilateral, whereas leg cellulitis is more often unilateral. Stasis dermatitis is characterized by scaling and mild-to-moderate erythema. If the erythema is fiery red, the redness is rapidly progressive, the patient is systemically ill, or there is a leukocytosis, cellulitis may be the presumptive diagnosis.

Allergic contact dermatitis, such as poison ivy dermatitis, may result in lesions that are intensely inflamed. The distribution of the lesions often suggests an exogenous cause. In plant dermatitis, linear erythema, often with blisters, is an indicator of where the plant has brushed against the skin. Antibiotic creams containing neomycin are another relatively common cause of allergic contact dermatitis. Because antibiotic creams often are used on wounds, it is easy to understand how allergic contact dermatitis caused by the cream may be mistaken for a potentially serious wound infection.

17. In which disease associated with leg ulceration is débridement generally contraindicated?

Pyoderma gangrenosum.

18. When should patients with dermatitis (eczema) be given systemic steroids?

Systemic steroids generally should not be given to patients with chronic dermatitis. Systemic steroids, although inexpensive and easy to use, do not correct what is often the underlying problem, that of a faulty skin barrier. This is especially the case when the skin is dry. Patients taking systemic steroids also may exhibit a rebound of disease when the steroids are tapered. Patients with acute dermatitis that is expected to be self-limited may be given systemic steroids if the severity of disease merits and there are no contraindications. An example is severe poison ivy dermatitis.

19. What are the divisions of the classes of topical corticosteroids, and on which areas of the skin are they appropriately applied?

Low-potency topical corticosteroids (class 6 or 7 topical steroids, such as 1% and 2.5% hydrocortisone, 0.05% desonide) are appropriate to use on the face, axillae, groin, breasts, and genitalia, where the skin is thinner and more prone to cutaneous side effects.

Moderate-potency topical corticosteroids (class 4 or 5 topical steroids, such as 0.025% fluocinolone, 0.1% triamcinolone, 0.2% hydrocortisone valerate) are useful on the neck and body, avoiding the more sensitive areas mentioned previously. This class is given most appropriately as first-line therapy for skin conditions diagnosed in the ED.

High-potency topical corticosteroids (class 2 or 3 topical steroids, such as 0.05% fluocinonide, 0.1% halcinonide, 0.25% desoxymethasone) should not be applied to the face, breasts, genitalia, axillae, or groin. Topicals in this class are more likely to produce side effects if used diffusely or for long periods (> 2 weeks). This class should be prescribed only if moderate-potency topical corticosteroids have not been effective or if the condition is limited to the particularly thick skin of the palms and soles.

Superpotency topical corticosteroids (class 1 topical steroids, such as 0.05% elobetasol, 0.05% betamethasone diproprionate in optimized vehicle, 0.05% halobetasol, 0.05% diflorasone) usually are reserved for chronic, recalcitrant conditions, often of the palms and soles. The risk of side effects is greatest with this class, and this class of steroid should be dispensed in a continuity-of-care, rather than an ED setting.

20. Does the vehicle of the topical corticosteroid affect potency?
Yes. The same corticosteroid may be significantly more or less potent, depending on the vehicle. For example, 0.1% mometasone cream is classified as medium potency, class 4, whereas 0.1% mometasone ointment is high potency, class 2. In general, ointments are most potent, followed by gels, emollients, creams, lotions, solutions, and sprays.

BIBLIOGRAPHY

1. Gable EK, Liu G, Morell DS: Pediatric exanthems. Prim Care 27:353–369, 2002.
2. Goldsmith LA, Lazarus GS, Tharp MD: Adult and Pediatric Dermatology: A Color Guide to Diagnosis and Treatment. Philadelphia, F.A. Davis, 1997.
3. Jain AM: Emergency department evaluation of child abuse. Emerg Med Clin North Am 17:575–593, 1999.
4. Pressel DM: Evaluation of physical abuse in children. Am Fam Physician 61:3057–3064, 2000.
5. Roujeau JC, Kelly JP, Naldi L, et al: Medication use and the risk of Stevens-Johnson syndrome or toxic epidermal necrolysis. N Engl J Med 333:1600–1607, 1995.
6. Sams HH, Dunnick CA, Smith ML, King LE Jr: Necrotic arachnidism. J Am Acad Dermatol 44:561–573, 2001.
7. Weston WL, Lane AT, Morelli JG: Color Textbook of Pediatric Dermatology. St. Louis, Mosby, 1996.
8. Zuberbier T, Greaves MW, Juhlin L, et al: Management of urticaria: A consensus report. J Invest Dermatol Symp Proc 6:128–131, 2001.

64. TROPICAL AND TRAVEL MEDICINE

Alexander Brough, M.D., and Gayle Galleta, M.D.

1. Why should I read this chapter? I don't travel overseas.
While many so-called tropical diseases are uncommon in North America, they are quite prevalent in other continents. Patients seen in an American ED recently may have been in a foreign country. Changing disease patterns abroad have a direct impact on the health of travelers and immigrants. Although tropical diseases may sound exotic, they are diagnosed in North America and often are evaluated first in the ED.

2. What is a tropical disease?
An illness acquired in the tropics. The field of tropical and travel medicine encompasses tropical and nontropical illness, however. Malaria, although considered to be a tropical disease, has a worldwide distribution that is far greater than the tropical regions. Some pathogens are domestic, such as Hantavirus, found mostly in the southwestern United States.

3. What is the most important diagnostic tool in evaluating a tropical disease?
Obtaining a **travel history**. Travel outside of the United States, or even to certain rural areas of the United States, should make one suspicious for an atypical illness, such as a tropical disease. Further history items that are helpful if one is considering a tropical pathogen are a vaccination history, the use of malaria prophylactic medications, and rural versus urban travel.

4. Will I ever see malaria?

Quite possibly. A total of 1,540 cases of malaria were reported from 47 states to the Centers for Disease Control (CDC) in 1999. Most infections were acquired overseas. The affected patients were mostly civilians on business and vacation travel. Three cases were due to acquisition within the United States. As recently as the mid-20th century, malaria was endemic to most of the United States.

5. What causes malaria?

There are four species of the protozoan *Plasmodium*: *P. falciparum*, *P. vivax*, *P. ovale*, and *P. malariae*. It usually is spread by the bite of an infected female *Anopheles* species mosquito, but it also may be spread by exposure to infected blood and via congenital transmission. *P. falciparum* causes the most severe and life-threatening form of infection. Failure to use or poor compliance with a prophylactic medication has been associated with most cases of traveler's acquired malaria seen in the United States.

6. Describe the clinical presentation of malaria.

The incubation period varies depending on the involved species. Symptoms develop after 10 to 14 days with *P. falciparum* and may be latent for 1 year with *P. vivax*. Patients present with fever, chills, headache, nausea, vomiting, abdominal pain, cough, and myalgias. The symptoms are often vague and easily attributable to common domestic ailments. Physical examination may reveal jaundice, hepatomegaly, and splenomegaly. Anemia and thrombocytopenia are common laboratories findings. Severe malaria is a true emergency. Patients may develop altered mental status, pulmonary edema, shock, disseminated intravascular coagulation, profound anemia, acidosis, and hypoglycemia. A diagnosis is made with light microscopy visualization of protozoa on blood smears. Antigen assay kits also are available. If malaria is suspected, prompt treatment should be initiated and admission considered. Because blood smears are often negative, they should be repeated every 12 hours on at least three occasions until a diagnosis can be made. Mainstays of treatment include chloroquine, mefloquine, and doxycycline, although multiple agents are available.

7. What is leptospirosis?

Leptospirosis gained national attention after an outbreak among several triathlon participants in Springfield, Illinois. Leptospirosis is caused by the spirochete *Leptospira interrogans*, which has several mammalian hosts, including cattle, dogs, and humans. It is transmitted through dermal abrasion and mucosal surfaces that have been in contact with water previously contaminated with spirochetes, discharged in infected mammalian urine. Leptospirosis is endemic to Central and South America.

8. Describe the clinical course of leptospirosis.

After an incubation period of 4 to 20 days, the initial phase develops with symptoms of sudden fever, chills, headache, and myalgias, especially of the lower extremities. Signs include lymphadenopathy, petechiae, and hepatosplenomegaly. After a period of ostensible resolution, a second phase manifests with fever, myalgias, and meningeal irritation. Laboratory evaluation reveals an aseptic meningitis. The diagnosis is made with a microscopic agglutination test or a serologic enzyme-linked immunosorbent assay (ELISA). Several antibiotics are effective in treating leptospirosis, including doxycycline, penicillin, ampicillin, and third-generation cephalosporins.

9. What is dengue fever and dengue hemorrhagic fever (DHF)?

Dengue fever and DHF are caused by any of four different types of dengue viruses of the flavivirus family. It is spread by the bite of an infected *Aedes aegypti* mosquito. The symptoms occur after a 4- to 7-day incubation period and last about 1 week. Initial symptoms characteristic of dengue fever include an acute fever, retro-orbital headache, nausea, vomiting, a maculopapular rash, severe myalgias, and arthralgias. With resolution of symptoms comes immunity to the offending virus serotype. However, it is possible to acquire an infection from another serotype. Dengue is endemic to tropical regions of Asia, Oceania, Central, and South America.

DHF is a more severe syndrome that is often fatal; it is characterized by dermal and mucosal hemorrhage and pleural and peritoneal effusions. DHF can develop into a severe syndrome known as **dengue shock syndrome**, in which massive amounts of intravascular fluid are lost over a short period. The mechanism of disease for DHF is not clear. It represents either an enhanced immune response to the dengue virus or perhaps a second infection from another viral serotype.

10. How do I diagnose and treat dengue fever?

The diagnosis can be confirmed with ELISA serology. Treatment consists of supportive care. Patients with DHF require intensive care.

11. What is West Nile viral encephalitis?

The West Nile virus is a flavivirus that is acquired through a mosquito vector. Previously endemic to Europe and Asia, it first was seen in an outbreak in New York City in 1999 and since has been reported in several states. The first series of infections initially were thought to be the result of an endemic viral infection, such as St. Louis encephalitis, but later were determined to be an infection imported from overseas. Infections are mostly asymptomatic. Symptomatic infection with the West Nile virus occurs after 3 to 15 days. Initial symptoms include fever, headache, weakness, nausea, vomiting, diarrhea, and a stiff neck. The physical examination shows hyporeflexia, decreased strength, and paralysis. Diagnosis is made with antibody assays, such as ELISA. Treatment consists of supportive care.

12. What is South American hemorrhagic fever (SAHF)?

SAHF is a type of viral hemorrhagic fever and refers to an illness caused by several viruses of the Arenaviridae family. Several offending viruses present with similar symptoms and are spread by the same mechanism of inhalation of viral particles aerosolized from rodent excrement. The geographic distribution of SAHF is South and Central America. The incubation period is 6 to 16 days. The syndrome consists of a sudden onset of fever, chills, dizziness, headache, nausea, vomiting, myalgias, and arthralgias. Later findings include altered mental status, hyporeflexia, and ataxia. The hemorrhagic component starts with facial flushing, conjunctival injection, and petechiae; then pulmonary edema; and finally shock. Thrombocytopenia, leukopenia, and proteinuria are found on laboratory evaluation. A definitive diagnosis is made with an ELISA. Treatment involves early intervention to maintain intravascular volume. Ribovarin has shown promise as an intervention. Mortality is 30% if untreated.

13. What is hantavirus?

A member of the Bunyaviridae family that is endemic to North America, but most cases originate in the Southwest United States. An infection with the hantavirus is contracted by inhaling viral particles aerosolized from rodent excrement. The incubation period is 7 to 28 days. The syndrome of infection with hantavirus is the hantavirus pulmonary syndrome.

14. Describe the clinical course of hantavirus pulmonary syndrome.

The initial phase consists of fever, headache, nausea, vomiting, diarrhea, and myalgias lasting 3 to 5 days. Increasing shortness of breath and cough due to pulmonary edema heralds the second, cardiopulmonary phase. The oxygen saturation is low, and later shock ensues. Laboratory findings include leukocytosis, thrombocytopenia, hemoconcentration, elevated lactate dehydrogenase, and increased partial thromboplastin time. The second phase lasts 24 to 48 hours. Clinical improvement is noted with diuresis. Diagnosis is made with ELISA and Western blot tests. Intensive care support is essential. The use of ribavirin is under investigation as an intervention.

15. Where can I go for help?

The Centers for Disease Control (CDC) and the World Health Organization (WHO) have informative websites: www.cdc.gov and www.who.int/home-page. The CDC has a traveler hotline: (877) 394-8747.

BIBLIOGRAPHY

1. Centers for Disease Control: Update: Leptospirosis and unexplained acute febrile illness among athletes participating in triathlons—Illinois and Wisconsin, 1998. MMWR Morb Mortal Wkly Rep 47:673–678, 1998.
2. Centers for Disease Control: Weekly update: West Nile Virus activity—United States, November 14–20, 2001. Morb Mortal Wkly Rep MMWR 50:1061–1062, 2001.
3. Doyle TJ, Bryan RT, Peters CJ: Viral hemorrhagic fevers and hantavirus infections in the Americas. Infect Dis Clin North Am 12:95–110, 1998.
4. Humar A, Keystone J: Evaluating fever in travelers returning from tropical countries. BMJ 312:953–956, 1996.
5. Humar A, Ohrt C, Harrington MA, et al: Parasight F test compared with polymerase chain reaction and microscopy for the diagnosis of *Plasmodium falciparum* malaria in travelers. Am J Trop Med Hyg 56:44–48, 1997.
6. Kain KC, Keystone JS: Malaria in travelers, epidemiology, disease, and prevention. Infect Dis Clin North Am 12:267–284, 1998.
7. Khan AS, Khabbaz RF, Armstrong LR, et al: Hantavirus pulmonary syndrome: The first 100 US cases. J Infect Dis 173:1297–1303, 1996.
8. Nash D, Mostashari F, Fine A, et al: The outbreak of West Nile virus infection in the New York City area in 1999. N Engl J Med 344:1807–1814, 2001.
9. Newman RD, Barber AM, Roberts J, et al: Malaria surveillance—United States, 1999. MMWR Morb MOrtal Wkly Rep 51:15–28, 2002.
10. Rigau-Perez JG, Clark GG, Gubler DJ, et al: Dengue and dengue hemorrhagic fever. Lancet 352:971–977, 1998.
11. Strickland GT: Hunter's Tropical Medicine and Emerging Infectious Diseases, 8th ed. Philadelphia, W.B. Saunders, 2000.
12. Vaughn DW, Nisalak A, Solomon T, et al: Rapid serologic diagnosis of dengue virus infection using a commercial capture ELISA that distinguishes primary and secondary infections. Am J Trop Med Hyg 60:693–698, 1999.

XII. Environmental Emergencies

65. ELECTRICAL AND LIGHTNING INJURIES
Samuel J. Killian, M.D.

ELECTRICAL INJURIES

1. Who is predisposed to electrical injuries and why?
There is a bimodal distribution. Children and work-related accidents account for most cases. Household injuries (low-voltage) usually are seen in children 1 to 6 years old. These injuries usually occur as a result of oral or digital contact with electrical cords, wall sockets, or extension cord outlets. Incidence declines until another resurgence between 15 and 40 years of age. Serious high-voltage electrical injuries are most common in the workplace among electrical, construction, and industrial workers. Electrocution is the fifth leading cause of fatal occupational injuries in the United States, accounting for approximately 800 deaths per year. These injuries and deaths are almost always accidental and preventable.

2. What are the basic definitions I need to know?
Volt: Unit of electrical force that causes current to flow. It is measured between two physical points, such as the two terminals of a battery.
Current: The flow of electrons per second. It is measured in **amperes**.
Direct current (DC): Unchanging direction of current flow (battery).
Alternating current (AC): Electrical source with changing direction of current flow.
Frequency: The number of transitions from positive to negative per second in AC.
Resistance: The tendency of a material to resist the flow of electrical current.
Ohm: Unit of resistance.

3. What is Ohm's law? Why is it important?
The quantity of current flowing through a tissue is often the main determinant of damage to that tissue. This can be calculated using Ohm's law:

$$\text{Current (I)} = \text{Voltage (V)}/\text{Resistance (R)}$$

An equivalent expression is Voltage (V) = Current (I) × Resistance (R). Greater resistance or lower voltage results in decreased current flow through the tissues and subsequently less injury.

4. What are the two main classifications of electrical injury?
Electrical injuries often are classified as high-voltage (> 1000 volts) or low-voltage (< 1000 volts). Voltage in high-tension transmission lines exceeds 100,000 volts. The voltage in distribution lines is reduced to 7000 to 8000 volts and further stepped down before delivery to homes. In general, high-voltage injuries are more serious than low-voltage injuries; however, other factors can affect profoundly the degree of injury.

5. List factors that determine the nature and severity of electrical injuries.

Voltage	Current pathway
Resistance of tissues	Duration of contact
Type of current (AC vs. DC)	Associated injuries such as falls
Amperage	

6. What is the voltage of household wiring?

In the United States, household wiring has 120 volts of AC current with a frequency of 60 Hz. In Europe, the standard is 220 volts. In the standard color coding of these wires, ground wires are green, neutral wires are white, and hot wires are black.

7. Explain the order of resistance of body tissues.

Nerves offer the least resistance, followed in order by blood vessels, mucous membranes, muscle, skin, tendon, fat, and bone. Skin resistance can be highly variable depending on its thickness, vascularity, and degree of resistance. The thick, dry skin of callused feet and hands is much more resistant to electrical current flow than the wet, thin skin found on the lips and tongue. Sweating and immersion in water greatly decrease the skin's resistance. Studies have shown that dry skin over the palms and soles has a resistance of approximately 100,000 ohms and drops to 2,500 ohms when moist. Immersion in water further drops skin resistance to 1500 ohms.

8. How do surface contact, current pathway, and duration of contact affect the seriousness of electrical injury?

As the cross-section diameter of the tissue through which a given current passes increases, less heat is generated, and less damage occurs. The pathway that a current takes is essential in determining which tissues are at risk. Current that takes a hand-to-hand pathway is more dangerous than current that takes a hand-to-foot pathway because of the potential for passage through the heart. A vertical pathway, parallel to the body's axis, is even more dangerous with higher incidences of ventricular fibrillation, central nervous system complications, and fetal death. A current pathway entirely below the symphysis pubis is unlikely to cause any life-threatening injury. The longer the contact with current flow, the greater the injury.

9. Why is AC more dangerous than DC?

AC is said to be about three times more dangerous than DC of the same voltage. AC is capable of producing ventricular fibrillation at a low voltage (50 to 100 mA) because it is a repetitive fibrillatory stimulus. AC causes continuous muscle contraction, or tetany, when muscle fibers are stimulated 40 to 110 times per second. With the 60-Hz frequency in the United States, tetany occurs even at low amperages, which may result in the victim being unable to release the current source voluntarily. DC tends to cause a single muscle spasm, often throwing the victim from the source, resulting in a shorter duration of exposure but increasing the likelihood of traumatic blunt injury. It can cause cardiac arrhythmias, particularly asystole.

10. Name five different mechanisms of electrical injury.

Direct contact, arc, flash, thermal, and traumatic. The last four are considered indirect mechanisms. In **direct contact injuries**, the victim becomes part of the circuit. The injury reflects the passage of current through the body and often is demarcated by entrance and exit wounds. The most destructive indirect injury occurs when the patient becomes part of an electrical arc, which is a current spark formed between two objects of different potential that are not in contact with each other. High temperatures often are generated (2500°C), which can cause deep thermal (fourth-degree) burns. An example is a small child who puts the power cord into his mouth. Electrical **flash burns** result when current strikes the skin but does not enter the body, usually causing superficial, partial-thickness burns. Secondary **thermal injuries** may occur when the victim's clothes ignite. **Traumatic injuries** may result from the violent tetanic muscle contraction associated with the AC sources or from being thrown from a DC source.

11. Which organ systems can be damaged by electrical injury?

Electrical Injuries by Organ System

SYSTEM	INJURY
Skin	Thermal burns such as entrance and exit wounds, flexor crease burns, mouth commissure burns (risk of delayed bleeding from labial artery when the eschar separates)
Cardiac	Cardiac arrest from asystole (DC) or ventricular fibrillation (AC), other arrhythmias, nonspecific ST-T changes (common), acute myocardia infarction (rare)
Vascular	Hemorrhage, arterial and venous thrombosis, ischemia
Nervous	Loss of consciousness, amnesia, confusion, disorientation, concentration and memory problems, suppression of respiratory center, seizures, paralysis, paresthesias
Musculoskeletal	Muscular pain, muscle necrosis (rhabdomyolysis), compartment syndrome, dislocations, fractures
Respiratory	Inhibition of the brainstem respiratory centers
Gastrointestinal	Hollow visceral and solid visceral injury (both rare), stress ulcers
Renal	Myoglobinuria, acute tubular necrosis, renal failure
Ophthalmologic	Cataracts

12. What are the most frequent causes of immediate death from electrical injury?

Cardiac arrhythmias and respiratory arrest. Asystole is more common from contact with a DC source. Ventricular fibrillation usually results after AC exposure.

13. What are some prehospital considerations in the treatment of electrical injuries?

Rescuer safety is the first priority. If possible, secure the area and turn off the power source. Next, attempt to remove the victim from the source. Extreme caution must be used near high-voltage sources because dry wood and other materials can conduct significant current with voltages greater than 30,000. Dry polypropylene ropes are safest for pulling wires off the victim. When the scene is secure, the basic rules of advanced cardiac life support (ACLS) and advanced trauma life support (ATLS) apply. Address the ABCs (airway, breathingm circulation); cardiac monitoring is essential. Assume traumatic injuries, and immobilize the spine as usual. Treat arrhythmias in the standard manner. Two large-bore IV catheters should be established, and aggressive fluid replacement needs to be initiated. Maintain resuscitation measures for extended periods because ultimate recovery may be achieved in cases that initially appear refractory.

14. What is the difference between fluid resuscitation in electrical burns compared with other thermal injuries?

Traditional formulas for estimating volume repletion, such as the Parkland formula, are not applicable to electrical injuries because surface damage in electrical injury does not reflect the degree of deeper tissue damage. What one visualizes may just be the "tip of the iceberg." The fluid rate should be titrated to ensure a urine output of 50 to 100 mL/h (1 to 2 mL/kg/h). The objective of early, aggressive fluid resuscitation is to prevent renal failure secondary to rhabdomyolysis. Alkalinization of the urine further prevents the precipitation of myoglobin in the renal tubules.

15. Which ancillary studies are helpful in the evaluation of an electrical injury?

The depth of evaluation depends on the extent of injury. Most patients sustaining a high-voltage injury should receive an ECG; electrolytes, BUN, and creatinine; urinalysis for myoglobin; complete blood cell count; and creatine phosphokinase. If the current may have passed through the heart, cardiac enzymes should be obtained. Radiographs and CT scans should be ordered as necessary for other injuries.

16. Are any tests necessary in the evaluation of household electrical injuries?
All cases should be considered on an individual basis, but studies have found that in the absence of loss of consciousness, tetany, wet skin, or current flow that crosses the heart region, an ECG, cardiac monitoring, and laboratory evaluation are unnecessary.

17. What are the most common ECG abnormalities seen?
Sinus tachycardia and nonspecific ST-T wave changes that resolve spontaneously. Other nonfatal arrhythmias seen include atrial and ventricular ectopy, atrial fibrillation, first-degree and second-degree heart blocks, bundle-branch blocks, and Q-T interval prolongation.

18. What should be the disposition of victims of electrical injury?
Purely thermal injuries should be handled as such and disposition made accordingly. Asymptomatic patients with low-voltage injury in the absence of significant burns, ECG changes, or myoglobinuria can be discharged home with appropriate follow-up. All other victims, including those with high-voltage injuries, significant burns, mouth-commissure burns, or ECG changes, need admission. Obstetric consultation is recommended for all pregnant patients with electrical injury, regardless of presentation.

19. Name common pitfalls in the evaluation and management of electrical injury.
Injuries to the rescuers resulting from failure to secure the scene
Neglecting the ABCs
Failure to assume the presence of spinal injury

LIGHTNING

20. Don't most people who are struck by lightning die?
No. The case fatality rate is 25% to 32%, with 74% of survivors suffering some type of permanent sequelae, including chronic pain syndromes, sympathetic nervous system injury, sleep disturbances, and neurocognitive deficits. It is estimated that lightning causes 50 to 300 deaths per year in the United States with several thousand more nonfatal injuries. Although exact numbers are unavailable, lightning causes more deaths most years than any other natural phenomenon with the possible exception of flash floods.

21. Who is most likely to be struck by lightning?
Sportsmen, campers, swimmers, farmers, sailors, construction workers, and rangers. Children playing outside are frequent victims. Men outnumber women 5 to 1. Because people who are struck by lightning are most often healthy and productive young adults, lightning strike injuries represent a significant source of disability.

22. When and where are you most likely to be struck by lightning?
Lightning injuries occur most commonly during the thunderstorm season (May to September) in the afternoon and early evening. Geographically, areas in the United States with frequent lightning strikes include mountainous regions; the South; along the Atlantic coast; and in the Hudson, Ohio, and Mississippi River valleys.

23. How often do lightning deaths occur in multiples?
Lightning strikes frequently involve more than one victim, with 15% of lightning deaths occurring in multiples of two and another 15% occurring in multiples of three or more.

24. What kind of current is lightning?
Although technically neither DC nor AC, lightning behaves most like DC. It is probably best defined as a unidirectional massive current impulse. The average energy may be 2000 to 2 billion volts and 2000 to 300,000 amps.

25. How is lightning different than other high-voltage injuries?

Although the average voltage may be massive, the actual amount of energy delivered to tissues is often much less than in other high-voltage injuries. This is because of the brief (1/10,000 to 1/1,000 second) duration of current flow and the fact that the pathway taken by the energy is different. Most of the lightning current travels over the outside of the victim. A small amount of current may leak internally causing asystole, respiratory arrest, nervous system dysfunction, seizures, and spasm of muscles and arteries. Lightning seldom causes significant burns, tissue destruction, or myoglobinuria. One study describes an 89% incidence of burns with lightning injury, but only 5% were noted to be deep or serious.

26. What is the most common cause of death from lightning strikes?

Cardiopulmonary arrest. Lightning tends to cause ventricular asystole rather than fibrillation. Internal propagation of the electrical potential acts as a DC countershock, depolarizing the entire myocardium and causing asystole. Cardiac automaticity may allow the heart to begin beating again, but the accompanying respiratory arrest may last long enough to cause secondary deterioration of the rhythm.

27. Describe the five major mechanisms of lightning injuries.

1. **Direct strike**: When lightning contacts the victim directly. Usually results in the highest mortality and morbidity.

2. **Contact**: Injury from contact occurs when lightning strikes an object or structure that is touching the victim.

3. **Side flash or "splash"**: Lightning jumps from its primary strike site to involve a nearby person on its way to the ground.

4. **Step voltage or ground current**: The lightning current strikes the ground, then spreads radially to involve the victim.

5. **Blunt trauma**: Blunt trauma may occur when a person is thrown by the explosive-implosive force as the lightning pathway is instantaneously superheated then rapidly cooled. A person also may be thrown by massive opisthotonic contraction caused by the current itself.

28. What is unique about the prehospital care and resuscitation of victims of lightning injury?

Because nearly all victims who do not have initial cardiopulmonary arrest survive, efforts should be directed toward those who appear "dead." This differs from the usual mass casualty triage scenario of caring for the victims who show signs of life first and bypassing the dead. Aggressive cardiopulmonary resuscitation (CPR) should be attempted in all victims of lightning strike because their chance for a successful resuscitation is greater than for those with other causes of cardiac arrest, even among patients with rhythms traditionally unresponsive to therapy. Aggressive volume resuscitation is not normally needed as it is for victims of electrical injuries because muscle necrosis is rare.

29. Which organ systems can be damaged by lightning?

Lightning Injuries by Organ System

SYSTEM	INJURY
Cardiac	Asystole, arrhythmias, nonspecific ST-T changes, acute myocardial infarction (rare)
Respiratory	Inhibition of the brainstem respiratory centers
Nervous	Loss of consciousness, confusion, disorientation, amnesia, autonomic dysfunction (with loss of pupillary function), coagulation of brain substance, epidural and subdural hematomas, intraventricular hemorrhage, skull fractures, seizures, transient or permanent paralysis

(Table continues on next page.)

Lightning Injuries by Organ System (cont.)

SYSTEM	INJURY
Skin	Feathering, linear burns, punctate burns, true thermal burns
Musculoskeletal	Muscle necrosis (rare), dislocations, fractures
Renal	Myoglobinuria (rare)
Gastrointestinal	Gastric atony, ileus, perforations (uncommon)
Ophthalmologic	Mydriasis, loss of light reflex, anisocoria, Horner's syndrome, cataracts
Otologic	Tinnitus, hearing loss, ruptured tympanic membranes

30. What should be the disposition of lightning victims?

All patients with cardiac or neurologic abnormalities require hospital admission. Patients with associated trauma or burns may need admission depending on the extent of the injury. All others may be discharged.

31. What kind of laboratory work or other studies do I need to order?

An ECG is essential and frequently shows Q-T prolongation even when the ECG is otherwise normal. Minimal laboratory evaluations include a complete blood count, creatine phosphokinase, and urinalysis (to look for myoglobin). In more severely injured patients, electrolytes, BUN, creatinine, and cardiac enzymes may be indicated. Other diagnostic studies should be directed toward specific injuries found on initial assessment.

32. What are the general recommendations for lightning safety?

In 1999, the Lightning Safety Group, a group of experts including meteorologists, atmospheric physicists, lightning protection experts, physicians, educators, athletic trainers, and National Aeronautic and Space Administration and National Oceanic and Atmospheric Administration's National Severe Storms Laboratory researchers met to form new lightning safety recommendations. These were based on expert opinion and new data revealing that lightning may travel much farther than traditionally thought—as far as 15 to 20 miles between inter-strike distances depending on terrain. These recommendations are:

• Have an evacuation plan and follow it.
• Be aware of weather predictions before outdoor activities.
• If bad weather is expected, have a designated lightning spotter.
• Danger still exists by the time lightning is a count of 30 seconds away.
• Seek shelter in a substantial building or an enclosed metal vehicle.
• Do not be the highest object, close to a high object, or connected to one.
• Do not resume activity until 30 minutes after the last flash of lightning or sound of thunder.

33. What is a common mistake made in the management of lightning injuries?

Failure to recognize that lightning injuries are different from other high-voltage electrical injuries.

BIBLIOGRAPHY

1. Bailey B, Gaudreault P, Thivierge RL, Turgeon JP: Cardiac monitoring of children with household electrical injuries. Ann Emerg Med 25:612–617, 1995.
2. Brighton P: Lightning injuries revisited. Ann Emerg Med 26:264–265, 1994.
3. Cherington M, Martorano FJ, Siebuhr LV, et al: Childhood lightning injuries on the playing field. J Emerg Med 12:39–41, 1994.
4. Cherington M: Lightning injuries. Ann Emerg Med 25:516–519, 1995.
5. Cooper MA: Electrical and lightning injuries. In Rosen P, Barkin RM (eds): Emergency Medicine: Concepts and Clinical Practice, 4th ed. St. Louis, Mosby, 1998, pp 1010–1021.
6. Cooper MA: Emergent care of lightning and electrical injuries. Semin Neurol 15:268–277, 1995.

7. Cooper MA, Andrews CJ: Lightning injuries. In Auerbach P (ed): Wilderness Medicine, 3rd ed. St. Louis, Mosby, 1995, pp 261–289.
8. Cooper MA, Holle R, Lopez R: Recommendations for lightning safety. JAMA 282:1132–1133, 1999.
9. Fish R: Electric shock: Part I. Physics and pathophysiology. J Emerg Med 11:309–312, 1993.
10. Fish R: Electric shock: Part II. Nature and mechanism of injury. J Emerg Med 11:457–462, 1993.
11. Fontanarosa PB: Electric shock and lightning strike. Ann Emerg Med 22:378–387, 1993.
12. Jain S, Bandi V: Electrical and lightning injuries. Crit Care Clin 15:319–331, 1999.
13. Martinez JA, Nguyen T: Electrical injuries. South Med J 93:1165–1168, 2000.

66. NEAR DROWNING

Jedd Roe, M.D., M.B.A.

1. Define terms associated with submersion accidents.

Drowning is death by suffocation from submersion in liquid.

Near drowning is survival (at least temporarily) after a submersion event.

Immersion syndrome is sudden death after submersion in very cold water, probably secondary to vagally mediated asystolic cardiac arrest.

Wet drownings are those in which aspiration of water occurred during the event; 80% to 90% of drownings are classified as wet drownings.

Dry drownings are those in which asphyxia is caused by laryngospasm without aspiration.

2. How many people drown?

Each year in the United States, more than 8000 persons die from drowning (> 500,000 worldwide). It is the third leading cause of accidental death in all ages. Drowning is the second leading cause of accidental death in persons between 5 and 44 years old, exceeded only by motor vehicle fatalities. An estimated 50,000 persons annually are near-drowning victims who survive an immersion event.

3. Who drowns and why?

The incidence of drowning peaks in two groups—teenagers and toddlers. In **teenagers** (ages 15 to 24), nearly 80% of drowning and near-drowning victims are male. Teenage boys are victims because of risk-taking behavior during swimming, boating, diving, or other water-related activities. Alcohol is a contributing factor in more than 60% of all teenage drownings.

Of all drowning victims, 40% are younger than 4 years old. **Toddlers** are at risk because of their inherently inquisitive nature and their physical inability to extricate themselves from hazards such as pools, buckets, tubs, toilets, or washers. Inadequate supervision, even for brief moments, is the primary cause of drowning in toddlers. One always must consider the possibility of abuse when evaluating a child drowning victim. An estimated 59% of drownings in persons younger than 1 year occur in bathtubs, and 56% of these are a result of child abuse.

Other risk factors in all age groups are as follows:

Inability to swim	Hot tubs/spas
Seizures	Hypothermia
Trauma	Cardiovascular disease
Ethanol	Child abuse/neglect
Hyperventilation	Diabetes
Drugs of abuse	Suicide

In the United States, 50,000 new pools are added annually to the 4.5 million pools that already exist. The increasing prevalence of hot tubs, pleasure craft, and outdoor sports has increased greatly the number of persons at risk of drowning. Of drownings, 90% occur tantalizingly close to safety, within 10 yards.

4. What kills a drowning victim?

Historically, emphasis has been placed incorrectly on the significance of drowning in salt water versus fresh water because of presumed differences in the pathophysiology of the aspirated water. In fresh-water aspirations, the hypotonic fluid was thought to diffuse into the circulation, increasing blood volume and decreasing the concentration of serum electrolytes. This also causes a loss of surfactant and results in alveolar collapse. Sea water was thought to pull fluid into the alveoli, decreasing the blood volume and increasing the electrolyte concentrations. This transudated fluid would cause a pathologic effect on pulmonary alveolar membranes, causing noncardiogenic pulmonary edema.

Of drowning victims, 10% to 20% have not aspirated water, and most victims of drowning do not aspirate enough fluid to cause a significant alteration in blood volume or electrolytes or a life-threatening pulmonary shunt secondary to perfusion of fluid-filled alveoli. Death is most often the result of asphyxia caused by laryngospasm and glottis closure. Although this mechanism is less common, more successful resuscitations (80% to 90% of all patients) occur in this group of patients. The aspirated water is a significant pulmonary irritant and contaminant, however, that may increase intrapulmonary shunting, resulting in hypoxemia.

5. What happens in a drowning?

The first event is an unexpected or prolonged immersion. The victim begins to struggle and panic. Fatigue begins, and air hunger develops. Reflex inspiration ultimately overrides breath holding. The victim swallows water, and aspiration occurs causing laryngospasm that may last for several minutes. Hypoxemia worsens, and unconsciousness ensues. If the victim is not rescued and resuscitated promptly, central nervous system damage begins within minutes.

6. Describe the presenting symptoms.

The presenting pulmonary symptoms are varied. The patient may be completely asymptomatic, have a mild cough, show mild dyspnea and tachypnea, or be in fulminant pulmonary edema. The clinical spectrum of central nervous system findings may range from confusion or lethargy to coma. Some patients may be found in cardiac arrest.

7. What is the pulmonary pathophysiology?

The central clinical feature of *all* drowning or near-drowning victims is hypoxemia caused by laryngospasm or aspiration. The PO_2 decreases, the PCO_2 increases, and there is a combined respiratory and metabolic acidosis. If the patient is successfully resuscitated, the recovery phase often is complicated by aspirated water or vomitus. Aspiration can cause airway obstruction by particulates, bronchospasm by direct irritation, pulmonary edema from parenchymal damage, atelectasis from loss of surfactant, and pulmonary bacterial infections. Some patients may later develop pulmonary abscesses or empyema.

8. How is the cardiac system affected in drowning?

Cardiac decompensation and arrhythmias are caused by hypoxemia and complicated by the ensuing acidosis. The heart is relatively resistant to hypoxic injury, and successful resumption of cardiac activity is common, but severe central nervous system damage often occurs. Response of the heart to therapy, particularly antiarrhythmic medications, may be limited by hypoxia, acidosis, and hypothermia. Primary therapy is aimed at reversal of these three problems.

9. What is the prehospital treatment?

The most important part of treatment of a near-drowning victim is delivered in the prehospital phase. If a drowning victim has appropriate airway management and ventilation is rapidly established, anoxic brain injury is avoided, and prompt and full recovery is anticipated. The patient without rapid airway management and ventilation suffers irreversible anoxic brain injury and either is unresponsive to resuscitation or has a progressively deteriorating course after initial resuscitation. Therapy must correct hypoxia, associated acidosis, and hypotension as rapidly as possible. Establish a patent airway using appropriate cervical spine precautions if indicated because diving injuries often are associated with cervical spine injury. Apply a nonrebreather oxygen mask to patients with spontaneous respirations. Initiate bag-valve-mask breathing or endotracheal intubation if indicated. Correct hypoxia and acidosis by hyperventilation with 100% oxygen. IV access is needed.

10. When is endotracheal intubation indicated?
Any person with altered mentation or an inability to protect the airway needs intubation. Presence of significant aspiration or secretions usually indicates such a need. In the initially stable patient, increased PCO_2 or low PO_2 with oxygen therapy indicates that extensive pulmonary compromise may exist, and early airway management with positive-pressure ventilation and positive end-expiratory pressure is appropriate.

One important point is to determine if the near-drowning event may have occurred as a result of diving into water. This patient may have suffered a cervical spine injury, and appropriate precautions should be taken with in-line stabilization of the neck during intubation.

11. If aspiration is suspected, what treatment is needed?
Pulmonary treatment is supportive. Close observation for signs of a developing pulmonary infection is needed. Some cases with significant aspirations may require bronchoscopy to remove particulate matter and tenacious secretions. Bronchodilator therapy with β-agonists is appropriate if bronchospasm is evident.

12. Does a normal chest radiograph rule out pulmonary injury?
No. A normal chest radiograph may be seen in 20% of cases. Typical findings include perihilar infiltrates and pulmonary edema, although these classic descriptors of acute respiratory distress syndrome (noncardiogenic pulmonary edema) may take hours to develop.

13. Is there a role for prophylactic antibiotics or glucocorticoids?
When contaminated water is involved (e.g., sewage), prophylactic antibiotics may be considered. In all other instances, prophylactic antibiotics are of no proven benefit. Glucocorticoids are of no proven benefit.

14. Is there an indication for the use of sodium bicarbonate during resuscitation?
No. Respiratory and metabolic acidosis should be treated by mechanical ventilation and hyperventilation.

15. Discuss the approach to patients with a decreased level of consciousness or coma.
Hypoxic injury leads to cerebral edema and a concomitant rise in intracranial pressure. Although there was initial enthusiasm for treatment of presumed elevated intracranial pressure with the usual modalities of muscle paralysis, hyperventilation, mannitol, barbiturate coma, hypothermia, and steroids, more recent studies have shown no improvement in outcome with these therapies. Supportive care is the mainstay of therapy. Be attentive to the possibility of cranial or spinal injuries in all boating or diving injuries. Do not forget the possibility of suicide or child abuse. If the history is in doubt, assume a cranial and a cervical injury. The possibility of toxicologic conditions also should be investigated with appropriate toxicologic screens performed.

16. Are glucocorticoids, barbiturate coma, or induced hypothermia indicated?
No. These therapies are unproven and remain controversial.

17. What is unique about cold-water drowning?
Cases in which victims of prolonged immersion in cold water have been resuscitated successfully without apparent neurologic sequelae are reported occasionally. The number remains small, however. Sudden submersion in cold water theoretically induces the mammalian diving

reflex, in which blood is shunted from the periphery to the central core. The induced hypothermia causes a decrease in metabolic demand, reducing potential hypoxic injury in prolonged asphyxia. Cold water does have potentially deleterious effects. Most significant are the induced cardiac irritability from hypothermia, exhaustion, and altered mental status. Resuscitation of hypothermic near-drowning victims should be continued until patients are adequately rewarmed (see Chapter 67, Hypothermia and Frostbite).

18. When should resuscitative efforts be withheld?

Generally, all patients should receive initial resuscitative efforts. One child recovered successfully from a 66-minute submersion in cold water, and other studies have reported that patients requiring CPR in the field may make a full recovery. When their core temperature has normalized and therapeutic efforts remain unsuccessful, patients can be pronounced dead.

19. What is the disposition of a near-drowning victim?

All drowning victims deserve aggressive in-hospital resuscitation until all reasonable efforts prove futile and the patient is near normothermic. All near-drowning victims require close evaluation. Some respiratory complications of drowning are delayed in presentation and usually appear within 8 hours. A patient with any respiratory complaints or symptoms, chest radiograph abnormalities, or a demonstrated oxygen requirement should be monitored closely in a hospital for at least 24 hours. Similarly, any patient who received resuscitative efforts or had a reported loss of consciousness, cyanosis, or apnea should be monitored closely. Patients without any symptoms and completely normal evaluation may be discharged with instructions to return immediately if respiratory distress ensues.

20. What are the most important factors in estimating prognosis?

The most important factor in determining outcome is the patient's response to resuscitation as measured by serial neurologic examinations. One study showed that a Glasgow Coma Scale improvement of 3 points on arrival to the intensive care unit portends 100% full recovery in the pediatric population. Poor prognostic factors include a Glasgow Coma Scale score less than or equal to 5, prolonged submersion (> 5 minutes), delay in initiating CPR, pH less than 7.0, water temperatures of 10°C (77°F), and asystole on arrival to the ED. Patients who arrive aware and alert have a 100% complete neurologic recovery, whereas 95% of arousable patients with altered mentation have a complete neurologic recovery.

BIBLIOGRAPHY

1. Batts JJ: Drowning. In Ferrera PC, Colucciello SA, Marx JA, et al (eds): Trauma Management: An Emergency Medicine Approach. St. Louis, Mosby, 2001, pp 594–607.
2. Bierens JJ, van der Velde EA, van Berkel M, van Zanten JJ: Submersion in the Netherlands: Prognostic indicators and results of resuscitation. Ann Emerg Med 19:1390–1395, 1990.
3. Braun R, Krishmel S: Environmental emergencies. Emerg Med Clin North Am 15:461–465, 1997.
4. Feldhaus KM, Knopp RK: Near-drowning. In Rosen P, Barkin RM (eds): Emergency Medicine: Concepts and Clinical Practice, 4th ed. St. Louis, Mosby, 1998, pp 1061–1066.
5. Flood TJ, et al: Childhood drownings and near drownings associated with swimming pools—Maricopa County, Arizona, 1988 and 1989. MMWR Morb Mortal Wkly Rep 39:441–442, 1990.
6. Modell JH: Drowning. N Engl J Med 328:253–256, 1993.
7. Orlowski JP: The hemodynamic and cardiovascular effects of near-drowning in hypotonic, isotonic, and hypertonic solutions. Ann Emerg Med 18:1044–1049, 1989.
8. Orlowski JP, Szpilman D: Drowning: Rescue, resuscitation, and reanimation. Pediatr Clin North Am 48:627–646, 2001.
9. Weinstein MD, Krieger BP: Near-drowning: Epidemiology, pathophysiology, and initial treatment. J Emerg Med 14:461–467, 1996.
10. Wintemute GJ: Childhood drowning and near-drowning in the United States. Am J Dis Child 144:663–669, 1990.

67. HYPOTHERMIA AND FROSTBITE

Daniel F. Danzl, M.D.

HYPERTHERMIA

1. What is accidental hypothermia?

The body's core temperature unintentionally decreases to less than 35°C (95°F). The preoptic anterior hypothalamus normally maintains a diurnal temperature variation within 1°C; significant pathophysiology develops at less than 35°C.

2. What factors are important in the epidemiology of hypothermia?

Primary accidental hypothermia results from direct exposure to the cold. Secondary hypothermia is a natural complication of many systemic disorders, including sepsis, cancer, and trauma. The mortality of secondary hypothermia is much higher. Outdoor exposure is not the only threat to thermostability. Many victims are found indoors, in particular, the elderly.

3. How is body temperature normally regulated?

The normal physiology of temperature regulation is activated by cold exposure, producing reflex vasoconstriction and stimulating the hypothalamic nuclei. Heat preservation mechanisms include shivering, autonomic and endocrinologic responses, and adaptive behavioral responses. Acclimatization to heat stress is efficient. Although birds migrate and bears hibernate, humans can't acclimate to a "three dog night."

4. What are the usual mechanisms of heat loss that predispose to hypothermia?

Radiation usually accounts for 55% to 65% of heat loss. Conduction and convection contribute another 15%. Moisture accelerates such heat loss; conductive losses increase 25 times in cold water. The usual baseline 20% to 30% heat loss from respiration and evaporation is affected by the relative humidity and the ambient temperature.

5. Describe the common findings in mild, moderate, and severe hypothermia.

Mild hypothermia (32.2°C to 35°C [90°F to 95°F]) depresses the central nervous system and increases the metabolic rate, pulse, and amount of shivering thermogenesis. Dysarthria, amnesia, ataxia, and apathy are common findings.

Moderate hypothermia (27°C to 32.2°C [80°F to 90°F]) progressively depresses the level of consciousness and the vital signs. Shivering is extinguished because arrhythmias commonly develop. The Q-T interval is prolonged, and a J wave (Osborn wave) may appear at the junction of the QRS complex and ST segment. Patients become poikilothermic and cannot rewarm spontaneously. A cold diuresis results from an initial central hypervolemia, which is caused by the peripheral vasoconstriction.

Severe hypothermia (< 27°C [80°F]) results in coma and areflexia, with profoundly depressed vital signs. Carbon dioxide production decreases 50% for each 8°C fall in temperature; there is little respiratory stimulation.

6. Which three categories do the factors predisposing to hypothermia fit into?

1. Decrease heat production
2. Increase heat loss
3. Impair thermoregulation

7. What decreases heat production?

Decreased heat production is common (1) at the age extremes, (2) with inadequate stored fuel, or (3) with endocrinologic or neuromuscular inefficiency. Neonates are poorly adapted for cold, even without being subjected to emergent deliveries and resuscitations. The elderly have progressively impaired thermal perception. Anything from simple hypoglycemia to more severe malnutrition represents a threat to the core temperature. Examples of endocrinologic failure are myxedema, hypopituitarism, and hypoadrenalism.

8. What are the common causes of increased heat loss?
Increased heat loss results mainly from exposure or dermatologic problems that interfere with the skin's integrity. Iatrogenic causes include emergency childbirth, cold infusions, and heat-stroke treatment.

9. How is thermoregulation impaired?
Centrally, peripherally, metabolically, or pharmacologically. A variety of **central nervous system** processes affect hypothalamic function. Traumatic or neoplastic lesions, degenerative processes, and congenital anomalies induce hypothermia. Acute spinal cord transection extinguishes **peripheral** vasoconstriction, which prevents heat conservation. The abnormal plasma osmolality common with **metabolic** derangements, including diabetic ketoacidosis and uremia, is an additional cause of hypothermia. There are innumerable **medications** and toxins that can impair central thermoregulation when present in either therapeutic or toxic doses.

10. When should hypothermia be suspected?
The diagnosis is simple when a history of exposure is obvious. The history may not be available or helpful, however, and subtle presentations are far more common in urban areas. Ataxia and dysarthria may mimic a cerebrovascular accident or intoxication. The only safe way to avoid missing the diagnosis is to measure the patient's temperature routinely.

11. Are there decoys that confuse the physical examination?
If there is a tachycardia disproportionate for the temperature, suspect hypoglycemia, hypovolemia, or an overdose. Hyperventilation, which is inappropriate during moderate or severe hypothermia, suggests a central nervous system lesion or one of the systemic acidoses, such as diabetic ketoacidosis or lactic acidosis. A cold-induced rectus spasm and ileus may mask or mimic an acute abdomen. Suspect an overdose or central nervous system insult whenever the level of consciousness is not consistent with the temperature.

12. What options are available to measure the core temperature?
Rectal, esophageal, tympanic, and bladder temperature measurements. Each has its limitations. The rectal temperature may lag or be falsely low if the probe is in cold feces. Esophageal temperature is falsely elevated during heated inhalation. The reliability of tympanic measurements is unclear.

13. How does temperature depression affect the hematologic evaluation of patients?
Anemia is masked because hematocrit increases 2%/1°C drop in temperature. Do not rely on leukocytosis to predict sepsis because the leukocytes often are sequestered. Always check the electrolytes because there are no safe predictors of the values. The increased viscosity seen with cold hemagglutination often results in either thrombosis or hemolysis, and a type of disseminated intravascular coagulation syndrome can occur. Coagulopathies are not reflected by the deceptively normal prothrombin or partial thromboplastin time because these tests are done routinely on blood rewarmed to 37°C.

14. Should arterial blood gases be corrected for temperature?
No. Correction implies acidosis is beneficial. An uncorrected pH of 7.4 and PCO_2 of 40 mmHg confirm acid-base balance at all temperatures.

15. State the key decision regarding how to rewarm a patient.
The primary initial decision is whether to rewarm the patient passively or actively. Passive rewarming is noninvasive and involves simply covering the patient in a warm environment. This technique is ideal for previously healthy patients with mild hypothermia.

16. List conditions that mandate active rewarming.
Cardiovascular instability
Temperature less than 32.2°C (90°F)
Age extremes
Neurologic or endocrinologic insufficiency

17. What is core temperature afterdrop?
The commonly observed continued drop in core temperature after initiation of rewarming. There are two explanations: (1) temperature equilibration between tissues and (2) the circulatory return of cold peripheral blood to the core.

18. Are there unique considerations and complications with active external rewarming?
The external transfer of heat to a patient is accomplished most safely when the heat is applied directly to the trunk. In chronically hypothermic patients, rapidly rewarming the vasoconstricted extremities may overwhelm a depressed cardiovascular system and result in cardiovascular collapse. Monitoring in a heated tub can be difficult, and vasoconstricted skin is burned easily by electric blankets.

19. What is arteriovenous anastomoses rewarming?
Heat is provided by immersing the lower parts of all extremities in 44°C to 45°C water. Heat opens the arteriovenous anastomoses, and warmed venous subcutaneous blood returns to the heart. A permutation is negative pressure rewarming, in which the forearm is inserted through an acrylic tubing sleeve. The efficacy of this technique is unclear.

20. What constitutes active core rewarming?
Techniques that deliver heat directly to the core. Options include heated inhalation, heated infusion, lavage, and extracorporeal rewarming.

21. When is airway rewarming indicated?
Heated, humidified oxygen is always helpful and can be administered via mask or endotracheal tube. Heat transfer is not as significant by mask, but respiratory heat loss is eliminated while the patient is rewarmed gradually.

22. What are the techniques for heated irrigation?
Heat transfer from irrigation of the gastrointestinal tract is minimal. Irrigation should be considered only in severe cases and in combination with other techniques. Thoracostomy tube irrigation is a more promising alternative in severe cases. IV fluids heated to 40°C to 42°C are particularly helpful during major volume resuscitations and generally should be given peripherally.

23. When should heated peritoneal lavage be considered?
Double-catheter peritoneal lavage can rewarm efficiently seriously hypothermic patients. This invasive technique generally should be reserved for severely hypothermic and unstable patients when extracorporeal rewarming techniques are unavailable. Infuse 2 L of isotonic dialysate at 40°C to 45°C, and suction after 20 minutes.

24. When is extracorporeal rewarming indicated?
Cardiopulmonary bypass, arteriovenous and venovenous rewarming, and hemodialysis can be lifesaving in cardiac arrest situations. Patients with completely frozen extremities, severe rhabdomyolysis, and major electrolyte fluxes also are easier to manage in this manner.

25. What are the contraindications to cardiopulmonary resuscitation (CPR) in accidental hypothermia?

CPR should be initiated, unless do-not-resuscitate status is verified, lethal injuries are identified, no vital signs of life are present, or the chest wall is frozen and cannot be compressed. Because a profoundly hypothermic patient may appear dead, and because vital signs may be difficult to obtain, a cardiac monitor should be applied for at least 60 seconds to ensure that there are no signs of life.

26. Are there unique pharmacologic considerations during hypothermia?

Because protein binding increases as body temperature drops, and most drugs become ineffective, pharmacologic manipulation of the pulse and blood pressure generally should be avoided.

27. What is the significance of atrial and ventricular arrhythmias?

Atrial arrhythmias normally have a slow ventricular response. They are innocent and should be left untreated. Preexistent ventricular ectopy may resurface during rewarming and can confuse the picture. Ventricular arrhythmia treatment is problematic. The class III agents bretylium and amiodarone offer the most ideal pharmacologic properties.

FROSTBITE

28. Define frostbite.

Frostbite is the most common freezing injury of tissue. It occurs whenever the tissue temperature decreases to less than 0°C. Ice crystal formation damages the cellular architecture, and stasis progresses to microvascular thrombosis.

29. Which factors predispose to frostbite?

Tissue rapidly freezes when in contact with good thermal conductors, including metal, water, and volatiles. Direct exposure to cold wind (wind-chill index) quickly freezes acral areas (fingers, toes, ears, nose). A variety of conditions can impair the peripheral circulation and predispose to frostbite. Constrictive clothing and immobility reduce heat delivery to the distal tissues. Vasoconstrictive medications, including nicotine, can exacerbate cold damage, especially when coupled with underlying vascular conditions, such as atherosclerosis.

30. What peripheral circulatory changes precede frostbite?

Humans possess a *life-versus-limb* mechanism that helps prevent systemic hypothermia. Arteriovenous anastomoses in the skin shunt blood away from acral areas to limit radiative heat loss.

31. Before frostbite occurs, what other cutaneous events take place in the prefreeze phase?

As tissue temperatures decrease to less than 10°C, anesthesia develops. Endothelial cells leak plasma, and microvascular vasoconstriction occurs. Crystallization is not seen as long as the deeper tissues conduct and radiate heat.

32. What happens during the freeze phase of frostbite?

The type of exposure determines the rate and location of ice crystal formation. Usually, ice initially forms extracellularly, causing water to exit the cell and inducing cellular dehydration, hyperosmolality, collapse, and death.

33. Immediately after thawing, what may occur?

In deep frostbite, progressive microvascular collapse develops. Sludging, stasis, and cessation of flow begin in the capillaries and progress to the venules and the arterioles. The tissues are deprived of oxygen and nutrients. Plasma leakage and arteriovenous shunting increase tissue pressures and result in thrombosis, ischemia, and necrosis.

34. What is progressive dermal ischemia?

An additional insult to potentially viable tissue that is partially mediated by thromboxane. Arachidonic acid breakdown products are released from underlying damaged tissue into the blister fluid. The prostaglandins and thromboxanes produce platelet aggregation and vasoconstriction.

35. Describe delayed physiologic events.

Edema progresses for 2 to 3 days. As the edema resolves, early necrosis becomes apparent if nonviable tissue is present. Final demarcation often is delayed for more than 60 to 90 days. Hence the aphorism, "Frostbite in January, amputate in July."

36. What are the symptoms of frostbite?

Sensory deficiencies are always present, affecting light-touch, pain, and temperature perception. *Frostnip* produces only a transient numbness and tingling. It is not true frostbite because there is no tissue destruction. In severe cases, patients report a "chunk of wood" sensation and clumsiness.

37. What are chilblains (pernio)?

Repetitive exposure to dry cold can induce chilblains (cold sores), especially in young women. Pruritus, erythema, and mild edema may evolve into plaques, blue nodules, and ulcerations. The face and dorsum of the hands and feet commonly are affected.

38. What is trench foot?

Prolonged exposure to wet cold above freezing results in trench foot (immersion foot). Initially the foot appears edematous, cold, and cyanotic. The subsequent development of vesiculation may mimic frostbite. Liquefaction gangrene is a more common sequela, however, with trench foot than with frostbite.

39. How should frostbite be classified?

Classification by degrees as is done with burns is unnecessary and is often prognostically incorrect. **Superficial** or **mild** frostbite does not result in actual tissue loss; **deep** or **severe** frostbite does.

40. What do the various signs of frostbite indicate?

The initial presentation of frostbite can be deceptively benign. Frozen tissues appear yellow, waxy, mottled, or violaceous-white. Favorable signs include normal sensation, warmth, and color after thawing. Early clear bleb formation is more favorable than delayed hemorrhagic blebs. These result from damage to the subdermal vascular plexus. Lack of edema formation also suggests major tissue damage.

41. How should frozen tissues be thawed?

Rapid, complete thawing by immersion in 40°C to 41°C circulating water is ideal. Reestablishment of perfusion is intensely painful, and parenteral narcotics are needed in severe cases. Premature termination of thawing is a common mistake because an incomplete thaw increases tissue loss. Never use dry heat or allow tissues to refreeze. Rubbing or friction massage may be harmful.

42. What steps should immediately follow thawing?

1. Handle tissues gently, and elevate the injured parts to minimize edema formation.
2. If cyanosis is still present after thawing, monitor the tissue compartment pressures.
3. Consider streptococcal and tetanus prophylaxis.
4. Avoid compressive dressings, and use daily whirlpool hydrotherapy.
5. Consider phenoxybenzamine (Dibenzyline) in severe cases.
6. Whenever possible, defer surgical decisions regarding amputation until clear demarcation, mummification, and sloughing are present.

43. How are blisters treated?

Clear blisters may be temporarily left intact. After débridement, topical aloe vera (Dermaide) applied directly to frostbitten areas is a specific thromboxane inhibitor. When coupled with systemic ibuprofen, this strategy can minimize accumulation of arachidonic acid breakdown products. In contrast, hemorrhagic blisters should be left intact to prevent tissue desiccation.

44. Are any ancillary treatment modalities really helpful?

A variety of antithrombotic and vasodilatory treatment regimens have been tried, including medical and surgical sympathectomies. These modalities, plus dextran, heparin, and a variety of antiinflammatory agents, have not conclusively increased tissue salvage.

45. What are some of the common sequelae of frostbite?

The most common symptomatic sequelae result from neuronal injury and abnormal sympathetic tone. Thermal misperception, paresthesias, and hyperhidrosis may become long-term complaints. Delayed findings also include epiphyseal damage, nail deformities, and cutaneous carcinomas.

BIBLIOGRAPHY

 1. Danzl DF: Accidental hypothermia. In Auerbach P (ed): Wilderness Medicine, 4th ed. St. Louis, Mosby, 2001, pp 135–177.
 2. Danzl DF, Pozos RS: Accidental hypothermia. N Engl J Med 331:1756–1760, 1994.
 3. Giesbrecht GG: Prehospital treatment of hypothermia. Wilder Environ Med 12:24–31, 2001.
 4. Gilbert M, Busund R, Skagseth A, et al: Resuscitation from accidental hypothermia of 13.7°C with circulatory arrest. Lancet 355:375–376, 2000.
 5. Goldberg BD, Robinson WA, Watson WA: Impact of delayed presentation on the efficacy of thromboxane inhibition in the treatment of frostbite. J Wilder Med 5:325–330, 1994.
 6. Lazar HL: The treatment of hypothermia. N Engl J Med 337:1545–1547, 1997.
 7. Lloyd EL: Accidental hypothermia. Resuscitation 32:111–124, 1995.
 8. McAdams TR, Swenson DR, Miller AR: Frostbite: An orthopedic perspective. Am J Orthop 28:21–26, 1999.
 9. Mills Jr WJ: Summary of treatment of the cold injured patient. Alaska Med 35:50–53, 1993.
10. Paton BC: "From-Larrey to Mills": The road to rapid rewarming—a commentary. Wilder Environ Med 9:223–225, 1998.

68. HEAT ILLNESS

Shawna J. Perry, M.D., and David J. Vukich, M.D.

1. What area of the brain is considered the body's thermostat for heat regulation?
The anterior hypothalamus.

2. List the four methods of transferring heat from the body to the environment.

1. **Radiation**. Infrared energy is radiated directly into the environment.

2. **Conduction**. Whenever the body touches a surface that is cooler than itself, heat is transferred to that object by conduction.

3. **Convection**. Air moving over the surface of the skin, even imperceptibly, carries heat away.

4. **Evaporation**. The water in perspiration changing from its liquid state to its gaseous state is the most effective means of heat loss to the environment.

3. List the three organ systems primarily responsible for heat loss.

1. **Skin**. Vasodilatation and perspiration make the surface of the skin the primary location for heat loss.

2. **Cardiovascular system**. The heart is responsible for providing a substantial increase in cardiac output to compensate for peripheral vasodilatation and increased volumes of blood being pumped to the periphery.

3. **Respiratory system**. Some degree of evaporation cooling occurs through respiration.

4. How does high humidity affect heat loss?

Evaporation of perspiration is the primary and most effective method of cooling, normally releasing 1 kcal for each 1.7 mL of perspiration. As humidity rises, perspiration evaporates more slowly, accumulating in clothing or rolling off the body. Less and less cooling is accomplished, and, eventually, at very high humidity, perspiration becomes totally ineffective.

5. What is the range of heat illness manifestations, from least to most serious?

- **Heat edema**. Seasonal, transient, nuisance only
- **Heat rash**. Miliaria, transient, uncomfortable, minor
- **Heat cramps**. Painful, easily treated, acclimation occurs
- **Heat exhaustion**. Serious but no organ damage, mild hyperpyrexia
- **Heatstroke**. Critical, organ damage, significant mortality, markedly elevated body temperature

6. What are heat cramps? What causes them?

Heat cramps are painful contractions of the larger muscle groups of the body, usually the calves and thighs, that occur during or shortly after strenuous exercise in the heat. These cramps are usually caused by the replacement of water without adequate salt, resulting in a hyponatremic state in the muscles and, eventually, painful large muscle contractions.

7. How are heat cramps treated?

The treatment of choice is fluid and electrolyte replacement by oral and/or intravenous administration of normal saline. Changes in mental status or fever are not associated with heat cramps and indicate more serious heat illness.

8. Define heat exhaustion.

Heat exhaustion is a more serious heat syndrome caused by either **water depletion** or **salt depletion** in the face of heat stress. It results in nausea, vomiting, light-headedness, mild hyperpyrexia, and signs of dehydration with only minimally altered mental status. The salt depletion type arises when fluid losses are replaced with only water, with subsequent hyponatremia and relatively decreased intravascular volume. The water depletion type is more dangerous, progressing rapidly to dehydration and heatstroke if not reversed. The prognosis for both types is good if treated promptly.

9. How is heat exhaustion treated?

Cooling is the primary therapy, and this can be accomplished simply by removing the patient from the heat source to recover in a cool area. Intravenous fluids also are required, and in most cases normal saline can be the initial choice regardless of whether water or salt depletion is predominant. Serum electrolyte levels should be determined, and those results should guide subsequent fluid therapy and electrolyte repletion if needed.

10. What is the basic pathophysiologic mechanism for heatstroke?

Heatstroke results from a failure of the body's thermoregulatory mechanisms to dissipate body heat, causing markedly elevated body temperature and resulting in multisystem organ damage and failure. The source of heat stress is exogenous. The risk for developing heatstroke increases when the heat index (how it "really feels" when air temperature is combined with humidity) is 105°F (40.5°C) or greater. Core body temperatures are in the range of 104.5°F (40.5°C) in heatstroke patients, but the range is wide. There are case reports of body temperatures as high as 114.8°F (46°C), some with full recovery. Marathon runners and other well-trained athletes may exceed a core temperature of 107°F (41.6°C) during exercise, but these individuals are acclimated to this and can tolerate these extremes successfully under favorable conditions.

11. Describe the types of heatstroke. How are they manifested?

Heatstroke may be categorized as classic or exertional. **Classic heatstroke** usually involves an elderly or debilitated patient, in an urban setting without access to air conditioning, who is exposed passively to significant thermal stress. These persons generally do not have the ability to remove themselves from the heat and are exposed to it over many hours or days. Their ability to respond to the heat stress is compromised, and their normal thermoregulatory mechanisms are overwhelmed. These victims frequently have been perspiring for a prolonged length of time, and they are extremely dehydrated. Other groups at risk are the very young (age < 4 years); those with cardiovascular diseases, neurologic diseases, or endocrine disorders; and those with previous heatstroke.

Exertional heatstroke occurs in a younger, usually physically fit population with normal thermoregulatory systems. Because of severe exogenous heat stress and concomitant exertional heat production, the body's heat loss mechanisms are rapidly overwhelmed. Frequently, these victims are not dehydrated and may be wet with perspiration when they are seen. Nonetheless, their body temperatures are elevated significantly.

Both forms of heat illness are associated with significant changes in mental status and involvement of multiple organ systems.

12. Which medications increase the risk of heatstroke?

Psychotropics (i.e., haloperidol), anti-Parkinson's agents, tranquilizers (i.e., phenothiazines), and diuretics all increase the risk of heatstroke. Caffeine, alcohol, and illicit drugs (i.e., ecstasy, cocaine) also lower the threshold for developing heat illness.

13. Which organ systems are primarily affected in heatstroke?

All organ systems may be affected but four predominate.

1. **Central nervous system**. Altered mental status is always present, sometimes with posturing, paralysis, or seizures. As the hyperpyrexia continues, coma eventually may ensue.

2. **Cardiovascular system**. High-output congestive heart failure, pulmonary edema, and, eventually, complete cardiovascular collapse occur.

3. **Hepatic system**. Central lobular hepatic necrosis occurs with high temperatures.

4. **Renal system**. Exertional heatstroke frequently leads to rhabdomyolysis and acute tubular necrosis. These effects are less common with classic heatstroke.

14. What abnormal laboratory values are expected with heatstroke?

Although nearly all organ systems and laboratory values eventually may be affected, elevation of hepatic enzymes is consistent and can occur early. Urinalysis frequently shows elevated specific gravity, many cells, and, in exertional heatstroke, myoglobin and lactic acidosis. Complete blood cell count (CBC) and clotting studies may indicate disseminated intravascular coagulation, and creatine phosphokinase (CPK) may be significantly elevated.

15. State the primary goal in the treatment of heatstroke.

In addition to supporting the **ABCs** (airway, breathing, and circulation), the most important therapeutic goal is to lower the patient's body temperature to less than 101°F (38.8°C) within 1 hour. At the extremely high temperatures of heatstroke, the heat directly damages cells and tissues; morbidity and mortality are directly affected by the duration of hyperpyrexia.

16. Describe the most effective means of lowering the body temperature in heatstroke.

The rapid cooling of heatstroke patients can be achieved by either immersion therapy or evaporation. Evaporation tends to be the most practical and effective in the ED setting. Treatment should begin immediately. The patient must be removed from the thermal heat stress, disrobed, and wrapped in wet towels during transport. In the ED, warm water mist is applied to the patient's exposed skin with a handheld spray bottle. While this is being done, a fan or fans should be directed for continuous airflow over the moistened skin surface, dramatically enhancing evaporation. Although simple, this method is effective at reducing body temperature. Ice packs may be applied to the groin and axilla but must be monitored to avoid cold damage to the skin.

Ice water baths or extremely cold cooling surfaces are effective but are controversial in the emergency setting. There is a risk of vasoconstriction of the periphery that can cause reflex shivering and greatly inhibit the ability of the body to lose heat. Internal or invasive cooling methods, such as gastric lavage, bladder irrigation, or peritoneal lavage, should be used only after there has been no response to external treatment.

17. What is the prognosis for heatstroke?

Prognosis varies greatly with the person's age and the setting of the heatstroke. The literature reveals that young military recruits who are treated aggressively have almost no mortality, whereas inner-city elderly persons with heatstroke have a high mortality rate (> 50%). Poor prognostic indicators include delay in cooling, coma lasting longer than 2 hours, elevated creatinine kinase, elevated lactate dehydrogenase, elevated liver enzymes, hypotension, and prolonged prothombin time. Permanent organ system damage frequently occurs, involving the heart, the central nervous system, or the kidneys through rhabdomyolysis and acute tubular necrosis.

BIBLIOGRAPHY

1. Armstrong LE: Whole body cooling of hyperthermic runners: A comparison of two field therapies. Am J Emerg Med 14:355–358, 1996.
2. Costrini A: Emergency treatment of exertional heat stroke and comparison of whole body cooling techniques. Med Sci Sports Exerc 22:15–18, 1990.
3. Hassanein T, Razack A, Gavaler J, Van Thiel DH: Heatstroke: Its clinical and pathological presentation with particular attention to the liver. Am J Gastroenterol 87:1382–1389, 1992.
4. Epstein Y, Sohar E, Shapiro Y: Exertional heatstroke: A preventable condition. Isr J Med Sci 31:454–462, 1995.
5. Hubbard RW: Heat stroke pathophysiology: The energy depletion model. Med Sci Sports Exerc 22:19–28, 1990.
6. Rydman RJ, Rumoro DP: The rate and risk of heat-related illness in hospital emergency departments during the 1995 Chicago heat disaster. J Med Systems 23:41–56, 1999.
8. Khosla R, Guntupalli K: Heat related illnesses. Crit Care Clin 15:251–263, 1999.
9. Royburt M, Epstein Y, Solomon Z, Shemer J: Long-term psychological and physiological effects of heat stroke. Physical Behav 54:265–267, 1993.

69. ALTITUDE ILLNESS

Benjamin Honigman, M.D., and Michael Yaron, M.D.

1. What is altitude illness?

A complex of symptoms brought on by the hypoxic conditions associated with travel to elevations usually greater than 8000 feet (barometric pressure < 560 mmHg). At this altitude, arterial blood oxygen saturation decreases to less than 90%. Extreme altitude is greater than 19,000 feet, whereas moderate altitude is 8000 to 12,000 feet.

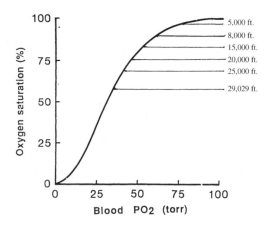

2. What are the characteristics of altitude illness?

Acute mountain sickness (AMS) is manifested by headache associated with fatigue, dizziness, nausea or vomiting, anorexia, and insomnia after a gain in altitude. Complications are high-altitude pulmonary edema (HAPE) and high-altitude cerebral edema (HACE).

3. What is the incidence of altitude illness?

AMS, 20% to 50%
HAPE, 1% to 6%
HACE, less than 1%.

4. What predisposing factors are associated with altitude illness?

Rate of ascent
Exertion on arrival
Younger age (HAPE)
Elevation attained
Previous symptoms of altitude illness
Individual physiologic susceptibility
Duration of stay at altitude
Recent upper respiratory infection (HAPE)

5. List the characteristics of HAPE.

Dyspnea at rest
Cough
Cyanosis
Rales on physical examination
Hypoxia
Alveolar infiltrates on chest film

6. What are the characteristics of HACE?

AMS with progressive neurologic symptoms such as ataxia (earliest symptom) and confusion, progressing to stupor and coma; CT scans may show cerebral edema.

7. What is the proposed mechanism of altitude illness?

Altitude illness is probably a spectrum of problems that share a common pathophysiologic mechanism. Hypoxemia at altitude occurs within minutes of arrival and leads to the clinical syndromes. The individual's response to hypoxemia is measured by the hypoxic ventilatory response, which in some individuals is low, producing relative hypoventilation during the acclimatization process. Hypoventilation ,altered fluid hemostasis resulting in fluid retention,pulmonary hypertension, and inflammatory mediated pulmonary edema exacerbates the hypoxemia and results in a shift of fluid into the alveoli in the lung (HAPE). Hypoxemia affects intracranial autoregulation, resulting in brain swelling and increased intracerebral pressures (HACE).

8. What is the natural course of AMS?

AMS may begin 1 to 12 hours after arrival at altitude but most commonly is seen 6 to 12 hours after ascent.Symptoms generally resolve within 24 to 48 hours with acclimatization. Rarely, AMS progresses to HACE or HAPE.

9. How can altitude illness be prevented?

(1) Slow graded ascent to allow for adaptation, (2) mild-to-moderate exercise on first day at altitude, and (3) sleeping at lower elevations. When above an altitude of 2500 m, the sleeping altitude should not be increased by more than 600 m in 24 hours, and an extra day of acclimatization should be taken for every 1200 m gained. Acetazolamide, *Ginko biloba*, and dexamethasone have been shown to be effective agents in the prophylaxis of AMS.

10. What are the dosages of acetazolamide and dexamethasone?

Acetazolamide: 125 mg twice a day for 1 day before arrival at altitude and continued for 2 days after arrival.

Dexamethasone: 4 mg every 6 hours for 48 hours before travel and 2 days after arrival.

11. What are the primary modes of therapy for AMS?

Acetazolamide is an effective treatment of moderate symptoms of AMS (250 mg twice a day for 2days). Dexamethasone (4 mg every 6 hours) also can be used. Ibuprofen can be used for headache, and antiemetics can be used for vomiting. If moderate symptoms occur, oxygen should be used for 24 to 48 hours. If these agents are ineffective or if symptoms progress, descent is mandatory.

12. If you are at extreme altitudes, have no oxygen, and cannot descend, is there an effective temporizing treatment for altitude illness?

Yes, a portable hyperbaric chamber (Gamow Bag).

13. What is the Gamow Bag? How does it work?

A portable neoprene bag that can be inflated to an 8-foot length. It can hold one or two persons and functions like a portable hyperbaric chamber. It should be inflated to 2 psi above atmospheric pressure and can simulate a descent of 4000 to 6000 feet, which is usually enough to improve symptoms.

14. What is the treatment for HAPE?

Descent and oxygen for severe cases; if neither is available, nifedipine, 10 mg orally followed by 30 mg extended release every 24 hours, can be used. For mild cases at altitudes of 8000 to 10,000 feet, oxygen and rest can be used as initial therapy to try to prevent the need for descent.

15. Are any pharmacologic modalities effective for HAPE?

Nifedipine has been used by some investigators. It improves pulmonary hemodynamics and respiratory function.

CONTROVERSIES

16. Should the general population of tourists use acetazolamide before altitude travel?

For: Acetazolamide is an effective prophylactic medication for AMS. Because AMS affects 25% of tourists traveling to resort communities between 8000 and 12,000 feet, and because vacations are usually only 7 to 10 days long, it is advisable to take this medication to provide the best opportunity to prevent AMS. It is cheap, inexpensive, safe, and effective

Against: At moderate elevations, 75% of individuals are not affected by altitude. Acetazolamide is sulfa-based, and allergies to sulfa are common. The side effects include diuresis and a metallic taste when eating or drinking. Carbonated beverages taste flat. AMS usually lasts for only 24 to 48 hours and generally can be prevented with judicious exercise on the first day of travel, avoiding medication.

BIBLIOGRAPHY

1. Bartsch P, Maggiorini M, Ritter M, et al: Prevention of high-altitude pulmonary edema by nifedipine. N Engl J Med 325:1284–1289, 1991.
2. Ellsworth AJ, Larson EB, Strickland D: A randomized trial of dexamethasone and acetazolamide for acute mountain sickness prophylaxis. Am J Med 83:1024–1030, 1987.
3. Grissom CK, Roach RC, Sarquist FH, Hackett PH: Acetazolamide in the treatment of acute mountain sickness: Clinical efficacy and effect on gas exchange. Ann Intern Med 116:461–465, 1992.
4. Hackett PH, Rennie D: The incidence, importance and prophylaxis of acute mountain sickness. Lancet 2:1149–1155, 1976.
5. Hackett PH, Roach RC: High Altitude illness. N Engl J Med 345:107–114, 2001.
6. Honigman B, Moore L, Yip R, et al: Acute mountain sickness in a general tourist population at moderate altitudes. Ann Intern Med 118:587–592, 1993.
7. Honigman B, Read M, Lezotte D, Roach R: Sea-level physical activity and acute mountain sickness at moderate altitude. West J Med 163:117–122, 1995.
8. Johnson TS, Rock PB: Acute mountain sickness. N Engl J Med 319:841–845, 1988.
9. Larson EB, Roach RC, Schoene RB, Hornbein TF: Acute mountain sickness and acetazolamide. JAMA 248:328–332, 1982.
10. Reeves JR, Schoene RB: When lungs on mountains leak: Studying pulmonary edema at high altitude. N Engl J Med 325:1306–1307, 1991.
11. Roach RC, Houston CS, Honigman B, et al: How well do older persons tolerate moderate altitude? West J Med 162:32–36, 1995.
12. Scoggin CH, Hyers TM, Reeves JT, Grover RF: High-altitude pulmonary edema in the children and young adults of Leadville, Colorado. N Engl J Med 297:1269–1272, 1977.
13. Singh I, Khanna PK, Srivasta ML, et al: Acute mountain sickness. N Engl J Med 280:175–184, 1969.
14. Yaron M, Honigman B: High altitude illness. In Marx JA, et al (eds): Rosen's Principles and Practice of Emergency Medicine: Concepts and Clinical Practice, 5th ed. St. Louis, Mosby, 2002.

70. DIVING EMERGENCIES AND DYSBARISMS

John McGoldrick, M.D.

1. Who is at risk for dysbaric injuries?

There are more than 5 million trained scuba divers in the United States. This group, in addition to caisson workers, commercial divers, and aviators, is most often subject to dysbaric injuries.

2. What are the most serious dysbaric emergencies?

Decompression sickness (DCS) and arterial gas embolism (AGE).

3. Why are scuba divers at risk for diving medical problems?

In compressed gas or scuba diving, the diver breathes air or other gas mixtures at elevated pressures underwater. Divers are exposed to a pressure environment, and the problems seen can be caused by the mechanical effects of increases or decreases of pressure on the diver's body or by the elevated partial pressures of the gases respired at depth.

4. Why do I need to understand the physics involved?

An understanding of the gas laws is helpful in understanding the pathophysiology of diving-related medical problems.

Gas Laws

Boyle's law: At a constant temperature, the volume of a perfect gas varies inversely with the pressure, and the pressure varies inversely with the volume. That is, the higher the pressure, the smaller the volume, and vice versa.

Charles' law: For any gas at a constant pressure, the volume of that gas varies directly with the absolute temperature. That is, change in either volume or pressure is directly related to change in temperature.

General gas law: A combination of the above two laws.

$$P_1 V_1 / T_1 = P_2 V_2 / T_2$$

where P_1 = initial pressure, V_1 = initial volume, T_1 = initial temperature, P_2 = final pressure, V_2 = final volume, and T_2 = final temperature.

Dalton's law (the law of partial pressure): The total pressure exerted by a mixture of gases is equal to the sum of the pressure of each of the different gases making up the mixture, with each gas acting as if it alone were present and occupying the total volume. That is, the whole is equal to the sum of its parts.

$$P_{total} = P_x + P_y + P_z \ldots$$

Henry's law: The amount of any given gas that will dissolve in a liquid at a given temperature is a function of the partial pressure of that gas in contact with the liquid. That is, as one dives deeper, more gas will dissolve in the body tissues.

---

5. Define pressure. What is the atmospheric pressure at sea level?

Pressure is force exerted on a given unit of area: pressure = force/area. Under standard conditions, atmospheric pressure at sea level is 14.7 psi.

6. What is atmospheric absolute (ATA)?

Another unit of pressure used, where 14.7 psi equals 1 ATA. Average sea water density is such that each 33 feet of depth equals an additional atmosphere of pressure.

1 ATA = 29.9 inches of mercury (in. Hg)
      = 760 millimeters of mercury (mmHg)
      = 33 feet of sea water (fsw)
      = 34 feet of fresh water
      = 14.7 pounds per square inch (psi)
      = 1033 grams per square centimeter (g/cm^2)
      = 10.08 meters of sea water (msw)
      = 1013.3 millibars (mbar)

7. What is nitrogen narcosis?

Nitrogen narcosis (also known as "rapture of the deep") is the anesthetic-like effect that nitrogen exerts on a diver as its partial pressure increases with depth. Each 50 fsw has been equated to having the effect of one martini—hence the "martini rule." With considerable individual variation, at 100 fsw, a diver may feel light-headed and euphoric, lose dexterity and reasoning ability, and have increased reaction times. At depths greater than 300 fsw, unconsciousness can occur.

8. Can carbon monoxide present a problem for scuba divers?

Carbon monoxide can be a problem only if the air supply is contaminated from improper placement of the compression engine exhaust, whereby carbon monoxide can be blown into the air intake of the pump when tanks are being filled.

9. What is the most common form of injury that affects divers? What causes it?

Barotrauma, which is caused by expansion or contraction of gas in or around the body secondary to changes in atmospheric pressure produced by ascending or descending in the water column (Boyle's law). These changes in volume in turn distort or damage the tissue surrounding the gas spaces. Barotrauma can occur during descent or ascent.

10. What is middle ear squeeze?

Middle ear squeeze occurs when there is a pressure differential across the tympanic membrane. A pressure differential develops as a diver descends (or ascends) unless air is able to enter (or exit) the middle ear via the eustachian tube. As the differential pressure increases, the middle ear mucosa becomes edematous and hemorrhagic. Tympanic membrane rupture can occur. When tympanic membrane rupture occurs in the water, vertigo may result from caloric vestibular stimulation.

11. Can middle ear squeeze be prevented?

Experienced divers use a Valsalva or Frenzel maneuver to equalize pressure in the middle ear as they descend.

12. What is the treatment for middle ear squeeze?

Depending on the severity, ear squeezes usually can be treated symptomatically with decongestants. Tympanic membrane perforations are an absolute contraindication to diving because of the risk of calorically induced vertigo.

13. What is external ear squeeze?

If air cannot freely enter or exit the external canal (because of cerumen impaction, ear plugs, or a tight-fitting wet suit hood), the resultant negative pressure in the canal causes the tympanic membrane to bulge outward. The lining of the canal becomes edematous and hemorrhagic, producing ear pain that does not resolve by middle ear pressure equalization.

14. What is the treatment for external ear squeeze?

Ascent and a topical corticosteroid antiinflammatory (Corticosporin Otic suspension) for any significant external ear canal trauma.

15. What is inner ear barotrauma?

Inner ear barotrauma can occur when a pressure differential between the inner and middle ear is created, causing either an implosive or explosive round or oval window rupture. The problem usually occurs close to the surface during a difficult descent, as the middle ear differential is accentuated by a forceful Valsalva-induced increase in inner ear pressure.

16. Name the symptoms of round or oval window rupture.

Sudden onset of severe vertigo not relieved by ascent, roaring tinnitus, nystagmus, a feeling of fullness in the affected ear, and sensorineural hearing loss. Inner ear barotrauma should be differentiated from alternobaric vertigo (which usually occurs during deep dives and is transitory) and inner ear decompression sickness (which usually is associated with deep dives using a helium and oxygen breathing mixture).

17. What is the treatment for round or oval window rupture?

Using antivertiginous drugs, such as prochlorperazine, diazepam, or meclizine. Patients should be referred to an ear, nose, and throat surgeon for follow-up.

18. What causes alternobaric vertigo?

This condition is thought to be caused by a unilateral pressure differential between the middle and inner ears. The symptoms are transient sudden vertigo and an overwhelming feeling of disorientation. Symptoms usually last less than 1 minute and occur more frequently during ascent than descent. The vertigo may persist on the surface and be accompanied by nausea, vomiting, and nystagmus without tinnitus.

19. What is the treatment for alternobaric vertigo?

Alternobaric vertigo is usually transitory and usually does not require treatment. Decongestants can hasten clearing. For persistent symptoms, antiemetic and antivertiginous drugs can be used. Occasionally a myringotomy may be necessary to relieve symptoms.

20. What other types of barotrauma are seen in diving accidents?

Pulmonary overinflation may occur when a diver is ascending in the water column and ascends too fast or fails to exhale. Constant exhalation is required to vent air from the lungs of an ascending diver to prevent pulmonary overinflation (Boyle's law). Failure to do so results in alveolar rupture with escape of air into one or more of three directions: into the mediastinum, causing pneumomediastinum and interstitial emphysema; into the pleural space, causing pneumothorax; or into the pulmonary venous system, causing arterial gas embolism.

21. What are the symptoms of interstitial emphysema?

Air escaping from alveolar rupture can dissect into the mediastinal space and, from there, into the pericardium, cephalad into the neck as subcutaneous air, or caudally as retroperitoneal air. Signs and symptoms include subcutaneous air (crepitus), change in voice, Hammond's crunch, pericardial air, and dyspnea.

22. What is the treatment for interstitial emphysema?

Interstitial emphysema is usually not life-threatening and can be treated symptomatically. Breathing 100% oxygen can hasten resolution. The presence of interstitial emphysema indicates escape of alveolar air, however, and mandates monitoring for other, more serious consequences of pulmonary overinflation.

23. What is AGE?

AGE is the most serious and the most fatal of all diving accidents and is second only to drowning as the leading cause of death in sport divers. Air bubbles that enter the pulmonary venous system coalesce and travel to the left side of the heart. From the left ventricle, they may enter the coronary arteries or the cerebral circulation, causing myocardial infarction and cerebral embolism.

24. How does AGE present?

AGE occurs on ascent, and the time from alveolar rupture to initiation of symptoms is usually less than 10 minutes. Neurologic symptoms can range from subtle changes in mood or affect, visual disturbances, and unilateral or bilateral muscular and sensory disturbances to immediate unconsciousness. Other manifestations include apnea, cardiac dysrhythmia, and cardiac arrest. Sudden loss of consciousness on surfacing must be assumed to be AGE until proved otherwise.

25. Describe the treatment for AGE.

Definitive treatment of any gas embolism requires a recompression chamber. During transport, an adequate airway and proper ventilation and circulation should be ensured; 100% oxygen is administered. Patients should be transported in a left-side-down position. Ground transport is preferred, but if air transport is used, cabin altitude should be kept as close to sea level as possible.

26. What is DCS?

DCS is the result of a series of pathophysiologic responses to the evolution of dissolved tissue gases, precipitated by a change in ambient pressure. Bubbles released from solution by a too-rapid reduction in ambient pressure obstruct blood flow, cause changes in blood chemistry, or stretch and damage tissue.

27. How do these bubbles form?

When a mixture of gases is inspired, the amount of each gas that becomes dissolved is proportional to the partial pressure of each gas (Henry's law). The eventual tissue concentration of gases also depends on the rate at which gases are removed or metabolized. When breathing air, the dissolved tissue gas of concern is nitrogen. The oxygen component is removed rapidly by metabolism, but nitrogen is inert. Tissues with an elevated nitrogen content must release nitrogen to the blood, which transports it to the lungs for elimination. If the ambient pressure is reduced too rapidly, nitrogen cannot diffuse from tissues fast enough, the tissues become supersaturated, and some of the nitrogen comes out of solution as bubbles.

28. What happens to these nitrogen bubbles?

These bubbles can be interstitial, intralymphatic, or intravascular. They can cause symptoms mechanically (blockage of vascular flow or distortion of tissues), indirectly (endothelial damage, protein denaturation, altered blood coagulation), or a combination of the two.

29. When does DCS present?

Symptoms usually are present within 12 hours after diving: 80% of patients in one study had symptoms within 1 hour of surfacing, and 95% had symptoms within 4 hours. Symptoms seldom occur after 12 hours but may not present for 24 hours or longer, making diagnosis difficult.

30. Can flying after diving contribute to symptoms of DCS?

Commercial aircraft are not pressurized to sea level, so flying adds a DCS risk to a diver who may have subclinical bubbles. It generally is recommended that divers wait at least 24 hours after diving before flying to decrease this risk.

31. What is the clinical presentation of DCS?

DCS has classically been divided into two groups: **Type 1 DCS** (musculoskeletal) presents as limb pain or with skin or lymphatic involvement. **Type 2 DCS** (neurologic) includes all other symptoms. DCS is an evolving condition; the patient who presents with type 1 symptoms can go on to develop more serious type 2 symptoms.

32. What is "the bends"?

Type 1 DCS, known as pain-only bends, presents as pain that is confined to the arms or legs and may be aggravated by movement and relieved by direct pressure on the area (as with a sphygmomanometer cuff). The pain is usually periarticular, involves the upper extremities three times as often as the lower extremities in divers, and ranges from mild discomfort (niggles) to severe pain. There should be no association with systemic symptoms, and the pain should not be referred or confused with paresthesias or hypesthesias.

33. How else can type 1 DCS present?

When there are skin and lymphatic manifestations, type 1 DCS can present as pruritus alone, skin marbling, or various rashes and lymphatic symptoms. Pruritus is usually encountered only after deep chamber dives in which the diver is surrounded by compressed air. Gas entering the sweat and sebaceous glands is thought to form pruritic bubbles as the diver surfaces. Pruritus is not considered a true form of DCS and resolves rapidly. It must be differentiated, however, from the tingling of paresthesias and hypesthesias of type 2 DCS.

34. How is type 1 DCS treated?

Symptoms of type 1 DCS indicate that tissue supersaturation has occurred and may progress to type 2 DCS. All type 1 DCS symptoms should be treated with recompression.

35. How does type 2 DCS present?

Type 2 DCS includes all other manifestations, such as pain in areas other than the extremities, central nervous system (CNS) signs or symptoms, and pulmonary manifestations ("chokes"). Pain other than in the extremities may represent referred pain from visceral sites or spinal cord involvement.

36. What is the most common type of DCS?

Spinal cord DCS is the most common type in sport scuba divers, whereas cerebral DCS is the most common in aviators.

37. How does spinal cord DCS present?

Paresthesia is a common presenting symptom of a spinal cord "hit" and may progress to ascending numbness, dermatomal distribution of pain, or paraplegia. Cord lesions are common in the lumbosacral area and may be associated with bladder paralysis, urinary retention, fecal incontinence, and, occasionally, priapism.

38. How does cerebral DCS present?

Cerebral DCS can present as seizures, hemiplegia, scotoma, diplopia, tunnel vision, or blurry vision. Headaches are common. Soft signs include unusual fatigue, a sense of detachment, and inappropriate or uncharacteristic behavior. Any neurologic symptom can be associated with the intravascular or extravascular evolution of bubbles anywhere in the nervous system.

39. What are "staggers" and "chokes"?

Divers may have labyrinthine or inner ear DCS ("staggers") or pulmonary DCS ("chokes").

40. List the usual symptoms of inner ear DCS.

Vertigo
Nausea
Vomiting
Hearing loss
Tinnitus
Nystagmus

41. How does pulmonary DCS present?

Pulmonary DCS usually occurs within minutes of surfacing. Accumulation of bubbles within the pulmonary arterial tree can cause substernal pain, cough, and dyspnea, which can progress to respiratory failure and shock.

42. How are the various types of type 2 DCS treated?

IV fluid therapy with crystalloid is necessary in all cases of type 2 DCS because fluid loss, hemoconcentration, and increased blood viscosity promote vascular occlusion. Diazepam or prochlorperazine is useful in controlling the vertigo, nausea, and vomiting associated with labyrinthine DCS. Definitive treatment is recompression as soon as possible.

43. How does recompression or hyperbaric therapy work?

The three objectives in recompression therapy are (1) to reduce the size of the bubble, (2) to promote bubble reabsorption, and (3) to prevent further bubble evolution. Reduction in size is accomplished by the increase in ambient pressure. Breathing 100% oxygen washes out tissue nitrogen, enhancing diffusion by widening the nitrogen partial pressure difference.

44. What is the disposition of a patient after recompression therapy is complete?

After recompression is complete, the patient should be evaluated for admission to the hospital for further observation. Any recurrent or new symptom is classified automatically as type 2 and treated with further recompression.

45. When can patients return to diving after recompression therapy?

The patient should not dive for 4 to 6 weeks after type 1 DCS and at least 3 to 6 months after type 2 DCS. A second incident of type 2 DCS should warrant critical evaluation of the patient's fitness for further diving.

46. Have respiratory symptoms been attributed to other disorders besides DCS and pulmonary barotrauma in recreational scuba divers?

Yes. A variety of disorders may cause respiratory symptoms, including barotrauma, pulmonary DCS, water aspiration, and inhalation of contaminated gases. More recently, a syndrome of pulmonary edema has been described in scuba divers. This syndrome is not associated with a decompression mechanism and presents with cough, weakness, expectoration of froth, chest discomfort, orthopnea, wheezing, hemoptysis, and dizziness. Reported cases of the syndrome have responded to standard medical therapy for pulmonary edema, including oxygen, diuresis, and positive-pressure ventilation.

CONTROVERSIES

47. How does one distinguish between DCS and AGE?

A detailed neurologic evaluation is required in all cases. Symptoms of DCS and AGE are often difficult to distinguish. There is currently a trend away from differentiation between DCS and AGE, approaching both as decompression illnesses that require recompression. Initial treatment includes 100% oxygen, rehydration with IV crystalloid, and expeditious transport to a recompression chamber.

48. How should patients be positioned for transport to a recompression chamber after they have suffered an AGE?

The proper positioning of an air embolism patient is controversial. The head-up position can distribute air to the cerebral circulation. The head-down position can distribute more air to the coronary circulation and can increase cerebral blood flow and further increase intracranial pressure. The best compromise may be to place the patient supine with the head in a neutral position to allow unrestricted arterial and venous blood flow from the head.

49. If symptoms of decompression illness resolve after the use of 100% oxygen, should the patient undergo recompression therapy?

Most physicians trained in hyperbaric medicine recommend that a washout recompression treatment be given even if the diver becomes totally asymptomatic after breathing 100% oxygen.

50. Does a patent foramen ovale (PFO) increase the risk of DCS?

In a metaanalysis of four studies of PFOs and divers, the risk ratio for DCS was increased by a factor of 5 for individuals with a PFO. The incidence of DCS in sport divers is low (about 0.03%), however, and the significance of this small increase in the risk ratio for divers with PFOs is questionable.

51. Should people with a PFO scuba dive?

The presence of asymptomatic PFOs in the general population is reported to be about 30%. There is no recommendation that people with asymptomatic PFOs should not scuba dive. It is recommended, however, that a workup for a hemodynamically significant PFO be done in any diver who develops unexplained AGE or type 2 DCS and wants to continue scuba diving.

52. Are there any new treatments being tried for refractory DCS?

Oxygen-helium recompression therapy has been advocated as an alternative to conventional United States Navy oxygen treatment tables. Theoretical benefits are thought to be related to the lower diffusion and solubility coefficients of helium in fatty tissue, allowing a greater outward flux of nitrogen. A further advantage is that higher treatment pressures may be maintained with less risk of oxygen toxicity.

There have been case reports of adjunctive IV lidocaine being beneficial in cases of refractory DCS. The exact pathophysiology of DCS is unclear. Current concepts support activation of the coagulation and complement systems, with promotion of interstitial edema and microvascular sludging, leading to progressive local ischemia. Lidocaine is theorized to ameliorate many of these local effects, to reduce intracranial hypertension associated with AGE, to increase spinal cord blood flow, and to preserve nerve conduction in isolated nerves.

BIBLIOGRAPHY

 1. Arthur DC: A short course in diving medicine. Ann Emerg Med 16:689–701, 1987.
 2. Bove F: Cardiovascular problems and diving. SPUMS J 26:178–186, 1996.
 3. Cogar WB: Intravenous lidocaine as adjunctive therapy in the treatment of decompression illness. Ann Emerg Med 29:284–286, 1997.
 4. Goldenberg I, Shupak A, Shoshani O: Oxy-helium treatment for refractory neurological decompression sickness: A case report. Aviat Space Environ Med 67:57–60, 1996.
 5. Hampson NB, Dunford RG: Pulmonary edema of scuba divers. Undersea Hyperb Med 24:29–33, 1997.
 6. Hardy KR: Diving-related emergencies. Emerg Med Clin North Am 15:223–240, 1997.
 7. Kerut EK, Norfleet WT, Plotnick GD, et al: Patent foramen ovale: A review of associated conditions and the impact of physiological size. J Am Coll Cardiol 38:613–623, 2001.
 8. Myers RA, Bray P: Delayed treatment of serious decompression sickness. Ann Emerg Med 14:254–257, 1985.
 9. Strauss MB, Borer RC: Diving medicine: Contemporary topics and their controversies. Am J Emerg Med 19:232–238, 2001.
10. Vane KD: Mechanisms and risks of decompression. In Bove AA, Davis JC (eds): Diving Medicine. Philadelphia, W.B. Saunders, 1997.

XIII. Neonatal and Childhood Disorders

71. FEVER IN CHILDREN YOUNGER THAN 3 YEARS

Ann B. Marshall, M.D.

1. What constitutes a fever?

38°C (100.4°F). A rectal temperature is the gold standard for determining body temperature in infants and children. Axillary and tympanic temperatures lack sensitivity; an afebrile temperature by these methods does not rule out a fever. A young infant with an infection may be afebrile.

2. How accurate are parents' assessments of fever in their child?

Tactile skin assessment of temperature by parents is correct in identifying the absence of fever 73% to 98% of the time. Parents who believed their children were febrile were correct 74% to 90% of the time. In general, a measured home temperature should be considered accurate.

3. An infant or young child has a fever; what's the big deal?

Most younger children have a clear source of infection (e.g., upper respiratory infection or otitis media). About 20% have no identifiable source (fever without a source [FWS]). Serious bacterial infection (SBI), such as bacteremia, meningitis, urinary tract infection, and bacterial enteritis, is difficult to distinguish from simple viral illness but is extremely important to recognize and treat.

4. At what temperature should I consider pursuing FWS in the febrile infant or young child?

SBI is present in about 3% to 11% of febrile children 3 months to 3 years of age with a temperature of 39°C (102.2°F) or greater. In studies of infants younger than 3 months old with FWS, the rate of SBI is 10% to 18.5% with temperatures of 38°C (100.4°F) or greater. Any child with a fever who is **toxic appearing**, regardless of temperature, should be evaluated for SBI.

5. What do you mean by *toxic appearing*?

Before, during, and after the physical examination, the physician should note the patient's level of alertness and activity, respiratory effort, muscle tone, eye contact, ability to feed, and interactiveness. Toxic-appearing children may show irritable behavior, poor feeding, lethargy, cyanosis, and unwillingness to interact with family members or the physician.

6. Which antipyretic agents should be used in the febrile child?

Aspirin has been associated with the development of Reye's syndrome in children with some febrile illnesses and should not be used in children for the treatment of fever. **Acetaminophen** is effective as an antipyretic and safe in recommended doses of 10 to 15 mg/kg. Liquid **ibuprofen** (10 mg/kg) also is an effective antipyretic in children.

7. Should I worry about masking a further rise in temperature with antipyretics?

No. Defervescence often results in improved feeding, increased activity levels, and a child who feels a whole lot better!

8. My patient has an FWS and a concerning temperature for his age group (see question 4); what do I do now?

Start your sepsis workup, which may include some or all of the following:

1. A catheterized urine specimen for urinalysis and culture
2. Blood for a complete blood count and culture
3. Cerebrospinal fluid for direct examination and culture
4. Stool specimen (if diarrhea)
5. Chest radiograph

9. Whoa! That seems awfully expensive (not to mention invasive). Can't I limit my workup?

Urine specimen: Urinary tract infection increasingly is recognized as a common SBI in young children. The catheterized specimen is necessary because bagged specimens have an unacceptable rate of contamination. You can be selective, however, based on patient gender and age. Current recommendations state urine cultures should be obtained in certain high-risk groups: all boys younger than age 6 months, uncircumcised boys younger than 12 months, and girls younger than 12 months. In everyone not in these groups but younger than 2 years old, urine microscopy can be used to determine need for culture.

Chest radiograph: Chest radiographs can be performed selectively. You may limit this study to patients with hypoxia, respiratory distress, focal findings on lung examination, or white blood cell (WBC) counts greater than 15,000/μL to 20,000/μL and no other source.

10. How should I approach the infant younger than 1 month of age with fever (temperature > 38°C)?

A conservative approach can be used in these patients consisting of a sepsis workup, including complete blood count with differential, blood culture, catheterized urinalysis and culture, and standard cerebrospinal fluid evaluation and culture. If the infant has diarrhea, stool should be examined for WBCs. If respiratory symptoms or hypoxia is present, a chest radiograph should be done. Generally, patients should be admitted for observation and parenteral antibiotics until all cultures are negative. Admitting these patients for observation but holding antibiotics (pending culture results) is also a reasonable approach in a well-appearing infant.

11. How should the 1- to 3-month-old (28 to 90 days) febrile child be managed?

In general, these patients also should undergo a sepsis workup. A toxic-appearing child should have the full workup and be admitted for intravenous antibiotics. For a low-risk, well-appearing infant with a reliable caregiver, outpatient management is an alternative to admission. Two main outpatient options exist: (1) a mandatory lumbar puncture and 50 mg/kg of ceftriaxone before discharge or (2) omit the lumbar puncture and antibiotics. Both options require extremely close follow-up (within 24 hours).

12. What do you mean by *low-risk* infant?

Three sets of criteria have been published with regard to what makes a febrile infant *low risk*. The individual clinician decides which to use. All three strategies include a well-appearing, previously healthy infant and require close follow-up for patients meeting low-risk criteria.

1. The **Rochester criteria** specify the following: no coincident otitis media, WBC count between 5,000/μL and 15,000/μL, absolute band count less than 1,500/μL, urinalysis with 10 or less WBCs/high-powered field (hpf), stool with 5 or less WBCs/hpf . If all criteria are met, patients are discharged home without antibiotics.

2. The **Boston criteria** include no evidence of otitis, WBCs less than 20,000/μL, urinalysis less than 10 WBCs/hpf, cerebrospinal fluid less than 10 WBCs, and normal chest radiograph (if obtained). Patients are discharged after antibiotics.

3. The **Philadelphia criteria** include WBCs less than 15,000/μL, band-to-neutrophil ratio less than 0.2, urinalysis less than 10 WBCs/hpf and negative Gram stain, cerebrospinal fluid less

than 8 WBCs and negative Gram stain, and negative chest radiograph and stool (if obtained). Patients are discharged without antibiotics.

13. What is the best approach to febrile infants and toddlers 3 to 36 months of age?

Children in this age group generally may be managed with less invasive evaluation and treatment. Children with fever greater than 39°C and no focal infection should have a complete blood count. If the WBCs are greater than 15,000/µL, a blood culture should be obtained. A urine culture should be obtained for boys younger than 6 months old and girls younger than 24 months old. In this age group, children with meningitis are more likely to have clinical signs and symptoms than those in the younger age group. The clinical impression of a child unlikely to have meningitis is more reliable. In this group, it is permissible to treat with empirical intramuscular ceftriaxone without obtaining a cerebrospinal fluid culture. The patients should be scheduled for a 24-hour follow-up visit.

14. What common bacterial pathogens occur in otherwise healthy infants and toddlers?

AGE	PATHOGEN
< 28 days	Group B streptococcus, *Escherichia coli*, other gram-negative enteric bacteria (*Klebsiella, Listeria*)
29–60 days	Group B streptococcus, *E. coli, Klebsiella*, occasionally *Listeria, Streptococcus pneumoniae, Haemophilus influenzae* type B, and *Neisseria meningitidis*
61–90 days	*S. pneumoniae, H. influenzae* type B,[*] *N. meningitidis*, occasionally group B streptococcus and gram-negative enteric bacteria
> 90 days	*S. pneumoniae*,[†] *H. influenzae* type B, *N. meningitidis*

[*] The incidence of *H. influenzae* has decreased greatly since the widespread use of the Hib vaccine.
[†] The results from a phase III U.S. trial of the conjugate pneumococcal vaccine are similar to those for the Hib vaccine. This ultimately may result in a significant change in clinical practice.

15. What is the natural history of occult bacteremia?

Bacteremia is not a benign illness. Approximately one third of infants with occult bacteremia secondary to pneumococcus, *H. influenzae* type B, and *N. meningitidis* improve clinically and have negative blood cultures within 72 hours without treatment. Bacteremia secondary to *H. influenzae* and *N. meningitidis* is much more likely to progress to serious illness than is bacteremia secondary to *S. pneumoniae. S. pneumoniae* is the leading pathogen in occult bacteremia. Among patients with occult pneumococcal bacteremia who do not receive antibiotics at initial evaluation, 10% to 25% develop complications (cellulitis, pneumonia, and sepsis), and 3% to 6% develop meningitis.

16. What antibiotics should be used for empirical treatment?

AGE	TREATMENT
Birth–4 weeks	Ampicillin, 100 mg/kg/24 h q 4–6 h IV, plus an aminoglycoside (gentamicin, 5 mg/kg/24 h q 8 h IV), or cefotaxime, 50–150 mg/kg/24 h q 6–8 h IV
4 weeks–3 months	Ampicillin, 200 mg/kg/24 h q 6 h IV, and cefotaxime, 150 mg/kg/24 h q 6–8 h IV
3 months–3 years	Ceftriaxone, 50 mg/kg IV or IM × 1 dose

17. Which children with fevers have to be hospitalized?

Febrile infants less than 28 days old
Children who appear ill on clinical assessment

Children with an unreliable caregiver or poor social situation
Children who are immunocompromised and have a fever

CONTROVERSIES

18. Do all febrile infants less than 28 days old have to be admitted to the hospital?

Clinical studies attempting to apply low-risk criteria to febrile neonates have found that it is safe to manage this subgroup as inpatients without antibiotic therapy. These protocols misclassify about 3% of febrile neonates who have SBI—an unacceptably high number. Until further studies are done to determine outcome in infants discharged with an SBI, the recommendation to admit these patients still stands.

19. What about a child with a high fever and otitis media?

According to the Rochester criteria, the presence of otitis media excludes the patient from being considered low risk. Most authorities agree that well-appearing infants with otitis media as the sole factor keeping them from meeting the low-risk criteria may be managed as outpatients with close follow-up and oral antibiotic therapy.

20. Do all patients with positive blood cultures require hospitalization for parenteral antibiotics?

In general, yes. One exception to this rule is the low-risk infant more than 28 days old with blood culture positive for penicillin-sensitive *S. pneumoniae*. If these patients are afebrile and well appearing, they can be managed as outpatients with oral penicillin with good follow-up. Infants whose blood culture turns positive after 24 hours (true pathogens are more likely to become positive within 24 hours) with a Gram stain suggestive of a contaminant can be treated as outpatients if afebrile and well appearing. They can be treated according to their initial outpatient strategy (i.e., with or without antibiotics).

BIBLIOGRAPHY

1. Bachur R, Harper M: Predictive model for serious bacterial infections among infants younger that 3 months of age. Pediatrics 108:311–316, 2001.
2. Baraff L: Management of fever without source in infants and children. Ann Emerg Med 36:602–614, 2000.
3. Baraff L: Management of febrile neonates: What to do with low-risk infants. Pediatr Infect Dis J 13:943–945, 1994.
4. Bonadio W: The history and physical assessment of the febrile infant. Pediatr Clin North Am 45:63–76, 1998.
5. Chiu C-H, Lin T-Y: Identification of febrile neonates unlikely to have bacterial infections. Pediatr Infect Dis J 16:59–63, 1997.
6. Kadish H, Loveridge B: Applying outpatient protocols to febrile infants 1–28 days of age: Can the threshold be lowered? Clin Pediatr 39:81–88, 2000.
7. Kupperman N, Flesher GR: Predictors of occult pneumococcal bacteremia in young febrile children. Ann Emerg Med 31:679–687, 1998.
8. Lopez J, McMillin K: Managing fever in infants and toddlers. Postgrad Med 101:241–251, 1997.
9. Rehm K: Fever in infants and children. Curr Opin Pediatr 13:83–88, 2001.

72. SEIZURES IN INFANCY AND CHILDHOOD

Patricia A. Braun, M.D.

1. List some common causes of pediatric seizures.
• Infection
• Trauma (epidural or subdural hematoma)
• Metabolic abnormalities (hypoglycemia, hypoxia, electrolyte abnormalities)
• Neoplasms
• Toxins (intoxication/ingestion, drug withdrawal)

2. What components of the history are important?
1. It is important to obtain details of the actual event: Was this a generalized seizure or did it start as a focal seizure? How long did it last? Was there incontinence, tongue biting, or a postictal period?
2. Inquire about possible factors that could have caused the seizure. A careful questioning for accidental or nonaccidental head trauma is essential. Is there a possibility of an ingestion? Has the child been ill with fever? Is the child prone to breath holding, or does he or she have pulmonary disease with resultant hypoxia?
3. Determine the past medical history and if there is a family history of seizures.
4. Assess the child's current neurologic status to determine whether or not it is at baseline.

3. What about the physical examination?
1. A careful neurologic examination establishes any focal deficits and determines new versus old findings.
2. Always look for evidence of head trauma and trauma to the rest of the body, which may clue you in to the possibility of abuse.
3. Do a funduscopic examination, looking for retinal hemorrhages, a sign of abuse.
4. In febrile seizures, look for the source of the fever.

4. Are there different causes of seizures in the neonate?
Seizures are more likely to be associated with inborn metabolic disorders (consider hypoglycemia, pyroxidine deficiency, or hypocalcemia), hypoxic injury, intracerebral hemorrhage, kernicterus, or drug withdrawal from maternal use. Seizures in neonates must be evaluated more aggressively than those in older children.

5. What is a febrile seizure?
A benign event usually occurring between the ages of 3 months and 5 years that is associated with fever but is without evidence of intracranial infection or another defined cause.

6. Are all febrile seizures the same?
Febrile seizures can be divided into two types. A **simple febrile seizure** is a generalized, tonic-clonic seizure that lasts fewer than 15 minutes and occurs only once in a 24-hour period in a febrile child who does not have a central nervous system infection or a severe metabolic abnormality. A **complex febrile seizure** is prolonged (i.e., lasting > 15 minutes), focal, or are multiple in a 24 hour period. A febrile seizure usually occurs within the first 24 hours of a febrile illness. There should be a return to a normal neurologic state after the seizure.

7. Is there a genetic predisposition to developing febrile seizures?
Febrile seizures run in families. Approximately 10% to 20% of younger siblings of patients who have had a febrile seizure also go on to have a febrile seizure. There is a greater chance if a parent has a history of febrile seizures.

8. What is the workup of the child with a simple febrile seizure?

If the event was a simple febrile seizure and the child's neurologic state has returned to normal, the workup should be no more than that for the evaluation of febrile illness.

9. What is the likelihood of further febrile seizures?

The risk of a first recurrence is 30%, even within the same febrile illness. The risk is 50% if the first seizure occurs in a child less than 12 months old or if the febrile seizure is a recurrence.

10. Is there a way to prevent febrile seizures?

In 1999, the American Academy of Pediatrics recognized that simple febrile seizures are a benign and common occurrence and stated that although there are a few therapies effective at preventing the recurrence of febrile seizures, the potential side effects of these drugs did not commensurate the benefit. Antipyretic medicines alone are not effective in preventing the recurrence of simple febrile seizures, although they may make the patient feel more comfortable.

11. Does a febrile seizure predict the development of epilepsy?

Only a few children who have suffered a febrile seizure go on to develop epilepsy. Children who have a family history of epilepsy, who have a history of preexisting neurologic disease, or who had a complex febrile seizure are more likely to develop epilepsy. Without these risk factors, a child has a 1% chance of developing epilepsy compared with a 0.4% chance for children who have never had a febrile seizure.

12. Which children should be considered for anticonvulsant therapy?

Because fewer than 50% of children with a single seizure have a second seizure, prophylaxis is not indicated in the ED. Prophylaxis should be considered in the presence of abnormal neurologic development or prolonged or focal seizures or in children with transient neurologic deficit.

13. What infections cause seizures?

Meningitis and **encephalitis** are associated often with seizures but, as discussed earlier, should be accompanied with other signs. *Shigella* gastroenteritis provoked seizures in 45% of patients via their endotoxins. These seizures are by definition *not* febrile seizures.

14. What is status epilepticus?

Continuous seizure activity or recurrent seizures lasting at least 30 minutes without the recovery of consciousness between attacks.

15. How should status epilepticus be treated?

Secure the airway; establish intravenous access; and obtain blood for complete blood count, electrolytes, glucose, and drug levels and toxicology screen. Administer 25% dextrose at 1 mL/kg if hypoglycemia is present. Administer 4 mL/kg of 3% normal saline for hyponatremia. The first-line agent is diazepam (0.1 to 0.5 mg/kg intravenously; maximal dose, 5 mg) or lorazepam (0.05 to 0.15 mg/kg intravenously; maximal dose, 4 mg). If a seizure lasts longer than 10 minutes, phenobarbital (20 mg/kg infused at a rate no faster than 30 mg/min) should be given. If the seizure continues, additional doses of diazepam or lorazepam may be given. If seizure activity persists, a second long-acting anticonvulsant, such as phenytoin (15 mg/kg), should be given.

16. What if there is no intravenous access?

Rectal administration of diazepam at 0.5 mg/kg of parenteral solution is absorbed rapidly. Use a tuberculin syringe to deliver the dose.

17. State the advantages of lorazepam over diazepam.

Lorazepam is a longer acting benzodiazepine than diazepam because it is less lipophilic and does not redistribute as quickly. It may have a 12- to 24-hour duration of action but does not reach peak serum concentration for 30 to 120 minutes. Lorazepam may be given intravenously, 0.05 to 0.15 mg/kg, or rectally, 0.1 to 0.4 mg/kg.

18. What if seizures continue after administration of benzodiazepines and phenytoin?
Phenobarbital is the next drug option, at a loading dose of 15 to 25 mg/kg, infusing no faster than 30 mg/min. At this point, the child should be intubated. Be sure to consider other possible causes (hypoglycemia, INH toxicity, intracerebral mass, or infection). If the seizure has not terminated, consider general anesthesia and neuromuscular blockade.

CONTROVERSY

19. Should a lumbar puncture be performed?
Most would say that in an older child without signs of meningitis, the presence of a seizure should not mandate a lumbar puncture. Because meningeal signs may be absent in children younger than 12 to 18 months, the threshold to do a lumbar puncture should be low. The threshold also should be low in a child who has had a complex febrile seizure.

BIBLIOGRAPHY

1. Baumann RJ, Duffner PK: Treatment of children with simple febrile seizures: The AAP practice parameter. Pediatr Neurol 23:11–17, 2000.
2. Bradford JC, Kyriakedes CG: Evaluation of the patient with seizures: An evidence based approach. Emerg Med Clin North Am 17:203–220, 1999.
3. Camfield PR, Camfield CS: Management and treatment of febrile seizures. Curr Probl Pediatr 27:6–14, 1997.
4. Committee on Quality Improvement, Subcommittee on Febrile Seizures, American Academy of Pediatrics: Practice parameter: Long-term treatment of the child with simple febrile seizures (AC9859). Pediatrics 103:1307–1309, 1999.
5. Hirtz DG: Febrile seizures. Pediatr Rev 18:5–8, 1997.
6. Knudsen FU: Febrile seizures: Treatment and prognosis. Epilepsia 41:2–9, 2000.
7. Mackowiak PA: Diagnostic implications and clinical consequences of antipyretic therapy. Clin Infect Dis 31(suppl 5):S230–233, 2000.
8. Pellock JM: Treatment of seizures and epilepsy in children and adolescents. Neurology 51(5 suppl 4):S8–14, 1998.
9. Sabo-Graham T, Seay AR: Management of status epilepticus in children. Pediatr Rev 19:306–309, 1998.

73. ACUTE UPPER AIRWAY OBSTRUCTION IN PEDIATRICS

Joan Bothner, M.D.

1. How common are upper airway emergencies in pediatric patients?
Upper airway obstruction is a common cause of pediatric ED visits, accounting for approximately 15% of all critically ill patients. Infectious causes account for 90% of these, with viral croup accounting for 80%. Epiglottitis accounts for 5% of severe cases. Other significant causes include other infectious pathogens (bacterial tracheitis, retropharyngeal space infections, tonsillar pathology, peritonsillar abscesses, mononucleosis, and diphtheria, which is rare today in the United States). Traumatic causes also must be considered, including foreign bodies, external trauma to the neck, burns, and iatrogenic causes (i.e., postintubation). Congenital causes must be considered in young infants. Less common causes are tumors and edema secondary to anaphylactic reactions.

2. Summarize the most common causes of upper airway emergencies in pediatric patients.

Causes of Upper Airway Obstruction

	ETIOLOGY	AGE RANGE	ONSET	TOX-ICITY	DROOL-ING	TREATMENT
Croup	Parainfluenza	6 months–3 years	URI prodrome	Mild	Absent	Mist, steroids, aerosolized epinephrine
Epiglottitis	*H. influenzae*	3–7 years	Acute	Marked	Frequent	Airway management, antibiotics
Retropharyngeal abscess	Multiple; anaerobes	Infancy–6 years	URI, sore throat	Variable	Variable	Antibiotics, drainage
Bacterial tracheitis	*S. aureus*	≥ 3 years	"Croup" prodrome	Moderate	Usually absent	Airway management, antibiotics

URI, upper respiratory infection.

3. Why are upper airway problems more serious in pediatric patients than in adults?

There are several important differences between the adult and the pediatric airway. The child's tongue is large, easily displaced, and the most common cause of airway obstruction in the obtunded child. The most narrow portion of the pediatric airway is at the cricoid ring, making obstruction with subglottic pathology more likely than in adults. The most significant contribution to increased resistance with obstruction is the small radius of the pediatric larynx (resistance is inversely related to the fourth power of the radius, or 1 mm of swelling in an infant airway causes big problems). A healthy child can tolerate moderate-to-severe airway obstruction and maintain tidal volume almost to the point of exhaustion, at which time hypoxemia, hypercapnia, and acidosis progress rapidly, leading to cardiorespiratory arrest.

4. How can you tell where the problem is?

Stridor, which is derived from the Greek word meaning "creaking," is caused by rapid, turbulent flow through a narrowed airway. The sound generated depends on the degree of constriction and the localization of the obstruction. Observation of the child often offers the best clue to localization before a cold stethoscope touches his or her chest. Supraglottic lesions, such as epiglottitis, present with inspiratory stridor, a prolonged inspiratory phase, and a muffled cry or voice. Glottic lesions lead to high-pitched inspiratory stridor and a voice that is weak or hoarse. Subglottic lesions cause expiratory stridor with a normal voice and a brassy cough. A child who assumes the *sniffing position* has a significant upper airway obstruction, as does the child who is dysphagic or drools. Expiration should be passive; active expiration with a prolonged expiratory time, recruitment of the accessory muscles, wheezing, and a *tripod* position is significant for severe lower airway obstruction. All patients who breathe noisily do not have asthma, and with a few seconds of observation one should be able to differentiate between upper and lower airway obstruction.

5. What are the signs and symptoms of respiratory distress in a child, and when should I get worried?

Tachycardia and tachypnea are common. **Tachypnea** can be defined roughly as a respiratory rate greater than 40 breaths/min in an infant and greater than 30 breaths/min in a child. **Suprasternal retractions** indicate more severe obstruction than do intercostal and subcostal retractions. Warning signs of impending respiratory failure include marked retractions, decreased or absent breath sounds, increasing tachycardia, decreasing respiratory effort or rate, decreasing stridor, and a worried or unsettled appearance. Ominous signs are decreasing level of consciousness, hypotonia, extreme pallor, head bobbing with each breath, and decreasing heart rate. **Cyanosis** is an extremely late sign in upper airway obstruction. Arterial blood gases are ancillary, are of limited value, and show only mild hypoxemia (as does pulse oximetry), until exhaustion causes hypoventilation. **Hypercapnia** and **respiratory acidosis** necessitate immediate intervention. Basically the clinical state of the child should dictate intervention, with the most important parameter being mental status. A child who does not cry is not being "good"—he or she is in big trouble.

6. Okay, the child is in trouble. What do I do?

Ensuring an adequate airway is the only priority. Supplemental oxygen should be provided, and the child needs to be allowed to assume a position of comfort. Almost all children with an upper airway obstruction can be bag-valve-mask ventilated, and this always should be tried first in a child with respiratory failure. Oral intubation is the method of choice in a child requiring assisted ventilation. Endotracheal tube size can be estimated in children older than 2 years of age by adding 16 to the child's age in years and dividing by 4. An alternative method is by using a length-based tape, which provides a more accurate estimation of correct endotracheal tube size than does the child's age. Estimation of tube size by looking at the child's little finger or nares is unreliable and no longer can be recommended. Uncuffed tubes generally are used in children younger than 8 to 10 years old because of the anatomic narrowing of the airway at the level of the cricoid cartilage. A smaller tube and stylet need to be readily available because of the possibility of significant airway edema. Assume that all children have just eaten, and pay careful attention to aspiration prevention. Also essential is a large, working suction catheter and cricoid pressure. A needle cricothyroidotomy can be done if an airway is otherwise unobtainable. Endotracheal tubes are uncuffed up to size 5.5. Nasogastric tubes are essential because children are diaphragmatic breathers and cannot ventilate with a stomach full of air.

7. Discuss the signs and symptoms of croup, who gets it, what causes it, and what the physician can do for it.

Croup, or **laryngotracheobronchitis**, is the most common cause of infectious acute upper airway obstruction. Of children seen with croup, 10% require admission, and 1% to 5% require intubation. Viral causes include parainfluenzae virus type 1 (60%), other parainfluenza viruses, influenza virus types A and B, respiratory syncytial virus, rhinoviruses, and measles. The mean age of affected patients is 18 months, with a slight male predominance, and there is a seasonal increase in cases in autumn and early winter. The classic presentation is a history of a mild upper respiratory infection, followed by increasing stridor with worsening at night. Temperature elevation may be significant, but toxicity is minimal. Drooling is uncommon, and hoarseness and a barking cough are frequent. Croup is a clinical diagnosis, and laboratory data are almost useless. The white blood cell count may be minimally elevated. Radiographic evidence, present in 40% to 50% of patients, includes a distended hypopharynx with a narrowed subglottic region or a steeple sign. Treatment includes humidified air or oxygen, and several studies have shown a positive effect of humidification. Hypoxemia correlates with respiratory rate. Antibiotics have no role in the management of uncomplicated croup. A child with a classic history, a barking cough, and no stridor at rest can be managed with humidified air and steroids and discharged home after a brief period of observation. Aerosolized epinephrine, given via nebulizer, is indicated for children with stridor at rest or with marked increase in work of breathing, and it has been shown to decrease airway obstruction. Racemic epinephrine containing L-isomers and D-isomers of epinephrine historically has been used, but L-epinephrine has been shown to be just as effective; 0.5 mL of 2.25% racemic epinephrine is equivalent to 5 mL of 1:1000 L-epinephrine. Maximal effect of nebulized epinephrine is seen within 30 minutes, with a rebound to baseline at 2 hours in some patients. Criteria for admission include stridor at rest, cyanosis or other signs of significant respiratory compromise, dehydration, questionable follow-up, and possibly extremes of age. Intubation rarely is needed but is the therapy of choice in respiratory failure.

8. What about steroids and croup?

The use of steroids results in clinical improvement and has been shown to decrease the need for hospitalization. This decrease in symptoms occurs 6 hours after administration even in children with mild-to-moderate croup. Oral dexamethasone has been shown to be as effective as parenteral (intramuscular) dexamethasone in reducing symptoms and in preventing need for reevaluation. Dosing of dexamethasone in published studies in outpatients varies from 0.15 mg/kg to 0.6 mg/kg with a maximal dose of 8 mg. Most studies used the 0.6 mg/kg dose. There is no evidence to suggest that repeat dosing is indicated or helpful. Nebulized budesonide also has been studied but has not been shown to be of any benefit over either intramuscular or oral dexamethasone and is more expensive, less available, and more difficult to administer.

9. How does croup differ from epiglottitis?

Epiglottitis classically occurs in children 3 to 7 years old. It has a rapid onset with a high fever, significant toxicity, leukocytosis, drooling, dysphagia, stridor, preference for the sitting position with the head extended, and no cough. *Haemophilus influenzae* is the most common cause, and positive blood cultures occur in 60% to 95% of patients. The incidence of epiglottitis decreased significantly after the introduction of the conjugate *H. influenzae* type B vaccine. Other implicated agents include group A β-hemolytic streptococcus, *Streptococcus pneumoniae*, *Staphylococcus aureus*, some viruses, allergic reactions, and physical and thermal injuries. Radiographic evidence of epiglottitis includes a swollen epiglottis (the *thumb* sign), thickened aryepiglottic folds, and obliteration of the vallecula. The absence of cough and the presence of agitation and drooling are highly predictive of epiglottitis, whereas presence of a cough strongly suggests croup. Epiglottitis is rare in very young patients (only 4% of cases present in patients < 1 year old), but it may present with different signs and symptoms. All studies are retrospective, but in younger patients cough is seen, there may be an upper respiratory infection prodrome, fever may be lacking, and there may be no drooling or preference for an upright posture.

10. What is the appropriate management of a patient with suspected epiglottitis?

Do not agitate the child in any way. Do not send the child for radiographs. Start high-flow oxygen via a nonrebreather bag reservoir mask, if possible. Establishment of an airway is paramount and ideally is done in a controlled manner by an anesthesiologist with a surgeon in attendance. Blood work, intravenous lines, and antibiotics can wait. Antibiotics need to be effective against *H. influenzae*; cefuroxime, ceftriaxone, and cefotaxime are recommended. If a child obstructs, bag-valve-mask ventilation should be attempted first. Elective intubation in the ED is **never** indicated.

11. Why do children with epiglottitis obstruct?

Fatigue, laryngospasm, progressive swelling of the supraglottic structures, and pooled secretions.

12. What about bacterial tracheitis (membranous laryngotracheobronchitis) and retropharyngeal space infections?

Bacterial tracheitis is an uncommon but significant cause of acute upper airway obstruction. Clinically, affected children resemble children with croup but are older (mean age 4 years in some studies), have a longer prodrome, and appear more toxic with significant cough and stridor. The clinical presentation is not as rapid as epiglottitis, and drooling usually is not seen. The cause is unclear, but secondary invasion of the airway after a viral insult, specifically parainfluenza, influenza, and respiratory syncytial virus, is suspected. The most common bacterial pathogen is *S. aureus*, but *H. influenzae*, *S. pneumoniae*, and *Moraxella (Branhamella) catarrhalis* also have been isolated. Leukocytosis is common, and radiography may show subglottic narrowing with irregular intratracheal densities and clouding of the tracheal air column. Airway management and broad-spectrum antibiotics are the mainstay of therapy. Endoscopy is the diagnostic method of choice; findings include edema of the supraglottis, ulceration, and pseudomembrane formation in the trachea. Because of tenacious secretions, 60% to 80% of affected patients require establishment of an artificial airway and meticulous suctioning. Plugged endotracheal tubes are the most common cause of deterioration, and common complications include pneumonia, atelectasis, and cardiopulmonary arrest caused by airway obstruction. Blood cultures are almost always negative. Racemic epinephrine is of no proven benefit, and some authors believe that a lack of response differentiates bacterial tracheitis from croup.

Retropharyngeal space infections rarely cause true upper airway obstruction, but they deserve mention because of the need to differentiate this problem from croup and epiglottitis and the concern for an increase in incidence of these infections, which seems to correlate with culture-positive group A β-hemolytic streptococcal abscesses. About 90% of all cases occur in patients younger than 6 years. Symptoms include dysphagia, drooling, fever, nuchal rigidity with neck extension, stridor, irritability, and varying degrees of respiratory distress. Neck swelling may be seen, specifically posterior adenopathy. A prodrome of an upper respiratory infection with a complaint of sore throat is common. This infection is believed to arise from an extension of an acute infection of the ear, nose, or throat with spread to the retropharyngeal space. Trauma to the nasopharynx (e.g., from accidents with pencils) is also a predisposing factor. Cellulitis, or inflammation of the lymph nodes in the prevertebral space, occurs first with progression to abscess formation and suppuration. Causative agents include gram-negative rods, anaerobes, β-lactamase-producing organisms, *S. aureus*, and various streptococci. Diagnosis can be difficult in young children who cannot localize pain to the retropharyngeal space, and a retropharyngeal *bulge* on physical examination often is not seen. Lateral neck films are diagnostic (90% sensitivity) but can be difficult to interpret depending on the phase of respiration and neck position. Findings include increase in the width of the prevertebral space to greater than the anteroposterior width of the adjacent cervical vertebral body, anterior displacement of the airway, and loss of the normal step-off at the level of the larynx. Air-fluid levels are seen after abscess formation. CT scanning is highly sensitive, is helpful in equivocal cases, and is used to differentiate abscess from phlegmon or soft tissue cellulitis.

Treatment includes hospital admission, parenteral antibiotic therapy, and incision and drainage if an abscess is present. Most children do not need acute airway intervention. The most common presentation is a young child who appears mildly toxic, has an upper respiratory infection and a fever, and is alert, but who is holding his head stiffly and slightly extended. Extension of the neck seems to be most painful, versus pain with flexion as seen in meningitis. The patient may be drooling but usually is not in much respiratory distress. This diagnosis can be difficult to make, and a high index of suspicion often pays off. Consider it in young children who present with a sore throat, significant cervical adenopathy, and reluctance to move their neck.

13. When should a foreign body be suspected?

Most patients who present with foreign-body aspiration are younger than 3 years old and rarely are younger than 5 months; most are male. A history of an aspiration event is lacking in 30% to 50% of patients. The most commonly aspirated object is food, and most ends up in the esophagus or in the lower airways. Signs and symptoms depend on the site of obstruction. Patients with upper airway foreign bodies present with tachypnea, stridor, retractions, voice changes, cough, and wheezing. Absence of a positive history often delays diagnosis, so foreign bodies should be suspected in children who do not respond to appropriate intervention. Plain radiographs in upper airway obstruction can be suggestive, showing narrowing of the subglottic airway with a minimal opacity in the narrowed lumen. Fluoroscopy reveals prominent overinflation of the hypopharynx, decreased trachea diameter on inspiration, and distention of the trachea and collapse of the hypopharynx with expiration. Endoscopy is diagnostic. Immediate management depends on the degree of respiratory distress, but it should be minimal unless respiratory failure is imminent. Basic life support measures should be tried first (back blows, chest thrusts, and abdominal thrusts). If unconsciousness occurs, direct laryngoscopy should follow with attempted removal of the foreign object with Magill forceps if it can be visualized. If this fails, bag-valve-mask ventilation and intubation should be attempted, which ideally push the offending object into a bronchus. If the child cannot be intubated, a needle cricothyroidotomy should be attempted.

14. What about the child who has stridor and wheezing?

Consider congenital lesions in patients younger than 4 months old, especially if they have recurrent problems. The causes of stridor and wheezing in older infants and children include foreign bodies in the airway and in the esophagus and combinations of infectious causes.

CONTROVERSIES

15. The incidence of epiglottitis has decreased dramatically, but what are the major areas of controversy in the management of this disease?

To look or not to look. For fear of inducing a vasovagal episode, respiratory obstruction, and cardiovascular collapse, ED visualization of the epiglottitis in a child with acute stridor and in whom the diagnosis of epiglottitis is considered is not usually advocated. A study that directly addressed the question found no complications in patients with epiglottitis and no missed cases, however, although the numbers were small. Visualization was done, in the presence of an anesthesiologist, in children in whom epiglottitis was strongly suspected. Visualization first was attempted simply by asking the child to open his or her mouth, then by using a tongue depressor in the sitting child, with careful attention not to touch the epiglottis. These maneuvers were successful in more than 50% of patients. Use of a laryngoscope with the child sitting up was successful in an additional 30% of patients, and having the child lie supine was necessary only in 15% of patients. This author has concluded that visualization is a safe and effective aid in the evaluation of children with acute stridor. Visualization is not advocated for children in whom epiglottitis is strongly suspected but more as an aid in the diagnosis of questionable cases in lieu of radiographs.

The role of radiographs. Children with epiglottitis may have a normal-appearing epiglottis with distention of the hypopharynx being the only finding. Radiographs are read as falsely abnormal 30% of the time by ED physicians and radiologists. Children obstruct and arrest in radiology departments. Radiographs should be ordered only when someone is available who can read them correctly, when the child can be accompanied at all times, and if the diagnosis is in doubt. Direct visualization saves time and money, is more sensitive and specific, and may be safer. Obtaining a radiograph in a patient who clinically has epiglottitis is not useful.

Transport. Is establishment of an airway before transport necessary? Some centers advocate elective intubation of all transported patients. Children with epiglottitis have been transported safely without intubation, whereas some others experienced significant problems. The answer depends on many factors, including the degree of respiratory distress, the length of time of transport, and, most importantly, the skill in pediatric airway evaluation and management by the transporting personnel. The same controversy applies to hospitalized patients. Some centers observe patients with *mild* epiglottitis without airway management, although large clinical trials of this approach are lacking.

16. Do all patients who receive aerosolized epinephrine for croup need to be hospitalized?

Clinical studies showed that the dogma of the *rebound phenomenon* after aerosolized epinephrine does not exist; children who receive aerosolized epinephrine tend to return to their baseline level of respiratory distress when the effects of the aerosol have worn off. Several studies documented that it is safe to send children with mild-to-moderate croup home after a 2- to 4-hour postepinephrine observation period. In all of these studies, the children also were given dexamethasone. All of these studies used the racemic form of epinephrine. Although this approach is becoming more common, other factors, including available appropriate caretakers, reliable transportation, and distance from the hospital, must be considered before discharging home after a short period of observation in the ED children whose symptoms warranted aerosolized epinephrine. Such children must be able to keep themselves hydrated, have no significant increased work of breathing, and have no stridor at rest.

17. What is heliox, and how is it used in croup?

Helium decreases turbulent flow and airway resistance and has been used for decades in the management of patients with upper airway obstruction. Heliox is typically a 70% helium/30%

oxygen mixture. Two studies evaluated the use of heliox in hospitalized patients with croup. In a retrospective report of 42 patients, a reduction in the work of breathing was documented. In a second prospective, randomized study comparing heliox with racemic epinephrine in children hospitalized with severe croup who already had received intramuscular dexamethasone and humidified oxygen, both therapies were associated with a significant reduction in the croup score, but neither heliox nor racemic epinephrine showed a clear benefit over the other. Larger, randomized clinical trials are warranted to evaluate this therapy further.

BIBLIOGRAPHY

1. American Academy of Pediatrics, American Heart Association: Pediatric Advanced Life Support Provider Manual. Dallas, AHA, 2002.
2. Ausejo M, Saenz A, Pham B, et al: Glucocorticoids for croup. Cochrane Database Syst Rev 2:CD001955, 2000.
3. Fleisher G, Ludwig S (eds): Textbook of Pediatric Emergency Medicine, 4th ed. Baltimore, Williams & Wilkins, 2000.
4. Grosz AH, Jacobs IN, Cho C, Schears GJ: Use of helium-oxygen mixtures to relieve upper airway obstruction in a pediatric population. Laryngoscope 111:1512–1514, 2001.
5. Kirse DJ, Roberson DW: Surgical management of retropharyngeal space infections in children. Laryngoscope 111:1413–1422, 2001.
6. Klaussen TP, Craig WR, Moher D, et al: Nebulized budesonide and oral dexamethasone for the treament of croup: A randomized controlled trial. JAMA 279:1629–1632, 1998.
7. Lee SS, Schwartz RH, Bahadori RS: Retropharyngeal abscess: Epiglottitis of the new millennium. J Pediatr 138:435–437, 2001.
8. Ritticher KK, Ledwith CA: Outpatient treatment of moderate croup with dexamethasone: Intramuscular versus oral dosing. Pediatrics 106:1344–1348, 2000.
9. Weber JE, Chudnofsky CR, Younger JG, et al: A randomized comparison of helium-oxygen mixture (Heliox) and racemic epinephrine for the treatment of moderate to severe croup. Pediatrics 107:96, 2001.
10. Wright RB, Pomerantz WJ, Luria JW: New approaches to respiratory infections in children. Emerg Med Clin North Am 20:93–114, 2002.

74. PEDIATRIC BRONCHIOLITIS AND ASTHMA

Julie Seaman, M.D.

BRONCHIOLITIS

1. In what age group does bronchiolitis usually occur?

Infants and toddlers. It is seen most frequently in children between the ages of 3 and 6 months. Although older children and adults acquire the same viral infection of the smaller airways, they do not develop the clinical picture of bronchiolitis because bronchiolar edema is tolerated better in adults.

2. Name the clinical signs and symptoms.

Tachypnea, wheezing, nasal flaring, and retractions. These symptoms are usually preceded by 1 to 2 days of rhinorrhea, cough, or low-grade fever. Auscultation may reveal diffuse wheezing, prolonged expiration, and rales. Young infants may present with apnea only. Expiration may be prolonged, as with other obstructive lower airway respiratory illnesses.

3. What are the causes of bronchiolitis?

Respiratory syncytial virus (RSV) is responsible for more than 50% of cases. Parainfluenza, adenovirus, and influenza cause most other cases.

4. How is RSV transmitted?

Peak outbreaks of RSV occur in winter and spring. It is highly contagious and is transmitted by direct contact with contaminated surfaces (fomites) or secretions of infected patients (large droplet aerosols).

5. What is the pathophysiology of bronchiolitis?

Invasion of the smaller bronchioles by virus leads to edema and mucus and cellular debris accumulation, which causes bronchiolar obstruction and ventilation-perfusion mismatching.

6. What is the differential diagnosis of wheezing?

Asthma, bronchiolitis, foreign-body aspiration, pneumonia, cystic fibrosis, bronchiectasis, gastroesophageal reflux, and heart failure. Bronchiolitis is confused most often with asthma and may be indistinguishable from the initial presentation of asthma accompanied by a viral illness. Asthma usually has a more pronounced and prompt response to bronchodilators and is more likely in a child with previous episodes of wheezing and risk factors for asthma.

7. Name the radiographic findings of bronchiolitis.

Hyperinflation and a flattened diaphragm caused by air trapping are the most common findings. Parahilar peribronchial infiltrates and atelectasis may be present and indistinguishable from bacterial pneumonia.

8. What is the role of bronchodilators in the treatment of bronchiolitis?

The utility of bronchodilators in bronchiolitis is unclear. Despite multiple randomized, controlled trials, conclusive evidence of efficacy is still lacking. Common practice is to initiate a trial of a β-agonist nebulizer in the ED. If the child responds with decreasing wheezes, decreasing respiratory effort, or decreasing respiratory rate, the bronchodilator is continued for at least the first 48 hours of illness.

9. Is there a role for steroids in bronchiolitis?

Steroids have no proven benefit and are not recommended.

10. When should ribavirin be used?

Most clinical trials show that early ribavirin therapy improves oxygenation, decreases the need for mechanical ventilation, shortens hopitalizations, and improves pulmonary function. Based on concerns of cost, efficacy, and safety, however, ribivarin is indicated only in specific cases. When RSV has been confirmed, ribivarin may be givin to patients in severe respiratory distress, patients with comorbid conditions (congenital heart disease, bronchopulmonary dysplasia, cystic fibrosis, immunodeficiencies, recent transplant recipients, and children undergoing chemotherapy), and patients younger than 6 weeks.

11. Is there a way to prevent RSV infection?

As always, good hand washing and surface cleaning go a long way to protect against transmission. So far, attempts to produce a useful vaccine have been unsuccessful. There are two prophylactic therapies of RSV. Passive immunity with intravenous immunoglobulin specifically against RSV (RSV-IGIV) has been shown to decrease hospitalization and severity of disease in high-risk children. Palivizumab is a monoclonal antibody directed against the F protien. It is administered by monthy intramuscular injections and has been shown to decrease hospitalizations. Both methods are considered safe and effective but are restricted to high-risk infants.

12. How does bronchiolitis caused by parainfluenza virus differ from that caused by RSV?

Parainfluenza type 3 is the second most common cause of bronchiolitis. Peak incidence is in spring and summer. Ribavirin seems to inhibit viral replication of parainfluenza but has not shown clinical benefit and is not recommended.

13. List the admission criteria for bronchiolitis.

Age younger than 2 months
Hypoxemia on room air
History of apnea
Moderate tachypnea with feeding difficulties
Respiratory distress
Underlying chronic cardiopulmonary disorders

14. Is an episode of bronchiolitis a risk factor for the development of asthma?

It is unclear whether episodes of bronchiolitis are a causative feature of asthma or whether children who go on to develop asthma have an abnormality of their pulmonary physiology causing them to be more susceptible to bronchiolitis. Many children (30% to 50%) with bronchiolitis later carry a diagnosis of asthma, however. These children are more likely to have a family history of asthma and allergy, a prolonged acute episode of bronchiolitis, and exposure to cigarette smoke.

ASTHMA

15. Define asthma.

Asthma is a lung disease with the following characteristics: airway obstruction, inflammation, and hyperresponsiveness. **Airway obstruction** (blocking) or narrowing is responsible for the wheezing noises and cough and is usually reversible spontaneously or with treatment. The obstruction or narrowing can be caused by swelling, excessive mucus, or muscle contraction. **Inflammation** is caused by special cells (mast cells, macrophages) that release substances that damage the lining of the airway. **Hyperresponsiveness** is constriction of the airway triggered by environmental irritants, viral respiratory infections, cold air, or exercise.

16. What children are at highest risk for development of asthma?

The incidence and mortality have been rising steadily, especially in inner-city children. The risk of death from asthma is roughly three times higher for black children compared with white children. Before puberty, boys outnumber girls 2:1. With advancing age, asthma is seen as often in girls as in boys.

17. What is the natural history of asthma?

Of all asthmatic children, 50% are virtually free of symptoms within 10 to 20 years. Of children with severe asthma, 95% are symptomatic as adults.

18. How are bronchodilators used in the management of acute asthma?

Selective β_2-agonists are the mainstay of medications to reverse bronchospasm. In children with moderate-to-severe asthma, inhaled anticholinergic therapy (ipatroprium bromide) has been shown to decrease severity and hospitalizaiton rate when given in conjunction with β_2-agonists (albuterol).

19. When and how should steroids be administered?

Controlling inflammation is the cornerstone of asthma treatment. Steroids are indicated in wheezing patients whose symptoms do not resolve rapidly with bronchodilator treatment. A common practice is to prescribe a 5-day course of prednisone or prednisolone. Typically, prescribe 2 mg/kg orally (maximum 60 mg), followed by 1 mg/kg/d for the next 4 days. Oral prednisone has been shown to be as effective as intravenous methylprednisolone. An alternative to prednisone is dexamethasone. At a dose of 0.6 mg/kg (maximum, 16 mg) as initial treatment followed by the same dose in 12 to 24 hours, dexamethasone has shown similar efficacy, improved compliance, and fewer side effects compared with 5 days of prednisone. Dexamethasone causes adrenal suppression more readily than prednisone. It should be used with caution in patients with frequent asthma exacerbations. To decrease relapse, prescribe inhaled steroids at discharge in addition to oral steroids. Some studies showed nearly a 50% decrease in relapse and a decreased need for β_2-agonist use when outpatient inhaled steroids are added.

20. When is an arterial blood gas evaluation indicated in the ED?

Rarely. Patients usually can be evaluated clinically for fatigue, change in mental status, and decreasing oxygenation via pulse oximetry. The decision to mechanically ventilate a patient is made clinically. Arterial blood gas evaluation may be useful, however, when there is clinical doubt regarding the presence or development of hypercapnia. Initially, hyperventilation causes a low PCO_2. As airway obstruction worsens, the PCO_2 rises to normal or higher. A PCO_2 of 40 to 45 mmHg in the presence of respiratory distress indicates impending respiratory failure. Hypoxemia is common but usually reverses after the patient has received oxygen. Persistent hypoxemia (oxygen saturation < 90% or PO_2 < 60 mmHg on high-flow oxygen) is another indicator of respiratory failure. Arterial blood gas evaluation is vital in managing patients with severe respiratory compromise who are mechanically ventilated.

21. What should I do if my patient is going into respiratory failure?

Consider treatment with heliox, terbutaline, and epinephrine. If intubation is necessary, ketamine and paralysis are useful adjuncts.

22. What initial ventilator settings would you recommend for a child with asthma and respiratory failure who requires mechanical ventilation?

A large tidal volume and a slow rate usually are needed to provide adequate time for exhalation, preventing breath stacking and the potential for pneumothorax. A tidal volume of 15 mL/kg with a rate of 20 to 25 breaths/min in infants or 8 to 12 breaths/min in adolescents is a general starting point. Positive end-expiratory pressure should be avoided to prevent further risk of barotrauma. Sedation and neuromuscular blockade usually are indicated.

23. During an exacerbation of asthma, when should a chest radiograph be obtained? What are the findings?

A chest radiograph is indicated if pneumonia, pneumothorax, pneumomediastinum, or foreign body is suspected clinically. Chest radiographs commonly show hyperinflation, atelectasis, and peribronchial thickening, indicating lower airway obstruction. Approximately 25% of radiographs taken during an acute asthma attack show an abnormality other than hyperinflation. Pneumothorax is rare. Pneumomediastinum is more common in older children (age > 10 years), whereas infiltrates are more common in younger children.

24. Outline the initial assessment, evaluation, and treatment of an asthma exacerbation in the ED.

Step 1: Initial assessment
- Evaluate vital signs with pulse oximetry, use of accessory muscles, retractions, alertness, auscultation, and peak flow measurement.

Step 2: Initial treatment
- Administer oxygen as needed to keep saturation in the normal range.
- Administer nebulized albuterol every 20 minutes or continuously, depending on severity.
- Consider nebulized ipratropium bromide and albuterol if severity is moderate to severe.
- Begin steroids if symptoms are not resolved after one nebulized albuterol treatment. Oral prednisone, 2 mg/kg up to 60 mg, usually is used as the first dose. If patient is unable to tolerate oral medication, methylprednisolone, 2 mg/kg intravenously, may be used. Dexamethasone, 0.6 mg/kg up to 16 mg orally or intramuscularly, is another alternative.

Step 3: Repeat assessment
- If peak expiratory flow rate is greater than 70% baseline and there is no wheezing, retractions, or accessory muscle use, observe the patient for at least 1 hour after the last nebulized treatment.

Step 4a: Discharge
- Discharge home with a reliable caretaker, patient education, medications, and follow-up instructions.
- Medications should include albuterol, nebulized or inhaled every 4 hours as needed for wheezing, and prednisone, 1 to 2 mg/kg/d divided once or twice daily for a total of 5 days, or dexamethasone, one dose of 0.6 mg/kg the following day.

Step 4b: Admission
- For severe exacerbations unresponsive to albuterol, ipratropium bromide, and steroids, consider terbutaline drip, magnesium, aminophylline, heliox, ketamine, and paralysis with intubation.

BIBLIOGRAPHY

1. Flores G, Horwitz R: Efficacy of β_2-agonists in bronchiolitis: A reappraisal and meta-analysis. Pediatrics 100:233–239, 1997.
2. Hay WW, Groothuis JR, Hayward AR, Levin MJ (eds): Current Pediatric Diagnosis and Treatment, 13th ed. Stamford, CT, Appleton & Lange, 1997.
3. Orenstein DM: Bronchiolitis. In Behrman RE, Kliegman RM, Arvin AM (eds): Nelson Textbook of Pediatrics, 15th ed. Philadelphia, W.B. Saunders, 1996.
4. Quireshi F, Pestian J, David P, Zaritsky A: Effect of nebulized ipratropium on the hospitalization rates of children with asthma. N Engl J Med 339:1030–1035, 1998.
5. Qureshi F, Zaritsky A, Poirier M: Comparative efficacy of oral dexamethasone versus oral prednisone in acute pediatric asthma. J Pediatr 139:20–26, 2001.
6. Rowe BH: Nebulized ipratropium bromide in acute pediatric asthma: Does it reduce hospital admissions among children presenting to the emergency department? Ann Emerg Med 34:75–85, 1999.
7. Rowe BH, Bota GW, Fabris L: Inhaled budesonide in addition to oral corticosteroids to prevent asthma relapse following discharge from the emergency department. JAMA 281:2119–2126, 1999.
8. Sandritter TL, Kraus DM: Respiratory syncytial virus-immunoglobulin intravenous (RSV-IGIV) for respiratory syncytial viral infections. J Pediatr Health Care 11:284–291, 1997.
9. Sly RM: Asthma. In Behrman RE, Kliegman RM, Arvin AM (eds): Nelson Textbook of Pediatrics, 15th ed. Philadelphia, W.B. Saunders, 1996, pp 628–640.
10. Werner HA: Status asthmaticus in children, a review. Chest 119:1913–1929, 2001.
11. Yamamoto LG, Wiebe RA, Matthews WJ: A one-year series of pediatric emergency department wheezing visits: The Hawaii EMS-C project. Pediatr Emerg Care 8:17–26, 1992.

75. PEDIATRIC GASTROINTESTINAL DISORDERS AND DEHYDRATION

Mark E. Anderson, M.D.

1. What are the most common causes of acute abdominal pain in children?

The most common cause of acute abdominal pain in children is **nonspecific abdominal pain** and a specific cause may never be identified. The next most common cause of abdominal pain among children is acute appendicitis (32%). Other causes are grouped more easily according to patient age. In infants younger than 2 years old, causes include colic, gastroenteritis, viral illness, and constipation. Older children may experience pain caused by functional disorders, gastroenteritis, constipation, urinary tract infection, appendicitis, pelvic inflammatory disease, ectopic pregnancy, and inflammatory bowel disease. Uncommon but serious causes of abdominal pain include intussusception, volvulus, pancreatitis, diabetes, Meckel's diverticulum, sickle cell disease, leukemia, lymphomas, and testicular or ovarian torsion.

2. How should I approach the workup of a pediatric patient with abdominal pain?

Children may pose unique challenges because of their inability to articulate their complaints; however, much can be gained by carefully observing the patient while taking the history from the caregivers. Allow the patient to describe his or her complaints by asking age-appropriate questions. An adolescent should be given more independence and the opportunity to answer some questions, especially those pertaining to sexual activity, without the caregiver present. History from the caregivers and the patient should address acuteness; progression; timing; quality; location; radiation; severity; effect on physical activity; aggravating or alleviating factors; and associated symptoms, such as nausea, vomiting, diarrhea, dysuria, vaginal discharge, and menstrual history. The physical examination should include vital signs and temperature, determination of hydration status, a chest examination, a thorough abdominal examination (auscultated bowel sounds, palpable masses, tenderness, guarding, or rebound), an external genital examination, and a rectal examination. A pelvic examination should be done in all pubescent girls with lower quadrant abdominal pain or symptoms of pelvic disease. Ancillary data may include urinalysis, complete blood cell count, electrolytes, amylase, cultures for gonorrhea and *Chlamydia*, and diagnostic imaging including a chest radiograph.

3. **List the most common causes of gastrointestinal (GI) bleeding in children.**

Common causes of GI bleeding are differentiated most easily by determining upper versus lower GI bleeding, then by grouping according to patient age.

Upper GI bleeding produces positive nasogastric aspirates and generally develops from a site above the ligament of Treitz. It may present as hematemesis, coffee-ground emesis, or melena.
- **Neonates**: Idiopathic, ingested maternal blood, gastritis, esophagitis, peptic ulcer disease, bleeding diathesis.
- **Infants**: Idiopathic, gastritis, esophagitis, peptic ulcer disease, foreign-body ingestion, caustic ingestion.
- **Children**: Esophageal varices, esophagitis, peptic ulcer disease, foreign-body ingestion, caustic ingestion.

Lower GI bleeding is distal to the ligament of Treitz and may present as hematochezia or melena.
- **Neonates**: Benign anorectal lesions, upper GI bleeding, milk allergy, midgut volvulus.
- **Infants**: Benign anorectal lesions (anal fissure), intussusception, Meckel's diverticulum, infectious diarrhea, upper GI bleeding, milk allergy, lymphonodular hyperplasia of the colon.
- **Children**: Juvenile colonic polyps, benign anorectal lesions, intussusception, Meckel's diverticulum, infectious diarrhea, upper GI bleeding, inflammatory bowel disease.

In small children, massive GI bleeds may lead to shock before the onset of hematemesis or melena.

4. **How does the character of blood help determine the location of GI bleeding?**
- **Bright red hematemesis**: Little or no contact with the gastric secretions, usually active bleeding at a site at or above the cardia of the stomach.
- **Coffee-ground hematemesis**: Altered by gastric secretions.
- **Melena and tarry stools**: Requires blood loss greater than 50 to 100 mL in 24 hours and usually originates proximal to the ileocecal valve.
- **Streaks of blood on stool**: Lesion in rectal ampulla or in the anal canal.
- **Hematochezia**: Brisk hemorrhage or hemorrhage distal to the ileocecal valve.

5. **What is the Apt test?**

A test used to evaluate suspected upper GI bleeding in the neonate to determine the presence of swallowed maternal blood. A sample of the nasogastric aspirate or vomitus is placed on filter paper with a 1% NaOH solution. Fetal hemoglobin is more resistant to reduction and remains pink or bright red, whereas adult hemoglobin reduces more easily and turns yellow or rusty brown.

6. **What causes newborn jaundice, and when is it worrisome?**

Newborns normally become jaundiced to the face and upper chest in the first few days of life as the liver develops a capacity to conjugate bilirubin. **Physiologic newborn jaundice** should not exceed a rise of 5 mg/dL per day of life and always should consist of **unconjugated** bilirubin. The conjugated portion should not exceed 20% of the total, and the newborn infant should not appear jaundiced in the first day of life. Entities that may result in red blood cell hemolysis, such as glucose-6-phosphate dehydrogenase deficiency or neonatal sepsis, may present as jaundice.

7. How do I perform anoscopy on a neonate?

By inserting the rounded, closed end of a test tube into the neonate's rectum, you can detect local bleeding or inflammation.

8. How should constipation be managed in the outpatient setting?

As a general rule in the outpatient treatment of constipation in children, **disimpaction** is necessary before the initiation of long-term therapy. This can be accomplished with one or two enemas, remembering to use smaller or *junior* enemas for children. Long-term therapy involves the addition of free water to the diet and fiber-rich or bulk foods. In some cases, mineral oil or another mild stool softener can be used to prevent the formation of hardened stool. Encopresis, or involuntary stooling behavior, can be a sign of constipation or of a behavioral problem.

9. What serious entities can present as constipation in infants and children?

Apparent constipation in an infant can be an early manifestation of Hirschsprung's disease, wherein a portion of the large bowel, usually the distal segment, is devoid of ganglion cells, rendering the bowel incapable of coordinated motility. In its severe form, toxic megacolon, this can be life-threatening. Diagnosis is made on colonic biopsy showing the absence of ganglionic cells in the affected portion of bowel. Cystic fibrosis also may present with a complaint of difficulty with stooling. Well-formed stools in a child with cystic fibrosis are produced with great effort; in many cases, the diagnosis may have been made already, either through a primary care provider or on newborn screening in some states. Growth failure is a typical concomitant feature. Diagnosis can be made by measurement of sweat chloride in a special but relatively straightforward laboratory test.

10. What are the symptoms of an esophageal foreign body?

A normal infant investigates most objects by placing the object in his or her mouth. This normal developmental behavior can cause an airway or esophageal foreign body. Most swallowed items pass through the GI tract when the object is moved into the stomach. Parents can be advised to expect a surprise in the infant's stool over the next few days. On acute presentation, an airway foreign body must be suspected and ruled out. Commonly swallowed items such as coins appear in their widest dimension on frontal radiographs because the coronal plane of the esophagus is more distensible. Extra airway noise is an ominous sign and should alert the practitioner to prepare for urgent airway manipulation or consultation to help manage the foreign body. The upper airway in an infant or child is more funnel shaped than the adult airway, and foreign objects typically are lodged in the upper airway; this causes stridor, or a high-pitched inspiratory noise.

11. Using a posteroanterior film, how can I determine whether a coin is in the esophagus or in the trachea?

A coin in the esophagus lies in the frontal plane and usually appears as a full circle on a posteroanterior film. A coin in the trachea lies in the sagittal plane because the incomplete cartilage rings of the posterior trachea offer more space with less resistance, and the coin usually appears end-on as a line. The presumed location should be confirmed by obtaining a lateral film.

12. When should a foreign body of the GI tract be removed?

Any foreign body causing symptoms should be removed. Foreign bodies also should be removed if they appear lodged in the esophagus. Some clinicians advocate observing ingested coins for 24 hours in the hope of spontaneous passage, provided that the patient is truly asymptomatic. A conservative approach is the general rule when objects have cleared the esophagus, and passage can require days to weeks. Follow-up is important, and parents should be instructed to return with concerns, abdominal pain, fever, vomiting, and hematemesis or melena.

Removal of disc batteries is controversial. In the past, routine removal was advocated because of the potential for alkaline material to leak out and cause mucosal damage. Some gastroenterologists now prefer to follow closely ingestion of disc batteries if the battery is smaller than 15 to 20 mm. GI consultation should be obtained to determine appropriate management.

13. Describe the typical findings in appendicitis.

The classic presentation is crampy, periumbilical pain that gradually shifts to the right lower quadrant over 4 to 12 hours. After the onset of pain, associated symptoms include nausea and vomiting, anorexia, and mild fever. The patient may prefer to lie on his or her side with flexion at the hips. Physical examination may show decreased bowel sounds, maximal tenderness at McBurney's point (located 4 to 6 cm from the iliac crest on a line drawn between the iliac crest and the umbilicus), and positive psoas or obturator signs. Laboratory analysis may reveal an elevated white blood cell count with a left-shifted differential. Younger children more often have perforated appendicitis (almost 100% of patients < 1 year old). This can be a difficult diagnosis to make in a young child or infant because the classic presenting symptoms and signs often are not present.

14. What is intussusception?

Intussusception occurs when a portion of bowel telescopes into a neighboring segment, compromising vascular integrity of the involved bowel. It is rare in children younger than 3 months old and decreases in frequency after 3 years of age. The classic presentation is with intermittent irritability in a child. The periods of irritability may be associated with the child drawing his or her legs up to the chest. Intussusception also can present simply as altered mental status. Older individuals with intussusception may have a pathologic lead point, such as lymphadenopathy from lymphoma, Meckel's diverticulum, or Henoch-Schönlein purpura. These cases also are more likely to recur. Males are affected more often than females, and the incidence is about 1 to 4 cases in 1,000 live births. The treatment is prompt reduction either by a radiologist with air contrast or barium enema or surgical reduction.

15. What is Meckel's diverticulum?

A persistence of the omphalomesenteric duct remnant. It is the most common congenital malformation of the intestine, occurring in 2% to 3% of the population. It is approximately 2 to 3 cm long and, in 50% of cases, contains heterotopic tissue (gastric mucosa, pancreatic tissue, or endometrium). It usually is found on the antimesenteric border of the distal small bowel, approximately 90 cm proximal to the ileocecal valve. It is estimated that only 5% of patients become symptomatic. These patients are usually boys with a peak incidence at 2 years of age. The presence of gastric mucosa is associated with the formation of bleeding ulcers in the diverticulum, which usually present as painless rectal bleeding. Meckel's diverticulum also may present as an obstruction secondary to intussusception or volvulus formation.

16. How is hypertrophic pyloric stenosis best diagnosed?

The classic clinical presentation is a first-born 2- to 6-week-old male infant with progressive projectile, nonbilious emesis and failure to gain weight if symptoms are prolonged. Examination findings may include visible peristaltic waves, dehydration, and a palpable olive-shaped mass. Diagnosis can be confirmed by ultrasound of the hypertrophied pylorus or by an upper GI barium swallow showing a narrowing of the distal antrum and pylorus (*string sign*). Many authors recommend starting with a barium swallow because this provides the ability to diagnose other problems that may be considered in the differential diagnosis of hypertrophic pyloric stenosis (e.g., reflux, antral web, pylorospasm, malrotation). The availability of these procedures in children may depend on the institution and may factor into the decision regarding which test to order.

17. What are the typical electrolyte abnormalities in hypertrophic pyloric stenosis?

The projectile vomiting of hypertrophic pyloric stenosis typically causes a hypochloremic, hypokalemic metabolic alkalosis. Any combination of electrolytes can be seen with this diagnosis, and the associated laboratory findings are nonspecific.

18. What is a volvulus?

A twisting of the bowel on its own axis, causing a closed-loop intraluminal obstruction and occlusion of its blood supply. It is more common in children older than 1 year of age and may involve gastric, midgut, transverse, or sigmoid colonic tissue with inadequate posterior peritoneal attachment. Patients typically present with abdominal pain and vomiting. On examination, they may be found to have abdominal distention and a palpable abdominal mass.

19. What are the usual causes of diarrhea in infants and children?

Most diarrheal illness in pediatric patients is viral induced and self-limited in otherwise healthy individuals. The cause is largely seasonal for the viral agents. Rotavirus is a common agent and is noteworthy as a cause of multiple (10 to 20) loose, watery stools per day. With this degree of fluid loss, attention to hydration status is the mainstay of outpatient and inpatient treatment. Many viral causes of diarrhea exist. Bacterial sources also may cause profuse, watery diarrhea, but the presence of pus or mucus in the stool may help delineate these from viral causes. *Shigella* is noteworthy for the associated tenesmus and small-volume squirts of diarrhea that are associated. Fevers can be seen with viral and bacterial causes, but the associated misery of the child may be worse with invasive bacterial enteritis. The peripheral white blood cell count may be normal or elevated.

20. A 10-month-old infant presents with a high fever and an associated 2-minute generalized tonic-clonic seizure; peripheral white blood cell count is 11,000/μL with 30% segmented forms and 40% bands; the child has notable watery diarrhea. What is the diagnosis?

Shigella.

21. How should diarrhea be managed?

The patient's hemodynamic stability should be assessed quickly and treated if necessary. The decision to rehydrate orally or intravenously is made by assessing the patient's degree of dehydration (recent urine output, any mental status changes). Fluid losses amounting to moderate or severe dehydration (easy to calculate if a recent weight is known or documented) generally require aggressive intravenous fluid therapy while monitoring the patient closely. Infants and children may improve rapidly, then show interest in taking fluids orally. Because most diarrheal illnesses are viral in nature, no specific therapy is indicated. The presence of gross blood should alert the physician to the possibility of hemolytic-uremic syndrome, and stool should be cultured in this instance. Microscopic blood can be present with viral and bacterial causes. The presence of pus or mucus should prompt a stool culture. Empirical antibiotics are not indicated if the patient is not immunocompromised, very young, or very ill. Certain bacterial causes, such as *Shigella*, require antibiotic treatment generally because this agent is so infectious. Conversely, *Salmonella* generally does not require specific treatment, and careful attention to prevent additional fecal and oral spread is the mainstay of therapy.

22. What are the three major categories of dehydration?

1. Isotonic
2. Hypotonic or hyponatremic
3. Hypertonic or hypernatremic

23. What is oral rehydration therapy, and when is it appropriate?

The administration of small volumes of oral fluid solution (Pedialyte, Rehydralyte, Infalyte) containing glucose and electrolytes to reverse dehydration. The oral glucose in these solutions facilitates absorption of sodium and water across the mucosal cells of the small intestine. This process may take 4 to 8 hours, and it may be instituted in any patient with mild-to-moderate dehydration, who can tolerate oral fluids, even if the patient continues to have diarrhea. Instruct the parent or provider to offer sips of fluid frequently and give precautions to monitor closely for urine output and changing mental status. Infants and children who fail a trial of oral rehydration subsequently may be treated with intravenous fluids.

24. How is intravenous therapy administered?

In pediatric resuscitation, isotonic fluids such as normal saline or lactated Ringer's are given in 20 mL/kg aliquots over short periods of time. Infants and children have extremely elastic cardiovascular systems and can constrict their vasculature to a degree greater than the adult. A child in compensated shock (with normal blood pressure) may require repeat boluses. Dextrose-containing fluids should not be given to children as a volume expanding bolus because the solute load to the kidneys can cause further diuresis. Hypoglycemia should be tested for specifically using a serum glucose measurement device or a rapid colorimetric dipstick. In the setting of hypoglycemia, the infant or child is treated with 2 to 4 mL/kg of dextrose 10% (if < 3 months old) or dextrose 25% (if > 3 months old). Obtain a follow-up serum glucose measurement after administering the dextrose.

25. How do I calculate maintenance intravenous therapy?

- 10 kg: 4 mL/kg/h
- 10–20 kg: Add the above amount to 2 mL/kg/h for each kg over 10
- > 20 kg: Add the above amount to 1 mL/kg/h for each kg over 20

A child weighing 26 kg should receive 66 mL/h [(10 × 4) + (10 × 2) + (6 × 1) = 66 mL/h] of 5% dextrose one-half normal saline with 20 to 30 mEq of potassium/L. Alternatively, maintenance 24-hour fluids are 100 mL/kg for the first 10 kg, 50 mL/kg for the next 10 kg (10 to 20 kg), and 20 mL/kg for greater than 20 kg.

26. How is hypernatremic dehydration treated?

Initial treatment is aimed at establishing hemodynamic stability. An initial 20 to 30 mL/kg body weight of fluid may be necessary as a bolus to achieve stability. Subsequent therapy aims to establish normal serum sodium values over the following 48 to 72 hours. The process involves calculating the free water deficit, accounting for fluid already administered, and adding in maintenance requirements. Careful attention to electrolytes and administered fluid is important to prevent sequelae as the serum sodium corrects.

27. How should hyponatremia be corrected?

If the patient is symptomatic with seizures and has severe hyponatremia (usually a sodium level < 120 mEq/dL), a hypertonic solution of 3% saline may be administered carefully at 4 mL/kg until symptoms resolve. Use hyperosmolar sodium with caution and generally only in the setting of documented or strongly suspected hyponatremia. Otherwise the preferred solution is 0.9% saline to correct the deficit no faster than 15 mEq/dL every 24 hours.

28. How do I estimate the amount of total body fluid deficit?

The fluid deficit of a child can be estimated by multiplying his or her weight in kilograms by the estimated percentage of dehydration (10 kg × 10% = 100 mL). If a recent weight is available, the acute weight loss generally represents fluid losses.

29. State the major complications of dehydration.

Shock and acute renal tubular necrosis. In severe cases, renal vein thrombosis or sinus thrombosis in the brain can occur.

30. Do umbilical hernias need surgical consultations?

Rarely. Most regress without treatment, although some may persist until school age. Incarceration of umbilical hernias is unusual. Covering the hernia and reducing it (e.g., with tape, coins, straps) does not change the natural course. Surgical consultation may be warranted if there is no resolution by school age or if cosmesis is a concern.

BIBLIOGRAPHY

1. American Heart Association and the American Academy of Pediatrics: Pediatric Advanced Life Support. Dallas, AHA, 1997.
2. Barkin RM, et al: Pediatric Emergency Medicine, 2nd ed. St. Louis, Mosby, 1997.
3. Behrman RE, Kleigman RM, Nelson WE (eds): Nelson Textbook of Pediatrics, 16th ed. Philadelphia, W.B. Saunders, 2001.
4. Paajanen H, Somppi E: Early childhood appendicitis is still a difficult diagnosis. Acta Pediatr 85:459–462, 1996.
5. Rothrock SG, et al: Clinical features of misdiagnosed appendicitis in children. Ann Emerg Med 20:45–50, 1991.

76. COMMON PEDIATRIC INFECTIOUS DISEASES

Elaine Norman Scholes, M.D.

1. Why are we still discussing measles (rubeola)? Isn't it a disease of the past?

In the 1990s, there were several outbreaks of measles in middle and high schools and on college campuses secondary to waning immunity in older children. More than 25,000 cases of measles occurred in the United States in 1991. It is now recommended that all children be revaccinated at 4 to 6 years of age.

2. What is the mode of transmission of the measles virus?

By direct contact with infectious droplets or by airborne dissemination.

3. What is the incubation period for measles?

From exposure to the onset of symptoms, 8 to 12 days. It is 14 days from exposure to the onset of the rash.

4. When are patients with measles contagious?

Patients are contagious 1 to 2 days before they become symptomatic. They are also contagious for 3 to 5 days before the rash appears until 4 days after the rash appears.

5. List the main signs and symptoms in patients with measles.

High fever
Conjunctivitis
Photophobia
Coryza
Cough
Rash
Koplik's spots

6. What are Koplik's spots, and when do they appear?

1- to 3-mm bluish white spots on a bright red surface that appear first on the buccal mucosa opposite the lower molars. They are a pathognomonic exanthema of measles. They appear approximately 10 days after exposure (within 48 hours after the onset of symptoms). The spots spread to involve the buccal and labial mucosa and disappear on the second day after the onset of the rash.

7. Describe the typical rash of rubeola or measles.

A discrete red maculopapular rash first appears on the forehead, becoming coalescent as it spreads down the trunk to the feet by the third day of the illness. The rash fades in the same head-to-feet pattern as it appeared.

8. Name two frequent complications of measles.

Middle ear infections and bronchopneumonia.

9. What is subacute sclerosing panencephalitis?

A rare degenerative central nervous system disease caused by a latent measles infection, occurring an average of 10 years after a primary measles illness. Patients have progressive intellectual and behavioral deterioration and convulsions. This disease is not contagious.

10. Why is a second dose of measles vaccine required?

There is a 5% vaccine failure after the first dose of measles vaccine even when given after age 12 months. After two doses of measles, vaccine failure is uncommon.

11. Describe the exanthem seen in rubella.

Numerous discrete rose-pink maculopapules first appear on the face and, as in rubeola, spread downward to involve the trunk and extremities. The rash on the face fades on day 2, and the rash on the trunk becomes coalescent. By the third day, the rash disappears, which is why rubella is also called *3-day measles*.

12. What are Forschheimer spots?

Pinpoint red macules on the soft palate seen early in rubella; however, in contrast to Koplik's spots, they are *not* pathognomonic.

13. What is the incubation period for mumps?

16 to 18 days.

14. When are patients with mumps considered contagious?

1 to 2 days (up to 7 days) before the onset of parotid swelling. Patients are no longer infectious 7 to 9 days after the onset of parotid swelling.

15. List the major complications of mumps.

- Meningoencephalitis in 0.5% of cases
- Orchitis after puberty
- Sterility (rare)
- Arthritis, renal involvement, thyroiditis, mastitis, and hearing impairment (all rare)

16. Name the causative agent in erythema infectiosum (fifth disease).

Human parvovirus B19.

17. Describe the characteristic rash in erythema infectiosum.

Erythematous ears and a maculopapular rash on the cheeks that coalesce to form the characteristic **slapped-cheek appearance** are the initial signs of illness. The rash spreads to the extremities 1 to 2 days later with a reticular, lacelike pattern caused by central clearing of the confluent rash.

18. What is the classic presentation of roseola (erythema subitum)?

Typically a child between 6 months and 2 years old (up to 4 years old) presents with a history of high fever of 3 days' duration and mild symptoms, if any. The fever abates abruptly, followed by the appearance of a macular rash on the trunk and thighs.

19. Name the causative agent in roseola.

Human herpesvirus-6.

20. What is the incubation period for varicella (chickenpox)?

10 to 20 days.

21. When is varicella contagious?

From 1 to 2 days before the appearance of the rash until no new lesions are forming (usually 7 to 10 days after the appearance of the rash). The lesions do not have to be completely resolved to be no longer contagious but should be crusted and dry.

22. Name the mode of transmission and the cause of infectious mononucleosis (IM)?

IM is transmitted through direct and prolonged contact with oropharyngeal secretions. It is caused by the Epstein-Barr virus.

23. List the clinical manifestations of IM.

• Fever lasting 1 to 2 weeks
• Lymphadenopathy (usually nontender, no overlying erythema, most often bilateral cervical location, with epitrochlear nodes being suggestive of IM)
• Tonsillopharyngitis (usually an exudate is present—need to obtain a throat culture)
• Spleen or liver enlargement

24. What clinical signs are seen in young children with IM?

Rashes, abdominal pain, upper respiratory infections with cough, failure to thrive, and early-onset otitis media.

25. In older children and adults with IM, administration of which antibiotic is correlated with a rash?

Ampicillin, by an unknown mechanism of action, can cause a rash in patients with IM. When treating streptococcal tonsillitis in patients with IM, use erythromycin instead.

26. What are the hematologic findings in IM?

A relative lymphocytosis of greater than 50% of all leukocytes and a relative atypical lymphocytosis of 10% of leukocytes are the typical findings, although the relative percentage of atypical lymphocytes in children may be lower than in adults.

27. What are heterophil antibodies?

Serum IgM antibodies with the capability to agglutinate horse (better than sheep or bovine) erythrocytes. The ability to absorb to beef red blood cells but not guinea pig kidney distinguishes heterophil antibodies in IM from both Forssman antibodies (found in normal serum) and the antibodies in serum sickness. A heterophil titer greater than 40 with a good clinical history for IM strongly supports the diagnosis. It is positive in 90% of cases of IM, with few false-positive results except in young children, in whom Epstein-Barr virus serology is needed to establish the diagnosis.

28. What is the monospot test?

This qualitative, rapid slide test is used to detect serum heterophil antibodies in IM. It is positive in 70% of patients during the first week of illness and in 85% to 90% of patients during the third week. In children younger than 4 years old, this test may be negative because of lower levels of detectable heterophil antibodies. Epstein-Barr virus serology, which is more sensitive, should be used with this age group.

29. Describe the treatment of uncomplicated IM.

Supportive therapy and rest are the mainstays of treatment, with emphasis on analgesia for sore throat, headaches, and myalgias; oral fluids to prevent dehydration secondary to discomfort with swallowing; and a decrease in normal activity. Patients should be given specific instructions about restriction of activity, which vary depending on the severity of the illness and the patient's tolerance. If there is splenic enlargement, contact sports should be avoided until it has resolved.

30. Summarize the complications of IM.

Respiratory	Airway obstruction
Hematologic	Thrombocytopenia
	Hemolytic anemia
	Granulocytopenia
Neurologic	Encephalitis, lymphocytic meningitis
	Cerebellar ataxia
	Guillain-Barré syndrome
	Transverse myelitis
	Bell's palsy
	Optic neuritis
Cardiac	Pericarditis, myocarditis
Other	Splenic rupture
	Uveitis, keratitis
	Fatal disease (familial, sporadic, other)
	Chronic disease
Infection	Tonsillar, peritonsillar abscess
	Sinusitis
	Pneumonia

From Nelson JD (ed): Current Therapy in Pediatric Infectious Disease. St. Louis, Mosby, 1986, p 158, with permission.

31. What is the role of corticosteroids in the treatment of IM?

The use of steroids in upper airway obstruction may decrease the need for more invasive procedures by reducing edema and hyperplasia of the lymphoid tissue in the nasooropharynx. There is usually improvement in 6 to 24 hours after administration of intravenous steroids. Steroids also may be useful for neurologic, hematologic, and cardiac complications. Corticosteroids have not been shown to reduce splenomegaly or the risk of rupture of the spleen. Dexamethasone can be given parenterally if the patient is unable to take oral medication. The initial loading dose is 1 mg/kg/d (maximum 10 mg), followed by a dose of 0.5 mg/kg every 6 hours. The patient can be switched to oral medication when it is tolerated: prednisone, 2 mg/kg/d (maximal dose, 60 to 80 mg/d), divided every 6 to 12 hours for 5 to 7 days.

32. Which analgesics should be recommended in patients with IM?

Acetaminophen and ibuprofen.

33. How long does the patient need to worry about the risk of splenic rupture?

Rupture of the spleen usually occurs during the second or third week of the illness, if at all. Patients must avoid contact sports while the spleen is enlarged. Follow-up examinations determine when it is safe to play contact sports.

BIBLIOGRAPHY

1. Asano Y, Nakashima T, Yoshikawa T, et al: Severity of human herpesvirus-6 viremia and clinical findings in infants with exanthem subitum. J Pediatr 118:891–895, 1991.
2. Behrman RE, Kliegman RM, Jenson HB (eds): Nelson Textbook of Pediatrics, 16th ed. Philadelphia, W.B. Saunders, 2001.
3. Chetham MM, Roberts KB: Infectious mononucleosis in adolescents. Pediatr Ann 20:208–213, 1991.
4. Feigin RD, Cherry JD (eds): Textbook of Pediatric Infectious Diseases, 4th ed. Philadelphia, W.B. Saunders, 1997.

5. Grose C: The many faces of infectious mononucleosis: The spectrum of Epstein-Barr virus infection in children. Pediatr Rev 7:35–44, 1985.
6. Hartley AH, Rasmussen JE: Infectious exanthems. Pediatr Rev 9:321–329, 1988.
7. Hay WW, Hayward AR, Levin MJ (eds): Current Pediatric Diagnosis and Treatment, 15th ed. New York, McGraw-Hill, 2001.
8. Mandell GL, Bennett JE, Dolin R (eds): Principles and Practice of Infectious Diseases, 5th ed. Philadelphia, Churchill Livingstone, 2000.
9. Nelson JD: Current Therapy in Pediatric Infectious Disease. St. Louis, Mosby, 1986.
10. Oski FA (ed): Principles and Practice of Pediatrics, 2nd ed. Philadelphia, J.B. Lippincott, 1994.
11. Pickering LK (ed): Report of the Committee on Infectious Diseases, 25th ed. Elk Grove Village, IL, American Academy of Pediatrics, 2000.
12. Sumaya CV: Epstein-Barr virus serologic testing: Diagnostic indications and interpretations. Pediatr Infect Dis 86:337–342, 1986.
13. Sumaya CV: New perspectives on infectious mononucleosis. Contemp Pediatr 6:58–76, 1989.
14. Yamanski K, Shiraki K, Kondo T, et al: Identification of human herpesvirus-6 as a causal agent for exanthem subitum. Lancet 1:1065–1067, 1988.

77. INFREQUENT INFECTIONS IN CHILDREN

Roger M. Barkin, M.D., M.P.H.

1. Is it true that infrequent means unimportant?

Infectious diseases account for a significant percentage of pediatric visits to the ED for acute illness. Although most conditions are self-limited and infrequent, some infections are significant in that they may be life-threatening and require consideration in the differential diagnosis of many presenting complaints. Many of these conditions are discussed in other sections of this book. Infections that are not multisystem are generally covered in organ-specific chapters.

2. What are the most common findings associated with botulism in children?

Botulism results from ingestion of preformed toxins (e.g., canned vegetables), ingestion of spores in infant botulism (honey), or spore contamination of open wounds. One third of the 100 annual cases in the United States are food-borne; the remainder are cases of infant botulism. *Clostridium botulinum* produces a neurotoxin that blocks the presynaptic release of acetylcholine after an incubation period of 12 to 48 hours. Clinically, patients develop symmetric descending paralysis with weakness and equal deep tendon reflexes associated with a normal sensorium. Pupils are fixed and dilated with oculomotor paralysis, blurred vision, diplopia, ptosis, and photophobia. Associated findings may include slurred speech, nausea, vomiting, constipation, vertigo, dry mouth, dysphagia, and urinary retention. Dyspnea and rales, progressing to respiratory failure, may be noted.

3. Are there specific measures that should be initiated in the patient with botulism?

Initial management must focus on support, airway maintenance, and monitoring. Botulism equine trivalent antitoxin (ABE) should be administered and is available from the Centers for Disease Control (404-639-3670/2888) or from local state health departments.

4. What are the distinct clinical presentations of diphtheria?

Corynebacterium diphtheriae, an unencapsulated, club-shaped gram-positive bacillus, produces an exotoxin that results in four patterns of clinical findings. The pharyngeal-tonsillar complex consists of a sore throat, fever, vomiting, dysphagia, and malaise associated with a gray, closely adherent pseudomembrane. Respiratory obstruction may develop. Less common presentations include laryngeal diphtheria with hoarseness and loss of voice; respiratory tract edema may lead to obstruction. Serosanguineous nasal discharge may persist for weeks, usually without systemic findings. A sharply demarcated ulcer may develop on the skin with a membranous base. This latter cutaneous form is found mostly in the tropics but may present in alcoholics and lower socioeconomic populations. The diagnosis is confirmed by Löffler's medium and tellurite agar cultures and Gram stain.

5. How is a child with diphtheria treated?

After ensuring stability of the airway and absence of associated cardiovascular dysfunction secondary to myocarditis, antitoxin should be initiated after intradermal or conjunctival tests for horse serum sensitivity. Concurrently, antibiotics should be initiated with penicillin or with erythromycin in a penicillin-allergic patient. Carriers should be treated with antibiotics.

6. What clinical findings must be present to make the diagnosis of Kawasaki disease?

A multisystem disease occurring predominantly in children younger than 5 years of age, Kawasaki disease also is known as *mucocutaneous lymph node syndrome*. The cause is thought to be related to lymphotropic retrovirus, although the epidemiology is undefined. The syndrome is triphasic in clinical presentation. An acute febrile episode (temperature > 38.5°C for at least 5 days) with the appearance of five major diagnostic criteria, at least four of which must be present for confirmation of the typical presentation.

1. Discrete bilateral, nonexudative, conjunctival infection, usually occurring within 2 days of the onset of fever and sometimes lasting 1 to 2 weeks.

2. Mouth changes appearing 1 to 3 days after onset and possibly lasting for 1 to 2 weeks. Erythema, fissuring, and crusting of the lips; a diffuse, oropharyngeal erythema; and strawberry tongue may be present.

3. Peripheral changes beginning after 3 to 5 days and lasting 1 to 2 weeks. The hands and feet may be indurated. Erythema of the palms and soles is present; desquamation of the tips of fingers and toes occurs 2 to 3 weeks after the onset of illness.

4. Erythematous, polymorphous rash occurs concurrently with the fever and spreads from the extremities to the trunk. It usually disappears within 1 week.

5. Enlarged lymph nodes, usually cervical and greater than 1.5 cm.

7. What is the most significant complication of Kawasaki disease?

The most significant complication is **coronary artery disease** caused by arteritis, aneurysm, or thrombosis. Other findings include diarrhea, vomiting, hydrops of the gallbladder, leukocytosis, cough, proteinuria, arthritis, meningismus, and cerebrospinal fluid pleocytosis.

8. What infectious conditions should be considered in a child presenting with diffuse erythroderma?

Several acute infectious entities may present with diffuse erythroderma: a scarlatiniform rash caused by group A streptococcus, *Staphylococcus aureus*, or a viral illness; scalded skin syndrome (*S. aureus*); toxic epidermal necrolysis or erythema multiforme caused by a variety of infections and drugs; Kawasaki disease; toxic shock syndrome (*S. aureus*); and leptospirosis.

9. How do young children present when they have infectious mononucleosis?

Caused by the Epstein-Barr virus, infectious mononucleosis most frequently occurs in adolescents and young adults. Young children may have fever, diarrhea, pharyngitis, otitis media, pneumonia, lymphadenopathy, hepatomegaly, and splenomegaly. In contrast, adults more commonly have a 3- to 5-day prodrome of malaise, anorexia, nausea, and vomiting, which is followed by high fevers, pharyngitis, lymphadenopathy (especially cervical), and splenomegaly. The monospot and heterophil antibody tests are usually negative in children younger than 5 years old, requiring specific Epstein-Barr virus titers to make a definitive diagnosis. Serologic diagnosis can be done by measuring antibody to viral capsid antigen, which rises above 1:160 during acute infection.

10. Summarize the clinical characteristics of a patient with toxic shock syndrome.

Toxic shock syndrome is usually associated with *S. aureus* secondary to a toxin elaborated by the coagulase-positive organism. Findings may include:

1. Fever greater than 38.9°C
2. Rash that is diffuse, blanching, macular, erythematous, nonpruritic
3. Desquamation 1 to 2 weeks after the onset of illness, particularly of the palms and soles
4. Hypotension
5. Involvement of three or more of the following organ systems: gastrointestinal (vomiting or diarrhea), muscular (myalgia), mucous membranes (vaginal, oropharyngeal, conjunctival hyperemia), renal (elevated blood urea nitrogen and creatinine, pyuria), hepatic (elevated liver function tests), hematologic (thrombocytopenia), or central nervous (disorientation, altered consciousness)

11. Describe the three stages of clinical progression of a child with pertussis.

Pertussis (or whooping cough) is caused by *Bordetella pertussis*, a gram-negative coccobacilli, occurring in all age groups. It peaks in late summer and early fall with an **incubation period** of 7 to 10 days. Initially patients have respiratory complaints of fever, rhinorrhea, and conjunctivitis lasting 2 weeks (catarrhal). The **paroxysmal phase** follows; severe cough, hypoxia, unremitting paroxysms, and vomiting may occur for 2 to 4 weeks. Apnea, pneumonia, pneumothorax, seizures, and hypoxia may complicate the illness. In the **convalescent phase**, there is an associated residual cough.

12. What are the typical stages of Reye's syndrome?

Reye's syndrome is an acute, noninflammatory encephalopathy with altered level of consciousness, cerebral edema without perivascular or meningeal inflammation, and fatty metamorphosis of the liver, probably secondary to mitochondrial dysfunction. It is a multisystem disease that probably has many associated causes, the findings often being referred to as *Reye-like syndrome*. Salicylate ingestion has been incriminated, especially when occurring in association with chickenpox or influenza. It is uncommon. Clinically, patients present with a respiratory or gastrointestinal prodrome followed in several days with an encephalopathic picture that is marked by behavioral changes and a deteriorating level of consciousness. Progression of brainstem dysfunction occurs in a cephalocaudal pattern:

0   Alert, wakeful

I   Lethargy. Follows verbal comments, normal posture, purposeful response to pain, brisk pupillary light reflex, and normal oculocephalic reflex

II   Combative or stuporous, inappropriate verbalizing, normal posture, purposeful or nonpurposeful response to pain, sluggish pupillary reaction, and conjugate deviation on doll's eye maneuver

III   Comatose, decorticate posture and decerebrate response to pain, sluggish pupillary reaction, conjugate deviation on doll's eye maneuver

IV   Comatose, decorticate posture and decerebrate response to pain, sluggish pupillary reflexes, and inconsistent or absent oculocephalic reflex

V   Comatose, flaccid, no response to pain, no pupillary response, no oculocephalic reflex

BIBLIOGRAPHY

1. American Academy of Pediatrics: Report of the Committee on Infectious Diseases. Elk Grove, IL, AAP, 2000.
2. Dajani A, Taubert K, Takahashi M, et al: Guidelines for long-term management of patients with Kawasaki disease. Circulation 89:916–922, 1994.
3. Galazka A: The changing epidemiology of diphtheria in the vaccine era. J Infect Dis 181(suppl 1):S2–S9, 2000.

4. Rowley AH, Shulman ST: Kawasaki syndrome. Pediatr Clin North Am 46:313–329, 1999.
5. Saiman L, Prince A, Gersony WM: Pediatric infective endocarditis in the modern era. J Pediatr 122:847–853, 1993.
6. Sato N, et al: Selective high dose gamma-globulin treatment in Kawasaki disease: Assessment of clinical aspects and cost effectiveness. Pediatr Int 41:1–7, 1999.
7. Schreiner MS, Field E, Ruddy R: Infant botulism: A review of 12 years' experience at the Children's Hospital of Philadelphia. Pediatrics 87:159–165, 1991.
8. Shapiro RL, Hatheway C, Swerdlow DL: Botulism in the United States: A clinical and epidemiologic review. Ann Intern Med 129:221–228, 1998.
9. Stevens DL: The toxic shock syndrome. Infect Dis Clin North Am 10:727–746, 1996.

78. EMERGENCY DEPARTMENT EVALUATION OF CHILD ABUSE

Ann B. Marshall, M.D.

1. How is child abuse defined?

The Child Abuse Prevention and Treatment Act (CAPTA) defines child abuse and neglect as an act (or failure to act) that results in risk of serious harm, death, physical or emotional harm, or sexual abuse or exploitation of a child younger than 18 years old by a parent or caregiver who is responsible for the child's welfare.

2. What is the prevalence of child abuse?

More than 3 million cases of child abuse or neglect are reported each year. In 1996, there were more than 1000 fatalities attributed to child abuse. Between 1986 and 1993, there was a 67% increase in documented abuse or neglect cases (a combination of improved reporting and an actual increase in incidence). A Gallup poll showed that parents admitted to a rate of physical abuse 16 times the reported incidence and a 10 times greater incidence of sexual abuse.

3. What is the epidemiology and sociology of child abuse?

Child abuse crosses all cultural, ethnic, socioeconomic, and racial lines. It is strongly associated, however, with poverty and financial stress. It also is highly correlated with less parental education, unemployment, poor housing, and single parenting. It tends to occur in multiproblem families, such as those plagued by domestic violence, substance abuse, and mental illness.

4. Name some of the important historical indicators of child abuse.

In addition to the family characteristics listed previously, historical indicators include multiple previous hospital visits, a history of untreated injuries, delay in seeking medical attention, cause of trauma unknown according to parents, cause of trauma inappropriate for developmental age of child, and history incompatible with physical findings.

5. Who are the perpetrators?

In most cases, the abuser is a parent. The National Center on Child Abuse and Neglect reported that 77% of victims were abused by a parent; 12% by other relatives; 5% by noncaretakers; and 2% by foster parents, facility staff, or child care staff. Of abusers, 70% are age 20 to 40 and slightly more likely to be women, although men are more likely to perpetrate sexual abuse.

6. Name the most common organ systems involved in ED presentation of an abused child.

Cutaneous, skeletal, and neurologic findings are most common. Of children hospitalized for abuse, 50% present with burns, bruises, or other dermatologic findings.

7. What in the patient's history should increase my concern for child abuse?

Be concerned if parents have expectations of their child that are developmentally inappropriate, if they express negative views of their child, or if they have little knowledge of different disciplining techniques beyond corporal punishment. Look for signs of depression and substance abuse in the caregiver.

8. List physical findings that are clues to child abuse.

- Multiple lesions in various stages of healing (bruises, fractures)
- Any bruises in young, nonmobile infants or bruises in older children over areas of the body that usually are protected (back, chest, genitalia, abdomen)
- Immersion burns (sharp demarcation, no splash marks)
- Patterned bruising or burns—hand print, loop marks (cord, rope), belt buckle imprints
- Bites—all bites inflicted on young children should arouse suspicion of abuse
- Retinal hemorrhages (dilate pupil for optimal examination)
- Sudden change in neurologic status
- Failure to thrive in absence of chronic disease (weight > 2 SD below mean expected for age)

9. How does the presence of bruising help make the diagnosis of child abuse?

The appearance of multiple bruises at different stages of healing is highly suggestive of physical abuse and must be documented.

0–2 days	Swollen, tender, red-blue
3–5 days	Blue-purple
5–7 days	Green
7–10 days	Yellow
10–14 days	Brown
14–28 days	Resolved

10. What fractures are suggestive of child abuse?

Of fractures in children younger than 1 year old, 56% are nonaccidental. Multiple fractures of different ages and spiral fractures in preambulatory children are characteristic of child abuse. Epiphyseal separation and metaphyseal chip fractures are associated with traction, rotation, and shaking injuries and are virtually diagnostic of nonaccidental trauma. Rib and spine fractures are considered strong evidence of abuse. Skeletal injuries with the highest specificity for abuse include metaphyseal lesions, posterior rib fractures, scapular fractures, spinous process fractures, and sternal fractures. Moderate-specificity fractures include multiple fractures (especially bilateral), epiphyseal separation, fractures of different ages, vertebral body fractures and subluxations, digital fractures, and complex skull fractures.

11. What is a skeletal survey, and who should receive one?

A true skeletal survey includes separate views of every bone, avoiding the attempts to view multiple areas on the same film (the *babygram*). It includes radiographs of the skull, chest, long bones, hands, and spine. Skeletal surveys should be done in all cases of suspected abuse in children younger than 2 years old. The radiologist should be informed of the reason for the examination. There is a high false-negative rate of skeletal surveys, and repeat films or bone scans may be necessary.

12. What is the leading cause of death in abused children?

Head injury is the most common cause of mortality in child abuse victims. The usual mechanisms are shaking and blunt trauma. Skull fractures can occur with mild or moderate trauma (usually linear and nondisplaced), but skull fractures associated with abuse are more likely bilateral, comminuted, and depressed. Subdural hematomas are correlated strongly with intentional trauma. Diffuse brain edema is seen commonly in infants who have been shaken or suffered major blunt impact leading to prolonged apnea.

13. What is *shaken baby syndrome*?

This terms refers to injury resulting when an infant is shaken vigorously. The acceleration/deceleration forces can lead to subdural hematomas, cerebral contusions, edema, and cervical spine hematomas. The most common chief complaint is respiratory distress. The diagnosis is suggested by retinal hemorrhages and xanthochromic or bloody spinal fluid. CT or MRI can confirm the diagnosis. Of children who present comatose after shaking, 50% die, and half of the survivors have significant neurologic sequelae.

14. Name other life-threatening injuries that are seen in child abuse.

Abdominal injuries usually are seen in children older than 1 year of age and are the second most common cause of death from abuse after head injuries. The mortality rate from visceral injuries has been reported to be 50%. The most common injuries include hollow viscus damage, mesenteric vascular injury, and injury to the pancreas and liver. Most of these injuries occur as a result of blunt trauma to the midabdomen.

15. When child abuse is suspected in the ED, what else should be considered in the differential diagnosis?

Coagulation disorders
Mongolian spots
Henoch-Schönlein purpura
Scurvy or rickets
Osteogenesis imperfecta
Folk remedies from different cultures, such as *coining* or *cupping*
Sudden infant death syndrome

16. When should sexual abuse be suspected?

Sexual abuse must be investigated if the child reports it. Changes in behavior, such as sleep disturbances, enuresis, poor school performance, and abdominal pain, have been observed in newly identified sexually abused children. Other signs of sexual abuse include sexually transmitted disease in a prepubescent child or genital trauma.

17. What data should be obtained in the ED when evaluating a sexually abused child?

For acute assault, the sexual assault forensic evidence kit should be used, including chlamydia test; gonorrhea cultures of the cervix, pharynx, and rectum (if indicated); vaginal swabs; saliva samples; pubic hair controls; blood for ABO typing; pregnancy test; and Venereal Disease Research Laboratory (VDRL) test.

18. Should sexually abused children be given antibiotic prophylaxis for sexually transmitted diseases?

Victims of sexual assault should be cultured initially, and antibiotic therapy should be guided by culture results. If parental anxiety is high for potential sexually transmitted disease or if the perpetrator is thought to be infected, prophylactic antibiotics may be offered.

19. Should all abused children be admitted to the hospital?

If medically indicated, such as for head trauma, abused children must be admitted. If admission is not medically indicated, child protective services should be able to assist in arranging a safe disposition for the patient. If placement is unavailable, the patient should be a *social admission* until another safe environment can be provided.

20. What is the extent of legal responsibility of an ED caregiver in caring for an abused child?

The chief responsibility of ED physicians is to recognize and report child abuse. Physicians are mandated by law to notify local child protection authorities of suspected child abuse cases.

Failure to do so is usually a fourth-degree misdemeanor and may be considered a malpractice of omission. The parents should be informed calmly of the report. The physician also is obligated to arrange a safe disposition for the child. For physicians reporting child abuse, every state provides immunity from any potential civil and criminal liability. The physician acting in good faith need not fear legal repercussions from the family or caregivers.

BIBLIOGRAPHY

1. Bernet W: Practice parameters for the forensic evaluation of children and adolescents who may have been sexually abused. J Am Acad Child Adolesc Psychiatry 36:423–442, 1997.
2. Freitag R, Lazoritz S, Kini N: Psychosocial aspects of child abuse for primary care pediatricians. Pediatr Clin North Am 45:391–402, 1998.
3. Jain AM: Emergency department evaluation of child abuse. Emerg Med Clin North Am 17:575–591, 1999.
4. Johnson CF: Abuse and neglect of children. In Berhrman RE, Kliegman RM, Arvin AM (eds): Nelson Textbook of Pediatrics, 15th ed. Philadelphia, W.B. Saunders, 1996, pp 112–120.
5. MacMillan HL, Fleming JE, Trocme N, et al: Prevalence of child physical and sexual abuse in the community. JAMA 278:131–135, 1997.
6. Nimkin K, Lleinman PK: Imaging of child abuse. Pediatr Clin North Am 44:615–635, 1997.
7. Paradise JE: The medical evaluation of the sexually abused child. Pediatr Clin North Am 37:839–862, 1990.
8. Tercier A: Child abuse. In Rosen P, Barkin RM (eds): Emergency Medicine: Concepts and Clinical Practice, 4th ed. St. Louis, Mosby, 1998, pp 1108–1123.

79. PROCEDURAL SEDATION OF THE PEDIATRIC PATIENT

F. Keith Battan, M.D.

1. Why would you want to sedate a child?

If you are reading this answer, you have never tried to do a procedure such as complicated laceration repair on a screaming, thrashing, uncooperative toddler! Children who may benefit from sedation are those undergoing painful or frightening procedures, including laceration repair, incision and drainage of abscesses, burn care, reduction of fractures or dislocations, examinations after sexual assault, and diagnostic procedures such as CT or MRI. Toddlers or preschool-age children benefit most from sedation, although older children sometimes require sedation for successful completion of a procedure. Effective ED sedation may enable an emergency physician to do a procedure that otherwise would require general anesthesia in the operating room. Sedation relieves excessive fear and anxiety, allows a more precisely performed procedure, decreases nociception, and may provide amnesia for the procedure.

2. What's wrong with "brutacaine"?

"Brutacaine" (i.e., simply holding the child down and doing the procedure) can result in a crying, thrashing patient whose injury is difficult to examine, explore, and repair. Continuous crying leaves the child, family, and staff exhausted and appears to onlookers as torture. The child is left with unpleasant memories and may fear return visits for care. This factor is particularly important for children requiring repeat procedures, such as lumbar punctures or burn care. There is no morbidity, other than psychological, associated with doing a procedure without sedation, and this approach may be appropriate for some short, simple, uncomplicated procedures. In general, providing sedation and analgesia for children is an accepted and expected part of emergency medicine.

3. What is the difference between a sedative and an analgesic?

An **analgesic** treats pain, whereas a **sedative** or **anxiolytic** relieves fear and anxiety. Some analgesics, particularly narcotics, have sedative and analgesic properties, which make them useful in certain procedures. If a procedure is painful and frightening (e.g., chest tube insertion), the child would benefit from sedation and analgesia, by multiple or single agents.

4. What is the difference between sedation and procedural sedation?

Sedation refers to blunting of the **level of consciousness** (LOC). Procedural or light sedation refers to a minimal depression of LOC, wherein the child is awake but may have droopy eyes and slightly slurred speech. The child should be able to respond to verbal command or physical stimulation and maintain protective airway reflexes. Deep sedation implies a depressed LOC from which the child is not easily aroused, and protective airway reflexes are partially or totally lost. General anesthesia represents the end of this continuum. Procedural or light sedation is the optimal state for sedation of children in the ED. Care must be taken because many sedatives can result in general anesthesia if given in sufficient doses, which is not desirable in the ED because of the risk of cardiorespiratory depression or aspiration.

5. List the characteristics of an ideal sedative.

• Produces effective anxiolysis, even during painful procedures.
• Safe; produces a predictable degree of sedation for a given dose and has minimal effects on airway reflexes and cardiorespiratory status.
• Movement is minimized.
• Amnesia is provided for the procedure.
• Produces no adverse interactions with other agents that may be used concurrently.
• Reversible.
• Can be administered painlessly.
• Has rapid onset, short duration, and rapid recovery (**most important**).

6. Why are the above-listed characteristics ideal for a pediatric sedative?

These factors allow the sedative to be administered incrementally over a short time span (i.e., **titrated**) until the desired level of sedation for the particular patient and procedure is reached. Children have tremendous variability in dosing requirements for a desired sedation level, and titration allows individualization of dosing.

7. What is a poor sedative?

One example is the combination DPT (Demerol [meperidine], Phenergan [promethazine], and Thorazine [chlorpromazine]). This combination, still used at some centers, has potential side effects that include oversedation (some children are sedated for 8 hours and are not normal for 36 hours), extrapyramidal reactions, and life-threatening side effects such as respiratory arrest and hypotension, even at less-than-recommended doses. A poor sedative requires painful intramuscular administration, has highly variable onset and sedative effects, and does not allow the clinician to titrate the dosage. The clinician has little control over and must accept the sedation level achieved, which may be either inadequate or excessive.

8. Discuss the risks and costs associated with sedation.

• With oversedation, there is risk for (1) aspiration, from vomiting and loss of airway reflexes; (2) hypoventilation with resultant hypoxia, hypercarbia, and cardiopulmonary arrest; (3) shock; and (4) laryngospasm.
• Use of sedative agents may entail additional costs for drugs, monitoring, and intravenous lines. Additional ED personnel and time sometimes are necessary during procedures involving sedation. If an operating room trip is avoided for optimal performance of a procedure under conscious sedation in the ED, however, there is overall savings and the best possible result.

• Postsedation, there is a recovery period, during which children may vomit, be agitated, be ataxic, and respond to commands poorly. Close observation continues to be essential.

• Because of the risks involved, at least verbal informed consent should be obtained and documented.

9. What monitoring is appropriate during procedural sedation?

The best monitor is a skilled, dedicated observer who is not involved in the procedure and who can observe the child's LOC, response to verbal and physical stimulation, airway patency, respiratory function, and perfusion. Sedated children should not be left unobserved.

The monitoring required depends on the patient and the medications used. The more potent the agent, the more complete the monitoring that is required. Some agents, such as chloral hydrate, do not require monitoring other than by clinical means. Full monitoring consists of continuous cardiopulmonary monitoring, including pulse oximetry and frequent assessments of perfusion, including blood pressure determinations. If single agents or combinations are used that have the possibility of serious side effects or if deep sedation is inadvertently reached, intravenous access should be established, and full monitoring and constant observation should be continued throughout the procedure.

Personnel and equipment to perform airway management and resuscitation must be readily available. Ideally, patients should be given nothing orally for several hours before the procedure if sedatives are to be used, but this is rarely possible in an ED setting. Keep in mind the general (and usually accurate) rule that children's stomachs are always full.

10. Are there any children who should not receive procedural sedation in the ED?

Relative contraindications to procedural sedation in the ED relate to the risk of complications, including aspiration and potential difficulty in managing the airway. Children who may be better candidates for operating room procedures under more controlled conditions include the following:

Unstable patients, such as children with abnormal mental status or hemodynamic instability
Infants younger than 6 months old
Children with craniofacial malformations, such as Pierre-Robin anomaly
Children with cerebral palsy and abnormal swallowing mechanisms
Children with snoring, stridor, apnea, or abnormal breathing regulation (rare)
Children with seizure disorders
Children with vomiting or gastroesophageal reflux

11. What should I do if a child experiences respiratory depression or becomes poorly perfused while sedated?

Specific treatment: For narcotics and benzodiazepines, specific reversing agents are available. Naloxone (0.1 mg/kg intravenously, intramuscularly, or endotracheally, up to 4 mg per dose) reverses narcotic effects, and flumazenil (0.01 mg/kg intravenously, up to 1.0 mg) reverses benzodiazepine overdose.

General measures: Discontinue sedative or narcotic administration. Maintain the airway and provide assisted ventilation, initially with bag-valve-mask ventilation, then with endotracheal intubation if necessary. If poor perfusion or shock is present (e.g., capillary refill time > 2 seconds, cool extremities, weak pulses, poor tone), obtain vascular access and initiate treatment with a bolus infusion of 20 mL/kg of crystalloid solution.

12. What are some options available for procedural sedation?

1. **Midazolam** (Versed), the first water-soluble benzodiazepine, has particular usefulness in pediatrics. Its rapid onset and short duration of action make it ideal for titration of sedation level. It can be given by oral, rectal, intranasal, intramuscular, or intravenous routes. The first three routes have the advantage of painless administration. Children fear injections and intravenous lines more than many illnesses or injuries. The pharmacokinetics of midazolam are nearly the same clinically when the drug is given intranasally, 0.3 mg/kg, as when given intravenously.

Although there is a burning sensation in the nasal mucosa, no injection is required. Oral and rectal administration result in relatively delayed onset, titration is difficult, and higher doses are required because of extensive first-pass hepatic metabolism. Intramuscular injections of midazolam can be combined with opioid analgesics in the same syringe if systemic analgesia is desired, or they can be given sequentially by intravenous infusion. Intravenous administration allows optimal ability to titrate the dose to the desired sedation level and provides a *lifeline* if resuscitation becomes necessary. Children expected to undergo complicated or prolonged procedures are best sedated by this route.

   2. **Barbiturates** minimize movement during the procedure, which makes them advantageous for diagnostic studies such as CT or MRI. Rectal administration of thiopental is safe and effective. Onset of action with intravenous administration is rapid. Potential side effects, although uncommon, include respiratory and cardiac depression and laryngospasm.

   3. **Narcotics**, such as morphine, meperidine, and fentanyl, are analgesics that also have sedative effects. They can be combined with anxiolytics such as the benzodiazepines and the newer analogs alfentanil and remifentanil. Desired and adverse effects, such as respiratory depression, are potentiated when given together; initial sedative doses should be reduced when combined. Fentanyl has particular usefulness in the ED because of its rapid onset, accurate dosing, and rapid recovery. Administration is generally intravenous. Similar to all narcotics, fentanyl has side effects of respiratory and cardiac depression, apnea, facial pruritus, nausea, and vomiting. When fentanyl is given rapidly or in high doses, the *wooden-chest syndrome* (thoracic and abdominal wall rigidity) can occur. This muscular rigidity can be reversed by naloxone or neuromuscular blockade, allowing the clinician to assist respiration (and relieve his or her own resultant hyperventilation!) A unique feature of fentanyl is that apnea can occur without the usual concomitant decrease in mental status. Because of these potent side effects, full monitoring by continuous clinical observation, cardiorespiratory monitor, and pulse oximetry is necessary. Blood pressure should be determined at frequent intervals.

   4. **Ketamine** is chemically related to the drug of abuse phencyclidine (PCP) but has advantages for pediatric sedation. It produces sedation, a dissociative amnesia, and weak analgesia and has the advantage of not causing cardiorespiratory depression. Time to onset of acceptable sedation is within 5 minutes in most children, and recovery time is usually reasonably rapid. Ketamine can be given intravenously or intramuscularly. Adverse effects can include random purposeless movements, nausea and vomiting, laryngospasm, and respiratory depression. Contrary to conventional wisdom, the rate of laryngospasm is low (0.017% in a review of 11,589 cases). Because of its sialagogue (salivation-enhancing) effects, ketamine frequently is given with glycopyrrolate or atropine in the same syringe. Ketamine should not be used in the presence of head injury, acute upper respiratory infection, pulmonary disease, hypertension, glaucoma, psychosis, thyroid disease, or porphyria. Unpleasant emergence reactions and nightmares can occur in children. Clinical observation and pulse oximetry and cardiac monitoring should be continuous when administering ketamine.

   5. **Nitrous oxide** is an excellent sedative and has weak analgesic properties. It has no significant side effects when used as a 50/50 nitrous oxide/oxygen mixture but should not be used in the presence of pneumothoraces or bowel obstruction. Emesis is a risk, as in all sedated patients. Clinical monitoring and oximetry are needed.

   6. **Propofol** is used increasingly, alone or in combination with fentanyl. It has ultra-rapid onset and fast emergence. Side effects are similar to the barbiturates.

13. Summarize selected agents for procedural sedation.

	INITIAL DOSE	ROUTE	MONITORING	NOTE
Midazolam	0.1 mg/kg	IV, IM	Cardiac monitor	Titrate to effect
	0.3 mg/kg	IN	Oximetry[*]	
	0.5 mg/kg	PR, PO	Blood pressure[†]	10 mg max

(*Table continued on next page.*)

	INITIAL DOSE	ROUTE	MONITORING	NOTE
Pentobarbital	4–6 mg/kg 2–6 mg/kg slowly	IM IV	Cardiac monitor	Fewer spontaneous movements
Fentanyl	2–4 μg/kg slowly	IV	Cardiac monitor Oximetry* Blood pressure†	Avoid rapid or high-dose infusions Use with caution
Ketamine	1 mg/kg 3–4 mg/kg	IV IM	Cardiac monitor Oximetry* Blood pressure†	Dissociative amnesia Many spontaneous movements
Nitrous oxide	30–50% NO$_2$	Inhalation	Clinical Oximetry*	Older children able to hold mask
Propofol	0.5–1.0 mg/kg	IV	Cardiac monitor	Can be given by continu- ous infusion: 25–150 μg/kg/min

PO, oral; PR, rectal; IN, intranasal; IM, intramuscular; IV, intravenous.
* Continuous pulse oximetry.
† Blood pressure taken every 10 minutes.

14. How can I successfully sedate a child?

Preparation is important. Provide a calm and quiet atmosphere. Careful explanation of the procedure and the avoidance of untruths help to allay the child's fears. Clinicians increasingly appreciate the fact that the presence of the parents in the room during the procedure decreases the child's anxiety and facilitates the procedure. After the sedative is given, the child should be allowed to remain in a quiet, calm atmosphere, with the parents present, until the full sedative effect is achieved. If the child becomes agitated, it subsequently becomes much more difficult to achieve the desired sedation level. A trained observer should monitor the child as he or she becomes sedated. After sufficient time for the expected sedative effects to appear, gently stimulate the child to ascertain his or her reaction. If the child reacts with agitation and crying and still has a normal mental status, administer additional sedative and continue to monitor. With intravenous or intranasal midazolam, if the LOC is normal and the child is still too agitated to start the procedure after 3 to 4 minutes, give half the initial dose and reassess the child in another 3 to 4 minutes. Although the initial dose of intravenous midazolam is 0.1 mg/kg, 0.7 to 0.8 mg/kg in repeated doses may be necessary to achieve adequate sedation. The risk of cardiorespiratory depression is generally proportional to the degree of mental status depression. Fentanyl is a notable exception. Only the amount necessary to achieve conscious sedation as described earlier should be used, and the child should be monitored fully for side effects. When the sedation level is judged adequate, proceed, keeping in mind that short-acting sedatives may require redosing during prolonged procedures.

15. When can children who have received sedatives be discharged from the ED?

The child should have normal vital signs, be reasonably alert, be able to sit without assistance, take liquids by mouth, and respond to commands given in a normal voice.

BIBLIOGRAPHY

1. American College of Emergency Physicians: Clinical policy for procedural sedation and analgesia in the emergency department. Ann Emerg Med 31:663–677, 1998.
2. Dachs RJ, Innes GM: Intravenous ketamine sedation of pediatric patients in the emergency department. Ann Emerg Med 29:146–150, 1997.
3. Graff KJ, Kennedy RM, Jaffe DM: Conscious sedation for pediatric orthopaedic emergencies. Pediatr Emerg Care 12:31–35, 1996.

4. Hoffman GM, Nowakowski R, et al: Risk reduction in pediatric procedural sedation by application of an American Academy of Pediatrics/American Society of Anesthesiologists process model. Pediatrics 109:236–243, 2002.
5. Krauss B, Green SM: Sedation and analgesia for procedures in children. N Engl J Med 342:938–945, 2000.
6. Litman RS: Conscious sedation with remifentanil and midazolam during painful medical procedures. Arch Pediatr Adolesc Med 153:1085–1088, 1999.
7. Luhmann JD, Kennedy RM, et al: A randomized clinical trial of continuous-flow nitrous oxide and midazolam for sedation of young children during laceration repair. Ann Emerg Med 37:20–27, 2001.

80. NEONATAL RESUSCITATION

Owen P. O'Meara, M.D.

1. I'm an ED physician. Why should I learn about neonatal resuscitation?

The resuscitation of newborn infants in the ED is a fact of life. The main objective should be a healthy infant and mother. Help should be sought from Pediatrics and Obstetrics as soon as it is evident that the delivery of an infant is going to occur in the ED. Most mistakes in the care of the newborn are made as the result of panic, which can be avoided if the guidelines presented here are followed. All ED personnel should be formally trained in basic newborn resuscitation. Almost all teaching programs have this training available.

2. What is the most important thing to learn from this chapter about neonatal resuscitation?

There are some differences in the process of resuscitation between adults and infants and between infants and older children.

3. How can you tell if an infant needs resuscitation?

Infants are cyanotic at birth as a result of the low partial pressure of oxygen in utero. More important criteria for determining the need for resuscitation include lack of spontaneous activity and respiratory effort in association with bradycardia despite stimulation, such as gentle rubbing over the thoracic spine and flicking of the soles of the feet.

4. What spontaneous activity should one expect in an infant following birth?

Most infants have a grimace-like facial expression and some spontaneous motor activity of the extremities. Almost all newborns make some effort to cry or breathe spontaneously within 15 to 20 seconds after delivery.

5. Define bradycardia in the newborn.

Heart rate less than 100 beats/min 30 seconds after birth.

6. When should central cyanosis resolve in a healthy newborn after delivery?

Central cyanosis and cyanosis of the membranes of the oral cavity should clear during the first minute of life. Peripheral cyanosis of the extremities may persist for several minutes in an otherwise healthy newborn. Persistent peripheral cyanosis of the hands and feet also is called **acrocyanosis**.

7. After delivery in the ED, what is the first priority in the care of the newborn?

First, warm the infant. The infant must be dried with a warm cloth and placed under a radiant warming unit that is left on in the ED or, at the very least, is turned on the moment the personnel are alerted to the fact that a woman in labor is on the way in. These measures to prevent evaporative heat loss avert many of the metabolic complications that can occur. It may be necessary to change toweling during the procedure to prevent the infant's skin from becoming wet again.

8. During delivery of the infant, the presence of meconium may be noted. How is this best dealt with after delivery of the head and after delivery of the rest of the body?

Meconium is a genuine risk for the infant. Aspiration of this material can cause a significant chemical injury to the respiratory tract, secondary to the presence of a variety of noxious substances in the meconium, such as bile acids. There should be an attempt to suction the infant's nasopharynx and mouth while the infant's head is still on the perineum and after delivery of the rest of the body. Positive-pressure ventilation should be avoided until after this is done. Direct suctioning of the infant's trachea should be avoided unless someone skilled in this procedure is present.

9. After the infant is dried, suctioned, and placed under a warmer, how do I decide whether further active intervention is needed?

If the infant is actively crying and has a heart rate of greater than 100 beats/min, further intervention is seldom needed in the ED. If the infant has apnea and bradycardia, the operator should begin with tactile stimulation as noted before. If the infant fails to respond to this within a few seconds and the heart rate remains less than 100 beats/min, bag-and-mask ventilation should be used. When the infant responds to this with a heart rate of greater than 100 beats/min, the operator should pause to see if the infant will begin to breathe spontaneously.

10. How many infants require intubation to provide adequate ventilation?

Almost all newborns can be ventilated by bag and mask alone. The newborn should be placed supine on the table of the warmer with the head tilted down and with the neck extended only slightly compared with an older child or adult. Ventilation of the newborn should be attempted only with a bag and mask designed for infants, with continuous oxygen flow through it. Most infants can be ventilated with a pressure of 20 cm H_2O. Almost all neonatal bags should have a blow-off valve and be of the self-inflating variety.

11. How can I be certain that I am ventilating the infant or that the position of the head is correct?

Someone other than the operator should be present to listen for heart rate and adequate breath sounds. If there is only one person present, watching for chest wall movement is the next best thing. If the lungs are not being ventilated, repositioning the head should be done until breath sounds are heard or chest wall movements are observed.

12. When should chest compressions begin in the course of this effort?

If, after 30 to 60 seconds of adequate ventilation, the infant's heart rate remains less than 80 beats/min, chest compressions should begin. Compressions should be at the rate of about 100 to 120/min and can be accomplished with no more effort than the tips of two fingers over the sternum. Avoid pressure over the infant's liver or xyphoid to avoid iatrogenic liver lacerations. After 20 to 30 seconds, the infant's heart rate should be ascertained, and the infant should be observed for spontaneous ventilation. In general, when heart rate is greater than 100 beats/min, chest compressions may be stopped. If bag-and-mask ventilation must continue, heart rate should be checked every 30 seconds to see if compressions should resume.

13. At what point in this process should Obstetrics and Pediatrics be notified?

Pediatrics and Obstetrics should be notified the moment that it is obvious a pregnant woman is going to deliver before transfer to Labor and Delivery. Their experience and assistance can be invaluable.

14. When should I attempt vascular access, and what vessel should I use?

As a general rule, the only vessel you should try to access in this setting is the umbilical vein, which is visualized easily in the cut umbilicus. An umbilical cut-down tray should be available in all EDs for this reason.

15. What drugs should be available for newborn resuscitation use, and when should they be given?

Drugs rarely are needed in the resuscitation of the newborn, especially if bag-and-mask ventilation is instituted early. When needed, usually no more than two agents are needed. **Epinephrine** 1:10,000 dilution is used if no heartbeat is noted for 6 to 10 seconds at any time during the resuscitation or if heart rate remains less than 60 to 80 beats/min after 30 seconds of *adequate* bag-and-mask ventilation and chest compressions. The usual dose is 0.1 to 0.3 mL. Epinephrine can be given via the endotracheal tube rather than trying to get vascular access and wasting time. The dose may be repeated every 5 minutes if the heart rate remains less than 100 beats/min.

A **volume expander** can be of use in the ED setting if there is evidence of blood loss. Newborn infants initially may have poor capillary refill even when they have adequate blood volume. Rapid volume replacement must be done with great caution in the very premature infant because of the risk of sudden increases in pressure in the cerebral vessels and the associated increased risk of intracranial bleeding. Albumin 5% solution and normal saline usually are all that is needed in this setting. Sodium bicarbonate 4.2% solution should be available, especially if cardiac arrest has occurred. This concentration solution delivers 0.5 mEq/mL, and the usual dose is 2 mEq/mL intravenously over a period of at least 2 minutes. This solution can be given through the umbilical vein but not the umbilical artery.

16. What is the best means of documentation of the results of resuscitation in the neonate?

The Apgar score, which makes use of five determinations and is done at 1 and 5 minutes in all births and every 5 minutes thereafter when resuscitation is in progress.

SIGN	0	1	2
Heart rate per minute	Absent	Slow (< 100)	> 100
Respirations	Absent	Slow, irregular	Good, crying
Muscle tone	Limp	Some flexion	Active motion
Reflex irritability (catheter in nares)	No response	Grimace	Cough or sneeze
Color	Blue or pale	Pink body with blue extremities	Completely pink

17. Is 100% oxygen safe to use in neonatal resuscitation?

There is a growing concern about reperfusion injury in neonates associated with the release of oxygen free radicals. Because the data are not definitive, 100% oxygen should be used.

BIBLIOGRAPHY

1. American Academy of Pediatrics, Committee on the Fetus and Newborn: Use and abuse of the Apgar score. Pediatrics 78:1148, 1986.
2. Bloom RS, Cropley C: AHA/AAP Neonatal Resuscitation Program Steering Committee: Textbook of Neonatal Resuscitation. Elk Grove Village, IL, American Heart Association and American Academy of Pediatrics, 2000.
3. Burchfield D, Erenburg, A, Mullett MD, et al: Why change the compression and ventilation rates during CPR in neonates? Pediatrics 93:1026, 1994.
4. Catlin EA, Carpenter MW, Brann BS, et al: The Apgar score revisited: Influence of gestational age. J Pediatr 109:865, 1986.
5. Yoder BA: Meconium-stained amniotic fluid and respiratory complications: Impact of selective tracheal suction. Obstet Gynecol 83:77, 1994.

XIV. Toxicologic Emergencies

81. GENERAL APPROACH TO POISONINGS

Katherine Hurlbut, M.D., and Ken Kulig, M.D.

1. List the 16 most common causes of death from acute poisoning reported to poison centers.

SUBSTANCE	%*
Analgesics	10.5
Cleaning substances	9.5
Cosmetics and personal care products	9.4
Foreign bodies	5.0
Plants	4.9
Cold and cough preparations	4.5
Bites/envenomations	4.2
Sedatives/hypnotics/antipsychotics	4.1
Topicals	4.1
Pesticides	4.0
Antidepressants	3.9
Food products, food poisoning	3.1
Alcohols	2.9
Hydrocarbons	2.8
Antihistamines	2.7
Antimicrobials	2.7

Note. Despite a high frequency of involvement, these substances are not the most toxic, but rather may be the most readily accessible.
* Percentages are based on the total number of human exposures rather than the total number of substances.
From Litovitz TL, Klein-Schwartz W, White S, et al: 2000 Annual report of the American Association of Poison Control Centers Toxic Exposure Surveillance System. Am J Emerg Med 19:337–396, 2001, with permission.

2. What is the current role of syrup of ipecac in treating acute poisoning?
Although syrup of ipecac induces vomiting within 20 to 30 minutes in most persons who are given a therapeutic dose, little poison is removed; there are more effective means of decontaminating the gastrointestinal (GI) tract. Ipecac may have a role in treating children at home, who frequently can be given a dose soon after ingestion. By the time most patients present to a hospital, however, too much time has elapsed for syrup of ipecac to be of benefit. Its use also delays the administration of activated charcoal, which needs to be given as quickly as possible for maximal benefit.

3. What is the current role of gastric lavage in treating acute poisonings?
Gastric lavage works faster than syrup of ipecac in emptying stomach contents, and activated charcoal can be administered down the lavage tube before it is pulled. Gastric lavage can be accomplished without prior tracheal intubation in most patients, but it is advised that airway equipment,

including suction, be immediately available at the bedside. Placing the patient on the left side in mild Trendelenburg position helps to prevent aspiration if vomiting occurs. Nasogastric tubes are too small to remove pills or large pill fragments; whenever gastric lavage is done, a large-bore tube (36F or 40F in adults) should be placed through the mouth. A bite-block with an oral airway prevents the patient from biting the tube. Proper location of the lavage tube in the stomach must be verified clinically or radiographically before lavage or administration of charcoal. Deaths have been reported resulting from charcoal instillation into the trachea by nasogastric tube. Gastric lavage generally is reserved for patients with potentially serious or life-threatening overdose who present within 1 or 2 hours after ingestion.

4. What is the current role of activated charcoal?

Activated charcoal has been shown in numerous studies to be superior to gastric emptying procedures for the treatment of acute overdose. Gastric emptying procedures involve time and some risk to the patient. The time involved in lavaging the patient or in inducing emesis with ipecac is time during which drugs are being actively absorbed. By giving a dose of activated charcoal immediately on patient presentation, the most effective means of GI decontamination already has been performed should the patient deteriorate. Not all drugs are adsorbed to charcoal, however. Drugs that are not adsorbed include lithium, acids and alkalis, potassium, iron, and perhaps others not yet studied. Patients with inadvertent trivial ingestions (generally children) do not require activated charcoal therapy.

5. What about the asymptomatic overdose patient?

It has been advocated by some that simple observation of asymptomatic overdose patients, with treatment only if symptoms develop, is a management option. Although this approach is safe for many patients who have ingested trivial overdoses, if a patient ingested something quite dangerous, an opportunity to prevent absorption may have been lost if nothing is done until symptoms develop. Administering a dose of activated charcoal to all patients with a history of deliberate drug overdose is done easily (although often messy) and helps to ensure safe and timely patient disposition.

6. Is there a role for cathartics in treating acute poisoning?

The theory behind cathartics is that they speed up GI transit time, allowing activated charcoal to catch up with pills in the bowel and prevent desorption of drug from activated charcoal. Cathartics have not been shown to reduce drug absorption or improve outcome significantly after overdose, but they can cause vomiting, abdominal pain, and electrolyte abnormalities. Use of cathartics is *not* warranted.

7. What is the current role of whole-bowel irrigation in the treatment of acute poisoning?

Whole-bowel irrigation uses a polyethylene glycol electrolyte solution such as GoLYTELY or Colyte, which is not adsorbed and flushes drugs or chemicals rapidly through the GI tract. This procedure seems to be most useful when radiopaque tablets or chemicals have been ingested because their progress through the GI tract can be monitored by radiography. This procedure also is commonly used when packets of street drugs, such as heroin or cocaine, have been ingested and need to be passed through the GI tract as quickly as possible and should be considered after overdose of sustained-release products. The limitations of the procedure are that unless the patient is awake, cooperative, and able to sit on a commode, there is a risk of vomiting and aspiration in addition to the logistical problem of having an unconscious patient in bed with massive diarrhea.

8. What is the role of multiple-dose charcoal in the treatment of acute poisoning?

Multiple-dose charcoal has been shown to enhance the elimination of many drugs that already have been absorbed from the GI tract or that are given intravenously. This process has been called **gastrointestinal dialysis** and has been shown to be effective for theophylline and perhaps phenobarbital poisoning. Numerous other drugs have been shown to have their pharmacokinetics altered by multiple-dose charcoal, but it is not clear if this makes a clinical difference. Many of these drugs have large volumes of distribution, and increasing elimination of the small amount present in the blood is unlikely to be of benefit. Multiple-dose activated charcoal is used most commonly after overdose of theophylline, phenobarbital, carbamazepine, and quinine.

9. Is forced diuresis of benefit in the treatment of acute poisoning?

Few drugs are excreted unchanged in the urine so that even increasing urine flow significantly above baseline is unlikely to be of benefit. By manipulating the pH of the urine by infusions of bicarbonate solution along with enhanced urine flow, however, in certain cases drug elimination can be increased. This most commonly is used for salicylates and phenobarbital. By placing three ampules of sodium bicarbonate in 1 L of D_5W along with potassium chloride and infusing this solution at rates sufficient to produce at least a normal urine flow and a urine pH of 7.5 or greater, the elimination of salicylate and phenobarbital can be increased. Intake and output and urine pH should be monitored hourly with a Foley catheter in place. In the presence of pulmonary or cerebral edema, which may occur in severe salicylate intoxication, alkaline diuresis is dangerous and should not be undertaken.

Alkaline diuresis also may work in a similar manner for chlorophenoxy herbicides, but acute poisonings by these agents are rare. The use of high-volume normal saline to treat lithium intoxication is common, and it is important to maintain adequate urine output and serum sodium in this scenario. It is not clear, however, that forced-saline diuresis for lithium intoxication is of extra benefit over simply ensuring normal renal flow.

10. When are extracorporeal techniques, such as hemodialysis or hemoperfusion, indicated?

Drugs can be removed successfully by extracorporeal maneuvers only if they have relatively small volumes of distribution and are found in significant quantities in the circulation, as opposed to having rapid and thorough tissue distribution. This is the case for only a few drugs. In practice, the drugs most commonly dialyzed after overdose include aspirin, lithium, and perhaps theophylline. Dialysis has the advantage over hemoperfusion in that it is frequently easier and faster to get started and can correct fluid and electrolyte abnormalities as it removes drugs. Charcoal hemoperfusion may be more effective at removing drugs that are highly bound to plasma proteins because the affinity for charcoal may be higher than the affinity for the protein carrier. The disadvantage of hemoperfusion is that unless frequently done in skilled hands, the procedure can result in frequent canister clotting. Hypocalcemia and a precipitous drop in platelet count are common. Drugs for which charcoal hemoperfusion is frequently employed include theophylline, phenobarbital, and a few other less common agents such as paraquat and amatoxin.

11. How can the diagnosis of a drug overdose be made when the patient is unconscious and history is unavailable?

The diagnosis of acute overdose is difficult to make sometimes and requires some detective work on the part of the physician. All unconscious patients should receive dextrose (or a rapid bedside serum glucose determination) and naloxone (Narcan); a positive response to either of these is diagnostic. Whenever possible, examination of the pill bottles available to the patient is important, and it is useful to call the pharmacies where the prescriptions were filled to determine if other prescriptions were filled there for different drugs. Discovering which chemical agents were available to the patient, including street drugs, is always important. If needle track marks are seen, consider street drugs commonly given intravenously, such as opiates, cocaine, and amphetamine. The physical examination is useful in narrowing the diagnosis to a class of drug or chemicals. This concept is commonly called **toxic syndromes.**

Most Common Toxic Syndromes

Anticholinergic
Common signs: Dementia with mumbling speech, tachycardia, dry flushed skin, dilated pupils, myoclonus, temperature slightly elevated, urinary retention, decreased bowel sounds. Seizures and arrhythmias may occur in severe cases

Common causes: Antihistamines, antiparkinsonism medication, atropine, scopolamine, amantadine, antipsychotics, antidepressants, antispasmodics, mydriatics, skeletal muscle relaxants, many plants (most notably jimson weed)

Sympathomimetic
Common signs: Delusions, paranoia, tachycardia, hypertension, hyperpyrexia, diaphoresis, piloerection, mydriasis, hyperreflexia. Seizures and arrhythmias may occur in severe cases

Common causes: Cocaine, amphetamine, methamphetamine (and derivatives MDA, MDMA, MDEA, DOB), over-the-counter decongestants (phenylpropanolamine, ephedrine, pseudoephedrine). Caffeine and theophylline overdoses cause similar findings secondary to catecholamine release except for the organic psychiatric signs

Opiate/Sedative
Common signs: Coma, respiratory depression, miosis, hypotension, bradycardia, hypothermia, pulmonary edema, decreased bowel sounds, hyporeflexia, needle marks

Common causes: Narcotics, barbiturates, benzodiazepines, ethchlorvynol, glutethimide, methyprylon, methaqualone, meprobamate

Cholinergic
Common signs: Confusion/central nervous system depression, weakness, salivation, lacrimation, urinary and fecal incontinence, GI cramping, emesis, diaphoresis, muscle fasciculations, pulmonary edema, miosis, bradycardia (or tachycardia), seizures

Common causes: Organophosphate and carbamate insecticides, physostigmine, edrophonium, some mushrooms (*Amanita muscaria, Amanita pantherina, Inocybe, Clitocybe*)

Serotonin
Common signs: Fever, tremor, uncoordination, agitation, mental status changes, diaphoresis, myoclonus, diarrhea, rigidity

Common causes: Fluoxetine, sertraline, paroxetine, venlafaxine, clomipramine; the preceding drugs in combination with monoamine oxidase inhibitors

---

12. How can a toxicology screen and other ancillary laboratory tests make the diagnosis of acute poisoning?

The blood and urine toxicology screen should be done on any patient who has significant toxicity and when the diagnosis is uncertain. Alternatives to a full toxicology screen include testing discrete serum levels of the toxins in question, doing a urine qualitative test for drugs of abuse, or drawing specimens but holding them until it is determined that a toxicology screen is definitely indicated. More drugs and chemicals are *not* found on typical toxicology screens than *are* found on the screens, although most drugs that commonly are ingested are found on comprehensive toxicology screens. It is important to communicate with the laboratory about which drugs are suspected, which drugs the patient takes therapeutically, and the clinical condition of the patient. Whenever there is a discrepancy between clinical suspicion and findings from the toxicology screen, it is useful to communicate with the toxicology laboratory personnel and assist them in determining if other tests are likely to be of benefit. Toxicology screens are expensive, frequently are inexact, and frequently do not give all the information that is expected by the clinician. It is important to interpret toxicology screens carefully and to know which drugs and chemicals were not screened for.

Nontoxicologic laboratory tests that are frequently useful include an ECG, which can help diagnose overdose of tricyclic antidepressants or cardiac medications; a chest radiograph, which if demonstrative of noncardiogenic pulmonary edema would make one think of salicylates or opiates; and a kidneys-ureters-bladder (KUB) screen, looking for radiopaque material, which would make one suspicious of ingestion of a heavy metal, including iron, phenothiazines, chloral hydrate, or chlorinated hydrocarbon solvents. Liver function tests may help to diagnose ingestion of hepatotoxins, such as acetaminophen or carbon tetrachloride. A urinalysis may show the presence of calcium oxalate crystals, suggesting the diagnosis of ethylene glycol poisoning. The acid-base status of the patient is important. Persistent unexplained metabolic acidosis always should prompt the search for other diagnostic clues to aspirin, methanol, or ethylene glycol poisoning. Many other drugs can cause a persistent, unexplained metabolic acidosis, including the ingestion of acids themselves, cyanide, carbon monoxide, theophylline, and others. In the workup of persistent acidosis, a serum osmolality done by freezing point depression can be useful if it is elevated. A difference between the measured osmolality and the calculated osmolality of greater than 10 is always significant, although a normal osmolol gap does not rule out toxic ingestion.

13. Discuss some other useful antidotes for common poisonings.

Naloxone and **dextrose** are the most common antidotes and should be given routinely to unconscious overdose patients. Intravenous administration of 2 mg of naloxone that results in awakening of the patient is diagnostic of acute opiate overdose. Lesser doses may be ineffective and should not be used, unless it is known that the patient is an opiate addict and that the 2-mg dose of naloxone will precipitate withdrawal. Many drugs and chemicals can cause hypoglycemia, including ethanol, and for this reason dextrose likewise should be given, unless it can be determined quickly that the blood glucose is normal.

Physostigmine is an antidote for the anticholinergic syndrome. Physostigmine can be diagnostically and therapeutically when the diagnosis of the anticholinergic syndrome is suspected. It should not be used to treat tricyclic antidepressant poisoning. Seizures and bradyarrhythmias have been reported when used in this setting. A dose of 1 to 2 mg given slowly intravenously to an adult is usually sufficient.

Digoxin immune Fab (Digibind) is a safe and effective antidote for digitalis glycoside poisoning and can rapidly reverse arrhythmias and hyperkalemia, which can be life-threatening. In contrast to naloxone, Digibind does not work immediately, and a full response to therapy may not be seen until approximately 20 minutes after administration. For a life-threatening digitalis overdose when the dose and the serum level are currently unknown, 10 vials of Digibind should be given.

Atropine and **pralidoxime (Protopam)** are antidotes used for cholinesterase inhibitor toxicity. This group of pesticides includes the organophosphates and carbamates, which commonly are found in household insecticides. Atropine is used to dry up secretions, primarily pulmonary, and pralidoxime is used primarily to reverse the skeletal muscle toxicity of these agents, including weakness and fasciculations.

Flumazenil is a benzodiazepine antagonist that has been shown to be useful in cases of acute benzodiazepine overdose resulting in significant toxicity. Its use may precipitate benzodiazepine withdrawal, including seizures. It should not be used when tricyclic antidepressants or other proconvulsants have been coingested with benzodiazepine. The usual adult dose is 0.2 mg followed in 30 seconds by 0.3 mg, followed in 30 seconds by 0.5 mg, repeated up to a total of 3 mg.

BIBLIOGRAPHY

1. Chyka PA, Seger D: Position statement: Single-dose activated charcoal. American Academy of Clinical Toxicology; European Association of Poisons Centres and Clinical Toxicologists. Clin Toxicol 35:721–36.
2. Hofer P, Scollo-Lavizzari G: Benzodiazepine antagonist Ro 15-1788 in self-poisoning: Diagnostic and therapeutic use. Arch Intern Med 145:663–664, 1985.
3. Hoffman RS, Smilkstein M, Goldfrank CR: Whole bowel irrigation and the cocaine body packer: A new approach to a common problem. Am J Emerg Med 8:523–527, 1990.
4. Kellerman AL, Fihn SD, Logerfro JP, et al: Impact of drug screening in suspected overdose. Ann Emerg Med 16:1206–1216, 1987.
5. Kulig KW, Bar-Or D, Cantrill SV, et al: Management of acutely poisoned patients without gastric emptying. Ann Emerg Med 14:562–567, 1985.
6. Litovitz TL, Klein-Schwartz W, White S, et al: 2000 Annual report of the American Association of Poison Control Centers Toxic Exposure Surveillance System. Am J Emerg Med 19:337–396, 2001.

7. Merigian KS, Woodard M, Hedges JR, et al: Prospective evaluation of gastric emptying in the self-poisoned patient. Am J Emerg Med 8:479–483, 1990.
8. Olson KR, Pentel PR, Kelley MT: Physical assessment and differential diagnosis of the poisoned patient. Med Toxicol 2:52–81, 1987.
9. Osterloh JD: Utility and reliability of emergency toxicologic testing. Emerg Med Clin North Am 8:693–723, 1990.
10. Pond SM, Lewis-Driver DJ, Williams GM, et al: Gastric emptying in acute overdose: A prospective randomised controlled trial. Med J Aust 163:345–349, 1995.
11. Tenenbein M: Position statement: Whole bowel irrigation. American Academy of Clinical Toxicology; European Association of Poisons Centres and Clinical Toxicologists. J Toxicol Clin Toxicol 35:753–762, 1997.
12. Vale JA: Position statement: Gastric lavage. American Academy of Clinical Toxicology; European Association of Poisons Centres and Clinical Toxicologists. J Toxicol Clin Toxicol 35:711–719, 1997.
13. Vale JA, Krenzelok EP, Barceloux GD: Position statement and practice guidelines on the use of multidose activated charcoal in the treatment of acute poisoning. J Toxicol Clin Toxicol 37:731–751, 1999.

82. THE ALCOHOLS: ETHYLENE GLYCOL, METHANOL, AND ISOPROPYL ALCOHOL

Louis J. Ling, M.D.

1. Why is it important to understand the metabolism of methanol?

The metabolites are the toxins and depend on alcohol dehydrogenase (ADH) for their conversion from the parent methanol. Ethanol saturates ADH and greatly decreases the amount of toxin. Folate is a cofactor in the breakdown of formic acid, and in monkeys (and other primates), folate supplementation maximizes its metabolism and decreases injury. Knowledge of the metabolism directs the treatment.

$$\text{Methanol} \quad \xrightarrow{\text{ADH}} \quad \underset{\text{(toxic)}}{\text{Formaldehyde}} \quad \to \quad \underset{\text{(toxic)}}{\text{Formic Acid}} \quad \xrightarrow{\text{folate}} \quad CO_2 + H_2O$$

2. Why is it important to understand the metabolism of ethylene glycol?

As with methanol, ethanol saturates ADH, inhibiting conversion of ethylene glycol into its harmful metabolites. Pyridoxine (vitamin B_6) and thiamine are cofactors in the final steps to form nonharmful end products and should be given to ensure maximal metabolism. Oxalate crystals may not appear until late in the course of the poisoning (see Figure, top of next page).

3. Why are the symptoms of ethylene glycol and methanol overdose often delayed?

Because the toxicity of methanol and ethylene glycol is the result of toxic metabolites, it may take 6 to 12 hours for sufficient quantities of these toxic metabolites to appear and cause symptoms. The delay in onset of symptoms is even greater with concurrent ethanol intoxication because the ethanol prevents the methanol metabolism.

4. How are methanol and ethylene glycol poisonings similar?

Methanol and ethylene glycol are metabolized initially by ADH. Methanol is metabolized further to formic acid, and ethylene glycol is metabolized to glycolic acid, glyoxylic acid, oxalate, and several nontoxic metabolites. Because of these end products, both poisons result in metabolic acidosis with an anion gap. Because of their low molecular weight, both increase the osmolar gap.

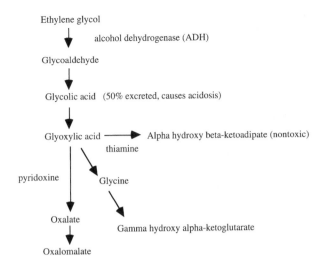

Ethylene glycol

alcohol dehydrogenase (ADH)

Glycoaldehyde

Glycolic acid   (50% excreted, causes acidosis)

Glyoxylic acid ⟶ Alpha hydroxy beta-ketoadipate (nontoxic)

thiamine

pyridoxine   Glycine

Oxalate

Gamma hydroxy alpha-ketoglutarate

Oxalomalate

(3% excreted)
crystallizes with calcium in urine, vessels

5. What is an anion gap?

Normal anion gap is the difference between unmeasured anions (e.g., various proteins, organic acids, phosphates) and unmeasured cations (e.g., potassium, calcium, and magnesium). The anion gap can be calculated from the formula:

$$\text{Anion gap} = (Na^+) - (HCO^{-3} + Cl^-)$$

6. What causes an increased anion gap?

When metabolic acidosis results from an ingestion or increase of nonvolatile acids, there are increased hydrogen ions with positive charges. Because there is an increase in unmeasured negatively charged anions and no increases in chloride, the difference between the measured cations and anions is increased, causing an increased anion gap. The normal anion gap is about 6 to 10 mEq/L. The cause of increased anion gap can be remembered by the mnemonic **A MUD PILES**.

A	= Alcohol	**P**	= Paraldehyde
		I	= Iron, Isoniazid (INH)
M	= Methanol	**L**	= Lactate
U	= Uremia	**E**	= Ethylene glycol
D	= Diabetic ketoacidosis	**S**	= Salicylate

7. What is an osmolal gap?

Small atoms and molecules in solution are osmotically active, and this activity can be measured by a depression in the freezing point or an elevation in the boiling point of the solution. If there is an increase in low-molecular-weight molecules, such as acetone, methanol, ethanol, mannitol, isopropyl alcohol, or ethylene glycol, the osmolality increases more than what is calculated from the usual serum molecules. The difference between the actual measured osmolality and the calculated osmolality is the osmolal gap, and a gap greater than 10 mOsm is considered abnormal.

8. How is an osmolal gap calculated?

$2 \times Na^+$ (mEq/L) + glucose (mg/dL)/18 + blood urea nitrogen (BUN) (mg/dL)/2.8 + ethanol (mg/dL)/4.3. The inclusion of the ethanol level excludes patients who have an elevated osmolal gap from ethanol ingestion alone. Using International System (SI) units, the calculated osmolality = $2 \times Na$ (mEq/L) + glucose (mmol/L) + BUN (mmol/L) + ethanol (mmol/L). The calculated osmolality is 285 ± 5 mOsm/L. A toxic ethylene glycol level of 25 mg/dL can be predicted to increase the osmolal gap 5 mOsm/L. Because of the small effects on the osmolality and the imprecision of the measurement, this test is not precise enough to be definitive. A normal osmolal gap does not exclude toxic levels of methanol or ethylene glycol. The laboratory must use the method of freezing-point depression so that volatile alcohols contributing to an osmolal gap are not boiled away during a boiling point elevation procedure.

9. How toxic are methanol and ethylene glycol?
  Death has been reported after 15 to 30 mL (1 to 2 tablespoons) of methanol. Others have survived larger ingestions, however. A minimal lethal dose for ethylene glycol is approximately 1 to 2 mL/kg.

10. List the signs and symptoms of methanol poisoning.
  Gastrointestinal toxicity
  Nausea
  Vomiting
  Abdominal pain
  Central nervous system toxicity
  Headache
  Decreased level of consciousness
  Confusion
  Ocular toxicity
  Retinal edema
  Hyperemia of the disc
  Decreased visual acuity
  Other toxicity
  Metabolic acidosis

11. What is the toxicity of ethylene glycol?
  There is central nervous system intoxication and gastrointestinal irritation early on followed by metabolic acidosis. Renal failure occurs frequently and typically is delayed in presentation. Cranial nerve deficits are a rare complication. Ethylene glycol is a frequent cause of death in animals who ingest antifreeze. Cause of death for these animals may not be apparent because toxicity is delayed.

12. Why does antifreeze have such a bright color?
  Antifreeze is a bright color that fluoresces with UV light so that leaks can be detected easier in the cooling system of a car. If the mouth and the urine are examined with a UV light, fluorescein can be detected in about 30% of patients with an ingestion. A positive test should encourage immediate treatment, but a negative test misses two thirds of ingestions.

13. How should patients with methanol and ethylene glycol poisoning be treated?
  Airway protection is paramount in patients with decreased level of consciousness or respiratory depression. Although gastric lavage might be helpful in large ingestions, small volumes and rapid absorption limit its effectiveness. Acidosis (pH < 7.2) should be treated aggressively with sodium bicarbonate. Ethanol and 4-methylpyrazole (4-MP) are antidotes that competitively block the conversion of methanol and ethylene glycol to their toxic metabolites, allowing for elimination of the unchanged poison without injury.

14. What are the indications for ethanol or 4-MP therapy?
  They should be used if ethylene glycol or methanol levels exceed 20 mg/dL; if acidosis is present, regardless of drug level; and if there is a history of a toxic ingestion while awaiting confirmatory blood methanol or ethylene glycol levels.

15. How is ethanol treatment started and maintained?

1. Maintain an ethanol level of 100 to 200 mg/dL
   Load   0.6–0.8 g/kg
   Maintenance   0.11 g/kg/h
   Dialysis   0.24 g/kg/h
2. Oral methods
   Load   20–50% solutions for load per nasogastric tube; 2 mL/kg of 50%
                        gives 0.8 g/kg
                        Use stock pharmacy solution and dilute 1:1
   Maintain   0.11–0.13 g/kg/h
                        0.16 mL/kg/h of 95% solutions but dilute with water 1:1 to avoid
                        gastritis and give 0.33 mL/kg/h
                        Increase proportionately with dialysis
3. Intravenous methods
   Load   10% concentration (used as standard treatment for stopping labor)
                        in D_5W through a central catheter at 10 mL/kg
   Maintain   1.6 mL/kg/h of 10% solution
                        Increase proportionately with dialysis

16. What are the problems with ethanol therapy?

Ethanol can be difficult to give consistently; ethanol blood levels are required to adjust the dose and avoid oversedation. Dialysis requires an increased dose and more blood levels. An infusion can cause pain resulting in the use of a central catheter. Ethanol may cause hypoglycemia, especially in children. These patients usually require the close monitoring of an ICU.

17. What is the role of 4-MP?

4-MP is replacing ethanol as a safe, easy-to-use antidote for methanol and ethylene glycol poisoning. 4-MP acts to inhibit ADH conversion of methanol and ethylene glycol to their toxic metabolites. The dose is 15 mg/kg every 12 hours and is increased to every 4 hours during dialysis. Typical treatment is for 48 hours.

18. What are the indications for hemodialysis?

Dialysis used to be the primary treatment for these poisons and should be done in patients with blood levels greater than 50 mg/dL, when the metabolic acidosis is not correctable, with pending renal failure, or with visual symptoms in a methanol overdose. Many clinicians recommend dialysis when blood levels exceed 25 mg/dL, if dialysis is readily available.

19. What if dialysis is unavailable?

Patients with ethylene glycol poisoning have been treated successfully with 4-MP alone without dialysis if there is no acidosis or renal failure. Because the half-life of ethylene glycol is prolonged, the treatment may be extended, but the invasive treatment of dialysis is avoided. As experience grows, the primary treatment for ethylene glycol may be 4-MP alone with limited dialysis use. In methanol poisoning, 4-MP slows the metabolism and increases the half-life of methanol, which has been measured at 30 to 52 hours. The use of 4-MP alone would not suffice for these patients.

20. How is isopropyl alcohol poisoning different from methanol and ethylene glycol poisoning?

Isopropyl alcohol is metabolized in the liver to acetone, which results in measurable ketonemia in the serum. Acetone is excreted by the kidney, resulting in ketonuria, and is exhaled through the lungs, giving patients an acetone aroma on their breath. Because these metabolites are not acidic, isopropyl alcohol poisoning does not result in metabolic acidosis and is far less toxic than either methanol or ethylene glycol poisoning.

21. What are the symptoms of isopropyl alcohol ingestion?

Isopropyl alcohol, commonly seen as rubbing alcohol, has a three-carbon chain rather than a two-carbon chain similar to ethanol. Because of this, it crosses the blood-brain barrier much faster and is about twice as intoxicating as ethanol. Because it commonly is found in concentrated solutions and is more potent, the central nervous system depression can occur rapidly and can continue from residual poison in the stomach. Isopropyl alcohol is much more irritating to the gastric mucosa and often causes abdominal pain, vomiting, and hematemesis.

22. What treatment is advisable for isopropyl alcohol poisoning?

Generally, patients need observation similar to that for patients intoxicated with ethanol to watch for respiratory depression. An isopropyl alcohol level is roughly equivalent to an ethanol level twice as high. An isopropyl level usually does not add greatly to clinical observation. In the rare, severe instance of coma or hypertension corresponding to isopropyl levels greater than 500 mg/dL, intubation and ventilation may be necessary, and hemodialysis may be helpful because it can greatly enhance removal of isopropyl alcohol from the body. An antidote is not available for isopropyl alcohol (nor is one needed).

BIBLIOGRAPHY

1. Barceloux DG, Krenzelok EP, Olson K, et al: American Academy of Clinical Toxicology practice guidelines on the treatment of ethylene glycol poisoning. Clin Toxicol 37:537–560, 1999.
2. Brent J, McMartin KE, Philips S, et al: Fomepizole for the treatment of ethylene glycol poisoning. N Engl J Med 340:832, 1999.
3. Brent J, McMartin KE, Philips S, et al: Fomepizole for the treatment of methanol poisoning. N Engl J Med 344:424–429, 2001.
4. Burkhart KK, Kulig KW: The other alcohols: Methanol, ethylene glycol, isopropanol. Emerg Med Clin North Am 8:913–918, 1990.
5. Dethlefs R, Naraqi S: Ocular manifestations and complications of acute methyl alcohol intoxication. Med J Aust 2:483–485, 1978.
6. Ford MD, McMartin K: Ethylene glycol and methanol. In Ford M, Delaney K, Ling L, et al (eds): Clinical Toxicology, Philadelphia, W.B. Saunders, 2001 pp 757–769.
7. Glaser DS: Utility of the serum osmol gap in the diagnosis of methanol or ethylene glycol ingestion. Ann Emerg Med 27:343–346, 1996.
8. Hylander B, Kjellstrand CM: Prognostic factors and treatment of severe ethylene glycol intoxication. Intensive Care Med 22:546–552, 1996.
9. Palatnick W, Redman LW, Sitar DS, Tenenbein M: Methanol half-life during ethanol administration: Implications for management of methanol poisoning. Ann Emerg Med 26:202–207, 1995.
10. Spillane L, Roberts JR, et al: Multiple cranial nerve deficits after ethylene glycol poisoning. Ann Emerg Med 20:208–210, 1991.

83. ALCOHOL-RELATED DISORDERS

John A. Marx, M.D.

1. Is a patient who smells of alcohol simply intoxicated?

Perhaps, and in most cases, yes. There is a clinically relevant differential of altered mentation in such a patient, however. It is crucial that every patient assumed to be drunk (only) receive careful initial and serial evaluations. This is neither time-consuming nor expensive.

2. List the differential diagnosis for altered mentation.

1. **Traumatic**
   Intracranial hemorrhage
   Hypotension secondary
   to hemorrhage

2. **Metabolic**
   Hypoglycemia
   Hepatic encephalopathy
   Hypoxia
3. **Toxicologic**
   Other alcohols
   Other toxins
   Disulfiram
   Disulfiram-ethanol reaction
4. **Infectious**
   Meningitis, meningoencephalitis
   Brain abscess
   Sepsis
5. **Neurologic**
   Postictal state
   Alcohol withdrawal
   Wernicke-Korsakoff syndrome

3. When should an acutely intoxicated patient be intubated?

Whenever you think it is indicated. No quantitative determinants (e.g., serum ethanol level) exist that serve as useful guidelines. Hypopnea and hypoventilation are rarely the issue, but the inability of the patient to protect the airway is. The odds against the stomach being empty approach infinity. For patients who are heavily intoxicated but not deemed to require intubation, lateral decubitus positioning is preferred. Restraining a patient supine or prone can be dangerous because of the risk of aspiration and airway compromise.

4. Which pharmacologic agents are best for management of alcohol withdrawal?

The most widely used and time-honored mainstay is the **benzodiazepine** class. Benzodiazepines should be given orally, intravenously, or in combination and titrated by clinical response. No single benzodiazepine has been proclaimed the best agent. Pharmacokinetics, the presence of intermediate metabolites, and mostly physician preference are deciding factors. Patients with mild withdrawal (normal vital signs, no hallucinosis) may be discharged with a 2- to 3-day course of a single agent (e.g., lorazepam, 1 to 2 mg twice a day). Haloperidol is an appropriate adjunct for hallucinosis. Theoretical concerns over lowering seizure threshold and exacerbating hemodynamic abnormalities in this class of patients have not been substantiated.

5. Describe an appropriate diagnostic workup for alcohol withdrawal seizures (AWDS).

Two issues are germane: (1) Is the story consistent with an AWDS? (2) Is this the initial presentation and workup for suspected AWDS?

Typically, AWDS occurs approximately 6 to 96 hours after the last drink and in clusters of one to four seizures. The seizures, usually grand mal, are self-limited. Coincident features of withdrawal may be lacking, and lateralizing findings during the seizure, the postictal state, or both are often present because of underlying structural pathology. In a first-time evaluation, other causes of or contributors to seizures should be sought. Routine laboratory studies (electrolytes, glucose, magnesium, calcium, toxicologic screen) are rarely useful unless history or physical examination is suggestive. Noncontrast CT helps guide management. Nearly 10% of patients show traumatic, infectious, vascular, or miscellaneous abnormalities. Generally, electroencephalography is not integral to the workup. Lumbar puncture is indicated when meningitis, meningoencephalitis, or subarachnoid hemorrhage is suspected. Subsequent visits demand scrupulous history and physical examination to ensure that other pathologic causes have not developed in the interim. If the presentation matches prior episodes and the findings on current neurologic examination are baseline, no other workup, including CT, is necessary. Lingering postictal confusion warrants a check of glucose and electrolytes. If the story or examination has changed significantly or is worrisome, the clinician should start from scratch.

6. How should AWDS be managed?

Acute. Active AWDS is handled in routine fashion (i.e., ensure patient safety and patent airway and administer D_{50}, naloxone, and intravenous benzodiazepines as needed). If diagnostic evaluation is unremarkable, an observation period of at least 6 hours is optimal because additional seizures are common and occur within this period. Use of benzodiazepines in the immediate postseizure observation period and for 2 days thereafter decreases the incidence of additional seizures during this vulnerable time.

Chronic. Patients whose seizures have an elliptogenic focus (e.g., old subdural) should receive anticonvulsant therapy such as **phenytoin**. Compliance is typically poor. In the patient with pure AWDS (CT is unremarkable), long-term anticonvulsant therapy is absolutely *contraindicated*. Physicians must resist the pharmacologic imperative to "prescribe something" long-term, unless there is clear justification to do so.

7. Can AWDS be prevented?

Data support prophylactic use of benzodiazepines in the acute withdrawal period, particularly in patients with a history of AWDS during abstinence and in patients who sustained a suspected AWDS as cause for their being brought to the ED or during their stay there.

8. Who is at risk for alcohol-induced hypoglycemia (AIH), and what is the clinical presentation?

AIH results from two pathophysiologic processes: insufficient glycogen stores and alcohol-induced impairment of gluconeogenesis. The three groups vulnerable to AIH are chronic alcoholics, binge drinkers, and young children. AIH may occur during intoxication or up to 20 hours after the last drink. Manifestations of neuroglycopenia (headache, depressed mental status, seizure, coma) predominate. Evidence of catecholamine excess, typical of insulin-induced hypoglycemia (tremulousness, diaphoresis, anxiety), is unusual. Two clinical caveats are important. Seizures are a frequent presentation in children. Localized central nervous system signs, including a strokelike picture, often occur in adults.

9. What causes alcoholic ketoacidosis?

This common metabolic disturbance occurs early after heavy binge drinking and is heralded by starvation and vomiting and occasionally shortness of breath (Kussmaul respirations) and abdominal pain. Ketoacidosis results from accumulation of acetoacetate and β-hydroxybutyrate. At presentation, serum pH and bicarbonate average 7.1 and 10. These values vary widely, however, because of the frequently overlapping conditions of withdrawal-related hyperventilation (respiratory alkalosis) and protracted emesis (metabolic alkalosis). When all three are coincident, the result is a triple acid-base disturbance. When in a clinical teaching situation, this allows you to interpret arterial blood gases and electrolytes pretty much any way you wish and still be at least partially correct. Be aware that depressed body stores of potassium and phosphate are typical. In alcoholic ketoacidosis, serum glucose is usually normal or may be low, a distinguishing feature from diabetic ketoacidosis.

10. How should alcoholic ketoacidosis be managed?

Treatment consists of rehydration with dextrose-containing crystalloid, antiemetics if needed, and benzodiazepines as dictated by symptoms of withdrawal. Vitamin, potassium, and phosphate supplementation is indicated. Bicarbonate administration is rarely required, and insulin therapy is proscribed. Normalization of metabolic abnormalities usually follows 12 to 16 hours of therapy.

11. What is the relationship between alcohol and metabolic acidosis?

Ethanol: Acute ethanol ingestion results in a mild increase in the lactate-to-pyruvate ratio. Clinically significant metabolic acidosis does not ensue.

Alcoholic ketoacidosis: This ethanol abstinence syndrome produces marked elevations in acetoacetate and β-hydroxybutyrate with resultant and occasionally profound increased anion gap metabolic acidosis. During the correction phase, a non-anion gap, hyperchloremic picture often develops (because some of the bicarbonate-bound ketoacids are excreted in the urine) on the road to normalization.

Ethylene glycol and methanol: Certain by-products of these highly toxic compounds produce increased anion gap metabolic acidosis.

Isopropyl alcohol: A significant portion of isopropyl alcohol is metabolized to acetone. This is a ketone but not a ketoacid. Exposure to this alcohol can cause ketosis and ketonuria but not acidosis.

12. Which coagulopathies should be anticipated in a chronic alcoholic?

Thrombocytopenia results from direct bone marrow depressant effects of ethanol, folate deficiency, and hypersplenism secondary to portal hypertension. Counts less than 30,000/μL resulting from alcohol usage alone are unlikely. Qualitative platelet defects also may occur.

Hepatocyte loss caused by chronic alcohol abuse depletes all coagulation factors except VIII, particularly II, VII, IX, and X. Alcoholics often have inadequate vitamin K stores because of hepatobiliary dysfunction and poor diet. Vitamin K is a requisite cofactor for the production of factors II, VII, IX, and X. When faced with gastrointestinal hemorrhage in a chronic alcoholic, an intravenous vitamin K supplementation trial is warranted. The far more likely culprit is hepatocellular destruction, however, for which vitamin K would not be helpful. Vitamin K does not begin to restore factor levels for 2 to 6 hours after administration. For emergent scenarios, fresh frozen plasma provides immediate factor supplementation.

13. How should the combative alcoholic patient be managed?

When the patient or staff is in jeopardy, the first step is mechanical containment of the patient. A sufficient number of competent personnel and restraint devices are necessary. A simple matter such as a closed head injury, hypoxia, or a full bladder may be the source of distress and should be excluded, managed, or relieved.

For chemical sedation, haloperidol is the preferred agent. It can be given quickly (initial dose, 5 to 10 mg intravenous push) and cause rapid onset of sedation (5 minutes). Repeat doses may be required. This agent is not detrimental to airway patency, ventilation, or hemodynamics. There is a 5% to 10% incidence of extrapyramidal reactions that usually occur 12 to 24 hours after administration; this compares favorably with the obvious dangers of benzodiazepines, narcotics, and paralytic agents.

14. When can an acutely intoxicated patient be safely discharged from the ED?

From a management perspective, there are two fundamental concerns: (1) Acute intoxication obfuscates the verification of certain diagnoses and the exclusion of others. (2) A physician who discharges an acutely intoxicated (i.e., incompetent) patient may be held accountable for the actions of that patient subsequent and proximate to discharge from the ED.

The conundrum lies in the definition of **intoxication**. Numerous tests provide tables that match serum alcohol levels with clinical findings. In truth, the degree of clinical intoxication at a specific serum alcohol level is variable in accordance with the patient's chronicity and severity of drinking. A veteran drinker with a level in excess of 500 mg/dL can look less drunk than a teenager at 100 mg/dL. The patient should undergo a scrupulous initial evaluation, then repeated examinations until the physician is comfortable that other medical concerns do not exist. Documentation of the discharge neurologic examination, including mental status, gait, and the fact that the patient is **clinically sober** is imperative. Particular attention should be paid to any patient in whom abdominal or closed head trauma may have occurred. The patient then may be discharged to an appropriate environment. Serum or breath alcohol determinations sometimes can be helpful at the outset of care but often are unneeded and can be problematic when obtained at discharge.

CONTROVERSIES

15. Must thiamine be administered before glucose in the alcoholic patient?

It has been widely held that delivery of glucose to a patient with marginal thiamine reserves would catapult that patient into Wernicke-Korsakoff syndrome. In an alcoholic patient, AIH or hypoglycemia of any cause is a far more likely cause of depressed level of consciousness than is Wernicke-Korsakoff syndrome. The use of a rapid glucose analyzer can avoid unneeded glucose administration to patients considered at risk for inadequate thiamine stores. Wernicke-Korsakoff syndrome develops over hours to days. The precipitous initiation of Wernicke-Korsakoff syndrome by dextrose has not been substantiated. The consequences of neuroglycopenia begin within 30 minutes, can be tremendously morbid, and are easily prevented. In alcoholic patients with known or strongly suspected hypoglycemia, administer glucose and deliver thiamine empirically as soon afterward as possible. Routine empirical administration of glucose and thiamine to all alcoholics is probably unnecessary.

16. Is it dangerous to administer thiamine intravenously?

Orally administered thiamine may be absorbed poorly in the alcoholic. The intramuscular route is painful and can result in hematomas or abscesses, particularly if the patient's coagulation status is impaired. The experience with intravenous thiamine is enormous, and the safety profile is exceptional. Thiamine may be given as part of fluid hydration and multivitamin preparations. It also can be given by bolus infusion.

17. Is there a cure for a hangover?

Probably not, at least not one with solid scientific credentials. There is no shortage of remedies, however, from the well-worn "hair of the dog that bit you" (i.e., start drinking again) to a more recently acclaimed concoction of vitamin B_6, nonsteroidal antiinflammatories, and hydration.

BIBLIOGRAPHY

1. D'Onofrio G, Rathlev NK, Ulrich AS, et al: Lorazepam for the prevention of recurrent seizures related to alcohol. N Engl J Med 341:609–610, 1999.
2. Earnest MD, Feldman H, Marx JA, et al: Intracranial lesions shown by CT in 259 cases of first alcohol-related seizures. Neurology 38:1561–1565, 1988.
3. Frommer DA, Marx JA: Wernicke's encephalopathy. N Engl J Med 313:637–638, 1985.
4. Marx JA, Berner J, Bar-Or D, Gorayeb MJ: Prophylaxis of alcohol withdrawal seizures: A prospective study [abstract]. Ann Emerg Med 15:637, 1986.
5. Mayo-Smith MF: Pharmacological management of alcohol withdrawal: A meta-analysis and evidence-based practice guideline. American Society of Addiction Medicine Working Group on Pharmacological Management of Alcohol Withdrawal. JAMA 278:144–151, 1997.
6. Rathlev NK, D'Onofrio G, Fish SS, et al: The lack of efficacy of phenytoin in the prevention of recurrent alcohol-related seizures. Ann Emerg Med 23:513–518, 1994.
7. Victor M, Adams RD, Collins GH: The Wernicke-Korsakoff Syndrome. Philadelphia, F.A. Davis, 1971.
8. Wrenn KD, Slovis CM, Minion G, Rotkowski R: The syndrome of alcoholic ketoacidosis. Am J Med 91:119–128, 1991.
9. Wiese JG, Shlipak MG, Browner WS: The alcohol hangover. Ann Intern Med 132:897–902, 2000.

84. ANTIPYRETIC POISONING

James C. Mitchiner, M.D., M.P.H.

SALICYLATE POISONING

1. What are the causes of salicylate overdose?

A salicylate overdose may be intentional or accidental. Parental administration of aspirin to a child using adult doses may cause toxicity. Bismuth subsalicylate (Pepto-Bismol), which contains 130 mg/tablespoon of salicylate, is often the culprit. In adults, simultaneous ingestion of proprietary aspirin and prescription medication may lead to unintentional overdose and to the formation of gastric concretions. Liquid methyl salicylate (oil of wintergreen) is especially toxic because of its high salicylate content (1 teaspoon = 7 g of salicylate) and rapid absorption. Dermal application of salicylic acid ointment is a rare cause of acute salicylism. The minimal acute toxic ingestion is 150 mg/kg.

2. What are the characteristics of a patient who presents with an acute salicylate overdose?

Patients may present with nausea, vomiting, tinnitus, fever, diaphoresis, and confusion. Hyperventilation may be ascribed mistakenly to anxiety. Patients also may present with headache or chronic pain, which prompted the ingestion of salicylate.

3. List some signs of salicylate intoxication.

Acid-base electrolyte disturbances
Dehydration
Hyperthermia
Gastrointestinal hemorrhage
Azotemia
Oliguria
Central nervous system alterations (ranging from mild confusion to seizures and coma)
Noncardiogenic pulmonary edema
Coagulopathy
Platelet dysfunction
Eyelid petechiae
Subconjunctival hemorrhage
Hypoglycemia (in children)
Rhabdomyolysis (rare)

4. Describe the acid-base disturbances.

Salicylates are capable of producing several types of acid-base disturbances. Acute **respiratory alkalosis**, without hypoxia, is due to salicylate stimulation of the respiratory center. If the patient is hypoxic, salicylate-induced noncardiogenic pulmonary edema should be considered. Within 12 to 24 hours after ingestion, the acid-base status in an untreated patient shifts toward an anion gap **metabolic acidosis**. A mixed respiratory alkalosis and metabolic acidosis typically is seen in adults. In patients presenting with **respiratory acidosis**, concomitant ingestion of a central nervous system depressant should be suspected. **Metabolic acidosis** is the predominant acid-base disturbance in children, in patients who take massive amounts of salicylates, and in patients (adults and children) who have chronic salicylate toxicity (see later).

5. What are some of the other metabolic disturbances seen in acute salicylate poisoning?

The patient may be dehydrated secondary to vomiting or to the diuretic effects of increased renal sodium excretion. Insensible losses are increased in patients with hyperventilation, and water and electrolyte losses may occur through diaphoresis in response to the hyperpyrexic state. Hypokalemia is due to renal excretion and respiratory and metabolic alkalemia (secondary to bicarbonate therapy).

6. I thought aspirin is an antipyretic. How does it cause a fever?

At a cellular level, salicylate poisoning leads to the uncoupling of oxidative phosphorylation. When this occurs, the energy obtained from oxygen reduction and reduced nicotinamide adenine dinucleotide oxidation that normally is captured to form adenosine triphosphate instead is released as heat.

7. Name some features of central nervous system dysfunction.

Irritability, confusion, delirium, tinnitus, vertigo, visual hallucinations, and disorientation may progress to seizures and coma secondary to cerebral edema.

8. Name some of the hematologic abnormalities.

These are rare in an acute overdose. Features include decreased production of prothrombin (factor II) and factor VII, an increase in capillary endothelial fragility, and a decrease in the quantity and function of platelets (i.e., decreased adhesiveness). Significant hemorrhage is unusual.

9. How is the severity of salicylate overdose assessed?

The **Done nomogram** was developed to determine the severity of salicylate poisoning. This nomogram is only a guideline, however, and applicable only to salicylate levels obtained 6 hours or more after **acute** ingestion. It should not be used for chronic overdoses, for ingestions of sustained-release or enteric-coated salicylates or methyl salicylate, in situations in which the time of ingestion is unknown, or in patients who are acidemic or azotemic. Salicylate levels should be repeated several hours apart, **while the patient is still in the ED**, so that the trend in the severity of poisoning can be assessed. The nomogram should be used with caution in the treatment of salicylate poisoning.

10. Which laboratory tests are indicated?

A serum salicylate level should be obtained in all cases. Arterial blood gases, complete blood cell count, electrolytes, blood urea nitrogen (BUN), creatinine, glucose, prothrombin time, international normalized ratio (INR), and urinalysis also should be considered. If the patient presents less than 6 hours after an acute ingestion, a salicylate level should be repeated at 6 hours. A quantitative acetaminophen level is recommended because many patients confuse these two antipyretics or mix both kinds in the same bottle. A limited toxicology screen, focusing on other treatable coingestions (opiates, barbiturates, ethanol, and cyclic antidepressants), should be done if clinically indicated.

11. How is an acute salicylate overdose treated?

If poisoning is through dermal contact, the skin should be washed copiously with tap water. For acute ingestions, gastric lavage should be done. A slurry of activated charcoal and cathartic (sorbitol or magnesium sulfate) should be given orally or by gastric lavage tube at a dose of 1 g of charcoal per kg body weight. Lavage may be useful even if the patient presents several hours after ingestion because large amounts of aspirin may form gastric concretions and delay absorption for 24 hours or longer. Isotonic intravenous fluids with bicarbonate (D_5W + 3 ampules $NaHCO_3$/L) should be administered at a rate of 10 to 15 mL/kg/h. After the patient has responded with diuresis, potassium loss should be replaced with potassium chloride at a dose of 20 to 40 mEq/L. Patients with hyperthermia should be cooled with a cooling blanket. Documented hypoglycemia should be treated with intravenous D_{50}. Patients with pulmonary edema should be treated in standard fashion, including oxygen, diuretics, intravenous nitroglycerin, and intubation, with respiratory support and positive end-expiratory pressure as needed. Sedation should be avoided because of the risk of respiratory depression leading to respiratory acidosis.

12. Is there a role for repetitive dosing of activated charcoal?

Because of aspirin release from the aspirin-charcoal complex in the gastrointestinal tract and subsequent absorption, salicylate levels may not decline significantly after a single dose of activated charcoal. Repeated doses of charcoal may be indicated to enhance elimination.

13. What is the rationale for alkaline diuresis?

Because aspirin is an organic acid, administration of bicarbonate intravenously raises the pH of the blood and *traps* salicylate ion, limiting the amount of salicylate that crosses the blood-brain barrier. Similarly, an alkalotic urine retains salicylate ion, preventing its reabsorption by the renal tubules. The use of **forced diuresis** is controversial, however, and has been reported to cause pulmonary edema. Many authorities believe that fluid replacement should be limited to fluids that have been lost through sweat, hyperventilation, and emesis.

14. Explain the paradox of a decreasing serum salicylate concentration and increasing clinical toxicity.

The serum salicylate level by itself does not reflect tissue distribution of the drug. If the patient's blood is acidemic, salicylate acid remains unionized, and more penetrates the blood-brain barrier, resulting in central nervous system toxicity. Salicylate levels should be interpreted in light of a concurrent blood pH; an acidotic pH is associated with toxicity regardless of the salicylate level.

15. What are the indications for hemodialysis?

Standard indications include persistent, refractory metabolic acidosis (pH < 7.10), renal failure with oliguria, cardiac dysfunction (congestive heart failure, arrhythmias, cardiac arrest), central nervous system deterioration (seizures, coma, cerebral edema), and an acute salicylate level greater than 130 mg/dL 6 hours after ingestion. Because ingestion of more than 300 mg/kg predicts severe toxicity, a nephrologist should be contacted early in anticipation of the possible need for dialysis.

16. What are the most common findings in chronic salicylate poisoning?

In contrast to acute salicylate poisoning, chronic salicylism is usually accidental. The principal diagnostic feature is a change in mental status manifested by weakness, tinnitus, lethargy, confusion, drowsiness, slurred speech, hallucinations, agitation, or seizures. Most patients are tachypneic, which is a compensatory response to metabolic acidosis. Because these signs are common to many other disorders, the diagnosis frequently is missed, resulting in a mortality rate of 25%. Many patients are older with a history of peptic ulcer disease, arthritis, or gastric surgery. Some have gastric outlet obstruction, resulting in delayed gastric emptying and, in some cases, formation of gastric bezoars. The latter is responsible for a slow leaching of salicylate compounds into the stomach. Serum electrolytes reveal an anion gap metabolic acidosis. The serum salicylate level may not be elevated, and the Done nomogram is of no use in chronic salicylate ingestions; if used, it often results in a false sense of security.

ACETAMINOPHEN POISONING

17. Is there anything new in acetaminophen toxicology?

Yes. The introduction of an extended-release acetaminophen formulation has compounded the difficulty in diagnosing acetaminophen poisoning. In such cases, serial acetaminophen levels should be obtained at 4 hours after ingestion and at 4-hour intervals. If any level is above the treatment line on the standard acetaminophen nomogram, antidote therapy with *N*-acetylcysteine (NAC) should be started.

18. What are the characteristics of acetaminophen overdose?

Acetaminophen is the drug most commonly involved in acute analgesic ingestions, either as a single agent or in combination with various cough, cold, or pain remedies. Early diagnosis of acute (phase I) acetaminophen toxicity is important because early symptoms may be subtle or absent; the onset of hepatotoxicity, the major manifestation, is delayed by several days after ingestion. Failure to recognize and treat toxicity within 16 hours of ingestion results in significant morbidity and mortality. *The main issue in treatment is the prevention of hepatotoxicity.*

19. Outline the four phases of acetaminophen overdose.

Phase I begins within hours of ingestion and is marked by anorexia, nausea, vomiting, and diaphoresis (some patients may be completely asymptomatic). These findings are associated with a multitude of other disorders, which accounts for the diagnostic difficulty in the recognition of occult acetaminophen poisoning.

Phase II begins 24 to 72 hours after ingestion and includes abnormalities in liver function tests and right upper quadrant abdominal pain.

Phase III starts 3 to 5 days after ingestion and includes features of advanced hepatotoxicity, including jaundice, hypoglycemia, coagulopathy, encephalopathy, and marked elevation of liver enzymes. Myocardiopathy and renal failure resulting from acute tubular necrosis also may be present.

Phase IV begins 1 week after ingestion if phase III damage is not permanent or lethal and for most patients is marked by a gradual return of laboratory values to normal levels.

20. What are the central nervous system manifestations of acute acetaminophen poisoning?

In the early stages, there are none, and abnormalities in mental status or level of consciousness should be attributed to other drugs (e.g., salicylates, opiates, sedatives) or to other disease states. Hepatic encephalopathy can occur in phase III.

21. Describe the pathophysiology of acetaminophen toxicity.

Acetaminophen is metabolized primarily by the liver. About 90% of it is conjugated with glucuronic or sulfuric acid to form nontoxic compounds that are excreted in the urine. About 2% of the drug is excreted unchanged in the urine. The remainder is metabolized by the cytochrome P-450 mixed-function oxidase system. This involves formation of a toxic intermediary compound, which is conjugated rapidly with hepatic glutathione. The resulting conjugate is metabolized further, and its by-products are excreted in the urine. Because the liver normally has a fixed amount of glutathione, this compound is depleted rapidly in an acute overdose. The toxic intermediary then accumulates, unmetabolized, and binds to the sulfhydryl groups of hepatic enzymes. The result is irreversible centrilobular hepatic necrosis.

22. How is hepatotoxicity predicted?

An acute ingestion of 7.5 g in an adult or 140 mg/kg in a child is generally predictive of hepatotoxicity. Certain drugs, such as cimetidine, compete with acetaminophen for metabolism by the P-450 pathway and theoretically offer some protection from hepatotoxicity. Certain drugs, such as phenytoin and phenobarbital, may induce the P-450 enzymes, allowing a greater percentage of acetaminophen to be metabolized to the toxic intermediary and increasing the risk of toxicity. The most accurate predictor of hepatotoxicity is the serum acetaminophen level obtained between 4 and 24 hours after **acute** ingestion. The **Rumack-Matthew nomogram**, which plots serum concentration against hours postingestion, is the standard reference for predicting hepatotoxicity in an acute overdose.

23. Why is hepatotoxicity in children rare?

No one knows. Toxicity in children is rare, even when toxic levels of acetaminophen are found. One theory holds that acetaminophen metabolism in children shows a preference for alternative pathways other than the P-450 system. The conversion from juvenile to adult metabolism is believed to occur between 6 and 9 years of age.

24. Are serial serum acetaminophen levels helpful?

If an accurate estimate of the time of ingestion cannot be obtained, the nomogram cannot be used, and serial levels should be obtained. Rising levels indicate potential hepatotoxicity.

25. Which laboratory tests are helpful?

If a serum acetaminophen level is in the toxic range on the nomogram, additional blood should be obtained for a complete blood cell count, electrolytes, BUN, glucose, prothrombin time, INR, and liver function tests. A **limited** toxicology screen also should be ordered, with attention to treatable concomitant ingestions, such as salicylates, opiates, barbiturates, ethanol, and cyclic antidepressants. If the acetaminophen level is within the toxic range, liver function tests, prothrombin time, and INR should be repeated daily while the patient is receiving treatment.

26. How is acetaminophen poisoning treated?

If the patient presents within 1 hour of ingestion, gastric lavage should be done. Activated charcoal (1 g/kg) mixed with sorbitol or magnesium sulfate should be administered by gastric lavage tube. If the patient presents more than 1 hour after ingestion, the charcoal and cathartic should be administered orally without lavage, unless there is another indication for gastric lavage (see Chapter 81, General Approach to Poisonings). The specific antidote is NAC (Mucomyst). This agent is a glutathione substitute with a high therapeutic-to-toxic safety ratio. It works best if given within 16 hours of ingestion. NAC should not be given indiscriminately and should be given only if the nomogram predicts toxicity on the basis of a timed serum acetaminophen level. It is given orally after dilution 1:5 with water or a beverage such as soda or juice. This dilution produces a 20% solution, which is given as a loading dose of 140 mg/kg, followed by a maintenance dose of 70 mg/kg every 4 hours for 17 additional doses. If the patient vomits a dose within 1 hour, the dose should be repeated. Intravenous antiemetics should be given if vomiting is persistent.

27. Is there a critical window in time to administer NAC?

Whenever possible, NAC should be given within 24 hours of acute acetaminophen overdose. NAC still may be of benefit if given more than 24 hours after acute ingestion in patients with detectable acetaminophen levels or elevated liver enzymes.

28. How does activated charcoal affect NAC absorption?

Although activated charcoal is capable of adsorbing NAC, the overall effect is probably clinically insignificant because there is usually an interval of several hours between the immediate administration of charcoal and the decision to administer NAC. Experimental coadministration of activated charcoal and NAC has not been shown to affect NAC pharmacokinetics.

29. What are the indications for intravenous NAC?

Because palatability of oral NAC is poor and vomiting is common, NAC sometimes is given by the intravenous route. Standard indications are (1) persistent vomiting unresponsive to antiemetics, such as ondansetron; (2) coingestion of an agent (e.g., iron) that necessitates ongoing gastrointestinal decontamination; (3) gastrointestinal bleeding or obstruction; (4) medical or surgical conditions precluding NAC administration; (5) hepatic encephalopathy; and (6) neonatal toxicity owing to maternal acetaminophen overdose.

30. How is intravenous NAC administered?

First, obtain informed consent. Have the pharmacy prepare a 3% solution by diluting the standard oral 20% solution with D_5W. A loading dose of 140 mg/kg is administered through a peripheral intravenous catheter over 1 hour, using a 0.2-μ millipore filter. Maintenance therapy is given at 4-hour intervals, at 70 mg/kg infused over 1 hour, beginning 4 hours after the loading dose, for a duration of 48 hours.

31. Should I be concerned about potential adverse reactions to intravenous NAC?

Yes, although such reactions are not as frequent as formerly believed (about 5%) and tend to occur during infusion of the loading dose. Flushing does not require specific treatment, and mild urticaria can be treated with diphenhydramine. Neither of these requires interruption of NAC therapy. More serious reactions, such as bronchospasm, angioedema, and hypotension, require aggressive therapy with antihistamines, steroids, and epinephrine, as needed, and discontinuation of the NAC.

32. What is the acetaminophen-alcohol syndrome?

Alcohol affects hepatic acetaminophen detoxification in two ways: (1) It lowers hepatic glutathione stores, resulting in a reduced capacity to detoxify the toxic intermediate compound, and (2) it induces the cytochrome P-450 system, increasing the proportion of ingested acetaminophen that is converted to the toxic intermediate. Diagnostic findings include a history of acetaminophen ingestion and elevated aspartate transaminase levels (usually > 800 IU/L) in patients with known or occult alcohol abuse who regularly take acetaminophen. The diagnosis initially is missed in one third of cases, and the mortality rate is greater than 30%. Treatment is generally supportive, although NAC has been tried, and liver transplantation is an option.

33. What is the treatment for chronic acetaminophen toxicity?

In chronic acetaminophen poisoning, the nomogram is not helpful in predicting toxicity. Repetitive ingestion is thought to be of serious concern only in alcoholics, patients on anticonvulsants, children with febrile illnesses, individuals taking large doses (e.g., > 10 g/d), and patients with symptoms of toxicity. NAC is recommended only for patients with detectable acetaminophen levels and evidence of liver injury.

IBUPROFEN POISONING

34. What are the characteristics of ibuprofen overdose?

Ibuprofen is readily available as an over-the-counter medication used in the treatment of mild-to-moderate pain and fever. Rapid absorption leads to peak drug levels within 2 hours. Symptoms usually are seen within 4 hours of ingestion and are more likely to be serious in children. Toxicity is limited in patients who ingest less than 100 mg/kg, whereas patients, primarily children, who ingest more than 400 mg/kg may be at risk for more severe symptoms.

35. List the primary symptoms of ibuprofen toxicity.

Gastrointestinal toxicity
Nausea
Vomiting
Abdominal pain
Hematemesis
Nephrotoxicity
Acute renal failure
Central nervous system toxicity (seen mostly in children)
Somnolence
Apnea
Seizures
Coma
Other toxicities
Severe metabolic acidosis
Thrombocytopenia

36. When should a serum ibuprofen level be obtained?

Because the serum ibuprofen level does not correlate with clinical symptoms, there is no role for this test in decision making.

37. Describe the treatment for ibuprofen toxicity.

Treatment is directed at alleviating symptoms and supportive care (see Chapter 81, General Approach to Poisonings). If hematemesis is present or there is blood in the stool, a nasogastric tube should be placed; if blood is present, the stomach should be irrigated with saline. A limited toxicology screen to search for other readily treatable toxins (salicylates, acetaminophen, opiates, barbiturates, cyclic antidepressants, and ethanol) is recommended. Seizures should be treated with intravenous diazepam. Renal and hepatic function tests should be ordered. Children with ingestions of greater than 400 mg/kg should be observed in the hospital. Forced diuresis, alkalinization, and hemodialysis are not indicated.

BIBLIOGRAPHY

1. Anderson RJ, Potts DE, Gabow PA, et al: Unrecognized adult salicylate intoxication. Ann Intern Med 85:745–748, 1976.
2. Bailey B, McGuigan MA: Management of anaphylactoid reactions to intravenous N-acetylcysteine. Ann Emerg Med 31:710–715, 1998.
3. Flomenbaum NE: Salicylates. In Goldfrank LR, Flomenbaum NE, Lewin NA, et al (eds): Goldfrank's Toxicologic Emergencies, 6th ed. Norwalk, CT, Appleton & Lange, 1998.
4. Hall AH, Smolinske SC, Kulig KW, et al: Ibuprofen overdose: A prospective study. West J Med 48:653–656, 1988.
5. Hillman RJ, Prescott LF: Treatment of salicylate poisoning with repeated oral charcoal. BMJ 291:1472, 1985.
6. Johnson SC, Pelletier LL: Enhanced hepatotoxicity of acetaminophen in the alcoholic patient: Two case reports and a review of the literature. Medicine 76:185–191, 1997.
7. Oker EE, Hermann L, Baum CR, et al: Serious toxicity in a young child due to ibuprofen. Acad Emerg Med 7:821–823, 2000.
8. Smilkstein MJ: Acetaminophen. In Goldfrank LR, Flomenbaum NE, Lewin NA, et al (eds): Goldfrank's Toxicologic Emergencies, 6th ed. Norwalk, CT, Appleton & Lange, 1998.
9. Smilkstein MJ, Knapp GL, Kulig KW, et al: Efficacy of oral N-acetylcysteine in the treatment of acetaminophen overdose: Analysis of the national multicenter study (1976–1985). N Engl J Med 319:1557–1562, 1988.
10. Yip L, Dart RC, Hurlbut KM: Intravenous administration of oral N-acetylcysteine. Crit Care Med 26:40–43, 1998.

85. SEDATIVES AND HYPNOTICS

James R. Miner, M.D.

1. What is the difference between a sedative and a hypnotic?

Sedatives are drugs that primarily cause relaxation and tranquilization. **Hypnotics** generally refer to drugs that put you to sleep. All of these agents tend to act by a similar mechanism, and the distinction between them is artificial. They are tranquilizing drugs and, in sufficient quantity, can cause depression of the central nervous system.

2. Which medications fall into this category?

Benzodiazepines, barbiturates, chloral hydrate, phenothiazines, antihistamines, buspirone, and zolpidem. Older drugs in this category but seen infrequently now include glutethimide, ethchlorvynol, meprobamate, and methaqualone. There are many agents, especially ethanol, that exhibit sedative/hypnotic effects, and it is a side effect of many drugs and toxins when given in toxic doses.

3. How do sedative/hypnotic overdoses present?

The specific effects can vary from drug to drug, but the characteristics shared by overdoses of all of these medications include a decreased level of consciousness. There are varying degrees of respiratory depression, decreased airway protection, and sometimes hypotension from sympatholysis.

4. Don't a lot of overdoses present this way?

Yes. This presentation is typical of ethanol, antihistamines, tricyclics, and a host of other drugs. The management of altered mental status in the setting of overdose is generally the same for all of these agents, but the differential diagnosis of altered mental status is huge, and as you treat the patient keep looking for the cause. Because many of these agents wear off with time, supportive care until the patient begins to improve usually shows that the patient had an overdose of an agent with sedative/hypnotic effects, although you may never know which agent it was.

5. How do I make the diagnosis of sedative/hypnotic overdose in a person with undifferentiated decreased level of consciousness?

After stabilizing the patient, examine him or her for clues to the cause of the decreased level of consciousness. Consider giving naloxone, D_{50}, thiamine, and flumazenil. Sudden improvements in the mental status after one of these treatments may help discern the cause of the change in mental status. Serial examinations can give an idea if the patient is getting better or worse. Patients who are improving may need little intervention other than supportive care until the drug clears from their system. Patients who are getting worse may require more aggressive therapy or a more aggressive search for alternative causes of a decreased mental status (e.g., a head CT scan to rule out an intracranial hemorrhage). Assume that all patients being treated for an overdose are suicidal until you can prove otherwise, and be sure they are treated appropriately for that.

6. Is there a role for drug screens or drug levels?

Sometimes. In an alert patient who can tell you what he or she took and whose condition is not worsening, there is no need for a drug level. With the exception of phenobarbital, the treatment for sedative/hypnotic overdose is supportive, and if the patient is improving, the drug is probably starting to wear off. The exception is in patients who are suicidal or who took the drug in a suicide attempt. All suicidal patients should have an acetaminophen level because toxic levels of this drug have few clinical manifestations early in the course of the overdose, and there is a useful antidote available.

In an unconscious patient, the use of drug screens and levels is more controversial. If you know the overdosed drug and are able to support the patient adequately, a level is unlikely to provide any benefit. If you do not know the nature of the overdose, a drug screen may elucidate the causative agent; however, if the patient is improving by your examination, knowing which sedative caused the change in mental status would not be likely to alter therapy. If the patient is not improving or is deteriorating, a drug screen may help confirm whether or not an overdose was the cause of the decreased level of consciousness. An acetaminophen level should be obtained on all unconscious overdose patients.

7. How do I treat these patients?

Airway: Assess the patient's airway and airway reflexes. Respiratory arrest is the major cause of early death. Is the airway clear? Does the patient swallow and cough? Is the gag reflex present? Appropriate corrective measures include supplemental oxygen, head tilt-chin lift, intubation, and assisted ventilation. If the patient cannot maintain his or her airway, he or she should be intubated immediately to protect against aspiration.

Breathing: Assess the patient's respiratory drive. Is the patient breathing? Is the patient having difficulty breathing? Are the lungs clear? What is the oxygen saturation? A patient who is barely breathing may have inadequate respiratory drive from the sedation, and a patient in respiratory distress may have aspirated gastric contents and now have respiratory compromise from aspiration pneumonia. If the patient cannot breathe adequately, he or she should be intubated to support respirations.

Circulation: Assess if the patient is hypotensive. How is the capillary refill? Does the patient feel cold or warm? What is the blood pressure? Patients who are hypotensive after overdose should receive volume expansion with normal saline and in rare instances may be placed on pressors if they are not responding to fluids or are exhibiting signs of fluid overload. (Remember to keep your differential diagnosis large, and don't forget that sometimes a sedative/hypnotic overdose is only part of the problem.)

Deficit: Determine how sedated the patient is. If awake, determine if the patient is oriented and whether or not he or she is confused. If the patient does not appear awake, figure out how sedated he or she is. It is important to assess how sedated a patient is so that during serial examinations you can determine if he or she is improving or deteriorating, which further guides management. Does the patient open his or her eyes to a normal voice, a loud voice, or gentle prodding, or is a maneuver such as sternal rubbing or gentle pressure below the ear along the posterior mandible necessary? Is the patient completely unarousable? Other signs that indicate the level of sedation include the degree of relaxation in the facial muscles (normal versus slack jawed) and in the eyes (open versus ptosis versus closed). Following these signs allows you to follow the progression of the patient's sedation.

8. How do I monitor these patients?

While patients are being observed for serial examinations, they should be assessed frequently to determine the pattern of changes in the mental status. A patient's respiratory status may deteriorate while being observed as a result of a toxic effect moving further toward its peak or as a result of decreased stimulation after the initial assessment has been completed. Patients can be monitored by continuous pulse oximetry, but in an otherwise healthy patient, if he or she is put on supplemental oxygen, the monitor is insensitive to changes in the patient's respirations and may not detect a declining respiratory status. Patients also can be monitored by end-tidal carbon dioxide, usually by a nasal cannula probe when not intubated. This probe displays a waveform of the patient's respirations, showing their rate and depth, which can be useful in the determination of how well a patient is breathing and quickly shows any changes in the quality of a patient's respirations. Blood pressure should be assessed regularly, and a cardiac monitor should be considered for patients who have taken drugs that also have toxic cardiac effects (chloral hydrate and rarely phenobarbital). Work indicates that bispectral electroencephalography analysis, which consists of a single forehead probe electroencephalography and gives a 1-to-100 analog score of a patient's level of consciousness (100, awake; 0, dead), is a useful monitor to follow the degree of sedation of patients and may prove to be a useful tool in monitoring changes in the degree of sedation of overdose patients.

9. What's the best way to decontaminate the gastrointestinal tract?

Activated charcoal can be given to prevent further drug absorption from the gastrointestinal tract at an initial dose of 1 g/kg. Cathartics, such as sorbitol, magnesium sulfate, or magnesium citrate, may be given with charcoal. If your patient has a decreased level of consciousness, he or she is likely to have decreased airway reflexes, and filling the stomach with charcoal may lead to an aspiration pneumonia far worse than the toxic effects of the drug taken. Always consider the need for airway management before charcoal is given; when indecisive, forego the charcoal, not the intubation.

Orogastric lavage may be of some benefit if accomplished early. Within 1 hour of the overdose, it is unlikely that much of the drug is left in the stomach, and there is little benefit from lavage.

10. Is there a way to enhance the clearance of sedatives/hypnotics?

Because most sedative/hypnotics are cleared by hepatic metabolism, there is little that can be done to enhance this short of supporting the patient and giving charcoal to prevent further absorption of the drug. The exception is phenobarbital. It is cleared predominately by urinary excretion, and this can be increased by alkalinizing the urine. Raising the urine pH to greater than 7.3 can increase the clearance of phenobarbital 10-fold. Raising the urine pH can be achieved by giving 1 ampule of $NaHCO_3$ intravenously, then 2 to 3 ampules of $NaHCO_3$ in 1 liter of 5% dextrose intravenously at 1 to 2 mL/kg/h. Hemodialysis generally is not useful because of the large volume of distribution of sedative/hypnotics. The exceptions are phenobarbital and chloral hydrate poisonings, which can be cleared in significant amounts by hemodialysis.

11. Are there any specific antidotes for sedative/hypnotic poisoning?
Flumazenil for benzodiazepine and zolpidem overdose.

12. How does flumazenil work?
It is a specific antagonist at the γ-aminobutyric acid A receptor. This is the receptor that benzodiazepines and zolpidem act on. Flumazenil antagonizes these drugs by completely inhibiting receptor occupancy. For symptomatic benzodiazepine overdose, 0.5 to 10 mg of flumazenil may be given intravenously in increasing doses.

13. Should flumazenil be given empirically to all patients with depressed mental status?
In general, no. Flumazenil is a relatively safe drug that may provide a diagnostic clue to benzodiazepine poisoning if a comatose patient has a response. This use may save an extensive and expensive workup and potentially may avoid the need for intubation before establishment of the diagnosis. Flumazenil has a half life of 1 hour, however, and the patient may develop a decreased level of consciousness again when it has worn off. A positive response to flumazenil does not guarantee a diagnosis of benzodiazepine poisoning. Awakening may occur in patients who have depressed mental status from either ethanol intoxication or hepatic coma. The response to flumazenil in these conditions is much less predictable, however, than it is in benzodiazepine poisoning.

14. What are contraindications to flumazenil?
Patients who have toxic amounts of tricyclic antidepressants in their systems may be more vulnerable to seizures if flumazenil is given, particularly if it is a mixed antidepressant and benzodiazepine overdose. An ECG should be obtained to rule out tricyclic antidepressant poisoning. If the ECG does not have a prominent R wave in lead AVR and a QRS duration of greater than 100 msec in the limb leads, it is safe to assume that dangerous levels of tricyclics are not present. If flumazenil is given inadvertently to a patient who is benzodiazepine dependent, acute withdrawal may occur, which often includes seizures. If the patient has a seizure disorder, flumazenil may provoke a seizure.

15. Should flumazenil be given to all patients with depressed mentation known to be secondary to an overdose of benzodiazepines or zolpidem?
Flumazenil reverses the toxidrome and wakes the patient. For patients with very depressed mentation, flumazenil can prevent the need for intubation. Flumazenil is expensive, however, and under certain circumstances (see question 14) could be dangerous. Most patients with benzodiazepine or zolpidem overdoses do well with supportive care. Few require intubation. Even patients who need to be intubated generally recover without sequelae.

16. What is Rohypnol?
Flunitrazepam (Rohypnol) is a benzodiazepine that is not available legally in the United States but is sold in Mexico. It has gained notoriety as the **date rape drug**. Similar to all benzodiazepines, flunitrazepam induces a depressed level of consciousness and amnesia. Although flunitrazepam has a reputation for its date rape utility, it is not clear if it is significantly different from other benzodiazepines. Street names for Rohypnol are *roshay*, *roofies*, and *roach*.

17. What is GHB?
An abbreviation for γ-**hydroxybutyrate**, which is a natural neurotransmitter that induces sleep. GHB has been sold as a muscle builder, a diet aid, and a sleep aid. It also is abused for a variety of other purposes. It is no longer legally available, but its synthesis is easy. GHB precursors and directions for its synthesis are widely available on the internet. Multiple precursors that are metabolized into GHB and have the same effects are available, including γ-butyrlactone and 1,4-butandiole.

18. How does GHB overdose present?

Patients generally have a decreased level of consciousness. In contrast to other sedative/hypnotic overdoses, the level of consciousness tends to fluctuate quickly between agitation and depression. Decisions about the airway management of these patients should be based on their status while their mental status is depressed. Death from GHB overdose, similar to other sedative/hypnotics, generally is related to respiratory compromise.

19. Are there any special considerations with chloral hydrate poisoning?

Chloral hydrate poisoning presents with signs and symptoms that are typical of sedative/hypnotic overdose. Atrial and ventricular arrhythmias, particularly tachyarrhythmias, may occur with chloral hydrate poisoning, and these patients need intensive cardiovascular monitoring.

20. A patient has depressed mental status and a vinyl-like odor on the breath. What does that mean?

A vinyl-like odor in association with a sedative/hypnotic overdose suggests poisoning by the drug **ethchlorvynol**. This drug is a sedative/hypnotic that is used much less commonly now than it was in the past. The clinical course of intoxication involves depressed mental status and coma, often lasting for a prolonged period. Treatment is supportive.

21. After a drug overdose, a patient is unconscious with widely dilated pupils. What drug should you think of?

Glutethimide. This drug is a sedative/hypnotic that was popular in the late 1950s but is now uncommon. Unusual features of glutethimide poisoning include prolonged and fluctuating coma and anticholinergic features such as widely dilated pupils.

22. How do patients die of sedative/hypnotic overdose?

There are a variety of toxic effects in this broad category of drugs, but generally sedation leading to respiratory compromise is the most lethal side effect. If respiratory compromise is prevented through airway management, patients generally survive with few sequelae.

BIBLIOGRAPHY

1. Chernik DA, et al: Validity and reliability of the Observer's Assessment of Alertness/Sedation Scale: Study with intravenous midazolam. J Clin Psychopharmacol 10:244–251, 1990.
2. Chin RL, Cullison B, Dyer JE, Wu TD: Clinical course of gamma-hydroxybutyrate overdose. Ann Emerg Med 31:716–722, 1998.
3. Poirier MP, et al: Utility of monitoring capnography, pulse oximetry, and vital signs in the detection of airway mishaps: A hyperoxemic animal model. Am J Emerg Med 16:350–352, 1998.
4. Rosow C, Manberg P: Bispectral index monitoring. Anesthesiol Clin North Am 2:89–107, 1998.
5. Sandler NA, Sparks BS: The use of bispectral analysis in patients undergoing intravenous sedation for third molar extractions. J Oral Maxillofac Surg 58:364–369, 2000.
6. Santos LJ, et al: Practical uses of end-tidal carbon dioxide monitoring in the emergency department. J Emerg Med 12:633–644, 1994.
7. Zvosec DL, McCutcheon JR, Spillane J, et al: Adverse events, including death, associated with the use of 1,4-butanediol. N Engl J Med 344:87–94, 2001.

86. MUSHROOMS, HALLUCINOGENS, AND STIMULANTS

Christina E. Hantsch, M.D., and Donna L. Seger, M.D.

MUSHROOMS

1. What are the symptoms and signs of mushroom poisoning?

Because each type of mushroom contains its own characteristic toxins, symptoms and signs depend on the species ingested. Mushroom species that contain cyclopeptides or orelline commonly cause gastrointestinal manifestations, such as nausea, vomiting, and diarrhea. Species containing monomethylhydrazine, muscimol, or psilocybin cause central nervous system manifestations, including hallucinations, seizures, and ataxia. Muscimol and psilocybin also can cause an anticholinergic syndrome. Muscarine-containing mushrooms produce a cholinergic syndrome.

2. Which mushrooms toxins cause the most concern?

Amatoxins, which are cyclopeptides found in *Amanita* and some *Galerina* species. The classic presentation of amatoxin poisoning includes an initial 6- to 12-hour period in which the patient remains asymptomatic. Subsequently, gastrointestinal symptoms develop. Severe hepatotoxicity becomes evident 24 hours to several days after the initial ingestion.

3. Do symptoms within 6 hours rule out amatoxin ingestion?

No. Not all patients exhibit the classic presentation. Mushroom ingestion often involves more than one species. The possibility of amatoxin ingestion needs to be considered in all cases.

4. Will boiling mushrooms destroy their toxins?

Not always. Although some toxins are heat-labile and can be deactivated by heating, amatoxin is not. Amatoxin is the most deadly mushroom toxin, and it is *not* destroyed by cooking.

5. Does coingestion of ethanol change the effects of mushrooms?

Coprine-containing mushrooms, when consumed in combination with ethanol, cause tachycardia, flushing, nausea, and vomiting. This is the same type of reaction as produced by disulfiram or metronidazole when combined with ethanol. Symptoms may occur when alcohol is consumed as late as 72 hours after mushroom ingestion. Coprine, similar to disulfiram and metronidazole, inhibits acetaldehyde dehydrogenase activity. Consequent accumulation of acetaldehyde causes the clinical manifestations.

6. How do I treat someone who has ingested mushrooms?

Treatment in all cases is primarily supportive to maintain circulation. Gastrointestinal decontamination is controversial. Charcoal administration may be considered. Seizures and hallucinations may be treated with diazepam.

HALLUCINOGENS

7. What are hallucinogens?

Typically the term *hallucinogen* refers to agents that are used recreationally for their mind-altering effects. Many substances (including mushrooms and stimulants) can cause hallucinations, perceptions without any basis in reality or alterations in the perception of reality.

8. List some examples of hallucinogens.
- Lysergic acid diethylamide (LSD)
- Marijuana
- 3,4-Methylenedioxyamphetamine (MDA)
- 3,4-Methylenedioxymethamphetamine (MDMA)
- 1-(1-Phenylcyclohexyl)piperidine (PCP)

9. Name the life-threatening effects of hallucinogens.
Seizures, hyperthermia, hypertension, or arrhythmias. Rhabdomyolysis can develop subsequently. Trauma frequently occurs as a result of the disinhibition and aggressiveness caused by hallucinogen abuse.

10. What is the treatment of hallucinogen toxicity?
There are no antidotes for hallucinogens. A benzodiazepine may be given to calm agitated patients. Haloperidol is another option. Haloperidol may be most appropriate for patients experiencing primarily the mind-altering effects of hallucinogens. Reassurance, a calm environment, avoidance of further trauma, and supportive care all are important. Occasionally, physical restraint, in addition to chemical restraint, may be necessary to protect the patient or staff from harm in cases of severe agitation.

STIMULANTS

11. How should one screen for cocaine?
Cocaine is metabolized rapidly, and detection of the parent compound in blood indicates recent use. The elimination half-life of cocaine after intravenous administration is 45 to 90 minutes. Cocaine undergoes nonenzymatic degradation to benzoylecgonine and ecgonine methyl ester. These substances are excreted renally and may be present in the urine for several days after the initial exposure. Routine urine (not blood) screening for cocaine abuse is done, and the samples are analyzed for the degradation products of cocaine.

12. What is free-base cocaine?
Cocaine usually arrives in the United States as cocaine hydrochloride. It often is converted back to its alkaloid form, or free-base, with an alkaline solution and a solvent. **Crack cocaine** is a form of free-base that is made with baking soda and water. Free-base cocaine is resistant to pyrolysis and can be smoked.

13. What is the significance of chest pain after use of cocaine?
Pneumothorax or pneumomediastinum may occur after a Valsalva maneuver when smoking cocaine. Myocardial infarction has followed intranasal, intravenous, and smoked cocaine, even in young patients with normal coronary arteries.

14. Does coingestion of ethanol change the effects of cocaine?
Yes. Cocaine and ethanol have synergistic cardiovascular effects. In the presence of ethanol, cocaine is metabolized to cocaethylene. Cocaethylene-enhanced catecholamine activity may explain these synergistic clinical effects.

15. What is *ice*?
A crystallized free-base methamphetamine that can be smoked. It is absorbed rapidly from the lungs. Similar to intravenous methamphetamine, it has the advantage of immediate euphoric effect without the risk attributed to intravenous drug administration. The clinical manifestations of methamphetamine are secondary to heightened catecholamine activity and are the same regardless of the route of administration. Potential adverse effects include hypertension, arrhythmias, intracranial hemorrhage, seizures, and hyperthermia.

16. What about *Adam* and *Eve*?

Adam is a street name for MDMA. *Ecstasy*, *E*, and *XTC* are other common names. *Eve* is a street name for MDEA. The euphoric effect of these **designer drugs** has made them increasingly popular recreational drugs. Designer drugs are so named because they were manufactured specifically to avoid illegal classification, although they are now illegal. Overdose of MDMA or MDEA, both amphetamine derivatives, clinically resembles amphetamine intoxication. Alteration in serotonin regulation is a known effect, but the exact mechanism of action of these agents is not known. Designer drugs are not detected on routine drug screens.

17. How should I treat someone with toxicity from stimulants?

Agitation or seizures can be treated with diazepam; large doses may be required. Hypertension from stimulant toxicity is usually short-lived; however, a true hypertensive emergency can be treated with nitroprusside. Routine cooling measures can be used to reduce body temperature in hyperthermic patients. Nitroglycerin and other cardiac interventions may be used in patients with ischemic chest pain from vasoconstriction or myocardial infarction. β-Blockers, such as propranolol, should be avoided because they may potentiate coronary artery vasoconstriction.

BIBLIOGRAPHY

1. Beebe DK, Walley E: Smokable methamphetamine ("Ice"): An old drug in a different form. Am Fam Physician 51:449–453, 1995.
2. Benowitz NL: Clinical pharmacology and toxicology of cocaine. Pharmacol Toxicol 72:3–12, 1993.
3. Brogan WC, Lange RA, Glamann B, Hillis LD: Recurrent coronary vasoconstriction caused by intranasal cocaine: Possible role for metabolites. Ann Intern Med 116:556–561, 1992.
4. Derlet RW, Heischober B: Methamphetamine—stimulant of the 1990s? West J Med 153:625–628, 1990.
5. Ellenhorn MJ: Ellenhorn's Medical Toxicology: Diagnosis and Treatment of Human Poisoning, 2nd ed. Baltimore, Williams & Wilkins, 1997.
6. Floersheim GL: Treatment of human amatoxin mushroom poisoning. Med Toxicol 2:1–9, 1987.
7. Goldfrank LR, Flomenbaum NE, Lewin NA, et al (eds): Goldfrank's Toxicologic Emergencies, 7th ed. New York, McGraw-Hill, 2002.
8. Henning RJ, Wilson LD, Glauser JM: Cocaine plus ethanol is more cardiotoxic than cocaine or ethanol alone. Crit Care Med 22:1896–1906, 1994.
9. Sternbach GL, Varon J: Designer drugs: Recognizing and managing their toxic effects. Postgrad Med 91:169–178, 1992.

87. OPIOIDS

Vikhyat Bebarta, M.D.

1. Aren't the numbers of heroin and other opioid abuse going down?

Actually, it is just the opposite. In the 1998 American Association of Poison Control Center's data, opioids were a coingestant in 11.6% of the 775 deaths reported that year. There has been an 80% increase in the abuse of opioids among high school youth from 1991 to 1998. The Drug Abuse Warning Network in the United States shows a 31% increase in ED visits from 1992 to 1998.

2. What receptors are activated with opioids?

Most analgesia results from the μ_1 receptors located in the brain. The μ_2 receptor is associated with some of the complications of opioids, including respiratory depression, constipation, euphoria, and pruritus. Miosis is caused by μ_2-related parasympathetic nerve excitation that innervates the pupil. κ receptors cause dysphoria and depersonalization. The δ receptors produce spinal analgesia.

3. **Define the terms** *opium*, *opiate*, *opioid*, **and** *narcotic*.

Opium is a mixture of alkaloids, including morphine and codeine, extracted from the opium poppy.

An **opiate** is a natural drug derived from opium (heroin, codeine, and morphine).

An **opioid** is any drug that has opium-like activity, including the opiates and all synthetic and semisynthetic drugs that interact with opioid receptors in the body.

The term **narcotic** is nonspecific; it originally meant any drug that could induce sleep.

4. **What is the typical presentation of opioid poisoning?**

The classic triad of opioid poisoning is **central nervous system (CNS) depression, respiratory depression**, and **miosis**. Patients who have overdosed on opioids are hyporeflexic and have decreased bowel sounds. They may be hypotensive, hypothermic, bradycardic, or cyanotic. The findings of miotic pupils, respiratory rate less than 12 breaths/min, and circumstantial evidence of drug use have a 92% sensitivity for responding to naloxone.

5. **Do all cases of opioid intoxication present with miosis?**

No. Mydriasis or normal pupils can occur in conjunction with opioid overdose with the following situations: diphenoxylate-atropine (Lomotil) poisoning; coingestion of other drugs; after the use of naloxone; hypoxia; prior use of mydriatic eye drops; or overdose of meperidine, morphine, propoxyphene, or pentazocine.

6. **Name other common non–opioid-related causes of miosis.**

Overdose or ingestion of clonidine, organophosphates, carbamates, phenothiazines, olanzapine, phencyclidine, or sedative/hypnotics. Pontine hemorrhage also causes CNS depression and miosis.

7. **How should a patient with respiratory compromise by opioid overdose be treated?**

Resuscitation takes precedence over the administration of naloxone. The patient's respiration must be supported with a bag-valve-mask until the opioid antagonist is given. If there is an inadequate response to naloxone, the patient should be intubated. Serum glucose levels should be checked and thiamine administered for almost all patients with altered consciousness. Activated charcoal should be given to patients with oral ingestions of opioids.

8. **What is the appropriate dose of naloxone?**

The recommended initial dose of naloxone for adults and children with CNS and respiratory depression is 2.0 mg intravenously. For children younger than 5 years old or less than 20 kg, 0.1 mg/kg should be administered. If a patient has CNS depression only, it is reasonable to start with a smaller dose (0.4 to 0.8 mg IV). If there is no response to a smaller dose, 2.0 mg can be given. Particularly for opioid abusers and patients who use opioids for chronic pain, even lower doses of 0.1 mg may be used, and additional doses can be given judiciously to prevent or attenuate withdrawal. Opioid withdrawal is unpleasant to the patient but is not life-threatening. It is sensible to titrate the dose of naloxone to reverse respiratory and CNS depression without precipitating withdrawal.

9. **Does naloxone have to be administered intravenously?**

No. If it is difficult to start in intravenous line, naloxone can be given intramuscularly if the patient does not have hypotension. A dose of 0.8 mg subcutaneously has an equal time to effect as 0.4 mg intravenously. It can be administered through the endotracheal tube or injected sublingually into the venous plexus under the tongue. The effectiveness of intranasal naloxone is being studied. Naloxone is not effective orally.

10. **Do all patients respond to 2.0 mg of naloxone?**

No. Larger doses of naloxone may be required to reverse the effects of codeine, diphenoxylate-atropine (Lomotil), propoxyphene (Darvon), pentazocine (Talwin), codeine, dextromethorphan, and the fentanyl derivatives. If an opioid overdose is suspected and the patient does not respond to an initial 2.0 mg of naloxone, repeat 2.0-mg doses of naloxone can be administered every 3 minutes until a response is noted or until 10 mg has been given. If there is no response to 10 mg of naloxone, it is unlikely that the diagnosis is an isolated opioid overdose.

11. How long does the clinical effect of naloxone last?

The duration of action of intravenous naloxone is 40 to 75 minutes. Many opioids produce clinical effects that last 3 to 6 hours. Although the duration of action of most opioids is much longer than that of naloxone, resedation is relatively uncommon.

12. Should naloxone be administered empirically to every patient with altered mental status?

Probably not. Although naloxone is a safe medication, it is not helpful in every patient who is altered, and often the response to naloxone has been shown to cloud the diagnostic picture. If a patient presents with an obvious sympathomimetic or anticholinergic syndrome, this agitated and stimulated patient probably would not benefit from naloxone. If the diagnosis of an opiate syndrome is obvious, and the patient's ventilatory status is adequate, naloxone may stimulate a withdrawal state that sometimes is more difficult to handle in a busy ED than a slightly sedated patient.

13. How should recurrent sedation and respiratory depression resulting from a long-acting opioid be treated?

A naloxone infusion should be started. Giving repeated doses of naloxone to an opioid-dependent patient may cause the patient to fluctuate between symptoms of withdrawal and CNS depression. A naloxone infusion is made to administer to the patient two thirds of the dose needed to reverse the patient's respiratory depression every hour. An easy approach is to mix the dose into 1 L of D_5W and run it at 100 mL/h. The infusion can be adjusted accordingly based on the patient's symptoms of withdrawal or sedation.

14. What is nalmefene, and is it better than naloxone?

Nalmefene is another opioid antagonist with a similar structure to naloxone but a longer duration of action (half-life of 4 to 10 hours). When compared in a randomized, double-blinded study with naloxone, it had similar clinical outcomes. Nalmefene has not become popular in most EDs because of the prolonged withdrawal symptoms that result and its high cost. Some opiate abusers may attempt to counter the antagonist by taking extra large doses of heroin, and when the nalmefene wears off, they may be at risk for opioid toxicity. A realistic indication of nalmefene may be with pediatric patients who have an accidental single ingestion and are admitted to the hospital for observation.

15. What about naltrexone?

Naltrexone is an oral opioid antagonist with a long duration of action. It is used for long-term detoxification therapy and has no significant role in management of acute opioid toxicity.

16. Who should be observed in the ED, and for how long?

Whether or not naloxone has been given, if the ventilatory drive is adequate, most patients can be observed for several hours until appropriately awake and discharged. Occasionally, patients may not respond to naloxone, have recurrent inadequate ventilation necessitating treatment, or develop complications of opioid use and must be admitted. Patients ingesting methadone may require admission for 24 to 48 hours. Most patients should be watched for at least 2 hours from use because the complication of noncardiogenic pulmonary edema would be manifest during this time. Most emergency physicians consider a conservative period of 4 hours after the last dose of naloxone adequate in an asymptomatic patient. This extended period may allow for recognition of potential coingestants and recurrent respiratory depression.

17. What are the signs of opioid withdrawal?

Anxiety, yawning, lacrimation, rhinorrhea, diaphoresis, mydriasis, nausea and vomiting, diarrhea, piloerection, abdominal pain, and diffuse myalgias. It typically occurs 12 hours after last heroin use and 30 hours after last methadone use.

18. How is opioid withdrawal best treated?

Treatment is symptomatic. Clonidine, 0.1 to 0.2 mg orally three times daily, may be helpful. Some patients may abuse clonidine, however, because it enhances the opioid euphoria. Also, intravenous fluids, antiemetics, and antidiarrheal agents may be used. If naloxone was given, the withdrawal symptoms resolve in 45 to 75 minutes, when the naloxone effect subsides.

19. How should body stuffers/packers be managed?

The packets can be seen on abdominal radiographs, radiographs with oral contrast material (Gastrografin), or abdominal CT. Lavage usually is not recommended because a cheap, safe antidote, naloxone, is available, and lavage has several potentially severe risks. Patients should receive activated charcoal and polyethylene glycol electrolyte solution (Colyte, GoLYTELY) to enhance elimination through the colon. Polyethylene glycol should be administered through a nasogastric tube at approximately 2 L/h until there is clear effluent rectally. Sometimes enemas may be used if the packets are in the distal colon or are felt on digital rectal examination.

20. What risk factors should I be aware of that are associated with death in heroin use?

Concomitant use of ethanol and benzodiazepines potentiates respiratory depression. Female gender, long-standing heroin use, and unmarried status are associated with increased death. Using heroin during the first 12 months after cessation of addiction treatment and the first 2 weeks after release from incarceration is associated with an increased death rate. Most deaths occur at home and with bystanders who often do not call for medical attention for fear of legal consequences.

21. List medical complications of intravenous opioid use.

Bacterial endocarditis
Septic pulmonary emboli
Nephropathy
Tetanus
Hepatitis
HIV infection
Cellulitis
Skin abscesses
Osteomyelitis
Wound botulism (especially with crude black tar heroin)
Compartment syndrome

22. How useful are toxicologic screens for opiates, and which opiates often are not detected?

Toxicologic screens are not generally helpful in the acute management of patients. Not only is there a significant delay in obtaining the results, but also the clinical presentation is most helpful and should be used to guide management. Opiate screens do not detect for methadone or propoxyphene, and specific screening tests are required. Fentanyl, pentazocine, meperidine, oxymorphone, oxycodone, and propoxyphene are not detected on most general opioid screens. Ingestion of poppy seeds can cause true-positive screens that are of no clinical significance. With further testing, this erroneous cause of positive screens can be ruled out.

23. Are there any other tests that should be checked with opiate ingestions?

Acetaminophen levels should be checked in all patients with oral exposures because it is often combined with hydrocodone, oxycodone, propoxyphene, and codeine.

Serum quantitative levels of specific opioids are of no benefit and should not be ordered.

24. What is the most common pulmonary complication of opioid use?

Noncardiogenic pulmonary edema, which occurs in approximately 3% of nonhospitalized patients, and approximately 50% of all opioid abusers develop it once in their life. The mechanism is unclear, but it is a result of capillary permeability and fluid leak. The patient presents with pink frothy sputum, cyanosis, and rales, and bilateral fluffy infiltrates are seen on the chest radiograph in the comatose patient. Naloxone does not reverse the process, and many patients may need mechanical ventilation. Heroin, methadone, morphine, and propoxyphene have been associated with noncardiogenic pulmonary edema.

25. In what situations can opioids cause seizures?

Intravenous use of fentanyl or sufentanil, overdose of propoxyphene or pentazocine, use of meperidine (especially oral doses), opioid withdrawal or high doses of intravenous morphine administered in neonates, and use of tramadol.

26. Is it appropriate to give dextromethorphan or meperidine to patients on antidepressant medications?

No. These combinations of drugs may precipitate the life-threatening serotonin syndrome. Any drug or combination of drugs can increase serotoninergic neurotransmission and precipitate the serotonin syndrome. Meperidine and dextromethorphan inhibit serotonin uptake. Many cyclic antidepressants and all the selective serotonin reuptake inhibitors inhibit serotonin reuptake. Monoamine oxidase inhibitors also are contraindicated because they decrease serotonin metabolism.

27. What is serotonin syndrome?

A syndrome characterized by alterations in cognition and behavior, autonomic nervous system function, and neuromuscular activity. The following symptoms and signs occur commonly: confusion, agitation, diaphoresis, sinus tachycardia, myoclonus, hyperreflexia, muscle rigidity, and tremor. Serotonin syndrome may be indistinguishable from malignant hyperthermia or the neuroleptic malignant syndrome, and it occurs unpredictably. Neuroleptic malignant syndrome often has a more gradual onset of days to weeks, it resolves over several days, it has more severe symptoms than serotonin syndrome, and it is uncommon to have hyperreflexia and myoclonus. Serotonin syndrome often begins within minutes to hours of starting a new medication.

Treatment is primarily supportive and includes rapid cooling, gastrointestinal decontamination in acute ingestions, benzodiazepines, fluids, and managing the airway. Neuromuscular paralysis may be necessary. Antiserotoninergic agents, such as cyproheptadine (Periactin), an oral agent, may be useful in some patients.

28. Why should I avoid prescribing meperidine (Demerol)?

Seizures may be caused by normeperidine, a metabolite of meperidine that is renally excreted. Normeperidine levels are elevated with repetitive administration of oral meperidine, renal failure, and concomitant use of drugs that induce hepatic enzymes, such as phenytoin, phenobarbital, and chlorpromazine. Naloxone does not relieve the seizures. Normeperidine can cause CNS agitation, tremors, and psychosis. The duration of action of meperidine is only 2 to 3 hours; in contrast to morphine, the half-life is prolonged by hepatic disease; and it can produce serotonin syndrome when combined with monoamine oxidase inhibitors.

29. Which antidiarrheal agent can cause significant toxicity if ingested?

Lomotil (diphenoxylate 2.5 mg + atropine 0.025 mg). Most overdoses occur in children. Classically the overdose is a two-phase toxicity: phase 1, anticholinergic symptoms (flushing, dry mouth), and phase 2, opioid effects. This pattern is uncommon, however. Delayed presentations have been reported, and all children should be observed in a monitored setting for a least 24 hours.

Loperamide is a nonprescription antidiarrheal agent derived from diphenoxylate. Acute overdoses usually produce only drowsiness but can cause coma, bradycardia, apnea, and miosis.

30. Which opioid can produce ventricular arrhythmias, a wide QRS complex, mydriasis, and seizures?

Propoxyphene has a quinidine-like effect that blocks sodium channels similar to cyclic antidepressants. Large doses of naloxone (10 mg) may reverse the CNS depression but not the cardiotoxic effects. Sodium bicarbonate has been used successfully for propoxyphene-induced arrhythmias. Propoxyphene has never been proved to be more effective for analgesia than salicylates, acetaminophen, or codeine.

31. What are designer drugs, and what are the two notorious designer drugs that have been used?

Designer drugs are drugs made as substitutes for other chemicals that are popular with illicit drug users. They are made inexpensively in "underground" laboratories. 3-Methylfentanyl is an analog of fentanyl known as *China White* or *Persian White* and is 2,000 times stronger than morphine and 20 times stronger than fentanyl. It can cause respiratory arrest quickly. It does not cause the "rush" of heroin, but instead offers a much longer euphoria. Various outbreaks in California, the East Coast, and more recently Europe have been reported. MPTP (1-methyl-4-phenyl-1,2,5,6 tetrahydropyridine) is a compound that was produced accidentally during the synthesis of MPPP, a meperidine analog. MPTP is cytotoxic for dopaminergic neurons in the substantia nigra. It produces a Parkinson-like syndrome that is permanent and occurs after a single ingestion of MPTP, but does respond to typical antiparkinsonism medications.

32. What over-the-counter cold remedy is sometimes abused by teenagers?

Dextromethorphan is the d-isomer of codeine. Its metabolite stimulates the release of serotonin and acts at the phencyclidine site, which accounts for its abuse as an hallucinogen. It may present with symptoms of opiate toxicity, but more commonly presents with slurred speech, nystagmus, hyperexcitability, and ataxia. Naloxone usually does not reverse the symptoms. Dextromethorphan does not cause false-positive results on urine toxicology screens.

33. Identify another analog of codeine.

Tramadol (Ultram) is a synthetic analog of codeine. Overdoses have been associated with seizures, hypertension, respiratory depression, and agitation. The seizures do not respond to naloxone. Although the drug has a low abuse potential, it is not recommended for patients with a history of opioid dependence.

BIBLIOGRAPHY

1. Brent J: Serotonin reuptake inhibitors, new antidepressants, and the serotonin syndrome. In Ford M, Delaney KA, Ling LJ, et al (eds): Clinical Toxicology. Philadelphia, W.B. Saunders, 2001, pp 522–531.
2. Clark RF, Wei EM, Anderson PO: Meperidine: Therapeutic use and toxicity. J Emerg Med 13:797–802, 1995.
3. Hoffman JR, Schriger DL, Luo JS: The empiric use of naloxone in patients with altered mental status: A reappraisal. Ann Emerg Med 20:246–252, 1991.
4. Kaplan JL, Marx JA, Calabro JJ, et al: Double-blind, randomized study of nalmefene and naloxone in emergency department patients with suspected narcotics overdose. Ann Emerg Med 34:42–50, 1999.
5. Kleinschmidt KC, Wainscott M, Ford MD: Opioids. In Ford M, Delaney KA, Ling LJ, et al (eds): Clinical Toxicology. Philadelphia, W.B. Saunders, 2001, pp 627–639.
6. Mills KC: Serotonin syndrome: A clinical update. Crit Care Clin 13:763–783, 1997.
7. Nelson LS: Opioids. In Goldfrank LR, Flomenbaum NE, Lewin NA, et al (eds): Goldfrank's Toxicologic Emergencies, 6th ed. New York, Appleton-Lange, 1998, pp 935–942.
8. Sporer KA: Acute heroin overdose. Ann Intern Med 130:584–590, 1999.
9. Wagner K, Brough L, Macmillan I, et al: Intravenous vs. subcutaneous naloxone for out-of-hospital management of presumed opioid overdose. Acad Emerg Med 5:293–299, 1998.

88. ANTIDEPRESSANTS: CYCLICS AND NEWER AGENTS

Shannon Sovndal, M.D., Eric Isaacs, M.D., and Russ Braun, M.D., M.P.H., M.B.A.

1. How are antidepressants classified, and what is their main mechanism of action?

Antidepressants can be divided into three broad categories that include **tricyclic antidepressants (TCAs), monoamine oxidase inhibitors (MAOIs)**, and newer agents often referred to as **atypical, heterocyclic, or second-generation antidepressants**. TCAs are classified as secondary or tertiary amines and contain a side chain with a varied number of methyl groups. They inhibit reuptake of neurotransmitters and antagonize postsynaptic serotonin receptors. MAOIs block the intracellular, mitochondrial enzyme monoamine oxidase, which normally deaminates biogenic amines, such as epinephrine, norepinephrine (NE), serotonin, and dopamine (DA). The atypicals are structurally diverse, but all have the common ability to inhibit presynaptic reuptake of serotonin (except bupropion, which is an NE and DA reuptake inhibitor). Many have additional actions, such as inhibition of DA or NE reuptake and serotonin or α-adrenergic blockade.

Mechanism of Action of Antidepressants

GROUP	MECHANISM OF ACTION	GENERIC EXAMPLES
Tricyclics	Blocks reuptake of NE	Amitriptyline (Elavil)
Tertiary		Doxepin (Sinequan)
Secondary amine		Nortriptyline (Pamelor)
Tetracyclic		Maprotiline (Ludiomil)
Dibenzoxazepine		Amoxapine (Ascendin)
Selective serotonin	Blocks reuptake of serotonin	Fluoxetine (Prozac)
reuptake inhibitors		Sertraline (Zoloft)
(SSRIs)		Paroxetine (Paxil)
Triazolopyridine	Serotonin receptor antagonist	Trazodone (Desyrel)
Monocyclic	Blocks reuptake of DA	Bupropion (Wellbutrin)
Monoamine oxidase	Increases CNS, NE, and DA levels	Phenelzine (Nardil)
inhibitors (MAOIs)		Tranylcypromine (Parnate)

CNS, central nervous system.

2. What are the epidemiologic characteristics associated with antidepressant overdoses?

Based on the American Association of Poison Control Centers' annual report, antidepressants are consistently second only to analgesics as the leading cause of poisoning death in the United States. There were more than 83,000 antidepressant toxic exposures in 2000, accounting for nearly 55,000 visits to health care facilities. Although overall mortality from antidepressants has fallen with the advent of the newer agents, 123 deaths were reported, with the largest number still due to TCA ingestion (amitriptyline in particular).

3. Compare the features of the newer agents versus TCAs and MAOIs.

The newer agents have fewer side effects, less toxicity, and a larger safety margin. The newer agents have little affinity for DA, γ-aminobutyric acid, acetylcholine, and β-adrenergic receptors, and as a result, there are fewer side effects. Atypicals have little action on cardiac sodium, potassium, and calcium channels and avoid much of the cardiotoxicity. In contrast to MAOIs, there is no risk of tyramine-like reactions, and there is no contraindication to the use of indirect sympathomimetics. With the exception of bupropion (high seizure risk), the newer agents are far safer than MAOIs and TCAs. The fatal toxicity index, which is the number of deaths per 1 million prescriptions, was 2.7 to 13.4 for SSRIs versus 19.1 to 231.8 for TCAs. Similarities include hepatic metabolism, futility of treatment with hemodialysis or hemoperfusion, and fast gut absorption (with the exception of TCAs secondary to their antimuscarinic effect on gut motility).

4. Describe the clinical presentation of atypical antidepressant ingestions.

Death secondary to SSRI overdose is extremely rare. In one large study, 45% of adults and 90% of children who overdosed on fluoxetine alone had no symptoms. In patients who are symptomatic, the most common complaints and findings are nausea, vomiting, tremor, decreased level of consciousness, seizures, and tachycardia. All SSRIs have the potential to produce the serotonin syndrome at toxic and therapeutic levels. This diagnosis is often difficult to recognize and should be kept in the differential when patients are taking newer antidepressants.

5. What is the serotonin syndrome?

The serotonin syndrome is a constellation of signs and symptoms manifesting as altered mental status, autonomic dysfunction, and neuromuscular hyperactivity.

Clinical Features of Serotonin Syndrome

Altered mental status	Diaphoresis
Myoclonus	Fever
Hyperreflexia	Shivering
Ataxia	Diarrhea

Agents Reported to Cause Serotonin Syndrome When Used in Combination

MAOIs	Meperidine
TCAs	Dextromethorphan
SSRIs	Tryptophan

6. What is the treatment of serotonin syndrome?

Supportive care and early recognition in the ED are paramount. Benzodiazepines are recommended by some and may have a protective role as a result of their inhibitory effects on serotoninergic transmission. Fever may be controlled with acetaminophen and external cooling measures. Cyproheptadine, a first-generation histamine-1 receptor blocker with nonspecific antagonism of serotonin receptors, has been approved by the Food and Drug Administration for use as an antihistamine and may be helpful in relieving serotoninergic symptoms.

7. List the signs and symptoms of TCA ingestions.

Initial signs and symptoms
  Sinus tachycardia
  Slurred speech
  Dry mouth
  Drowsiness

Later signs and symptoms
  Lethargy
  Hallucinations
  Coma
  Seizures
  Hypotension
  Arrhythmias

8. Name the four mechanisms of TCA toxicity.

1. **Anticholinergic**: The anticholinergic effects of TCA ingestions include supraventricular tachycardia, hallucinations, seizures, and hyperthermia.

2. **Quinidine-like**: The quinidine-like effects, manifested by decreased cardiac contractility, hypotension, and ventricular arrhythmias, are characteristic of all type 1a antiarrhythmics (e.g., quinidine, procainamide, and disopyramide)

3. **α-Adrenergic blockade**: Peripheral α-receptor blockade may lead to hypotension.

4. **Antihistamine**: Some TCAs (doxepin) are more potent than many of the newer histamine H_1 antagonists. These agents can cause sedation and coma.

9. Summarize the clinical presentations of TCA overdose.

	CARDIOVASCULAR	CNS	ANTICHOLINERGIC
Symptoms	Dizziness	Confusion	Blurred vision Dry mouth
Signs	Tachycardia Conduction blocks QRS widening Hypotension Arrhythmias Cardiac arrest	Delirium Agitation Hyperreflexia Myoclonus Seizures Sedation Coma	Mydriasis Decreased bowel sounds Urinary retention Hyperthermia Hypothermia

10. What is the anticholinergic syndrome?

Hyperthermia, blurred vision, dry mouth, skin flushing, hallucinations, and tachycardia. These effects may be summarized by the phrase "Hot as a hare, blind as a bat, dry as a bone, red as a beet, and mad as a hatter." Other substances that can cause anticholinergic symptoms are antihistamines, phenothiazines, scopolamine, belladonna, jimsonweed, nightshade, and *Amanita muscaria* mushrooms.

11. Are there any reliable indicators that identify toxicity risk early after antidepressant overdose?

Antidepressant overdose can cause life-threatening emergencies, such as shock, hypotension, cardiac arrhythmias, seizures, and multiple organ system failure, within hours of presentation. Most patients do not suffer such complications, however, and subsequently do not need expensive critical care resources. Multiple studies have used the **Antidepressant Overdose Risk Assessment** (ADORA) criteria to determine probable outcome. These criteria include QRS interval greater than 0.10 second, arrhythmias, altered mental status, seizures, respiratory depression, and hypotension. Patients are classified as low risk (absence of criteria) or high risk (presence of ≥ 1 of the criteria) based on development of signs or symptoms within 6 hours. One study showed 100% sensitivity in identifying patients who developed significant toxicity problems. If no signs or symptoms are observed by 6 hours, patients may be discharged from the ED for psychiatric evaluation.

12. What is the general approach to management of antidepressant overdoses?

Patient stabilization after an acute ingestion is paramount, including management of the ABCs (airway, breathing, and circulation) and supportive care. The patient should be given oxygen and the altered mental status protocol of glucose and naloxone (if indicated). After stabilization, gastrointestinal decontamination followed by administration of charcoal with a cathartic is recommended. Persons with TCA overdose are at risk of developing an ileus from anticholinergic effects. The use of serial-dosed charcoal is controversial and may put the patient at risk for bowel obstruction. It is important to be cautious during stabilization and gastrointestinal decontamination because patients can lose consciousness rapidly, placing them at risk for aspiration. For this reason, ipecac is contraindicated, and endotracheal intubation should be considered before gastric lavage in patients with a decreased level of consciousness. These patients require constant cardiac monitoring with intravenous access. A Foley catheter may be necessary because of the risk of urinary retention. Flumazenil use is contraindicated due to increased seizure risk.

13. What diagnostic testing is helpful with an antidepressant overdose?

An ECG is essential in the evaluation of a patient with TCA overdose. Any prolongation of the ECG intervals should be considered a sign of TCA cardiotoxicity. Because of the potential for polydrug ingestions with any overdose, you need to consider other toxins. Testing for acetaminophen and aspirin (or anion gap) levels is recommended. A full urine and serum toxicology screen generally is not indicated because of low yield and cost-ineffectiveness. Results of toxicology screens are often delayed and rarely change patient management.

14. Summarize the treatment recommendations for cardiovascular system toxicity.

Arrhythmias. Sodium bicarbonate is the drug of choice for treatment of ventricular arrhythmias. The mechanism of action of sodium bicarbonate is thought to be the result of increased sodium conductance through myocardial fast sodium channels and of increased plasma protein binding of TCAs (decreasing the amount of circulating free drug). Hypertonic saline may be beneficial, and hyperventilation is useful as an adjunctive measure to increase plasma pH. The dose of bicarbonate is 1 to 2 mEq/kg and may be repeated to maintain an arterial pH of 7.5. Alkalinization may be maintained through administration of repeated bicarbonate boluses or constant intravenous infusion of sodium bicarbonate added to maintenance fluids. Bicarbonate infusions are made by adding 3 ampules of sodium bicarbonate to 1 L of D_5W, which results in 132 mEq Na/L. Lidocaine is effective for ventricular tachycardia but may decrease cardiac contractility. Phenytoin has been used in first-degree atrioventricular block and intraventricular conduction defects; however, it also has been found by some authors to increase the frequency and duration of ventricular tachycardia. Group 1a antiarrhythmics (quinidine, procainamide, and disopyramide) are contraindicated because of their synergistic effects on cell membranes, which enhance antidepressant toxicity. Physostigmine is contraindicated for the treatment of ventricular arrhythmias. Sinus tachycardia and supraventricular arrhythmias usually do not require any specific treatment beyond supportive care.

Hypotension. Hypotension should be treated initially with fluids and Trendelenburg positioning; bicarbonate may be useful if hypotension does not respond. Vasopressors should be used with caution because they may increase ventricular irritability. NE and phenylephrine are the vasopressors of choice because of their primary α-adrenergic effect.

Widened QRS. Bicarbonate is useful in narrowing a widened QRS (> 120 msec), which may confer a cardioprotective effect.

15. Summarize the treatment recommendations for CNS toxicity.

Hallucinations. Physostigmine has been shown to reverse hallucinations; however, because it may precipitate seizures and asystole, it is not recommended. Neuroleptics should be avoided because they may lower the seizure threshold.

Coma. Imipramine, amitriptyline, doxepin, and trazodone are the most sedating of the antidepressants. Supportive care with aggressive airway management is fundamental. Coma lasting longer than 24 hours is rare and suggests further complications of a coingestant or inadequate gastrointestinal decontamination. Flumazenil use is contraindicated.

Seizures. Seizure activity related to TCA toxicity is usually brief. Benzodiazepines and phenobarbital are recommended for seizure management. Phenytoin can be used as a third-line drug but may exacerbate Q-T prolongation.

16. What other drug ingestions can mimic those of TCAs?

Cyclobenzaprine (Flexeril), structurally similar to amitriptyline, was developed in 1961 as an antidepressant and is now prescribed as a muscle relaxant. **Carbamazepine (Tegretol)** is structurally similar to imipramine but causes less cardiac toxicity in cases of overdose.

BIBLIOGRAPHY

1. Benson BE, Mathiason M, et al: Toxicities and outcomes associated with nefazodone poisoning: An analysis of 1,338 exposures. Am J Emerg Med 18:587–592, 2000.

2. Bosse GM, Barefoot JA, Pfeifer MP, Rodgers GC: Comparison of three methods of gut decontamination in tricyclic antidepressant overdose. J Emerg Med 13:203–209, 1995.
3. Callaham M, Kasrel D: Epidemiology of fatal tricyclic antidepressants: Implications for management. Ann Emerg Med 14:1–9, 1985.
4. Foulke GE: Identifying toxicity risk early after antidepressant overdose. Am J Emerg Med 13:123–126, 1995.
5. Graudins A, Vossler C, Wang R: Flouxetine-induced cardiotoxicity with response to bicarbonate therapy. Am J Emerg Med 15:501–503, 1997.
6. Graudins A, Stearman A, Chan B: Treatment of the serotonin syndrome with cyproheptadine. J Emerg Med 16:615–619, 1998.
7. Harrigan RA, Brady WJ: ECG abnormalities in tricyclic antidepressant ingestion. Am J Emerg Med 17:387–393, 1999.
8. Heard K, Cain BS, Dart RC, Cairns CB: Tricyclic antidepressants directly depress human myocardial mechanical function independent of effects on the conduction system. Acad Emerg Med 8:1122–1127, 2001.
9. Klein-Schwartz W, Anderson B: Analysis of sertaline-only overdoses. Am J Emerg Med 14:456–458, 1996.
10. Kolecki P: Isolated Venlafaxine-induced serotonin syndrome. J Emerg Med 15:491–493, 1997.
11. Liebelt EL, Francis PD, Woolf AD: ECG lead aVR versus QRS interval in predicitng seizures and arrhythmias in acute tricyclic antidepressant toxicity. Ann Emerg Med 26:195–201, 1995.
12. Litovitz TL, Klein-Schwartz W, et al: 2000 Annual report of the American Association of Poison Control Centers Toxic Exposure Surveillance System. J Emerg Med 19:337–395, 2001.
13. Mehta NJ, Alexandrou NA: Tricyclic antidepressant overdose and electrocardiographic changes. J Emerg Med 18:463–464, 2000.
14. Phillips S, Brent J, Kulig K, et al: The Antidepressant Study Group: Fluoxetine versus tricyclic antidepressants: A prospective multicenter study of antidepressant drug overdoses. J Emerg Med 15:439–445, 1997.
15. Sarko J: Antidepressants, old and new: A review of their adverse effects and toxicity in overdose. Emerg Med Clin North Am 18:637–654, 2000.
16. Sporer KA: The serotonin syndrome. Drug Safe 13:94–104, 1995.

89. HYDROCARBON POISONING (PETROLEUM DISTILLATES)

Louis J. Ling, M.D., and Stacey Bangh, Pharm.D.

1. What are the hydrocarbon agents?

Hydrocarbons are distillation products of crude oil. Although all petroleum distillates are hydrocarbons, all hydrocarbons are not derived from petroleum. They may be produced synthetically or distilled from other sources, such as wood tars (i.e., pine oils). They are classified as **aliphatic**, which are straight or branched-chain carbon links that are fully or incompletely saturated to hydrogen atoms; **aromatic**, which contain cyclic benzene rings; or **halogenated**, in which hydrogen atoms have been substituted with halide anions (Br, Cl, F, or I).

2. What types of symptoms do hydrocarbons cause?

Aspiration may lead to a **chemical pneumonitis**. Gastrointestinal absorption of hydrocarbons plays a minimal role in the development of pulmonary toxicity. Pulmonary toxicity is the result of direct tracheal instillation of the hydrocarbon. Attempts at swallowing a hydrocarbon may produce gagging and impair protective airway reflexes, resulting in influx of the agent into the trachea. Further migration down the airways produces acute inflammation, hemorrhage, edema, and loss of surfactant activity. Progression of the inflammatory response may lead to excessive intraluminal secretions, peribronchial edema and cellular infiltration, nonuniform atelectasis, obstructive emphysema, bronchospasm, interstitial edema, and alveolar consolidation.

These anatomic abnormalities contribute to ventilation-perfusion (V/Q) mismatch and resultant hypoxemia. Certain hydrocarbons cause unique toxicity if systemically absorbed. Toxic effects include transfer across the blood-brain barrier producing central nervous system (CNS) depression or excitation, bone marrow suppression, hepatic or renal toxicity, and cardiac arrhythmias. Hydrocarbons, when coupled with heavy metals (i.e., lead), may produce heavy metal intoxication.

3. Which characteristics of a hydrocarbon most increase the risk of aspiration?

Hydrocarbons are classified according to viscosity and volatility. **Viscosity** is the property that most increases the risk of aspiration. The viscosity of a hydrocarbon is determined by the time it takes to flow a specified distance through a calibrated diameter, measured in SSU units (Sabolt seconds universal). Low-viscosity agents (< 60 SSU) have less resistance to flow and are capable of spreading over the epiglottis and into the larynx. Agents most likely to be aspirated include mineral seal oils, mineral spirits, kerosene, turpentine, naphtha, gasoline, and aromatics. Less likely to be aspirated are high-viscosity agents (> 100 SSU), including waxes, paraffins, jellies, greases, and lubricating oils.

Volatility refers to the tendency of a liquid to become a gas. Vapors released from highly volatile hydrocarbons (primarily with low molecular weight and aromatics) may displace oxygen, resulting in a diminished inspired oxygen. Individuals working in enclosed areas with volatile hydrocarbons may experience symptoms from hypoxia.

4. How often does exposure to hydrocarbons result in clinical toxicity, and who is at greatest risk?

The American Association of Poison Control Centers collected data on 2,168,248 human exposures in 2000. Exposures to hydrocarbons (fuels and oils) accounted for 2.8% of all human exposures, or 59,889 cases. Children younger than 6 years old accounted for 23,418 cases. Accidental ingestion by toddlers is the number one cause of human exposure to hydrocarbon agents reported to poison control centers. Of the 33,192 cases with known outcomes in 2000, approximately 90% had no symptoms or minimal symptoms directly attributable to the exposure. A total of 16 deaths and 213 cases developed major toxicity.

5. What are the signs and symptoms of hydrocarbon poisoning?

The severity of symptoms depends on the degree of pulmonary aspiration. After attempts at oral ingestion, patients may experience paroxysmal coughing immediately in an effort to clear the airway. Nausea, emesis, and variable degrees of respiratory distress may ensue. Physical signs initially may be absent yet progress to cyanosis, mottling or dusky appearance of the skin, tachycardia, tachypnea, stridor, salivation, grunting, nasal flaring, retractions, hemoptysis, fever, rales, or wheezing. The presence or absence of hydrocarbon odor on the breath is not a reliable sign of aspiration. Symptoms may resolve or progress rapidly to significant respiratory distress. Hypoxia may lead to CNS excitation (hallucinations, agitation, confusion) or CNS depression (lethargy, coma). Direct pulmonary toxicity (V/Q mismatch) is the primary cause of hypoxia; however, volatilization of hydrocarbons may produce hypoxia from oxygen displacement. Extreme hypoxia may lead to arrhythmias, hypotension, seizures, and cardiopulmonary arrest.

6. How likely are patients to require hospitalization?

Most patients who ingest hydrocarbons do not develop clinical or x-ray evidence of pneumonia. Of 950 cases of hydrocarbon ingestion in children, 800 were asymptomatic at first physical examination and remained asymptomatic during a 6- to 8-hour observation period, with none developing x-ray evidence of pneumonitis. Of these, 150 patients were admitted to the hospital for at least 24 hours. Only 79 were initially symptomatic. Symptoms included paroxysmal coughing or choking, an elevated respiratory rate and tachycardia, lethargy or irritability, persistent emesis, and respiratory distress. Initial chest radiographs were abnormal in 90% of these patients. Only 7 cases progressed to worsening pulmonary disease, however. Two patients died. None of the initial

71 asymptomatic patients who were admitted developed significant pulmonary complications, despite 50% of them having initial abnormal chest radiographs. The development of symptoms or an abnormal chest radiograph occurred within 6 to 8 hours of the ingestion in all these patients.

7. What types of x-ray changes are most likely?

Initial chest radiographs may be normal in 60% of patients who later develop symptomatic pulmonary disease. Radiographic abnormalities may be present within 30 minutes of aspiration and include perihilar densities, extension of interstitial infiltrate, lobar consolidation, linear/basilar atelectasis, early alveolar infiltrate, and lobar atelectasis. Early (6 to 8 hours) abnormalities may lead to further progression. Pleural effusions, pneumothorax, pneumomediastinum, pneumopericardium, and pneumatoceles may develop.

8. Which patients should be admitted?

• All symptomatic patients (respiratory, CNS, and gastrointestinal symptoms mentioned earlier)
• All patients who develop abnormalities on chest radiograph in the first 6 to 8 hours
• All patients who develop desaturation or hypoxemia within 6 to 8 hours after ingestion

Other reasons for admission may include suicidal intent or ingestion of a hydrocarbon with unique systemic toxicity (i.e., pesticides or carbon tetrachloride). Patients who remain asymptomatic, have no radiographic evidence of pulmonary abnormality, and maintain normal oxygen saturations in a 6- to 8-hour observation period after hydrocarbon ingestion may be discharged, provided that adequate follow-up can be ensured. A 24-hour follow-up for discharged patients should be arranged.

9. Can laboratory evaluations help diagnose hydrocarbon pneumonitis?

Standard toxicology screens do not identify hydrocarbon agents and are not helpful in the diagnosis of hydrocarbon pneumonitis. Pulse oximetry is useful for following these patients. Patients who develop desaturation during the observation period require supplemental oxygen and admission. Serial arterial blood gases can be used to follow severely symptomatic patients. Secondary bacterial infections may occur in addition to the primary chemical pneumonitis. An initial cell count with differential may be elevated solely on the basis of the chemical pneumonitis. Serial cell counts with respiratory tract cultures (endotracheal tube aspirate, sputum) and blood cultures may help to diagnose a secondary bacterial infection.

10. Describe the appropriate management of a patient with hydrocarbon pneumonitis.

All symptomatic individuals should be referred to a health care facility for evaluation and treatment. The goal of initial treatment is to assess pulmonary symptoms and oxygen saturations. After assessment and stabilization of a secure airway, a chest radiograph should be obtained. Supraglottitis with upper respiratory tract obstruction may occur, particularly if the hydrocarbon was heated. Otherwise, treatment is primarily supportive. Oxygen should be administered to patients with desaturation or respiratory difficulty. Increased oropharyngeal secretions or gastric emesis may develop from chemical irritation and require suctioning and clearing from the airway. Petroleum distillates are not caustic, so upper airway and esophageal burns are unlikely. Development of bronchospasm may be treated with aerosolized and parenteral bronchodilating agents. Other supportive measures include intravenous fluids to maintain fluid and electrolyte balance; circulatory support, which may require pressors; and treatment of cardiac arrhythmias and seizures.

11. What means of respiratory support should be considered?

Indications for controlled endotracheal intubation include severe respiratory distress, a persistent alveolar-arterial oxygen gradient despite high-flow oxygen administration, and CNS depression leading to respiratory acidosis or an inability to maintain airway protective reflexes. Obstructive and restrictive lung disease may occur with chemical pneumonitis. Ventilatory management may require frequent reassessment and change. The development of edema, consolidation, and atelectasis may worsen V/Q mismatch. Positive end-expiratory pressure (PEEP) may be useful for ventilating patients. The restoration of functional residual capacity by PEEP may allow for lower inspired FiO_2 concentrations. Excessive PEEP may lead to pneumothorax and pneumo-mediastinum in individuals with obstructive lung disease.

12. Is hydrocarbon toxicity ever complicated by other toxic agents?
Hydrocarbons should be assessed for the presence of additives that may induce another toxi-city (e.g., the isopropyl alcohol in pine oil cleaners may lead to CNS depression and ketosis). Specific hydrocarbons may have unique toxicities requiring antidotal administration (e.g., ni-trobenzene leading to methemoglobinemia; methylene blue antidote). Toxicologic consultation can be obtained to help manage such complicated agents.

13. How are hydrocarbons abused?
Hydrocarbons may be poured into a container for **sniffing**, sprayed into a plastic or paper bag for **bagging**, or soaked onto a rag for **huffing**. They have a rapid onset of action and are well absorbed through the lungs with rapid distribution into the CNS.

14. List the most commonly abused substances and the chemicals they contain.

COMMON SOURCES	CHEMICAL INGREDIENTS
Spray paint	Toluene, butane, propane
Gasoline	Benzene, aliphatic and aromatic hydrocarbons
Cigarette lighter fluid	Butane, isopropane
Hair spray, deodorants, room fresheners	Butane, propane
Paint strippers	Methylene chloride
Model glues, rubber cement	n-Hexane, toluene, benzene
Whipped cream cans	Nitrous oxide
Varnishes, lacquers, resins	Benzene
Spot remover, typewriter correction fluid	Trichloroethane, trichloroethylene, carbon tetrachloride
Wood glues, lacquer thinner	Xylene

15. Which of the inhalants listed in the previous table is not a hydrocarbon?
Nitrous oxide, also known as **laughing gas**, is not a hydrocarbon. It is abused by inhaling the propellant from cans of whipped cream.

16. Why do spray paint abusers prefer metallic colored paint?
The toluene content is generally higher in metallic-based paints such as gold, copper, and silver.

17. What are signs and symptoms of hydrocarbon abuse?
Cardiovascular toxicity is the most serious complicaton in abusers. Hydrocarbons sensitize the myocardium to catecholamines, leading to an increased risk of arrhythmia augmented by the substance-associated hypoxia. This has come to be known as **sudden sniffing death**. After acute abuse of hydrocarbons, respiratory symptoms, salivation, and erythema may be seen. As the dose increases, slurred speech, diplopia, ataxia, disorientation, and hallucinations can be observed. This may progress to severe CNS depression, coma, seizure, or death. Chronic abuse can lead to cogni-tive impairment, personality changes, depression, anxiety, and renal and hepatic damage.

18. Is there any special treatment for hydrocarbon abusers?
Avoiding stimulation of these patients is important. Benzodiazepines can be used for agita-tion or hallucinations. Use catecholamines cautiously because they may exacerbate the cardiotoxicity

of inhaled hydrocarbons. Theoretically, bretyllium should be avoided in the treatment of ventricular arrhythmias because it promotes the release of endogenous catecholamines.

CONTROVERSIES

19. Does gastrointestinal decontamination help prevent pulmonary toxicity?

Gastric absorption of hydrocarbon does not lead to chemical pneumonitis. Only when extremely large quantities (> 18 mL/kg) of hydrocarbon are placed in an animal's stomach does enough gastric absorption occur to produce pneumonitis. The oral-to-tracheal LD_{50} for hydrocarbons in animal studies are 40:1 to 140:1. Direct instillation of hydrocarbon into the portal vein also failed to produce pneumonitis.

Induced emesis and gastric lavage carry the risk of aspiration of gastric contents. Activated charcoal does not bind well to petroleum distillates. The risks of induced emesis and gastric lavage probably outweigh the benefits with ingestion of a simple petroleum distillate.

As previously stated, hydrocarbons may possess the potential for serious systemic toxicity or may contain toxic additives. If a toxic quantity of such a substance is ingested, gastric lavage with a controlled airway may be beneficial. Such hydrocarbons can be remembered with the mnemonic **CHAMP**.

C = Camphor
H = Halogenated (10 mL of CCl_4 may lead to acute hepatic failure)
A = Aromatics
M = Metals
P = Pesticides

20. Should prophylactic antibiotics and steroids be given to patients who develop hydrocarbon pneumonitis?

Prophylactic administration of steroids and antibiotics is not currently recommended. In animal research studies, bacterial contamination of kerosene-aspirated animals compared with control animals was not significantly different. Antibiotic treatment did not change the rate or the type of bacterial organisms recovered from lung tissue. Groups that received dexamethasone had a significant increase in bacterial lung contamination. In a human clinical study, 71 children with a history of hydrocarbon ingestion and hospital admission with radiographic evidence of pulmonary abnormalities were randomized to placebo or methylprednisolone/penicillin for 3 days. No differences in respiratory rate, pulse rate, length of hospitalization, or radiographic changes were found. There were three cases of severe pneumonitis. There were no deaths. Large prospective, controlled human trials are lacking. With the available data, however, it seems that the prophylactic use of steroids and antibiotics is not warranted after hydrocarbon aspiration.

BIBLIOGRAPHY

1. Kurtzman T, Otsuka K, Wahl R: Inhalant abuse by adolescents. J Adolesc Health 28:170–180, 2001.
2. Litovitz TL, Klein-Schwartz W, White J, et al: 2000 Annual Report of the American Association of Poison Control Centers Toxic Exposure Surveillance System. Am J Med 19:337–396, 2001.
3. Machado B, Cross K, Snodgrass WR: Accidental hydrocarbon ingestion cases telephoned to a regional poison center. Ann Emerg Med 17:804–807, 1988.
4. Marks MI, Chicione L, Legere G, et al: Adrenocorticosteroid treatment of hydrocarbon pneumonia in children—a cooperative study. J Pediatr 81:366–369, 1972.
5. Mullin LS, Ader AW, Daughtrey WC, et al: Toxicology update isoparrafinic hydrocarbons: A summary of physical properties, toxicity studies and human exposure data. J Appl Toxicol 10:135–142, 1990.
6. Reyes de la Rocha S, Cunningham JC, Fox E: Lipoid pneumonia secondary to baby oil aspiration: A case report and review of the literature. Pediatr Emerg Care 1:74–80, 1985.
7. Scalzo AJ, Weber TR, Jaeger RW, et al: Extracorporeal membrane oxygenation for hydrocarbon aspiration. Am J Dis Child 144:867–871, 1990.

8. Steele RW, Conklin RH, Mark HM: Corticosteroids and antibiotics for the treatment of fulminant hydrocarbon aspiration. JAMA 219:1434–1437, 1972.
9. Taussig LM, Castro O, Landau LI: Pulmonary function 8 to 10 years after hydrocarbon pneumonitis. Clin Pediatr 16:57–59, 1977.
10. Truemper E, Reyes de la Rocha S, Atkinson SD: Clinical characteristics, pathophysiology, and management of hydrocarbon ingestion: Case report and review of the literature. Pediatr Emerg Care 3:187–193, 1987.

90. CHOLINERGIC INSECTICIDES

Gregory W. Burcham, M.D.

1. What are cholinergic insecticides?

Common poisons that are the most frequently used insecticides in the world. They act by inhibiting the enzyme **acetylcholinesterase (AChE)**. Because of their widespread use and their high toxicity, cholinergic insecticides account for more cases of serious human poisoning than any other insecticide. The two classes of cholinergic insecticides are organophosphates and carbamates. **Organophosphates** are divided into three groups, based on their toxicity. High-toxicity compounds include Parathion and Phosdrin and are used in commercial agriculture. The nerve agents Sarin, Soman, and Tabun are derivatives of these compounds. Intermediate-toxicity compounds are used as animal insecticides. Low-toxicity agents are used commonly in households and gardens and include Malathion and Vapona. **Carbamates** also vary by toxicity with aldecarb (Temik) being the most toxic and carbaryl (Sevin) being the least. Several carbamates have been used in medicine for years. Physostigmine is used for anticholinergic poisoning, and pyridostigmine and edrophonium (Tensilon) are used in myasthenia gravis.

2. How do organophosphates and cabamates differ?

They differ in their structures and binding mechanisms. Organophosphates can bind irreversibly to AChE, which permanently inactivates the enzyme. Acute toxic effects last until more AChE is synthesized, which can be more than 1 week. Carbamate binding is reversible, so toxicity lasts only until the toxin is degraded, usually in 6 to 8 hours. Carbamates do not penetrate the central nervous system (CNS) well and show little to no CNS toxicity.

3. Who is most at risk for cholinergic insecticide poisoning?

Migrant farm workers and other agricultural workers. Children are at an increased risk and usually come in contact the poison in a garage or shed at home where it is stored.

4. If I work in an urban area, do I need to know about cholinergic insecticides?

Yes. Although cholinergic insecticide poisoning is seen most frequently in commercial agricultural settings, these products are readily available over-the-counter and are used commonly in private homes and gardens. Organophosphates are ingredients in flea collars, ant traps, and flypaper. They are used occasionally in suicide attempts. There were nearly 16,000 organophosphate exposures in the United States in 2001. Even in treated patients, mortality is 10% for adults and 50% for children. Also, an understanding of cholinergic insecticide poisoning and treatment is directly applicable to management of nerve agent exposure.

5. How can a person get poisoned by these agents?

Organophosphates are highly lipid soluble and are well absorbed by all routes, including transdermally. Commercially the insecticides are stored as a powder or liquid and usually applied as an aerosol. Most occupational exposures occur via the skin or the airway. Intentional poisoning and poisoning in children usually occurs orally. Carbamates are not well absorbed through the skin, and these poisonings are primarily inhalational or oral.

6. Explain how cholinergic insecticides cause their toxic effects.

Cholinergic insecticide poisoning results in an excess of acetylcholine-mediated activity. Acetylcholine is a neurotransmitter that binds to nicotinic receptors in preganglionic parasympathetic and sympathetic synapses and motor end plates, muscarinic receptors in postganglionic synapses, and certain synapses in the CNS. Normally, acetylcholine is degraded by the enzymes AChE or pseudocholinesterase. Organophosphates and cabamates inactivate both enzymes, resulting in an overabundance of acetylcholine. This leads to overactivation, then paralysis of the cholinergic receptors, with the end result being an overstimulation of the autonomic nervous system, somatic musculature, and CNS. Organophosphate poisoning is more dangerous than carbamate poisoning. Both agents immediately bind to AChE. In 24 to 48 hours, organophosphate binding becomes irreversible and results in permanent inactivation of the enzyme. This process is known as *aging*. This delay between exposure and permanent inactivation provides a window for antidote therapy.

7. How does cholinergic poisoning appear clinically?

The clinical effects are logical if you consider the synapses affected by excess acetylcholine. Acetylcholine works at muscarinic, nicotinic, and central receptor sites.

Stimulation of the **muscarinic receptors** leads to increased exocrine gland secretions and smooth muscle contraction. This results in bronchorrhea and bronchospasm in the respiratory tree; salivation, nausea, vomiting, diarrhea, abdominal cramping, and incontinence in the gastrointestinal tract; diaphoresis in the skin; miosis and lacrimation in the eyes; and bradycardia and hypotension in the cardiovascular system.

Stimulation of the **nicotinic receptors** causes adrenal gland secretion of epinephrine and norepinephrine and activation at the motor end plates. This results in tachycardia and hypertension in the cardiovascular system; breakdown of glycogen into glucose in the liver; and in muscle fasciculations, cramps, weakness, and paralysis in the somatic muscles.

Cholinergic effects on the **CNS** include agitation, headache, ataxia, dysarthria, altered mental status, respiratory depression, seizures, and coma. Any of these symptoms may be delayed 6 hours after exposure.

8. What are the two mnemonics for muscarinic and nicotinic effects of organophosphate?

SLUDGE for muscarinic effects and the **days of the week (M, T, W, tH, F, S)** for nicotinic effects.

	Muscarinic		**Nicotinic**
S	Salivation	M	Muscle cramps
L	Lacrimation	T	Tachycardia
U	Urination	W	Weakness
D	Diarrhea	tH	Hypertension
G	Gastrointestinal upset and pain	F	Fasciculations
E	Emesis	S	Sugar (hyperglycemia)

9. How do I diagnose cholinergic insecticide poisoning?

The signs and symptoms of cholinergic toxicity should suggest cholinergic insecticide poisoning immediately. Clinically, tachycardia commonly predominates over bradycardia in acute poisoning, and miosis usually predominates over mydriasis. A garlic-like odor is typical of organophosphates and may be present. The absence of CNS symptoms may suggest carbamate poisoning. A history of exposure or symptoms in a person at risk for exposure should raise the index of suspicion. Because of their highly toxic effects, a lack of anticholinergic response to anticholinergic agents is strong evidence of cholinergic insecticide poisoning.

10. List the differential diagnosis.

Poisoning
Opiates
Phenothiazines
Nicotine
Muscarine-containing mushrooms
Rattlesnake venom
Scorpion venom
Infections
Meningitis
Encephalitis
Botulism
Gastroenteritis
Sepsis
Tetanus

CNS processes
Epilepsy
Subarachnoid or subdural hemorrhage
Alcohol withdrawal
Cerebral vasculitis
Metabolic disorders
Hypoglycemia
Diabetic ketoacidosis
Myxedema coma
Neuroleptic malignant syndrome
Thyrotoxicosis

11. Are there any tests that I should do?

- **Laboratory tests** should include complete blood count, liver function tests, electrolytes, blood urea nitrogen and creatinine, glucose, amylase, blood gas, cholinesterase activity, and urinalysis.
- A **chest radiograph** is important because pulmonary edema or evidence of aspiration is an ominous finding.
- An **ECG** should be obtained because arrhythmias such as heart block and torsades de pointes can occur.
- Other laboratory tests and imaging studies may be needed to help exclude other diagnoses.

12. Can any of the laboratory tests confirm cholinergic poisoning?

Although the diagnosis is primarily a clinical one, a decrease in red blood cell or plasma cholinesterase activity is seen in nearly all cases of cholinergic insecticide poisoning; this may require knowledge of the patient's baseline cholinesterase activity, however, which makes the test less useful acutely. AChE activity also can be reduced in liver disease, alcoholism, malnutrition, and dermatomyositis and by an autosomal recessive trait in normal individuals. Nevertheless, although it may not affect initial management, red blood cell and plasma cholinesterase activity should be measured because they may be helpful if the patient is hospitalized or when other diagnoses are being considered.

13. What emergencies exist with cholinergic poisonings?

Most early deaths occur when the combination of bronchospasm, bronchorrhea, respiratory muscle weakness, and depressed respiratory drive lead to respiratory failure. Atrioventricular blocks, bradycardia, hypotension, and torsades de pointes occasionally can lead to cardiac failure. Vomiting and diarrhea can lead to severe dehydration and electrolyte abnormalities. Seizures and coma can occur.

14. How do I treat someone with acute organophosphate poisoning?

There are many cases of secondary poisoning in health care providers treating such patients. Medical staff should be especially careful to avoid cutaneous or respiratory exposure while treating a patient with cholinergic insecticide poisoning. Decontamination should begin in the prehospital setting, and contact and respiratory precautions should be used. Begin treatment with the ABCDs (airway, breathing, circulation, and decontamination). Frequent aggressive suctioning of the airway is necessary to remove bronchial secretions. Oxygen should be administered. Intubation and mechanical ventilation may be required for persistent hypoxia, pulmonary edema, respiratory depression, or weakness. Cardiac monitoring is mandatory. For decontamination, all clothing should be removed, and the skin and hair should be washed with warm soapy water to remove any remaining insecticide and to prevent continued absorption. If the poisoning was by oral ingestion, gastric lavage followed by charcoal is indicated. If the patient already has diarrhea, a cathartic is not necessary. Succinylcholine, morphine, phenothiazines, barbiturates, furosemide, and theophylline are contraindicated in organophosphate poisoning. In any symptomatic patient, ICU admission for at least 24 hours is warranted. Prompt administration of atropine and pralidoxime are crucial.

15. Is there an antidote?

Specific treatment of organophosphate poisoning consists of the administration of atropine and pralidoxime (Protopam, 2-PAM). Atropine specifically counteracts the muscarinic effects of poisoning by blocking the muscarinic receptors. It should not be given until hypoxia has been resolved, however, because it can induce ventricular tachycardia or fibrillation. An initial dose of 2 to 4 mg intravenously should be given to adults and 0.015 to 0.05 mg/kg to pediatric patients. Drying secretions and mydriasis indicate adequate blockade of the muscarinic receptors, and atropine dosing should be guided by these findings. Be prepared to give what may seem like huge amounts of atropine. Doses of more than 1 g in 24 hours have been required, and atropine drips have been used. Most treatment failures occur from underdosing atropine. Atropine treatment alone is sufficient for managing carbamate poisoning. Pralidoxime can reactivate AChE and restore normal activity of the enzyme if it is administered before aging is complete. It is most efficacious when given within the first 24 to 48 hours after exposure but should be continued as long as necessary. Pralidoxime alleviates the nicotinic and CNS effects of organophosphate toxicity. The dose is 1 to 2 g over 30 minutes in adults and 25 to 50 mg/kg over 30 minutes in children. Clinical improvement can occur within minutes after administration. Doses can be repeated as necessary. Pralidoxime is not necessary for carbamate poisoning.

16. Are there delayed effects of cholinergic insecticide poisoning?

- Discontinuation of atropine or pralidoxime therapy prematurely can cause rebound symptoms.
- An intermediate syndrome can occur 24 to 96 hours after recovery from the acute cholinergic effects of organophosphate poisoning. It is manifested by specific weakness of the respiratory muscles, proximal limbs, and neck flexors. It is not responsive to atropine or pralidoxime, and ventilatory support may be necessary.
- Organophosphate-induced neurotoxicity can occur 10 to 21 days after exposure. It consists of a distal polyneuropathy, beginning with flaccidity and weakness and progressing to spasticity, hyperreflexia, and hypertonia.
- Neuropsychopathologic changes in behavior, cognition, and visual and motor functions have been described. These changes may persist for several months after symptomatic organophosphate toxicity.

Controversy exists over whether asymptomatic or chronic exposure causes effects as well.

BIBLIOGRAPHY

1. Aaron CK, Vance MV: Pesticides. In Marx JA, et al (eds): Rosen's Emergency Medicine: Concepts and Clinical Practice, 5th ed. St. Louis, Mosby, 2002.
2. Bardin PG, van Eeden SF, et al: Organophosphate and carbamate poisoning. Arch Intern Med 154:1433–1441, 1994.
3. Bryson PD: Comprehensive Review in Toxicology for Emergency Clinicians, 3rd ed. Taylor & Francis, 1997.
4. Clark RF: Insecticides: Organic phosphorous compounds and carbamates. In Goldfrank LR, et al (eds): Goldfrank's Toxicologic Emergencies, 7th ed. New York, McGraw-Hill, 2002.
5. Dart RC, et al (eds): The 5 Minute Toxicology Consult. Philadelphia, Lippincott Williams & Wilkins, 2002.
6. Eyer P: Neuropsychopathological changes by organophosphorus compounds—a review. Hum Exp Toxicol 14:857–864, 1995.
7. Henretig FM: Special considerations in the poisoned pediatric patient. Emerg Med Clin North Am 12:549–567, 1994.

8. Litovitz A, et al: 2000 Annual Report of the American Association of Poison Control Centers Toxic Exposure Surveillance System. Am J Emerg Med 19:337–395, 2001.
9. O'Malley M: Clinical evaluation of pesticide exposure and poisonings. Lancet 349:1161–1166, 1997.
10. Tafuri J, Roberts J: Organophosphate poisoning. Ann Emerg Med 16:193–202, 1987.
11. Woo OF: Organophosphates and carbamates. In Olson KR (ed): Poisoning and Drug Overdose, 3rd ed. Norwalk, CT, Appleton & Lange, 1994.

91. CORROSIVES

Christopher J. Ott, M.D.

1. Which agents are classified as corrosives and can cause injury?

In the United States, ingestion of strong alkaline or strong acidic materials produces most caustic injuries to the gastrointestinal (GI) tract. Alkaline substances are bases that release hydroxide ions on dissociation in water and are more frequently the reported causes of corrosive burns. Acids liberate hydronium ions with water contact. The alkaline and acidic materials may be in either liquid or solid form.

2. What tissue injuries are caused by alkaline corrosive preparations?

Alkalis produce liquefaction necrosis, with destruction of protein and collagen, tissue dehydration, saponification of fat, and blood vessel thrombosis, and most frequently affect the oropharynx and esophagus. This process can penetrate some or all layers of the esophagus and stomach with perforation and infection as early causes of morbidity and mortality. Strictures with altered motility occur as late complications of alkali ingestion. The injuries are classified by endoscopists according to the degree of penetration:

First-degree burns: Superficial erythema, edema
Second-degree burns: Erythema, blistering, superficial ulceration, fibrinous exudate
Third-degree burns: Deep ulceration, friability, eschar formation, perforation

3. What tissue injuries are caused by acidic corrosive preparations?

Acids produce coagulation necrosis, with damage to the columnar epithelium, submucosa, and muscularis mucosa. The injury is covered by a coagulum consisting of damaged tissue and thrombosed blood vessels. In mild-to-moderate cases, this coagulum or eschar may inhibit further penetration of acid and protect the deeper muscular layers. This facilitates passage of acid further down the GI tract with frequent involvement of the stomach and occasionally the proximal small intestine. In severe cases, full-thickness injuries with perforation can occur. Acid burns are classified using a five-grade system:

Grade 0:   Normal
Grade 1:   Edema, mucosal hyperemia
Grade 2a: Superficial ulcerations, mucosal friability, blisters
Grade 2b: Grade 2a findings plus circumferential ulceration
Grade 3:   Multiple, deep ulcerations and extensive necrosis

4. Are injuries produced by alkaline caustic agents limited to the esophagus?

No. Many studies suggesting a relative sparing of the stomach in ingestions of alkalis were performed in children, in whom the ingestions were accidental and involved small amounts of material. Hemorrhage and perforation of the stomach and small intestine have been reported with ingestion of large amounts of alkaline caustic substances. When the ingestion is known or suspected to be large, the stomach and small intestine also must be evaluated.

5. What injuries have been reported with the ingestion of household ammonia or bleach?

These common household cleaners generally cause problems only if aspirated or ingested in large amounts. Ingestion of household bleach (sodium hypochlorite) usually produces no injury or mild esophageal burns. Two cases of esophageal injury requiring surgical repair were reported in patients who were reexposed to the sodium hypochlorite when they vomited. Complications reported with large ingestions of household ammonia include severe esophageal burns and perforation, adult respiratory distress syndrome, gastric necrosis, airway obstruction resulting from supraglottic edema, and death.

6. What clinical signs and symptoms indicate the presence of a significant (greater than first-degree or grade I) GI tract injury?

The presence or absence of oropharyngeal burns cannot be used to determine the presence or absence of a significant upper GI tract lesion.

Alkalis: In small children suspected or known to have ingested a caustic alkaline substance, the presence of drooling, vomiting, or stridor may indicate a significant esophageal lesion. In a retrospective study of 79 pediatric patients by Crain et al, the presence of two or more of these signs predicted all the patients who were found to have significant esophageal lesions on endoscopy. All patients who presented with stridor had a significant esophageal lesion. These findings may be used as general guidelines to determine the need for endoscopy in the pediatric population, although the decision ultimately depends on the clinician's suspicion of a significant upper GI tract burn. Endoscopy is recommended for all adult patients regardless of the presence or absence of symptoms because these ingestions are often deliberate and may involve large amounts of caustic substance, and these patients may have significant injuries with few or no symptoms immediately apparent.

Acids: Dysphagia and odynophagia have been closely associated with acid-induced esophagitis. Signs and symptoms referable to significant gastric injuries are less reliable, with epigastric pain, tenderness, or both being reported in fewer than half of patients. GI tract hemorrhage and perforation may occur rapidly. Systemic effects, such as metabolic acidosis, disseminated intravascular coagulation, hyponatremia, and hypotension, may develop. Aspiration of acid can produce stridor, upper airway obstruction, and adult respiratory distress syndrome.

7. How should patients with suspected caustic injury be managed initially?

Airway management is the first priority because pharyngeal or laryngeal burns can compromise airway patency. Immediate endotracheal intubation should be performed for life-threatening respiratory compromise; cricothyrotomy or tracheotomy can be done when endotracheal intubation is unsuccessful. Nasotracheal intubation is contraindicated and should never be done. Less acute cases without stridor need ear, nose, and throat examination to evaluate the hypopharynx, cords, and larynx, basing the decision to intubate on the presence and severity of burns. Patients should not be given anything orally and should be given intravenous crystalloids and opioid analgesics for pain control. Corticosteroids may decrease laryngeal edema.

Alkalis: Gastric evacuation or neutralization therapies are contraindicated. The efficacy of H_2-blocker drugs is unknown, and antibiotics should be used only for known infection or concomitantly with corticosteroid therapy (see question 13). Patients with second-degree and third-degree burns should be admitted.

Acids: Gastric emptying is recommended via a nasogastric tube to decrease gastric mucosal exposure and systemic absorption of acids. The patient should remain gastrically intubated for continued decompression. Neutralization is contraindicated. Corticosteroids and antibiotics should not be given because their efficacy is unproved. Laboratory tests include coagulation studies and blood type and crossmatch.

8. Which laboratory or radiographic studies should be considered in suspected or known corrosive ingestion?

A complete blood cell count, blood type and crossmatch, arterial blood, and disseminated intravascular coagulation panel should be considered in all hemodynamically unstable patients or in patients with suspected severe burns or perforation. Chest and abdominal radiographs can aid in the diagnosis of GI perforations by exhibiting free air in the mediastinum or peritoneal cavity. Radiographs may identify ingested batteries or other radiopaque foreign bodies or material in the GI tract.

9. Summarize the indications for emergency endoscopy.

Alkalis: All pediatric patients with presenting signs and symptoms indicative of upper GI tract burns more serious than first degree should undergo endoscopy within 12 to 24 hours after ingestion. All adults with known or suspected alkali ingestion should have endoscopy during the same time frame.

Acids: Endoscopy should be done immediately in all cases of known or suspected acid ingestion because the findings help to determine the necessity of acute surgical intervention. Endoscopy also aids in lavage and evacuation of any remaining acid from incomplete nasogastric emptying and decompression.

10. Discuss the contraindications and potential complications of endoscopy.

For injuries caused by acids and alkalis, evidence of GI tract perforation rules out the use of diagnostic endoscopy. In the presence of severe hypopharyngeal burns, a flexible scope may be inserted through a rigid endoscope to minimize the risk of hypopharyngeal perforation. Alternatively, limited evaluation may be accomplished with a water-soluble contrast radiographic study.

Alkalis: Traditionally, diagnostic endoscopy is terminated at the first deep, penetrating, or circumferential burn of the esophagus. Development of the flexible endoscope and realization that alkaline caustic substances can produce life-threatening gastric and small intestinal injuries have led to more aggressive endoscopic examination. Panendoscopy of the upper GI tract, including stomach and duodenum, should be done in all cases of alkali ingestion that meet the criteria for endoscopy. The skill of the endoscopist determines whether endoscopy proceeds past the level of a deep esophageal burn.

Acids: Panendoscopy of the upper GI tract is the standard, given the predilection of acids to produce life-threatening gastric burns.

11. When is immediate surgical intervention indicated?

Alkalis: Surgery may be required for life-threatening GI hemorrhage or GI tract perforation, although some esophageal perforations have been managed successfully with drainage and antibiotics. Exploratory laparotomy for direct visualization of the stomach may be necessary when severe gastric injury is suspected and severe esophageal burns preclude gastric endoscopic examination.

Acids: Immediate surgery is indicated for GI tract perforation and when endoscopy reveals grade 3 burns with full-thickness necrosis of the esophagus or stomach. In the latter case, surgical drainage of the acid remaining in the stomach, with resection of nonviable tissue, may prevent further tissue damage and the systemic complications that may occur with perforation.

12. What complications and clinical sequelae may occur?

Ingestions of alkalis and acids may be complicated by GI tract perforation or hemorrhage, chemical pneumonitis, adult respiratory distress syndrome, and strictures of the upper respiratory or GI tract.

Alkalis: Esophageal squamous cell carcinoma may develop at the site of the stricture, with a latency period of 9 to 71 years. Patients who develop strictures must be monitored throughout their lives for the development of carcinoma.

Acids: Metabolic acidosis, hypotension, or disseminated intravascular coagulation can complicate these ingestions. As with alkali ingestions, malignancies can arise in stricture sites, mandating lifelong monitoring. Severe gastric burns with subsequent scarring can result in (1) achlorhydria and diminished or absent intrinsic factor and (2) dumping syndrome secondary to a small, immobile stomach.

13. Discuss unique issues involved with managing hydrofluoric acid (HFA) exposure and ingestion.

HFA can cause delayed presentation of burns and significant metabolic abnormalities associated with the calcium-leeching properties if free fluoride ions. It is used mainly in industrial glass etching, metal cleaning, electronics manufacturing, and rust removal. If the acid is of a low concentration ($\leq$ 12.5%), the tissue damage and symptoms may be delayed by 8 to 12 hours. The main local symptom is severe pain and can be managed by copious irrigation and the use of calcium-based gels and paste with local arterial infusions of calcium chloride to neutralize the fluoride ions. The other management issues associated with acidic burns should be addressed as in any exposure.

The most important issue affecting patients exposed to HFA is the systemic electrolyte abnormalities. Significant hypocalcemia, hypomagnesemia, and hyperkalemia may result from relatively small exposures. ECG monitoring for prolonged Q-T intervals, arrhythmias, and classic ECG findings of hyperkalemia is important. Treatment of hypocalcemia is paramount to ensure patient survival. The intravenous use of large amounts of calcium chloride is indicated until the patient's ECG normalizes and the serum calcium is normal. Do not wait to obtain serum calcium levels on patients to initiate or maintain treatment.

For ingestions, gastric installations of 20 mmol of calcium chloride in 1 L of normal saline through a nasogastric tube may be beneficial to prevent cardiovascular collapse in HFA ingestions. No evidence was found of increased gastric perforation with use of a nasogastric tube. For inhalation injury, which is often fatal, there is some case-based evidence that a 2.5% calcium gluconate nebulizer with systemic calcium replacement may be beneficial. It takes less than 10 mL of 100% HFA to bind all of the calcium in a 70-kg man. Strong consideration should be given to admitting and monitoring all moderate-to-significant HFA exposures for 24 to 48 hours to ensure adequate cardiac and electrolyte monitoring.

CONTROVERSY

14. Should corticosteroids be used in the treatment of alkali-induced esophageal burns?

For: When used in conjunction with esophageal dilation therapy for established strictures, corticosteroids begun immediately after injury may decrease the incidence of surgical repair of the esophagus. In studies by Haller and Tewfik, using a combination of corticosteroid and esophageal dilation therapies, no surgical repair was required in 14 patients who developed esophageal strictures. In Anderson et al's study, which used dilation therapy for all esophageal strictures, a trend toward less surgical repair of the esophagus was noted in the corticosteroid-treated group.

Against: Traditionally, early corticosteroid therapy was thought to decrease esophageal stricture formation. Analysis of comparable studies in the literature reveals the severity of the burn, rather than the use of corticosteroids, to be the major determinant of stricture formation. Anderson et al prospectively randomized 60 children with alkali-induced esophageal burns to treatment with or without corticosteroids. In this study, the development of strictures correlated better with burn severity than with the therapeutic regimen, and they concluded corticosteroids were of no benefit in preventing stricture formation.

BIBLIOGRAPHY

1. Anderson KD, Rouse TM, Randolph JG: A controlled trial of corticosteroids in children with corrosive injury of the esophagus. N Engl J Med 323:637, 1990.
2. Chan BS, Duggin GG, et al: Survival after massive hydrofluoric acid ingestion. J Toxicol Clin Toxicol 35:307–309, 1997.
3. Crain EF, Gershel JC, Mezey AP: Caustic ingestions: Symptoms as predictors of esophageal injury. Am J Dis Child 138:863, 1984.
4. Dilawari JB, Singh S, Rao PN, et al: Corrosive acid ingestion in man: A clinical and endoscopic study. Gut 25:183, 1984.

5. Ford M: Alkali and acid injuries of the upper gastrointestinal tract. In Hoffman RS, Goldfrank LR (eds): Critical Care Toxicology. New York, Contemporary Management in Critical Care, 1991, pp 225–244.
6. Hawkins DB, Demeter MJ, Barnett TE: Caustic ingestion: Controversies in management: A review of 214 cases. Laryngoscope 90:98, 1980.
7. Litovitz TL, Clark LR, Soloway RA: 1993 Annual report of the American Association of Poison Control Centers Toxic Exposure Surveillance System. Am J Emerg Med 12:546–584, 1994.
8. Middelkamp JN, Ferguson TB, Roper CL, et al: The management and problems of caustic burns in children. J Thorac Cardiovasc Surg 57:341, 1969.
9. Tewfik TL, Schloss MD: Ingestion of lye and other corrosive agents: A study of 86 infant and child cases. J Otolaryngol 9:72, 1980.
10. Wilkes G, et al: Hydrofluoric acid burns. EMedicine Journal 2, 2001.
11. Zargar SA, Kochhar R, Nagi B, et al: Ingestion of corrosive acids: Spectrum of injury to upper gastrointestinal tract and natural history. Gastroenterology 97:702, 1989.

92. BITES AND STINGS

Lee W. Shockley, M.D.

Always carry a flagon of whiskey in case of snakebite and furthermore always carry a small snake.
—W.C. Fields (1880?–1946)

SNAKEBITES

1. What is a snakebite?

A snakebite is Yukon Jack and Rose's Lime Juice although some experts make a snakebite with ale or lager and hard cider. A rattlesnake is (1) a pit viper or (2) the combination of blended whiskey, lemon juice, sugar, egg white, and Pernod. This chapter is concerning animal bites and stings, however.

2. Crotalid, crotaline, crotalus, crotaloid?

In the United States, there are two families of indigenous venomous snakes: Elapidae and Viperidae (subfamily Crotalinae). Elapidae species in the United States are represented by the coral snakes.

Rattlesnakes, cottonmouth, and copperhead snakes previously were categorized as the crotalid snakes (family Crotalidae). The classification for the pit vipers changed in the mid-1980s. The classification nomenclature is now family Viperidae, subfamily Crotalinae; the more appropriate term *crotaline* is used to refer to the Crotalinae subfamily, which includes North American species of *Agkistrodon* (copperhead, cottonmouth, and water moccasin snakes), *Crotalus* (rattlesnakes), and *Sistrurus* (massasauga and pigmy rattlesnakes). The crotaline snakes are the pit vipers.

3. What is the *pit* that distinguishes the pit viper?

A thermoreceptor organ located halfway between the snake's eye and nostril. It appears as a small indentation. If you are close enough to notice this feature, you're too close.

4. What is a dry snakebite?

A bite in which no venom was introduced.

5. What are the chances of a bite from a snake causing a dry bite? How can you tell?

About 25% of all bites from venomous snakes in the United States do not result in envenomation. Quick observations helpful in determining whether envenomation has taken place include the presence of fang marks that ooze nonclotting blood with surrounding ecchymosis and severe burning pain. These signs combined with microhematuria are characteristic of severe envenomation and a poor prognosis.

6. *True or false*: **Snakebites are uncommon but are highly lethal.**
   True *and* false. In the United States, snakebites are uncommon; however, mortality is rare. In their 1999 report, the American Association of Poison Control Centers (AAPCC) documented 5,766 snakebites (venomous and nonvenomous). The AAPCC database for 1999 had 2,201,156 human exposure cases and was believed to represent 95.7% of the total human toxic exposure cases that occurred in the United States in 1999. Snakebites made up only 0.26% of the reported human exposure cases. In 1999, there were two deaths attributed to snakebites in the United States (one from a rattlesnake, one from an unknown snake). The case-fatality rate was less than 0.035%. Of all the venomous snakebites in the United States, 98% are from pit vipers. If one examines only the venomous bites, mortality is still rare: rattlesnake bites, 0.1%; copperhead, cottonmouth, and coral snake bites, none in 1999.

7. **What about morbidity?**
   Morbidity is much more common:

SNAKE	MODERATE MORBIDITY (%)	LIFE-THREATENING MORBIDITY (%)
Rattlesnake (n = 993)	41	12
Copperhead (n = 579)	43	4
Cottonmouth (n = 111)	34	3
Coral snake (n = 46)	15	6

From Litovitz TL, Klein-Schwartz W, White S, et al: 1999 Annual Report of the American Association of Poison Control Centers Toxic Exposure Surveillance System. Am J Emerg Med 18:517–574, 2000, with permission.

8. **List some of the epidemiologic characteristics of snakebites in the United States.**
   • 90% occur from April to October
   • 50% occur between the hours of 2 P.M. and 9 P.M.
   • Male-to-female victim ratio is 9:1
   • 50% of victims are age 18 to 28 years
   • 80% of bites are on the fingers or hand; 15% involve the foot or ankle
   • Ethanol intoxication is a common risk factor for the victim

9. **What is in rattlesnake venom?**
   It is a soup of toxins that allows the snake to capture and consume its prey. Venom contains cytotoxic enzymes (good to help the snake digest its prey), neurotoxins (good to keep prey from fighting back or running away), and thrombin-like hemotoxins (good to get the prey to exsanguinate).

10. **List the clinical signs of Crotalidae (pit viper) envenomation.**
    Rapid onset of slow spreading edema (80%)
    Pain out of proportion to the puncture (72%)
    Weakness (65%)
    Light-headedness (52%)
    Nausea (48%)
    Erythema at the bite site (53%)
    Bleeding diathesis (52%)
    Lymphangitis, hypotension, shock, diaphoresis, chills (58%)
    Paresthesias, taste changes, fasciculations (33%)

11. Is there a validated scoring system to grade (and subsequently follow) crotaline envenomation?

Yes, the **Snakebite Severity Score**. It is a point system that scores signs and symptoms from the pulmonary system, cardiovascular system, local wound, gastrointestinal system, hematologic system, and central nervous system. It is detailed and beyond the scope of this text. (See reference 7.)

12. Compare Antivenin (Crotalidae) Polyvalent (ACP) (Wyeth-Ayerst Laboratories) with Crotalidae Polyvalent Immune Fab (Ovine) (CroFab) (Altana, Inc).

ACP is a horse serum-derived antivenin. Because it is a partially purified product of horse serum, ACP retains large amounts of proteins that do not neutralize venom. CroFab is produced from the serum of sheep immunized with one of four crotaline snake venoms, then digested with papain to produce antibody fragments (Fab and Fc). The more immunogenic Fc portion of the antibody is eliminated during purification. The four individual monospecific Fab preparations are combined to form the final antivenin product. Both products are provided as lyophilized powders and must reconstituted. The median time for reconstitution of ACP is greater than 90 minutes; the mean time for reconstitution of CroFab is 30 to 40 minutes. Neither ACP nor CroFab has been tested in the treatment of copperhead snakebite. Since the Food and Drug Administration (FDA) approval of CroFab, Wyeth has ceased manufacture of ACP (although many institutions have stocks of ACP that have not yet been used).

13. Why would one have to retreat with CroFab after initial control is achieved? What is *late recurrence*?

Probably because of the relatively small molecule size and consequent renal clearing, the effective half-life of CroFab may be insufficient for one-dose treatment of crotaline envenomation. Scheduled retreatment is recommended. Even so, late recurrence (2 to 14 days after envenomation) of symptoms is possible. Local recurrence occurs in 27% of patients. Coagulopathy recurs in 53% of patients (69% of patients with initial coagulopathy). Retreatment with CroFab is recommended for recurrent coagulopathy manifested by:

Fibrinogen < 50 µg/mL
Platelet count < 25,000/mm^3
International normalized ratio > 3.0
Activated partial thromboplastin time > 50 seconds
Multicomponent coagulopathy
Worsening trend in a patient with prior severe coagulopathy
High-risk behavior for trauma
Comorbid conditions that increase hemorrhagic risk

14. Can a crotaline bite cause a compartment syndrome?

It can, but it is unlikely. In most cases, venom is deposited in the subcutaneous tissue, not in fascial compartments. Documented elevated compartment pressures are rare. Compartment syndrome cannot be diagnosed reliably in an envenomated patient without directly measuring compartment pressures because the signs and symptoms of compartment syndrome (paresthesias, decreased pulses, and pain on motion) are similar to signs and symptoms of envenomation. The only way to determine whether compartment syndrome has developed is to measure the intracompartmental pressure. Because treatment with antivenin may improve compartment pressure, if the pressure is found to be elevated initially, you should monitor the compartment pressure while administering antivenin and perform fasciotomy only when pressures remain persistently elevated above 30 to 40 mm Hg.

One exception is the **envenomated finger**. A tense, blue or pale envenomated finger with absent or poor capillary refill may be treated by **digit dermotomy** on clinical grounds alone. To make the dermotomy, incise the skin (only) longitudinally, on the medial or lateral aspect of the digit from the web to the midportion of the distal phalanx. A digit dermotomy should not be used routinely in all finger bites; it is not appropriate for prophylactic treatment to prevent a digital compartment syndrome.

15. How is antivenin dosing altered for children, and why?

The amount of venom children receive is the same amount that adults receive; they receive a greater toxic load per body weight, have less body water to dilute the toxin, and have less inherent resistance to the effects of the venom. The dose of antivenin per kilogram needs to be higher for children than for adults. Some recommend increasing the dose by 50% in children weighing less than 45 kg.

16. How about baby rattlesnakes?

Venomous snakes hatch with their envenomation apparatus fully formed and potent.

17. What is the importance of the coloring of coral snakes, and what are the active components of its venom?

This small, thin, brightly colored snake is venomous; however, the king snake, which is non-venomous, has similar but not identical coloration. Remember:

"Red on yellow, kill a fellow" (coral snake)
"Red on black, venom lack" (harmless snake)

This rhyme helps only with the identification of North American snakes. Coral snake venom contains a neurotoxin that irreversibly binds to presynaptic nerve terminals and blocks acetyl-choline receptors. It may take weeks or months to regenerate the receptors. The clinical effects are slurred speech, ptosis, dilated pupils, dysphagia, and myalgias. Death results from progressive paralysis and respiratory failure. There is virtually no local tissue toxicity.

18. How is coral snake envenomation treated?

Neostigmine (2.5 mg every 30 to 60 minutes) and equine antivenin (Wyeth). Four to 6 vials of the coral snake antivenin are recommended for envenomations from the eastern coral snake or the Texas coral snake; envenomations from the western coral snake need not be treated with antivenin.

19. What treatments have been advocated for rattlesnake bites that are now considered to be ineffective or harmful? What nonantivenin treatments do make sense?

Incising the wound and attempting to extract the poison by oral suction (**cut and suck**), electric shock to denature the toxin proteins, carbolic acid, strychnine, enemas, urine, cauterization, prophylactic antibiotics, ice packs (cryotherapy), and arterial tourniquets are probably ineffective or harmful. In the early 1900s, whiskey was advocated as an antidote (see W.C. Fields's advice at the beginning of the chapter). The use of constriction bands, splints, and venom removal with The Extractor (a mechanical suction device that produces about 1 atm of negative pressure and may remove 30% of the injected venom if used within 3 minutes of the bite) are controversial, with proponents and opponents.

A constriction band (broad and flat band as opposed to a ropelike tourniquet) can be applied to exert a pressure great enough to occlude superficial veins and lymphatic channels (typically > 20 mm Hg) but loose enough to admit one or two fingers. It has been shown in experimental models to delay the systemic absorption of venom and may have use in cases with prolonged transport time.

A competing technique originating in Australia is the pressure-immobilization method. By firmly wrapping the bitten extremity with an elastic bandage (for pressures 40 to 70 mm Hg) and splinting the entire extremity, the onset of significant systemic toxicity may be delayed until the patient can be treated in a facility where antivenin therapy is available. Theoretically, however, **trapping** the venom in the bitten extremity may worsen local necrosis. Releasing the pressure could allow a bolus of venom to be released into the systemic circulation. The relative merits of the constriction band versus the pressure-immobilization technique have not been directly compared.

In an animal model, the time to death after injection of venom can be prolonged, and the median lethal dose of venom can be increased simply by immobilizing all four limbs (including the unbitten extremity). This technique also has not been studied clinically.

Nonsteroidal antiinflammatory drugs may compound a crotaline venom-induced thrombocytopenic bleeding diathesis and probably should be avoided.

20. What about some of the more exotic snakes (at least exotic by North American standards)?

In 1999, the AAPCC reported 2,252 cases of exposure to exotic snakes (poisonous, nonpoisonous, and "unknown if poisonous"). Although there were no deaths reported, there were seven patients with life-threatening morbidity and 78 with moderate morbidity. There are probably several thousand cobras brought into the United States annually. Their venom is neurotoxic. Cranial nerve dysfunction (ptosis, blurred vision, difficulty swallowing), mental status changes, respiratory muscle paralysis, paresthesias, weakness or paralysis, and hypotension can be some of the effects.

21. Where can I obtain information about antivenin for the treatment of bites from exotic snakes?

There is an **Antivenom Index** that is sent to all of the Poison Control Centers in the United States. It includes a catalog of all of the antivenoms stocked by North American zoos and aquariums. Possession of exotic venomous snakes may be restricted by law, and these cases should be reported to the authorities.

22. What is *snake oil*?

It's a term for a medication of dubious value, sold by charlatans. A naturally occurring "rock oil" (raw petroleum) was used by the Native Americans of the Seneca tribe in the Allegheny region of Pennsylvania as a topical ointment for burns and scratches. As early as 1792, opportunists bottled and sold the viscid, smelly, amber substance as Seneca Oil, with claims of miraculous cures for a wide variety of ills. Seneca was often mispronounced as "Sen-*ake*-a," and *Seneca Oil* became *snake oil*.

SPIDER BITES

23. State the incidence, mortality, and morbidity of spider bites in the United States.

There are two venomous spiders in the United States: *Latrodectus* (black widow) and *Loxosceles* (brown recluse or fiddleback). In 1999, the AAPCC reported 2,471 and 2,402 bites from each species. No deaths were attributed to *Latrodectus* bites. Two deaths were attributed to *Loxosceles* bites (one in a 6-year-old girl and one in a 42-year-old woman) giving a case-fatality rate of 0.08%. The *Latrodectus* bites produced moderate morbidity in 15% of patients and life-threatening morbidity in 0.7%. The *Loxosceles* bites produced moderate morbidity in 24% of patients and life-threatening morbidity in 1.5%.

24. What are the clinical signs of *Latrodectus* envenomation (black widow spider bite)?

The initial bite is usually not painful. The systemic signs and symptoms begin after a latent period of 10 to 60 minutes. Muscle cramps and spasms accompanied by pain and fever are typical manifestations. Diffuse abdominal muscle spasms may mimic the boardlike rigidity of an acute, surgical abdomen. Facial muscle spasm, lacrimation, photophobia, and swollen eyelids can cause the characteristic *facies latrodectisima*. There may be headache, light-headedness, nausea, vomiting, diaphoresis, and dysphagia in severe envenomations. Hypertensive crisis may be precipitated.

25. What is the treatment for the muscle spasms caused by *Latrodectus* envenomation?

Narcotics, benzodiazepines, and muscle relaxants, sometimes in large doses, may give symptomatic relief. The slow intravenous injection of 10 mL of 10% calcium gluconate has been advocated to relieve the muscle cramps, headache, and paresthesias. This treatment has become controversial because some *ex vivo* studies have shown a greater neurotransmitter release in the presence of extracellular calcium. There are no good clinical studies to settle the issue. There is an equine antivenin available (Merck). Its use is controversial, however, given the low mortality and morbidity of the bite compared with the risk of reactions to the horse serum.

26. What are the characteristic signs of a *Loxosceles* (brown recluse or fiddleback spider) bite?

After the bite, which often may not be painful, there is a latent period of 1 to 4 hours, followed by the development of a painful reddish blister surrounded by a blue-white halo (the **bull's eye lesion**). There may be chills, malaise, and a scarlatiniform rash. During the next 3 to 6 days, the lesion becomes hemorrhagic and spreads with a central area of necrosis. Healing is slow and may require débridement and skin grafting to treat large areas of skin necrosis. Cases of intravascular hemolysis have followed such bites.

27. What is the treatment for *Loxosceles* envenomation?

Local wound care. Some of these bites cause enough tissue loss to require skin grafting. Several adjunctive therapies, including hyperbaric oxygen, dapsone, steroids, antibiotics, colchicines, electric shock, phentolamine, dextran, diphenhydramine, and cyproheptadine, have been studied. None of these therapies has been proved effective, and they should be considered investigational.

28. Are mygalomorph spider bites (tarantulas) particularly dangerous?

On the whole, these bites tend to be of low toxicity with a mild, briefly active venom causing local symptoms only. The most dangerous mygalomorphs are the funnel-web spiders of southeastern Australia. These spiders can cause significant envenomation with intense local pain, nausea, vomiting, diaphoresis, salivation, muscle twitching, confusion, and severe dyspnea. Coma, cardiopulmonary failure, and death have been known to occur after such bites.

LIZARD BITES

29. Are there any venomous lizards in the world?

Yes, two species: the Mexican beaded lizard (*Heloderma horridum*) and the Gila monster (*Heloderma suspectum*). Both animals live in the desert areas of the southwestern United States and in Mexico. The venom of these lizards is similar to Crotalidae venom, although the clinical course is typically milder. The more serious problem with these reptiles is their powerful jaws and their tendency to hold onto their victims. They deliver their venom by chewing and dripping the venom into the lacerations created by their teeth. Their teeth also commonly break off in the wounds and become foreign bodies and a nidus for infection if not removed. The teeth, by the way, are radiolucent.

JELLYFISH STINGS

30. How do I treat jellyfish or other coelenterate stings?

Apply acetic acid (vinegar) continuously for at least 30 minutes. If acetic acid is not immediately available, saltwater lavage is a good start. Alcohol in the form of 40% isopropyl alcohol, perfume, aftershave lotion, or high-proof liquor may be a second choice to acetic acid. Alcohol treatment is controversial, however, because it may stimulate the nematocysts to release their venom, but this has not been shown to be clinically significant. Immersion of the affected extremity in hot water may be of some benefit (after alcohol or acetic acid decontamination). The nematocysts that remain in the skin can be removed by applying shaving cream, talc, baking soda, or flour and by shaving the area. The same treatment can be used for the stings from sea anemones or fire coral. There is an Australian box jellyfish (*Chironex flecker*) antivenin available. The recommended dosage for the antivenom is 1 to 3 ampules.

VENOMOUS FISH

31. Name some venomous fish, and state what their venoms have in common. How can that feature of their venom be used in treatment?

Stingray, scorpion fish, stonefish, catfish (freshwater catfish, sea catfish, coral catfish), old-wife fish, lionfish, zebrafish, butterfly cod, spiny dogfish, rabbit fish, ratfish, stargazer fish, surgeon fish, toadfish, weaver fish, bullrout, sculpin, and stinging sharks all have heat-labile toxins (heating destroys the toxin). The venom can be rendered nontoxic by placing the affected extremity of the victim (usually the foot) into hot water (≤ 45°C) for 90 minutes.

32. What else do I need to know about treatment of venomous fish wounds?

There is a stonefish antivenom available. It is a hyperimmune Fab2 horse serum preparation. There are three places in the United States that stock it: Sea World San Diego, Sea World Ohio, and the Steinhardt Aquarium in San Francisco.

Barbs and spines may remain embedded in the wound and should be removed.

SCORPION STINGS

33. What are the chances of envenomation from a scorpion bite? What are the active components of its venom?

There is no chance of envenomation from the bite (trick question); they do not envenomate by their bite but rather by their sting. Most scorpions that inhabit the United States are of low toxicity with stings comparable to bee stings. In 1999, the AAPCC reported 13,642 patients with scorpion stings. There was moderate morbidity in 3.7% of patients, life-threatening morbidity in 0.15%, and no deaths. The paired venom glands are located in the last of the five abdominal segments (the *tail*). The principal toxins are polypeptides and low-molecular-weight proteins, histamine, and indole compounds (including serotonin). The venom causes an increase in the sodium permeability of presynaptic neurons, which leads to continuous depolarization.

34. What are the signs of envenomation?

The sting is acutely painful. Later, systemic manifestations may develop:

Salivation	Diaphoresis	Perioral paresthesias
Dysphagia	Tongue fasciculations	Gastric distention
Hyperactivity	Diplopia	Mydriasis
Nystagmus	Roving eye movements	Visual loss
Incontinence	Penile erection	Hyperreflexia
Opisthotonos	Seizures	Hypertension
Pulmonary edema	Respiratory arrest	

35. What is the treatment for a scorpion sting?

The recommended treatment of scorpion stings consists mainly of local wound care, analgesia, and possibly parenteral benzodiazepines (intravenous medazolam) for the neuromuscular symptoms. There is a *Centuroides* scorpion antivenin, but its use is controversial given the low mortality and morbidity associated with most of these bites. The exception may be in the treatment of young children, however, because the mortality rate among children younger than 5 years old with severe scorpion envenomation may be 2.5 times that of adults. The antivenin is not FDA approved and is available only in Arizona through Arizona State University.

HYMENOPTERA STINGS

36. Are bee stings particularly dangerous?

They can be. Three people died in the United States from Hymenoptera stings in 1999 (AAPCC data).

37. What types of reactions occur from Hymenoptera stings (bees, wasps, and ants)?

There are four types of reactions: (1) toxic reactions, (2) anaphylactic reactions, (3) delayed reactions, and (4) unusual reactions. The **toxic reaction** is a nonantigenic response to the venom characterized by local irritation at the sting site and, potentially, vomiting, diarrhea, light-headedness, and syncope. There may be headache, fever, drowsiness, involuntary muscle spasms, edema without urticaria, and occasionally convulsions. Local toxic reactions are treated with supportive care, including cool packs and analgesics. Information about **anaphylactic reactions** can be found elsewhere in this book. **Delayed reactions** present as a serum sickness-like syndrome 10 to 14 days after the sting. Delayed reactions are treated with antihistamines and corticosteroids. **Unusual reactions** reported after Hymenoptera stings include encephalitis, neuritis, vasculitis, and nephritis.

38. How should a honeybee stinger be removed?

Honeybees almost always leave their stinger and venom sac in the victim. It may be best to remove the stinger by scraping it out with a credit card rather than by pinching and plucking it with fingers or tweezers and risking the inadvertent injection of more venom. Removal of the stinger should be done as soon as possible because the venom sac continues to pulse venom after it has detached from the bee.

39. What about *killer bees*?

Africanized bees (killer bees) may be encountered in South and Central America and in southern and southwestern portions of the United States. There is little difference between the Africanized bees and European bees in terms of appearance, the nature of their venom, and the amount of venom that they carry. The difference is in their aggressive behavior. Victims typically receive multiple stings during a swarming attack and a greater venom burden. Studies from Mexico reported 15% mortality from massive attacks.

40. After a patient has survived an anaphylactic reaction to a bee sting, what should be done to prepare the patient in case he or she is stung again?

The first step is avoidance of bees and wasps. It would be prudent for the patient to carry medical identification describing his or her bee-sting allergy, such as a MedicAlert bracelet. The patient should be given prescriptions for self-injection of epinephrine (the Ana-Kit or the EpiPen) and instructed in the use of these devices, which can be life-saving in a future anaphylactic reaction.

DOG AND CAT BITES

41. How many dog and cat bites occur annually? What is the risk of infection? What is the mortality from these bites?

We have no idea how many bites there are because most are inflicted by household pets, are not particularly serious, and are not reported. There are, however, more than 1 million patients in the United States who seek care in an ED for dog or cat bites. The infection rates are about 10% for dog bites and 50% for cat bites; this may represent a large selection bias, however, with more dog bite victims than cat bite victims presenting for treatment. There are 10 to 20 dog attacks in the United States annually that result in the death of the victim (10 to 20 times the number of venomous snakebite fatalities). The fatalities are most often small children.

42. Should I give prophylactic antibiotics to the victim of a dog or cat bite?

Low-risk wounds (immunocompetent patients with nonpuncture wounds that do not involve the hand or foot, which are treated within 12 hours and show no signs of infection) probably do not benefit from antibiotics. High-risk wounds may do better with antibiotics in addition to meticulous wound care. When choosing antibiotics, consider the polymicrobial nature of these infections (e.g., *Staphylococcus*, *Streptococcus*, *Pasteurella multocida*, anaerobes) (see Chapter 120, Wound Management). *Capnocytophaga canimorus* (DF2) is a fastidious gram-negative rod that can cause sepsis after a dog bite. Of patients who become seriously ill from this infection, 80% are immunocompromised (splenectomy, hematologic malignancy, or cirrhosis). It is a rare infection, but it carries a 25% to 36% mortality.[13]

HUMAN BITES

43. In an urban ED, what is the most commonly encountered bite wound, and why is it potentially very dangerous?

The most common bite wound is that caused by another person. A human bite that occurs when the fist of one opponent strikes the teeth of a second opponent is known as a **fight bite**. This usually involves the knuckles of the dominant hand. The importance of this injury is that the laceration can involve the extensor tendon and its bursa, the superficial and deep fascia, and the joint capsule. These structures are contaminated with oral flora at the time of injury and are notorious for becoming infected. There are at least 42 species of bacteria in human saliva. The most frequently cultured organisms from fight bites are *Streptococcus* and *Staphylococcus aureus* (usually penicillin resistant); 31% of these wound infections are due to gram-negative organisms, and 43% are due to mixed gram-negative and gram-positive organisms. Of these infections, 29% may be due to a facultatively anaerobic gram-negative rod, *Eikenella corrodens*.

44. How should a human bite wound be treated?

E. corrodens is typically resistant to the semisynthetic penicillins, clindamycin, and the first-generation cephalosporins. It is usually sensitive to penicillin and ampicillin, however. These wounds should be meticulously cared for, with special attention given to a thorough exploration and irrigation. Consider the polymicrobial nature of these infections when choosing antibiotics.

RABIES

45. What is rabies?

A disease caused by an RNA rhabdovirus transmitted by inoculation with infectious saliva. It is prevalent in parts of Latin America, Asia, Africa, South America, Europe, the Middle East, India, and Southeast Asia. Hawaii, England, Australia, Japan, and parts of the Caribbean are rabies-free. The virus primarily affects the central nervous system and is almost always fatal.

46. What types of animals are particularly high risk?

Immediate postexposure prophylaxis is recommended for patients who suffer bites from skunks, raccoons, bats, foxes, woodchucks, and most other carnivores, unless the area is known to be free of rabies or laboratory testing shows that the animal is nonrabid. Exposures from livestock, rodents, and lagomorphs should be considered individually but rarely require postexposure prophylaxis. Consult your state health department for local recommendations.

47. What does postexposure prophylaxis for rabies consist of?

Postexposure prophylaxis means trying to prevent the disease before it becomes manifest after a high-risk exposure. It begins with a thorough cleansing of the wound. After cleansing, 20 IU/kg of human rabies immunoglobulin is administered (50% injected in and around the wound, if possible, and 50% given intramuscularly in the gluteal). Human diploid cell vaccine (1.0 mL) is injected into the deltoid muscle (or the anterolateral thigh in young children) on days 0, 3, 7, 14, and 28. **Tip**: Do not administer the rabies vaccine and the rabies immunoglobulin in the same site.

SHARK BITES

48. How many people are bitten by sharks worldwide annually?

About 25. The odds of being bitten by a shark are about 1 in 5 million (less than being struck by lightning but greater than winning the Powerball lottery). If you swim with a buddy, it decreases your risk by 50%.

49. How do you make a shark bite?

Swim in shark-infested waters through schools of bait fish, disguised as a seal. Alternatively, mix dark rum, orange juice, sour mix, and grenadine.

TICK-BORNE DISEASES

50. What diseases can be transmitted through tick bites?

Tick paralysis, Lyme disease, Rocky Mountain spotted fever, tularemia, Colorado tick fever, and Q fever (see Chapter 61, Tick-borne Illnesses of North America).[10]

51. How do you remove a tick?

It seems that everyone has a favorite method for tick removal, including gentle traction, *unscrewing* the tick in a counterclockwise fashion, heat, and *smothering* the tick with alcohol or ointments. The most important part of tick removal is in being certain that the tick's head and mouth parts are not dislodged and left behind in the skin.

MOSQUITOES

52. They're annoying, but how deadly could mosquitos be?

Very deadly. One in every 17 people now alive on Earth will die of a mosquito-borne disease.

53. What diseases can mosquitos carry?

Eastern equine encephalitis, western equine encephalitis, St. Louis encephalitis, La Crosse encephalitis, Japanese encephalitis, Venezuelan equine encephalitis, malaria, yellow fever, Dengue fever, Bancroftian filariasis, epidemic polyarthritis (Ross River virus), Chikungunya fever, and Rift Valley fever, to name a few.

54. What is malaria, and how is it diagnosed?

A protozoan disease transmitted by the bite of the *Anopheles* mosquito. Annually, more than 200 million people contract malaria, and more than 1.5 million die. Consider the diagnosis in patients with recent travel to endemic areas and an unexplained febrile illness. There are clinical and laboratory features that suggest malaria, but the definitive diagnosis is made by seeing the parasites on Giemsa-stained thick and thin blood smears.

55. How is malaria treated?

Treatment decisions are based on the severity of the illness and the likelihood of infection with drug-resistant strains of *Plasmodium*. The Centers for Disease Control and Prevention maintains a 24-hour malaria hotline at (404) 322-4555.

INTERNET

56. Is there an e-mail list devoted to this topic?

Yes, at the Venom-L List, an Internet mailing list for venom researchers and medical professionals. To subscribe:

1. Address an e-mail message to majordomo@icomm.ca.
2. Leave the subject line blank.
3. In the body of the message, type: subscribe venom-l.

These instructions and a description of the mailing list are on their Web site: http://www.xmission.com/~gastown/herpmed/venom-l.htm

BIBLIOGRAPHY

1. Alagiakrishnan K, Gupta N: Treatment of aquarium fish sting injuries. Resident Staff Physician 47:27–28, 2001.

2. Auerbach PS: Envenomation by aquatic invertebrates. In Auerbach PS (ed): Wilderness Medicine, 4th ed. St. Louis, Mosby, 2001, pp 1450–1487.
3. Auerbach PS: Envenomation by aquatic vertebrates. In Auerbach PS (ed): Wilderness Medicine, 4th ed. St. Louis, Mosby, 2001, pp 1488–1506.
4. Auerbach PS, Halstead BW: Injuries from nonvenomous aquatic animals. In Auerbach PS (ed): Wilderness Medicine, 4th ed. St. Louis, Mosby, 2001, pp 1418–1449.
5. Boyer LV, McNally JT, Binford GJ: Spider bites. In Auerbach PS (ed): Wilderness Medicine, 4th ed. St. Louis, Mosby, 2001, pp 807–838.
6. Boyer LV, Seifert SA, Cain JS: Recurrence phenomena after immunoglobulin therapy for snake envenomations: Part 2. Guidelines for clinical management with crotaline Fab antivenom. Ann Emerg Med 37:196–201, 2001.
7. Dart RC, Hurlbut KM, Garcia R, Boren J: Validation of a severity score for the assessment of crotalid snakebite. Ann Emerg Med 28:371–372, 1996.
8. Dart RC, McNally J: Efficacy, safety, and use of snake antivenoms in the United States. Ann Emerg Med 37:181–188, 2001.
9. Dart RC, Waeckerle JF: Introduction: Advances in the management of snakebite symposium. Ann Emerg Med 37:166–167, 2001.
10. Gentile DA, Lang JE: Tick-borne diseases. In Auerbach PS (ed): Wilderness Medicine, 4th ed. St. Louis, Mosby, 2001, pp 769–806.
11. Hall EL: Role of surgical intervention in the management of crotaline snake envenomation. Ann Emerg Med 37:175–180, 2001.
12. Horowitz RS, Dart RC: Antivenins and immunologicals: Immunotherapeutics of envenomation. In Auerbach PS (ed): Wilderness Medicine, 4th ed. St. Louis, Mosby, 2001, pp 952–960.
13. Keogh S, Callaham ML: Bites and injuries inflicted by domestic animals. In Auerbach PS (ed): Wilderness Medicine, 4th ed. St. Louis, Mosby, 2001, pp 961–978.
14. Litovitz TL, Klein-Schwartz W, White S, et al: 1999 Annual Report of the American Association of Poison Control Centers Toxic Exposure Surveillance System. Am J Emerg Med 18:517–574, 2000.
15. Mckinney PE: Out-of-hospital and interhospital management of crotalins snakebite. Ann Emerg Med 37:168–174, 2001.
16. Minton SA, Bechtel B, Erickson TB: North American arthropod envenomation and parasitism. In Auerbach PS (ed): Wilderness Medicine, 4th ed. St. Louis, Mosby, 2001, pp 863–887.
17. Norris RL, Bush SP: North American venomous reptile bites. In Auerbach PS (ed): Wilderness Medicine, 4th ed. St. Louis, Mosby, 2001, pp 896–926.
18. Seifert SA, Boyer LV: Recurrence phenomena after immunoglobulin therapy for snake envenomatlons: Part 1. Pharmacokinetics and pharmacodynamics of immunoglobulin antivenoms and related antibodies. Ann Emerg Med 37:189, 2001.
19. Suchard JR, Connor DA: Scorpion envenomation. In Auerbach PS (ed): Wilderness Medicine, 4th ed. St. Louis, Mosby, 2001, pp 839–862.

93. SMOKE INHALATION

Richard E. Wolfe, M.D.

1. What is the principal cause of death in fire victims?

Smoke inhalation.

2. Does smoke cause thermal injury to the lungs?

Not usually. Air has such a low heat capacity that it rarely produces lower airway damage. The upper respiratory tract generally cools hot air before it reaches the vocal cords. The greater heat capacities of steam or heated soot can cause injury deep within the respiratory tract.

3. Why is smoke so lethal?

Carbon dioxide and carbon monoxide, the major components of smoke, are responsible for a drop in the concentration of ambient oxygen from 22% to 5–10%. Carbon monoxide and, more rarely, hydrogen cyanide block the uptake and use of oxygen, leading to severe tissue cellular hypoxemia. Depending on the fuel, temperature, and rate of heating, smoke contains a wide variety of toxins. Soot may act as a vehicle in transporting these toxic gases to the lower respiratory tract, where they dissolve to form acids and alkali. Removal of the soot is impaired by action of certain of these toxins on respiratory cilia, leading to severe, delayed pneumonia.

4. Name the four clinical stages of smoke inhalation.

Stage 1: Acute respiratory distress occurs 1 to 12 hours postinjury and is due to bronchospasm, laryngeal edema, and bronchorrhea.

Stage 2: Noncardiogenic pulmonary edema (adult respiratory distress syndrome) occurs 6 to 72 hours postinjury secondary to increased capillary permeability.

Stage 3: Strangulation occurs 60 to 120 hours postinjury from cervical eschar formation in patients with circumferential neck burns.

Stage 4: Onset of pneumonia 72 hours after injury, usually from *Staphylococcus aureus*, *Pseudomonas aeruginosa*, or gram-negative organisms.

5. How should smoke inhalation victims be managed in the field?

All victims should be placed on a 100% nonrebreather mask, even if they are asymptomatic. Oxygen dramatically accelerates the washout of carbon monoxide, shortening the half-life from 4 hours at room air to about 90 minutes. Endotracheal intubation is indicated for patients in respiratory distress. When intubated, the patient should be suctioned aggressively to remove inhaled soot. Patients with a loss of consciousness or altered mental status should be transported to a facility capable of providing hyperbaric oxygen (HBO) therapy.

6. Why is HBO therapy theoretically beneficial in smoke inhalation?

1. HBO therapy provides increased oxygen to poorly functioning mitochondrial enzymes inhibited by carbon monoxide and cyanide.

2. HBO therapy at 3 atm decreases the half-life of carbon monoxide to 23 minutes.

3. HBO therapy has been shown to reduce smoke-induced pulmonary edema.

4. At a cellular level, HBO therapy decreases the formation of intercellular adhesion molecule-1 on the endothelial membrane, which prevents neutrophils from infiltrating the central nervous system and causing a damaging inflammatory reaction and permanent neurologic sequelae.

7. What should I ask about the fire?

Ask if the patient was trapped in a closed space because significant inhalation injury would not occur in an open area. Try to determine what material was burning. The fuel is of primary importance in determining the composition of smoke and the risk to the patient.

8. Name some fuels and the materials from which they derive.

Hydrogen cyanide: combustion of wool, silk, nylons, and polyurethanes found commonly in furniture and paper.

Aldehydes, acrolein: wood, cotton, paper, and plastic materials.

Hydrogen chloride, phosgene: pyrolysis of chlorinated polymers; polyvinyl chloride (wire insulation materials); chlorinated acrylics; and wall, floor, and furniture coverings.

Oxides of nitrogen: nitrocellulose film.

Sulfur dioxide, hydrogen sulfide: rubber

9. How helpful is the physical examination in determining which patients have significant injury from smoke inhalation?

Not very helpful. Singed nasal hair is present in only 13% of patients with smoke inhalation. Although facial burns occur in 66% of patients with pulmonary burns, 86% of hospitalized patients with facial burns have no pulmonary injuries. Auscultatory findings and bronchorrhea are often absent initially. Sooty sputum is present in only 50% of smoke inhalation victims. Hoarseness is present in less than 25%. In other words, a normal physical examination does not rule out significant smoke inhalation.

10. How do I make the diagnosis of smoke inhalation injury?

Bronchoscopy is needed to confirm the presence of inhalation injury. Soot deposition in the airway, extensive edema, mucosal erythema, hemorrhage, and ulceration confirm that smoke inhalation has occurred. The initial bronchoscopy may be relatively normal because hyperemia and edema formation may take some time to evolve. A normal proximal airway does not rule out more distal injury.

11. How should asymptomatic patients be managed?

Provide comprehensive discharge instructions on when to return. Although the physical examination cannot reliably rule out complications such as delayed noncardiogenic pulmonary edema or pneumonia, ancillary studies and ED or in-hospital observation are not cost-effective. The patient should be instructed to return to the ED if shortness of breath, chest pain, or fever occurs.

12. If the patient's pulse oximetry is normal, would arterial blood gas analysis yield additional information?

In the presence of carboxyhemoglobin (CO), pulse oximetry may yield a falsely elevated reading. Arterial blood gases are of limited use and may be helpful only if the oxygen saturation is measured directly and not derived from the PaO_2 measurement. Although an increased alveolar-arterial gradient may correlate with smoke inhalation injury, it does not predict the severity of injury. Arterial blood gases are most useful in determining hypoventilation (increased PCO_2) and the presence of a metabolic or respiratory acidosis.

13. Should I get a chest radiograph on all patients with a history of smoke inhalation?

No. A chest radiograph offers little benefit in the ED. Chest radiographs are normal immediately after smoke inhalation injury, and abnormalities appear only on a delayed basis. A chest radiograph is not indicated in asymptomatic patients, and in most instances, it is useful only as a baseline in symptomatic patients.

14. Can I use the standard burn formula for intravenous fluids if smoke inhalation is present?

Patients with cutaneous and inhalation injuries pose a difficult problem because their fluid requirements are usually greater, but because of leaky capillaries, they are much more likely to develop membrane permeable pulmonary edema. Intravenous fluids must be guided by regular clinical reevaluation (breath sounds, oxygen saturation, urinary output, vital signs) rather than by formulas. Swan-Ganz monitoring may be required.

15. Is HBO therapy the only available therapy for cyanide poisoning?

No. All EDs should stock the Lilly cyanide antidote kit. Hydroxycobalamin (vitamin B_{12}) reduces cyanide concentrations and is available in Europe, although it has not yet been approved for use in the United States.

16. How does the Lilly cyanide antidote kit work?

Cyanide binds to the ferric ions, blocking the mitochondrial cytochrome oxidase pathway and cellular respiration. The cyanide antidote kit acts in two ways to limit this. (1) Nitrites generate methemoglobin, creating heme-ferric ions to compete with cyanide with mitochondrial ferric ions. (2) Sulfur transferase (rhodanase) binds cyanide molecules to sulfur-forming thiocyanate, which is nontoxic and eliminated in the urine. Thiosulfate accelerates this process by increasing available sulfur molecules. (See figure, top of next page.)

17. When should I use the cyanide antidote kit?

Symptomatic patients can have carbon monoxide or cyanide toxicity. Inducing methemoglobinemia with amyl nitrite capsules and sodium nitrite in patients with high CO levels must be avoided until the patient is in the HBO chamber. Until then, if measured oxygen saturation is low, use the sodium thiosulfate portion of the kit. High lactate levels can help distinguish cyanide from CO because elevations in serum lactate correlate well with cyanide toxicity. This can provide an indication for administration of sodium nitrite when HBO therapy is unavailable.

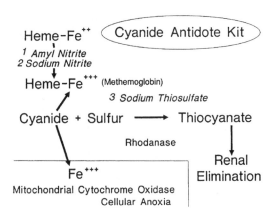

18. How do I administer the cyanide antidote kit?

Amyl nitrite **inhalers** are used in patients without intravenous access. These can be used every 3 to 4 minutes but are less effective than intravenous sodium nitrite. If a patient is apneic, break one of the amyl nitrite inhalants inside the resuscitation bag. When an intravenous line is established, the full amount of a 10-mL ampule or 5 to 10 mg/kg of sodium nitrite should be administered intravenously over 4 minutes. This is followed by 12.5 g of intravenous thiosulfate.

CONTROVERSY

19. Are steroids indicated in smoke inhalation?

It initially was assumed that if the tracheobronchial inflammatory response could be prevented or at least decreased by the antiinflammatory action of steroids, edema would be decreased, and surfactant would be maintained. It also was postulated that pulmonary fibrosis would be reduced after the acute injury. These beliefs initially were supported by early experimental studies. Later animal experiments and clinical trials could not show increased survival with the use of steroids. Moylan and Alexander, in a randomized prospective trial, showed a fourfold increase in mortality in the steroid-treated group. Other retrospective studies added to the argument against steroids. At present, routine administration of steroids in the ED is not indicated.

BIBLIOGRAPHY

1. Blinn DL, Slater H, Goldfarb W: Inhalation injury with burns: A lethal combination. J Emerg Med 6:471–473, 1988.
2. Cohen MA: Inhalation of products of combustion. Ann Emerg Med 12:628–631, 1983.
3. Kirk MA, Gerace R, Kulig KW: Cyanide and methemoglobin kinetics in smoke inhalation victims treated with the cyanide antidote kit. Ann Emerg Med 22:1413–1418, 1993.
4. Moylan JA, Alexander LG: Diagnosis and treatment of inhalation injury. World J Surg 2:185–191, 1978.
5. Nelson L, Hoffman R: Toxic inhalations. In Marx JA, et al (eds): Rosen's Emergency Medicine: Concepts and Current Practice, 5th ed. St. Louis, Mosby, 2002, pp 2163–2171.
6. Ramzy PI, Barret JP, Herndon DN: Thermal injury. Crit Care Clin 15:333–352, 1999.
7. Robinson NB, Hudson LD, Riem M: Steroid therapy following isolated smoke inhalation injury. J Trauma 22:876–879, 1982.
8. Stewart RJ, Mason SW, Taira MT, et al: Effect of radical scavengers and hyperbaric oxygen on smoke-induced pulmonary edema. Undersea Hyperb Med 21:21–30, 1994.
9. Zerbe NF, Wagner BK: Use of vitamin B12 in the treatment and prevention of nitroprusside-induced cyanide toxicity. Crit Care Med 21:465–467, 1993.

94. NUCLEAR, BIOLOGIC, AND CHEMICAL WEAPONS OF MASS DESTRUCTION

Jonathan D. Apfelbaum, M.D.

1. What is so terrifying about nuclear, biologic, and chemical (NBC) weapons?

NBC weapons are designed to kill or injure as many people as possible in the most efficient manner. These are the weapons of mass destruction. They are pathogenic to humans, animals, or plants. They are environmentally stable and effective at low dose. Most of them are cheap and easy to make. Recipes are available on the Internet. They are easy to transport and disperse. Compared with traditional explosives or other devices, NBC weapons may be silent, odorless, and colorless, and they can be difficult to detect. They can be disseminated easily in the air, providing an easy method to attack targets with enclosed spaces (such as the Tokyo sarin gas subway attack and the lesser known Dalles, Oregon, contamination of a salad bar with *Samonella typhimurium*).

People may not know they have been exposed, and there may be a significant delay before symptoms develop. When people become affected, the presenting symptoms may be nonspecific, leading to delay in diagnosis and treatment. Patients may require special precautions to prevent cross-contamination of responding personnel and specialized treatment to minimize injury. NBC weapons may involve agents with which medical personnel are unfamiliar and which they are poorly equipped to handle.

Because of the high toxicity of many NBC weapons and the devastating effects, terrorists have been more willing and able to use these weapons against civilian populations. The ability of medical providers to respond effectively to such a threat has lagged behind.

2. Aren't existing hazardous materials (HAZMAT) incident plans sufficient for NBC weapons?

No. Attack with NBC weapons and HAZMAT accidents occur rapidly and have the potential for involving large segments of a community. In both situations, responders need to wear appropriate personal protective equipment (PPE) and take appropriate precautions. HAZMAT plans may not anticipate the needs and contingencies, however, that must be addressed to deal with an attack with NBC weapons effectively. During more than 200 bioterrorism threats in the United States in recent years, the emergency medical services (EMS) and HAZMAT response has been disorganized, uninformed, and generally poor. The lessons learned from these threats include:

- There should be a uniform response to bioterrorist threats by local, state, and federal EMS, law enforcement, and health agencies.
- There should be a clear chain of command and delegation of authority.
- Undressing and showering after a mailed or telephoned threat should not be part of the routine response. Anthrax and other biologic agents can be dangerous if inhaled; if the organisms already have been inhaled, washing skin and clothing would have no effect.
- Spores that may have settled on the skin or clothing do not pose an inhalation threat. Surface cleaning can be addressed by washing the hands, face, and any other exposed skin with soap and water and placing clothes in plastic bags.
- Psychological help should be available in the aftermath of such events.
- Every attempt should be made to protect the modesty of the potential victims. In several well-documented cases, victims have been made to undress and shower in public or semi-public places, where they were watched by bystanders and filmed by members of the media.
- Laboratory data should be made available as soon as possible to confirm the presence or absence of a bioagent.

3. What is unique about an NBC terrorist attack compared with other mass disasters?

An NBC incident would be similar to a HAZMAT event in that it involves dangerous materials that may not be encountered everyday and that require special precautions and protective gear. In a terrorist attack, the potential exists for secondary devices designed to go off after the primary device, placing responding personnel at increased risk for injury or exposure. More than a HAZMAT event, an NBC attack could create a large number of injured or dead casualties. The level of violence associated with terrorist acts produces more victims and has a higher mortality than natural disasters or HAZMAT accidents. Contingency plans need to be developed to handle large numbers of dead victims. EMS systems and hospitals may become overwhelmed and need to anticipate such an event to plan for an effective emergency response.

The psychological impact of such an attack would create large numbers of psychological casualties. The unexpected nature of such an attack, the loss of security and safety, and the concern of death or injury from a unknown source creates significant concern and anxiety. Of the 5,500 patients from the 1995 Tokyo Aum Shinrikyo cult terrorist attack, 4,500 were psychological casualties. Their presenting complaints and symptoms may confuse the clinical picture. When injury has been ruled out, a psychological crisis team should be used to address and treat their concerns.

An intentional attack is a criminal event, and everything becomes evidence. The law enforcement agencies involved may cross many jurisdictions, including local police agencies, federal law enforcement groups (such as the FBI), special response teams, medical response teams, the Centers for Disease Control (CDC), the Public Health Service, and others. Each group has special needs that have to be addressed.

4. Aren't these types of terrorist attacks uncommon?

With the willingness of countries to sponsor terrorist organizations and the availability of the technology to make such devices, attacks with NBC weapons have become more common worldwide. Terrorists seem to be more willing to use such devices against civilian populations. Although the overall number of terrorist acts decreased worldwide over the last several years, the lethality of these attacks increased. With terrorism being the main venue for groups with ideologic differences to strike at the United States, NBC weapons are a prime choice to implement these attacks.

5. Why don't traditional mass casualty incident preparations work effectively for NBC assaults?

Because they do not anticipate and they are not prepared to deal with a situation involving NBC weapons. In NBC drills nationwide, first responders to scenes were killed or contaminated equipment and hospitals because they lacked the knowledge and preparation to deal with such an event. Lack of information or improper information has marked the scene of many NBC weapon threats or hoaxes, leading to delays, ineffective containment, multiple redundant decontaminations, improper care, misinformation being delivered to crews and patients, and general mishandling of the event.

6. What is the Nunn-Lugar-Domenici legislation?

The 1996 Defense Against Weapons of Mass Destruction Act. This Act recognized the lack of preparedness of most medical responders and provided funding and authority to train personnel in 120 cities in the United States to respond safely to acts of terrorism.

7. Describe some disaster planning misconceptions?

The disaster response requires the mobilization of large amounts of resources. Most problems in disaster response are not caused by a shortage of medical resources, but by the failure to coordinate their distribution and use.

Most of the care for the victims is provided by the prehospital personnel. Lack of prehospital care is the norm in most HAZMAT incidents. Patients triage themselves to the nearest available hospital. They arrive contaminated, unevaluated, and unstabilized. Only approximately

18% of patients are decontaminated in the field. Hospital personnel need to be prepared to perform decontamination at their facility (without contaminating or compromising their hospital) and manage their resources (such as bed space). Most prehospital personnel are not trained in the administration of antidotes or other definitive care for NBC attack victims.

A disaster plan is equivalent to disaster planning. Few disaster planners have actual experience because such events are uncommon. Generic plans often lack input from local response personnel. Training and practice need to be provided on a regular basis to maintain proficiency. Coordination with responding agencies and supporting medical resources needs to be addressed and confirmed. Any disaster plan needs to devote considerable effort to motivation and preparedness. Apathy and lack of administrative support doom a plan. Disaster drills need to be emphasized; procedures and policies need to be confirmed, familiar to the personnel who will be using them, and ungraded as needed; and the administration needs to support the ongoing review necessary for preparedness.

8. Explain the levels of PPE.

Level A: Required for exposure to areas of chemical release (**hot zones**), if air concentrations exceed those that are immediately dangerous to life or health. This level includes a self-contained breathing apparatus and fully encapsulated suits that are resistant to liquid and vapor penetration.

Level B: Required for exposures that pose a potential inhalation danger. This suit is less protective than the level A suit, but when used with a self-contained breathing apparatus or a supplied air respirator, it provides adequate vapor and liquid protection. This is the level of protection necessary for hospital personnel involved in decontamination.

Level C: Required when the contaminant is identified and an air-purifying respirator is appropriate for the agent involved. This level includes clothing protective for liquid and vapor and an ambient air-purifying respirator.

9. Summarize what should be included in a disaster plan.

Planning phase: All responsible personnel and agencies should be included. The plan should be simple, affordable, and similar to current protocols and responsibilities. Problems likely to occur should be anticipated and addressed. Joint planning sessions with all agencies involved should occur to coordinate effectively with the community disaster plan. Mutual aid agreements should be developed and implemented. Policies and procedures for decontamination and disaster management should be developed.

Topic to address should include:
- Communication between triage, receiving facilities, personnel, and the command center
- Coordination to share information
- Security and traffic control
- Congestion in treatment areas
- Proper identification of personnel and command structure
- Triage, patient tracking, and decontamination
- Information to families, police, and media
- Staff rotation
- Stress management
- Stockpiles of antidotes and antibiotics
- Backup plans to ensure the security and viability of the hospital, such as backup communication systems and alternative sites to provide medical care
- Acquisition of and training with protective equipment

Readiness phase: Personnel and agencies must take an honest inventory of their capabilities and address areas of deficiencies. Personnel must be made aware of the disaster plan, which should be practiced in realistic drills that include decontamination, large numbers of patients, and full equipment usage (e.g., protective gear). Plans should be reviewed regularly and updated as appropriate. The disaster plan needs to evolve as technology, weapons, and capabilities change.

Recovery phase: After an event has taken place, the focus shifts back from the needs caused by the disaster and the return to normal. The impacted population may have increased needs for food, shelter, medication, water, clothing, and emotional support that must be addressed. Hospitals and agencies must meet the emotional needs and fatigue of their personnel.

RADIATION

10. Describe the different types of radiation and what sort of shielding is required for each.

Alpha particles are two neutrons and two protons. These can be a componenet of nuclear fallout. They travel short distances and are stopped by paper or the outer layer of skin. They can cause local cell damage if they are ingested or inhaled.

Beta particles are high-energy electrons emitted from a nucleus. These particles can penetrate to the germinal layer of skin and cause cellular damage. They are stopped by wood or some PPE garments. Contact with skin or ingestion can cause tissue injury.

Gamma rays are photons and function similar to x-rays. These can penetrate deeply into tissue and constitute a significant hazard. They can be blocked with concrete or lead. Gamma radiation frequently accompanies the emission of alpha and beta radiation.

Ionized radiation comprises neutrons emitted from the nucleus of an atom. These neutrons are tissue penetrating and require significant amounts of lead or concrete or other special considerations for shielding.

11. What type of nuclear devices might be used by a terrorist?
- **Simple radiation device**. This is the exposure to radioactive materials without an explosive.
- **Radiologic dispersion device**. This involves an explosive that is contaminated with nuclear material ("a dirty bomb") or a failed nuclear weapon detonation. People are injured by the initial explosion, and survivors and rescue personnel are contaminated by the radioactive material.
- **Reactor**. The potential for nuclear reactor accident sabotage is extremely low; however, accidents have happened (Three Mile Island and Chernobyl).
- **Improvised nuclear device**. Construction of such a device, although theoretically possible, is difficult and unlikely. Detonation either would be a nuclear blast or act as a radiologic dispersal device without the nuclear material exploding.
- **Nuclear weapon**. The likelihood of stealing a nuclear weapon (James Bond notwithstanding) is extremely unlikely in the Western world. The collapse of the Soviet Union has resulted in compromised security of nuclear weapons and technology, however.

12. List types of radiation injury.
- **External irradiation**: The whole body, or part of it, is exposed to penetrating radiation from an external source. After external radiation exposure, the individual is not radioactive and can be treated like any other patient.
- **Contamination**: Radioactive materials are deposited externally, internally, or both. Radioactive materials can be inhaled, ingested, or deposited in wounds. These patients are radioactive and require decontamination.
- **Incorporation**: Radioactive materials are taken up by cells and incorporated into tissues or target organs. Contamination has to occur first for incorporation to occur.

13. State some radiation protection principles.
- Set up a controlled area large enough to hold the anticipated victims.
- Prevent tracking and spread of contaminants by covering floor area.
- Restrict access to controlled area.
- Monitor anyone or anything leaving the area. Check with a Geiger counter or other radiation detection device to ensure contaminants are not being moved out of the area.
- Use strict isolation precautions.

- Control waste and ventilation.
- Use waterproof materials to limit the spread of contaminants.
- Have all personnel wear dosimetry badges to keep track of their exposure.
- Set up decontamination areas with control of water runoff.
- Involve the institution radiation safety officer early.
- Consider medications for internal decontamination (such as DTPA for plutonium).
- Patient care comes first. Additional areas, personnel, and equipment can be decontaminated if need be.

14. What clinical effects do you see with radiation injury?

The structural damage to a cell's DNA can take place in less than 1 second. The clinical manifestation can take hours to years to present, however. Cell division might be impaired, or cell destruction might take place. In significant exposures, a fairly predictable course of acute radiation syndrome can occur. Factors associated with acute radiation syndrome are high dose, high dose rate, whole-body exposure, and penetrating irradiation. Acute radiation syndrome progresses through four clinical phases:

1. **Prodromal phase**. Symptoms are related to total radiation absorbed and include loss of appetite, nausea, vomiting, fatigue, diarrhea, fever, respiratory difficulties, and agitation.

2. **Latent phase**. This transitional period, when the initial symptoms resolve, may last 3 weeks but is shorter with increased radiation exposure.

3. **Illness phase**. Overt clinical manifestations occur, including infection, bleeding, diarrhea, electrolyte imbalances, altered mental status, and shock.

4. **Recovery or death phase**. Recovery takes weeks to months.

The phases of acute radiation syndrome are related to cell reproduction. The fastest dividing cells are affected earliest, specifically the cells in the **hematopoietic** and the gastrointestinal systems. These can be used as markers for prognosis. The absolute lymphocyte count at 48 hours after exposure is a good predictor for prognosis. If it is greater than 1,200, the patient likely received a nonlethal dose. If it is between 300 and 1,200, a significant exposure has occurred and the patient should be hospitalized. Less than 300 absolute lymphocyte count, the patient is critically ill and should be hospitalized and considered for colony-stimulating factors.

Symptoms in the **gastrointestinal** system are seen in acute doses greater than 600 rad. The higher the exposure, the sooner nausea, vomiting, and diarrhea develop. These symptoms coincide with the hematologic abnormalities. Sepsis, dehydration from loss of fluid, and electrolyte imbalances are the natural clinical course. At 10 days, severe bloody diarrhea is an ominous sign.

Neurologic sequelae can develop. Acute radiation doses of greater than 1,000 rad can cause diffuse microvascular leaks in the central nervous system, leading to edema, increased intracranial pressure, and death. This injury is usually rapidly fatal.

Dermal involvement can range from mild transient erythema, local pain, blister formation, necrosis, and loss of tissue. It is important to observe changes in the skin because this can help estimate the dose of radiation received. Because of the effect on dividing cells, if a radiation patient requires emergency surgery, it should be done within the first 24 to 48 hours after the radiation injury; otherwise it should be delayed for 3 months.

BIOLOGIC AGENTS

15. What is biologic warfare?

The use of microorganisms or toxins to produce death or disease in humans, animals, or plants. It is the oldest of the NBC triad, has been in use for at least 2,500 years, and is the most deadly per weight compared with chemical agents.

16. What comprises an ideal biologic warfare agent?

One that is cheap, is easy to make, is easy to aerosolize, is 1 to 5 μ in size so that is inhaled into the alveoli, has a high disease-to-infection ratio, maintains viability or infectivity in the environment, and has a vaccine or other prophylaxis to protect the attacker.

17. List some bacterial agents and their effects.

Anthrax: upper respiratory infection (URI) symptoms, mediastinitis, respiratory distress, pulmonary edema, meningitis

Plague (*Yersinia pestis*): URI symptoms, lymphadenopathy, pneumonia (pneumonic plague), septicemia

Tularemia: URI symptoms, pulmonary necrosis and inflammation, liver and renal injury

Q fever: URI symptoms, pneumonia, meningitis

Cholera: Nausea, vomiting, diarrhea, headache, dehydration

18. Can viruses be used as biologic warfare agents?

Yes. Some examples are smallpox, Venezuelan equine encephalitis (VEE), and viral hemorrhagic fevers (e.g., Ebola).

19. What am I most likely to see?

Well, it depends. According to Soviet scientists, as of 1997, the most likely agents in descending probability of use are:

- Smallpox virus
- *Y. pestis*
- *Bacillus anthracis*
- Botulinum toxin
- VEE virus
- *Francisella tularensis*
- *Coxiella burnetii*
- Marburg virus
- Influenza virus
- *Burkholderia mallei*
- *Rickettsia typhi*

20. How do I protect myself from becoming ill while taking care of these patients?

Universal precautions and prophylactic antibiotics (most of the bacterial agents are sensitive to doxycycline, streptomycin, gentamicin, tetracycline, or penicillin, depending on the organism). Some vaccines are available for anthrax, cholera, plague (not effective against aerosolized version), tularemia (experimental), Q fever, smallpox, VEE, and yellow fever (one of the viral hemorrhagic fevers).

21. What is the time course for these biologic agents?

For some of the toxins, symptoms occur 3 to 12 hours after inhalation (staphylococcal enterotoxin B [SEB]), with a rapid fulminant course. Most agents produce symptoms in 1 to 3 days, with clinical courses lasting 3 weeks (smallpox). This is important in understanding how patients will present. There will not be a mad rush (immediately) on the ED with people screaming they were exposed to anthrax. Instead, people with URI symptoms start presenting, then more with worsening symptoms. Gradually over several days, a pattern develops of significantly ill patients in local hospitals, which should start providers wondering about a common exposure. By the time the picture of a biologic attack becomes clear, the terrorist is long gone, and many people may be exposed, ill, or dead.

22. So far, the biologic agents have been infectious. What about the toxins?

Toxins are naturally produced poisons that are more toxic per weight than manmade chemicals (botulism is 15,000 more potent than VX). They tend to be nonvolatile, with minimal absorption through skin; this means you have to inhale or ingest them. They are not prone to person-to-person transmission. Toxicity varies by route, and victims may present with sudden onset of severe symptoms or death. Mechanisms of action include interfering with nerve conduction, interactions with the immune system, and inhibiting protein synthesis.

23. List some toxins and how they present.

Botulism: Blocks the release of acetylcholine. Patients present with descending paralysis and bulbar palsies. Progresses to respiratory failure with clear mental status.

Ricin: A potent cytotoxin made from castor beans. Blocks protein synthesis and causes nausea, vomiting, diarrhea, liver and renal failure, airway necrosis if inhaled, and multiple organ failure.

SEB: Stimulates the immune system and produces cytokines. Causes fevers, chills, headache, nausea, vomiting, cough, myalgias, arthralgias, dyspnea, chest pain, and adult respiratory distress syndrome. May be severely incapacitating if nonfatal.

24. Can biologic agents be detected in a time-effective manner?

The military has Biological Integrated Detection Systems, which sample air and can identify toxins. Long-Range and Short-Range Standoff Detection Systems, which use lasers to detect aerosol clouds, serve as early warning devices in combat. Currently there are few systems in place for civilian monitoring or detection.

25. How do I treat patients who have been exposed to biologic toxins?

Supportive therapy, early airway intervention, intravenous fluids, and comfort care. Patients suffering from botulism require prolonged intubation and ventilatory support (months).

26. Is there any prophylaxis against these toxins?

There is a vaccine available for botulism A through E and botulism antitoxin for strains A, B, and E, which may be effective if administered within the first 24 hours. Studies in animals showed promise for a Ricin vaccine, but it is not currently available. PPE with respiratory filters is the best protection at this time.

CHEMICAL AGENTS

27. What was the weapon in the Tokyo terrorist attack in 1995?

Sarin.

28. Was this the first attack by the Aum Shinrikyo cult?

No. In 1994, they field tested their crudely manufactured sarin, killing 7 people and injuring 200.

29. Why are chemical agents effective terrorist weapons?

They are cheap, are easy to make, and have delayed or immediate effects. They can be delivered by a variety of methods and are transported easily. Most countries are poorly prepared to deal with a terrorist chemical attack.

30. List some chemical warfare agents.

Nerve agents	GA (tabun), GB (sarin), GD (soman), VX
Cyanide	Hydrogen cyanide, cyanogen chloride
Pulmonary intoxicants	Phosgene, chlorine
Vesicants	Mustard, lewisite
Riot control agents	Mace, pepper spray
Miscellaneous	Ammonia

31. What effects do you see with chemical warfare agents?

It depends on the agent. **Nerve agents** are based on organophosphate pesticides and block muscarinic and nicotinic receptors. They may cause salivation, lacrimation, rhinorrhea, bronchial secretions, diarrhea, vomiting, sweating, miosis, fasciculation, muscle twitching, weakness, paralysis, and bronchoconstriction. Tachycardia, heart blocks, and other arrhythmias; seizures;

altered mental status; and other respiratory effects can be seen. **Cyanide** causes anxiety, hyperventilation, headache, vomiting, dizziness, cherry-red skin, seizures, apnea, and death.

Pulmonary intoxicants cause pulmonary irritation and damage and may lead to adult respiratory distress syndrome. **Vesicants** cause skin blistering and irritation and systemic effects, such as nausea, vomiting, diarrhea, ocular complications, and pulmonary distress. **Riot control agents** cause burning of the eyes, tearing, and pulmonary irritation.

32. What can I do about nerve agents? Is there an effective antidote?

The first part of treatment is self-protection. Use of PPE and decontamination is mandatory. Decontamination is with soap and water or a 1:10 solution of household bleach after all clothing has been removed. Removing the patient's clothing removes 80% of the contamination. Treatment of the basic ABCs with airway support as needed is the next step. The pharmacologic treatment, or antidote, is atropine and pralidoxime chloride (2-PAM). Initial dosing is 2 to 6 mg of atropine intramuscularly, intravenously, or via endotracheal tube and 300 to 1,000 mg of 2-PAM intravenously or intramuscularly. Total dosage required may be significantly higher. The military Mark I autoinjector, used for nerve agent exposure, has two autoinjectors, one with 2 mg of atropine, the other with 600 mg of 2-PAM. Dosing is guided by the patient's clinical response, and repeat doses are given until the patient is easier to ventilate, secretions are drying, or the patient is otherwise improving. Diazepam also is used to control seizures if they occur.

The current recommendations for treatment after nerve agent exposure is as follows:

EXPOSURE	CLINICAL CONDITION	TREATMENT
Latent	No complaints	None. Observe 1 h if inhaled, 18 h if dermal contact
Mild	Miosis, rhinorrhea, mild dyspnea	1 Mark I and observe
Moderate	More severe complaints, vomiting, diarrhea	1 Mark I, repeat atropine, 2 mg IV/IM at 5- to 10-min intervals until symptoms diminish
Severe	As above, plus altered mental status, coma, seizures, paralysis, cyanosis, or severe effects in ≥ 2 organ systems	ABCs, oxygen, 3 Mark I kits IM. Atropine, 2 mg IV at 3- to 5-min intervals until improving. Repeat 2-PAM, 1 g IV twice at hourly intervals. Diazepam for seizures

33. What about mustard gas? Wasn't that a World War I chemical weapon?

Yes, it was. In 1917, it was used by the Germans at Ypres, Belgium. In 16 months, there were more than 125,000 British casualties; however, most survived. Mustard is a vesicant (blister) agent that is toxic if inhaled or contacted. It caused injury to eyes, mucus membranes, airways, and gastrointestinal tract; blistering of skin; and bone marrow suppression. It is absorbed quickly, within several minutes of contact, and causes cellular damage, but clinical effects may not present for 2 to 8 hours. It mimics radiation injury and attacks rapidly dividing cell lines. Although it can cause significant tissue loss, treatment is with irrigation and topical lotions, not with aggressive hydration as with thermal injury. Other treatment includes ophthalmology consultation, respiratory support, and supportive care.

34. List some other antidotes for chemical weapons.

Mustard	Decontamination and supportive care
Lewisite	Decontamination, BAL, and supportive care
Cyanide	Decontamination, oxygen, amyl nitrite, sodium nitrite, and sodium thiosulfate

Phosgene   Decontamination and supportive care
Ammonia   Decontamination and supportive care
Chlorine   Decontamination and supportive care
CN (Mace), CS (tear   Decontamination and supportive care
  gas), and pepper spray

35. Is pepper spray a chemical agent? The same stuff everyone is carrying on their keychain?
Absolutely. Although it is milder than the CN and CS varieties, it can still cause tearing, eye irritation, blepharospasm, rhinorrhea, coughing, dyspnea, bronchospasm, and dermal irritation.

36. How can you detect these chemical agents?
In most cases, recognition is based on clinical signs and symptoms. Chemical detection equipment is available and useful for determining need for PPE and hazard assessment and to confirm adequate decontamination. The military has a categorization algorithm that helps break down symptoms and agents. Although it is not all-inclusive, it is helpful and can help direct therapy.

Rapid-onset (< 4 hours) respiratory casualties: Nerve agents, cyanide, mustard, lewisite, phosgene, and SEB inhalation.

Delayed-onset respiratory casualties: Inhaled anthrax, pneumonic plague, pneumonic tularemia, Q fever, SEB inhalation, Ricin inhalation, mustard, lewisite, and phosgene.

Rapid-onset (< 4 hours) neurologic casualties: Nerve agents and cyanide.

Delayed-onset neurologic casualties: Botulism (peripheral nervous system symptoms) and VEE (central nervous system symptoms).

37. State the cornerstones of management for dealing with a chemical weapons attack.
- Protect yourself. Use PPE and prevent contamination of medical personnel.
- Decontaminate.
- Treat patients based on clinical appearance and with supportive care until the agent has been identified. If victims appear as if they have been exposed to nerve agents, treat them as such until you can confirm the diagnosis. Most initial treatment in such an attack is based on the clinical presentation.

MULTIPLE CASUALTY INCIDENTS

38. What should the triage system for a multiple casualty incident (MCI) include?
It should parallel the triage system already in place so that in the event of an MCI respondents are not trying to use an unfamiliar plan. Practice regularly to ensure familiarity. Triage is a continual process requiring frequent reevaluation. On arrival to the ED, victims need to be re-triaged. A secure, shielded, accessible area near the ED entrance needs to be set up for the arriving patients.

There are two major triage systems. One is composed of **color-coded tags**:

Red: Immediate treatment/transportation. Seriously injured or ill with a reasonable chance for survival with medical attention.

Yellow: Delayed transportation/treatment. Requires care but can wait.

Green: The so-called walking wounded with minimal injuries, requiring no immediate care.

Black: Dead or expected to die soon.

The other system is the **START (Simple Triage And Rapid Treatment)**:

If someone can walk, they are directed to the **minimal** or walking wounded area.

Patients are evaluated for respirations, perfusion, and neurologic status.

Any condition deemed life-threatening, such as respirations greater than 30 breaths/min or inability to maintain airway, hypotension or delayed capillary refill, or altered mental status, are tagged **immediate**.

Normal findings are considered **delayed**.

39. So what are we doing to prevent or manage MCIs (remind me why I pay taxes)?

The Department of Health and Human Services (DHHS) in 1999 received $170 million specifically to fund this strategic need. This was increased to $285 million in 2000. DHHS activities have focused on five main areas:

1. Deterrence of biologic terrorism
2. Public health surveillance
3. Medical and public health response
4. Development of national pharmaceutical stockpiles
5. Research and development

40. What is the upside of all this increased preparedness?

The West Nile virus outbreak that occurred in New York City in August 1999 was controlled using many of the same resources. It involved the initial identification of unusual cases of encephalitis; surveillance and control by local public health departments; ruling out of bioterrorism by the FBI; laboratory and technical support at the local, state, federal, and military levels; and a collaborative response by the various agencies involved.

41. Are there any special issues hospitals need to consider in NBC MCIs?

Plans must be made to control the influx of patients, decontaminate them without contaminating the ED, and keep patients from leaving before they are safe or decontaminated. Most patients come themselves or are brought by bystanders to the hospital. They may not understand the delay in setting up equipment required for decontamination. The potential is for a sudden, large influx of patients who need to be directed and managed. PPE equipment must be maintained and available, and personnel must be trained in its use. Stockpiles of antidotes should be accessible. Information of available resources also should be accessible.

42. What are decontamination challenges at the receiving hospitals?

Hospital administrator and ED personnel need to evaluate their facility for their ability to secure the facility, decontaminate patients, train staff for performing such procedures, have available PPE, have security for patient's personal effects, and contain the decontamination runoff. Each facility is unique. These factors should be anticipated and a plan worked out within the limitations of each physical plant.

43. List key points to remember when planning a system for dealing with NBC events.

- Involve everyone.
- Tasks should parallel normal daily activities.
- Avoid activities for which people are not trained.
- Always wear PPE.
- Triage area should be secured, visible, and accessible.
- Use standard triage method.
- Review and revise on a regular basis and make improvements where needed.
- Practice, practice, practice.

44. Where can I get more information?
Medical and Scientific Web Sites

www.jama.ama-assn.org
www.nejm.org
www.thelancet.com
www.bmj.com
www.newscientist.com
www.medscape.com
www.sciam.com

Government Sites	Nongovernment Sites
www.cdc.gov	www.fas.org
www.nih.gov	www.hopkins-biodefense.org
www.fema.com	www.laskerfoundation.org
www.usamriid.army.mil	www.stimson.org
www.ncbi.nlm.nih.gov	www.potomacinstitute.com
	www.terrorism.com
	www.emergency.com

BIBLIOGRAPHY

1. Bradley RN: Health care facility preparation for weapons of mass destruction. Prehosp Emerg Med 4:261–269, 2000.
2. Cieslak TJ, Eitzen EM: Bioterrorism: Agents of concern. J Public Health Pract 6:19–29, 2000.
3. Cieslak TJ, et al: A field-expedient algorithmic approach to the clinical management of chemical and biological casualties. Milit Med 165:659–662, 2000.
4. Cole LA: Bioterrorism threats: Learning for inappropriate responses. J Public Health Pract 6:8–18, 2000.
5. Gallo RJ, Campbell D: Bioterrorism: Challenges and opportunities for local health departments. J Public Health Pract 6:57–62, 2000.
6. Hamburg MA: Bioterrorism: A challenge to public health and medicine. J Public Health Pract 6:38–44, 2000.
7. Hood E: Chemical and biological weapons: New questions, new answers. Environ Health Perspect 107: 931–932, 1999.
8. Macintyre AG, et al: Weapons of mass destruction events with contaminated casualties. JAMA 283:242–249, 2000.
9. Markovchick VJ: Radiation injuries. In Marx JA, Hockberger RS (eds): Rosen's Emergency Medicine: Concepts and Clinical Practice, 5th ed. St. Louis, Mosby, 2002, pp 1066–1074.
10. Medical Management of Biological Casualties Handbook, 2nd ed. Operational Medicine Department, U.S. Army Medical Research Institute of Infectious Diseases, 1996.
11. Medical Management of Chemical Casualties Handbook, 2nd ed. Chemical Casualty Care Office, U.S. Army Medical Research Institute of Chemical Defense, 1995.
12. Rotz LD, et al: Bioterrorism preparedness: Planning for the future. J Public Health Pract 6:45–49, 2000.
13. Silber SH, et al: Y2K medical disaster preparedness in New York City: Confidence of emergency department directors in their ability to respond. Prehosp Disaster Med 16:88–95, 2001.
14. Wetter DC, et al: Hospital preparedness for victims of chemical or biological terrorism. Am J Public Health 91:710–715, 2001.

95. CARDIOVASCULAR TOXICOLOGY

Christopher Dewitt, M.D., and Kennon Heard, M.D.

1. What effects do different poisons have on the heart rate, blood pressure, and QRS duration?
Bradycardia with:
  Hypertension: Phenylpropanolamine causes a reflex bradycardia because of its vasoconstrictive and hypertensive effects.
  Hypotension:
   Narrow-complex QRS:
   • α_2-Agonists (clonidine) inhibit the release of norepinephrine in the central nervous system, resulting in vasodilation, bradycardia, and somnolence.
   • β-Blockers (BBs) without sodium channel effects (see later).
   • Calcium channel blockers (CCBs) (see later).
   • Cardiac glycosides (see later).

Wide-complex QRS:
- BBs with sodium channel effects (propranolol, acebutolol, metoprolol).
- Severe CCB or cardiac glycoside toxicity causes ventricular escape rhythms.
- Propafenone has mainly sodium channel effects, but also has some β-blocking effects.
- Hyperkalemia from cardiac glycosides, BBs, and potassium-sparing diuretics.

Tachycardia with:

Hypertension:
- Sympathomimetics (amphetamines, cocaine, LSD, marijuana)
- Anticholinergics
- Monoamine oxidase inhibitors inhibit the breakdown of catecholamines in central nervous system synapses.

Hypotension:

Narrow-complex QRS:
- Angiotensin-converting enzyme inhibitors cause vasodilation and reflex tachycardia.
- α_1-Antagonists (prazosin, terazosin, doxazosin) cause vasodilation and reflex tachycardia.
- Diuretics cause tachycardia and hypotension secondary to dehydration.
- Nitrates cause vasodilation and reflex tachycardia.

Wide-complex QRS:
- Tricyclic antidepressants have effects on sodium channels causing widening of the QRS complex. In severe toxicity, this can lead to hypotension despite tachycardia from anticholinergic effects.
- Cocaine has sodium channel effects that late in the course override the ability to maintain blood pressure from tachycardia and vasoconstriction.
- Sotalol is a nonselective BB that also blocks potassium channels causing Q-T prolongation and risk for torsades de pointes.
- Class 1A antiarrhythmics (quinidine, disopyramide, procainamide) and 1C drugs (flecainide, encainide) owing to sodium channel blockade.

2. How do patients with a CCB overdose present?

CCBs decrease calcium influx into cardiac tissue and vascular smooth muscle. The heart depends on calcium for automaticity, conduction through the atrioventricular node, and contractility. Vascular smooth muscle requires calcium to maintain tone. Patients with CCB overdose present with hypotension (owing to decreased contractility and decreased vascular tone), bradycardia, and atrioventricular blocks. If hypotension is significant, patients may have altered mental status, organ ischemia, and acidosis.

3. Describe the treatment for CCB overdose.

Begin treatment with the ABCs (airway, breathing, circulation). Start an intravenous line, administer oxygen, institute cardiac monitoring, and obtain a thorough history. Other ingestions should be ruled out. Decontamination with gastric lavage, charcoal, and whole-bowel irrigation should be carried out. Hypotension initially should be treated with fluid boluses (2 L), and symptomatic bradycardia should be treated with atropine. Calcium is usually the next step in treatment for toxicity. Calcium chloride is preferred over calcium gluconate. The dose is 1 to 2 ampules intravenously and may be repeated every 10 minutes three to four times. Occasionally an infusion of calcium may be needed. Inotropic agents, such as dopamine, norepinephrine, or epinephrine, sometimes at high doses, are used next. Glucagon also can be used. Often an intravenous pacer is needed for continued bradycardia. Heroic measures, such as extracorporeal membrane oxygenation, intraaortic balloon pump, and cardiopulmonary bypass, have been used in severe refractory cases. Dialysis is not useful for CCBs.

4. How do patients with BB overdose present?

BBs compete with endogenous catecholamines for receptor sites; this blunts the normal adrenergic response, leading to bradycardia, atrioventricular blocks, and hypotension from decreased contractility. Patients suffering from BB toxicity present similarly to patients with CCB overdose. There can be a few differences, however, depending on which BB is involved. Some BBs, such as propranolol, are lipid soluble. This allows entry into the central nervous system, leading to seizures and altered mental status unrelated to blood pressure. Some BBs (propranolol, acebutolol, alprenolol, oxprenolol) antagonize sodium channels leading to a widened QRS. Sotalol also blocks potassium channels causing a prolonged Q-T interval and torsades de pointes.

5. Describe the treatment for BB toxicity.

Treatment is similar to that for CCB overdose. Glucagon is the drug of choice for treatment after fluids and atropine. Calcium has not been well studied for treatment of BB overdose. Seizures unrelated to hypotension should be treated with benzodiazepines; sodium bicarbonate is used for QRS widening.

6. How does acute digoxin toxicity differ from chronic digoxin toxicity?

Acute digoxin toxicity occurs after accidental or intentional ingestion of a supratherapeutic amount of digoxin-containing products. The dose usually considered possibly toxic is greater than 1 mg in a child and greater than 3 mg in an adult. Patients with acute digoxin toxicity often develop gastrointestinal symptoms, such as nausea or vomiting. The most common cardiac effects are bradycardia and heart block. After acute digoxin ingestion, blockade of the cellular sodium/potassium exchange pump leads to systemic hyperkalemia. Severe hyperkalemia (serum level > 5.5 mEq/L) is associated with a mortality of greater than 50% if untreated.

Chronic digoxin toxicity occurs when the dose or clearance of digoxin changes in a patient who is receiving long-term digoxin therapy. Initiation of quinidine, amiodarone, spironolactone, or verapamil may change the steady-state clearance of digoxin and result in toxicity. Decreased renal clearance of digoxin is seen commonly when a patient develops renal insufficiency. Symptoms of chronic digoxin toxicity are often subtle and nonspecific, including confusion, anorexia, vomiting, visual changes, and abdominal pain. The patient is often in bradycardia with varying degrees of heart block, but myocardial irritability is much more prominent than in acute poisoning. Patients often develop premature atrial and ventricular contractions, supraventricular tachycardia, ventricular tachycardia, or ventricular fibrillation. In contrast to acute digoxin toxicity, serum potassium is often normal or depressed unless the patient has hyperkalemia from renal insufficiency.

7. What are the indications for digoxin immune antibody fragments (Fab)?

Digoxin immune Fab is considered the drug of choice for treatment of life-threatening effects from either acute or chronic digoxin poisoning. The most common indications are symptomatic bradycardia, complete heart block, ventricular tachycardia, or ventricular fibrillation. Often, digoxin immune Fab must be administered to critically ill patients without laboratory confirmation of elevated digoxin levels. Patients with acute ingestion and a serum potassium of greater than 5.5 mEq/L have a poor prognosis and should be treated. Because serum digoxin levels correlate poorly with symptoms, there is no serum digoxin level that is considered an absolute indication for digoxin immune Fab.

8. How is digoxin Fab dosed?

Digoxin Fab may be dosed in one of several ways depending on the information available to the clinician:

1. If the patient is critically ill, 10 to 20 vials should be given empirically.

2. If the amount ingested is known, the following formula should be used: Dose (mg) × 1.4 = number of vials.

3. If the steady-state serum level is known, the following formula should be used: Serum level (ng/mL) × patient wt (kg)/100 = number of vials. (This normally results in a patient with chronic toxicity receiving 1 to 3 vials.)

9. What drugs cause cardiovascular toxicity by blocking cardiac sodium channels?

Many drugs bind to sodium channels when studied *in vitro*; however, some of these drugs rarely show cardiac effects or show these effects only in massive overdose. The major clinical manifestation of sodium channel blockade is prolongation of the QRS duration and ventricular arrhythmias.

Drugs with **primary toxic effects on sodium channel** include quinidine, flecainide, mexiletine, disopyramide, and procainamide. Patients poisoned with these agents are likely to present with prolonged QRS duration or arrhythmias as a primary problem but may have other toxic effects as well.

Drugs with **sodium channel effects and other serious effects** include sotalol, propranolol, tricyclic antidepressants, cocaine, chloroquine, propafenone, and thioridazine. Patients poisoned with these agents often present with other symptoms, but it is common to see prolonged QRS duration or arrhythmias as a toxic effect.

Drugs that have **sodium channel effects that are seen only in massive ingestions** include diphenhydramine, dimenhydrinate, carbamazepine, lidocaine, and norpropoxyphene (a metabolite of propoxyphene). Patients poisoned with these agents present with other symptoms but should be observed and treated if prolonged QRS duration or arrhythmias develop.

10. What is the antidote for drugs that cause sodium channel blockade?

Sodium bicarbonate (1 to 2 mEq/kg as a bolus) is used for the treatment of arrhythmias or prolongation of the QRS duration (> 120 msec) that occurs after the ingestion of any of these agents. If the QRS duration does not narrow after administration of sodium bicarbonate, a second bolus should be given. Hyperventilation should be initiated to induce a serum pH of 7.5 to 7.55. In addition to bicarbonate, patients with cardiovascular toxicity also likely require fluids and vasopressors for hypotension and endotracheal intubation for altered mental status.

BIBLIOGRAPHY

1. Antman EM, Wenger TL, Butler VP: Treatment of 150 cases of life threatening digitalis intoxication with digoxin specific Fab antibody fragments: Final report of a multi-center study. Circulation 81:1744–1752, 1990.
2. Kerns W, Kline J, Ford MD: Beta blocker and calcium channel blocker toxicity. Emerg Med Clin North Am 12:365–390, 1994.
3. Lewin NA: Cardiac glycosides. In Goldfrank LR, Flomenbaum NE, Lewin NA, et al (eds): Goldfrank's Toxicologic Emergencies, 6th ed. Stamford, CT, Appleton-Lange, 1998, pp 791–809.
4. Wax PM: Sodium bicarbonate. In Goldfrank LR, Flomenbaum NE, Lewin NA, et al (eds): Goldfrank's Toxicologic Emergencies, 6th ed. Stamford, CT, Appleton-Lange, 1998, pp 582–591.

XV. Gynecology and Obstetrics

96. PELVIC INFLAMMATORY DISEASE

Alexander T. Trott, M.D.

1. What is pelvic inflammatory disease (PID)?

An acute clinical syndrome caused by the spread of microorganisms from the vagina and cervix to reproductive organs. The organisms are most commonly sexually transmitted. PID can involve endometrium (endometritis), fallopian tubes (acute salpingitis), ovaries (oophoritis), and surrounding pelvic peritoneum (peritonitis). Any structure can be involved either alone or in combination. Inflammatory response can range from mild to severe.

2. Who is at risk for PID?

Sexually active women, between the ages of 15 and 19, who use no method of contraception are at highest risk. The risk is increased significantly if there have been recent encounters with multiple partners. Natural barriers to infection with sexually transmitted disease (STD) organisms are reduced during menses and by douching. Women in lower socioeconomic groups are at greatest risk, but the disease strikes at all levels of society. Although oral contraceptives are associated with a higher rate of chlamydial infection of the cervix, oral contraceptives lower the risk and the severity of disease if it does occur. The intrauterine device increases the risk for PID. Operative procedures such as dilation and curettage, hysterosalpingography, and legal abortion may increase the risk of PID.

3. What are the microbiologic causes?

A complex interplay between multiple organisms exists in the setting of PID. *Chlamydia trachomatis* and *Neisseria gonorrhoeae* are the most common organisms found, with 30% of cases having both organisms present. Facultative aerobes, such as *Escherichia coli*, group B streptococcus, and *Haemophilus influenzae*, and anaerobes may be recovered as well. Other implicated organisms include *Mycoplasma hominis* and *Ureaplasma urealyticum*.

4. Can patients have more than one STD?

The presence of one STD does not preclude another. Patients with PID can have syphilis or may be infected with human immunodeficiency virus (HIV). All patients being evaluated for an STD should have a serologic test for syphilis. Testing for HIV should be considered. Vaginitis, a mild vaginal infection caused by *Candida*, *Trichomonas*, or *Gardnerella*, may be associated with PID. Women who have vaginal discharge or itching require testing for chlamydia and gonorrhea, and a microscopic examination of vaginal secretions for the common causes of vaginitis should be ordered.

5. Describe the signs and symptoms of PID.

There are no reliable signs or symptoms clearly diagnostic of PID. The minimal criteria for empirical treatment is adnexal tenderness, the most sensitive physical examination finding for this condition. Additional criteria are cervical motion tenderness, vaginal discharge, and abdominal tenderness. Maintain a low threshold of suspicion for PID, particularly in patients with risk factors (see question 2). Extensive tubal inflammation and damage can occur in the face of mild clinical presentation, most commonly when the infection is due to *C. trachomatis*. Abnormal uterine bleeding or dysuria alone may be the only clinical evidence of PID.

6. What other diseases should be considered?

Of all patients admitted to the hospital for PID, 25% are found to have other conditions. The most important of these conditions are ectopic pregnancy and acute appendicitis. Ruptured corpus luteum cysts, pelvic endometriosis, ovarian torsion, and pelvic adhesion are included in the differential diagnosis. In a few patients, the cause of pelvic pain is never diagnosed despite extensive testing.

7. Which diagnostic tests should be performed?

- A β-human chorionic gonadotropin pregnancy test is recommended.
- If the pregnancy test is positive, an ultrasound is necessary to diagnose or rule out an ectopic pregnancy.
- A urinalysis may reveal a urinary tract infection as a possible cause of the patient's symptoms or a coexistent infection.
- A white blood cell count can help to indicate the severity of infection.
- Whenever a tuboovarian abscess is suspected, ultrasound is recommended.
- Cultures for *C. trachomatis* and *N. gonorrhoeae* are obtained in all patients with PID.
- Short of laparoscopy, there is no reliable test to exclude PID.

8. What are the consequences of PID, particularly if it is unrecognized or untreated?

All of the serious consequences of PID result from tubal inflammation and scarring. Acutely, PID can progress to tuboovarian abscess that may require surgical intervention. Ectopic pregnancy, the most serious consequence, is two to seven times more likely to occur in women with prior PID. Infertility is another serious sequela and is directly proportional to number of pelvic infections and severity of infection. One of the most troublesome sequelae of PID is chronic abdominal pain, which eventually may require a hysterectomy to resolve.

9. Who should be treated?

Because the consequences of unrecognized and untreated PID can be severe, **overtreatment** of sexually active women with pelvic organ symptoms is recommended. Only 30% of patients with PID have the classic textbook symptoms. Women with mild or atypical symptoms, especially if they fit the risk profile, should be treated empirically with a full course of antibiotics. In the setting of PID, the consequences of overtreatment greatly outweigh the risks of undertreatment. Response to antibiotics and close follow-up help resolve the diagnosis.

10. Who should be hospitalized?

The main reasons to hospitalize a patient with PID are to protect future fertility and to treat moderate-to-serious disease. Most authorities agree that young, nulligravida women, regardless of infection severity, require hospitalization for the first episode.

The Centers for Disease Control's Guidelines for Hospital Admission

1. Diagnosis is uncertain (appendicitis cannot be ruled out)

2. Pelvic abscess is suspected

3. Pregnancy

4. Severe illness present (high fever, peritoneal signs, vomiting)

5. Patient is an adolescent

6. Failure of outpatient therapy

7. Presence of HIV infection

11. Summarize the recommended antibiotic regimens for PID treatment.

Outpatient Treatment of PID

Regimen A

Ofloxacin, 400 mg PO b.i.d. for 14 d

Plus

Metronidazole, 500 mg PO b.i.d. for 14 d

Regimen B

One of following: (1) ceftriaxone, 250 mg IM once; (2) cefoxitin, 2 g IM, plus probenecid, 1 g PO in
a single dose concurrently once; *or* (3) other parenteral third-generation cephalosporin (e.g., ceftizoxime or cefotaxime)

Plus

Doxycycline, 100 mg PO b.i.d. for 14 d

Adapted from Centers for Disease Control: Sexually transmitted diseases treatment guidelines. MMWR
Morb Mortal Wkly Rep 47(RR-1):82, 1998.

Inpatient Treatment of PID

Parenteral Regimen A

Cefotetan, 2 g IV q 12 h; *or* cefoxitin, 2 g IV q 6 h

Plus

Doxycycline, 100 mg IV or PO q 12 h

Note: Because of pain associated with infusion, doxycycline should be given orally when possible,
even when patient is hospitalized. Oral and intravenous administration of doxycycline provide similar
bioavailability. If intravenous administration is necessary, lidocaine or another short-acting local
anesthetic, heparin, or steroids with a steel needle or extension of the infusion time may reduce infusion complications. Parenteral therapy may be discontinued 24 hours after a patient improves clinically, and oral therapy with doxycycline (100 mg b.i.d.) should continue for 14 days. When
tuboovarian abscess is present, clindamycin or metronidazole may be used with doxycycline for continued therapy rather than doxycycline alone because it provides more effective anaerobic coverage.

Parenteral Regimen B

Clindamycin, 900 mg IV q 8 h

Plus

Gentamicin, loading dose IV or IM (2 mg/kg body weight), followed by a maintenance dose (1.5
mg/kg) q 8 h. Single daily dosing may be substituted.

Note: Although use of one daily dose of gentamicin has not been evaluated for the treatment of PID, it
is efficacious in analogous situations. Parenteral therapy may be discontinued 24 hours after a patient improves clinically, and continuing oral therapy should consist of doxycycline, 100 mg PO
b.i.d., or clindamycin, 450 mg PO q.i.d., to complete 14 days of therapy. When tuboovarian abscess
is present, clindamycin may be used for continued therapy rather than doxycycline because clindamycin provides more effective anaerobic coverage.

Adapted from Centers for Disease Control: Sexually transmitted diseases treatment guidelines. MMWR
Morb Mortal Wkly Rep 47(RR-1):83, 1998.

12. Does the presence of an intrauterine pregnancy effectively rule out PID?

A common misconception is that PID cannot occur in a pregnant woman. It can occur, most
commonly in the first trimester in primigravidas. Infection can take place concurrently with fertilization or throughout the first trimester, after which the uterine cavity is obliterated by the
pregnancy. Although PID can occur under these conditions, it is uncommon.

13. Does a history of tubal ligation preclude the diagnosis of PID?

Bilateral tubal ligation (BTL) does not preclude PID. Of patients hospitalized with PID, 10%
have BTL. The symptoms and course of patients with PID and BTL are less severe. Patients with

BTL and PID have lower white blood cell counts, have shorter hospitalizations, and are rarely admitted with complications such as tuboovarian abscess or hydrosalpinx.

14. What is the appropriate follow-up for patients with PID?
Patients treated as outpatients need close follow-up. Response to treatment should be assessed within 48 to 72 hours. The patient can return to the ED, see a primary care provider, or be evaluated by a gynecologist. For reliable patients, a phone contact can suffice. For all patients, a test of cure by repeat examination and cervical cultures is recommended 2 to 4 weeks after the initial intervention.

15. Summarize the principles of management of acute PID.
• Rule out pregnancy
• Treat early and with broad- spectrum antibiotics
• Screen and treat lower genital infections in men and women
• Use standard clinical criteria to guide (not dictate) diagnosis
• Reassess patient 48 to 72 hours after initiating treatment
• Err on side of overdiagnosis of PID to prevent sequelae
• Encourage the use of a barrier contraceptive with spermicide
• Identify and treat or refer sexual partners
From Shafer MA, Sweet RL: Pelvic inflammatory disease in adolescent females. Adolesc Med State Art Rev 1:545–564, 1990.

BIBLIOGRAPHY

1. Abbuhl SB, Muskin EB, Shofer FS: Pelvic inflammatory disease in patients with bilateral tubal ligation. Am J Emerg Med 15:271–274, 1997.
2. Acquavella AP, Rubin A, Angelo LJD: The coincident diagnosis of pelvic inflammatory disease and pregnancy: Are they compatible? J Pediatr Adolesc Gynecol 9:129–132, 1996.
3. Barbosa C, Macasaet M, Brockmann S, et al: Pelvic inflammatory disease and human immunodeficiency virus infection. Obstet Gynecol 89:65–70, 1997.
4. Centers for Disease Control: Sexually transmitted diseases treatment guidelines. MMWR Morb Mortal Wkly Rep 47(RR-1):83, 1998.
5. Eschenbach DA, Wolner-Hanssen P, Hawes SE, et al: Acute pelvic inflammatory disease: Associations of clinical and laboratory findings with laparoscopic findings. Obstet Gynecol 89:184–192, 1997.
6. Hemsel DL, Ledger WJ, Martens M, et al: Concerns regarding the Centers for Disease Control's published guidelines for pelvic inflammatory disease. Clin Infect Dis 32:103–107, 2001.
7. Jossens MO, Eskenazi B, Schachter J, Sweet RL: Risk factors for pelvic inflammatory disease: A case control study. Sex Transm Dis 23:239–247, 1996.
8. Peipert JF, Ness RB, Blume J, et al: Clinical predictors of endometritis in women with symptoms and signs of pelvic inflammatory disease. Am J Obstet Gynecol 184:856–864, 2001.
9. Sweet R: Role of bacterial vaginosis in pelvic inflammatory disease. Clin Infect Dis 20(suppl 2):S271–S275, 1995.

97. SEXUAL ASSAULT

Kim M. Feldhaus, M.D.

1. What is the legal definition of sexual assault?
The carnal knowledge of a victim (male or female) without consent by the use of fear, force, threat of force, or fraud. Carnal knowledge can consist of complete vaginal, anal, or oral intercourse; incomplete penile or digital penetration; intentional fondling or touching; or coercion of the victim to fondle or touch the assailant's genitals. Lack of consent is an important aspect of the crime; nonconsenting victims include minors and victims who are intoxicated, drugged, asleep, or mentally incompetent.

2. How common is sexual assault?

Because of underreporting, the exact incidence of sexual assault is difficult to determine. The National Institute of Justice and the Centers for Disease Control estimate that 18% of women have been raped at some point during their lifetime; half of all victims were younger than age 18 when they experienced their first sexual assault. Of victims, 10% report the crime to law enforcement; approximately one third of women who suffer injuries from a sexual assault seek medical attention. Of victims who contact rape crisis centers, 70% to 80% are victims of acquaintance rape.

3. Why is it important for the ED physician to be knowledgeable about sexual assault?

The ED is the most common place for a sexual assault victim to present for acute medical care and forensic evidence gathering. A comprehensive ED sexual assault protocol that addresses medical care and the evidentiary examination is necessary for optimal patient care.

4. What information should be elicited in the patient history?

1. Information regarding the patient's general health, medications, and allergies should be obtained and a complete gynecologic history, including birth control usage, date and time of last consensual intercourse, last menstrual period, and history of recent gynecologic symptoms before the assault.

2. A directed history of the assault includes the date, time, and location of the assault; information concerning the assailants; and the type and details of the sexual acts, including type of force or threats used. The history must be obtained in a private setting; law enforcement personnel should not be present.

5. What should the physical examination consist of?

The purpose of the physical examination is to detect injuries requiring treatment and to record and gather forensic evidence for prosecution. A complete head-to-toe medical examination should be done regardless of whether the patient has consented to the evidentiary examination. Nongenital injuries, usually minor abrasions or contusions, occur more frequently than do genital injuries. Patients should be examined carefully for evidence of scratches, bruises, lacerations, teeth marks, or other signs of trauma. The gynecologic examination should include a thorough search for contusions, abrasions, lacerations, bleeding, or tenderness. A Wood's lamp fluoresces most semen stains, and toluidine blue dye reveals minor traumatic genital tears. A colposcopic examination may identify cervical injuries. A careful rectal examination should be done in cases of rectal penetration, and if blood is present, anoscopy or sigmoidoscopy should be done to identify internal injuries.

6. What evidence should be gathered as part of the forensic examination?

Specimens to detect sperm or semen may serve as evidence to prove sexual contact and possibly, to indicate the assailant's identity through DNA testing. Vaginal, oral, and rectal samples should be obtained when appropriate. Swabs of semen deposits on the skin should be collected; a Wood's lamp fluoresces semen. Samples of any foreign material should be gathered, and the clothing the victim wore should be collected. Saliva and hair samples should be gathered for comparison to saliva samples taken from the victim's skin and to loose hairs found at the crime scene or on the victim. Wet mount slides may be studied for motile sperm, depending on individual protocols. It is crucial to have a system in place to preserve the chain of evidence. If the history is suggestive for a drug-facilitated rape, urine specimens for toxicologic testing may be appropriate.

7. What laboratory studies are indicated?

A serum pregnancy test should be done to rule out a preexisting pregnancy; if a preexisting pregnancy is present, the patient should be reassured that this pregnancy was not the result of the assault. The routine collection of gonorrhea or chlamydia cultures is debatable. A preexisting infection is present in approximately 5% of assault victims (the same as the general population); identification of these patients allows for treatment of their regular partners. If the victim does not receive prophylactic antibiotics in the ED, chlamydia and gonorrhea cultures should be repeated in 2 weeks. Compliance with medical follow-up is historically poor, however. From a medicolegal perspective, positive cultures indicating preexisting sexually transmitted diseases (STDs) have been used by defense attorneys as evidence of the victim's sexual promiscuity. Human immunodeficiency virus (HIV) testing is not routinely indicated in the ED, but all victims should be referred to the health department or other agencies where counseling and confidential HIV antibody testing are available.

8. What is the risk of contracting a STD from a sexual assault?

Studies suggest that the risk of contracting a new chlamydia or gonorrhea infection from a sexual assault is 4% to 17%. The risk of contracting HIV infection is unknown but is believed to be significantly less than 1%.

9. Is empirical antibiotic treatment of sexual assault victims indicated?

For many sexual assault victims, the possibility of contracting a STD as a result of the assault is disturbing. Because of historically poor follow-up rates by sexual assault victims, prophylaxis for STDs should be offered to all sexual assault victims. Effective regimens include ceftriaxone, 125 mg intramuscularly in a single dose; cefixime, 400 mg orally in a single dose; or ciprofloxacin, 500 mg orally in a single dose, for gonorrhea coverage. Patients also should be given azithromycin, 1 g orally in a single dose, or doxycycline, 100 mg orally twice a day for 7 to 10 days, for chlamydia prophylaxis. The Centers for Disease Control also recommend a single 2-g metronidazole dose to treat *Trichomonas* and bacterial vaginosis. Hepatitis B prophylaxis should be considered if the assailant is believed to belong to a high-risk group for this disease.

10. State the risk of pregnancy after sexual assault.

The risk is about 1%. The presence of a preexisting pregnancy must be identified in the ED.

11. What are the current options for pregnancy prophylaxis?

When a preexisting pregnancy has been ruled out, various estrogen or progesterone preparations can be used to prevent pregnancy by delaying ovulation, preventing fertilization, or preventing implantation. These preparations should be given within 72 hours of the assault. The most widely used estrogen and progesterone combination is oral norgestrel and ethinyl estradiol (Ovral), 2 tablets at presentation followed by 2 tablets in 12 hours. A progesterone-only preparation is Plan B; 1 tablet is taken at presentation followed by 1 tablet in 12 hours. Patients should be warned about nausea as a side effect and possible vaginal spotting. The failure rate with Ovral and Plan B is less than 2%; however, patients should be advised to seek medical attention if menses is delayed.

12. What are the special characteristics of male sexual assault?

The male sexual assault victim should be treated similarly to a female victim. Special attention should be paid to the mouth, genitals, anus, and rectum. Men represent approximately 5% of reported sexual assault victims.

13. Discuss the special characteristics of pediatric sexual assault.

In pediatric sexual assault, the assailant is often known to the victim, and there is often a history of repetitive assaults. In addition to documenting signs of acute trauma, the physician should look for signs of recurrent abuse, such as healed hymenal tears, a large vaginal opening, vaginal discharge, or relaxed rectal sphincter tone. The gynecologic examination should take into account the nature of the assault and the age of the child. In the evaluation of a small child in whom a speculum examination is indicated, a nasal speculum may be used in place of a vaginal speculum. Sometimes the vaginal or rectal examination must be done under general anesthesia because of the emotional state of the child. The child should be protected from further abuse by admission to the hospital or by immediate referral to the appropriate social service agency.

14. Should pediatric patients be given prophylactic antibiotics?

Prophylactic antibiotics are not generally indicated when sexual abuse of children is suspected. The baseline infection rate in children is significantly lower than in adults, and the presence of a STD in a child is strong evidence that abuse has occurred. It is important to document the presence of the infection before treatment. In the child, chlamydia and gonorrhea cultures should be obtained from the vagina instead of the cervix.

15. State the important aspects of follow-up care for any victim of sexual assault.

Follow-up medical care should ensure that any physical injuries have healed properly, adequate pregnancy prophylaxis has been administered, STDs have been treated properly, and the victim has accessed supportive counseling. Provision of written aftercare instructions and information on community resources is essential.

16. What types of emotional trauma might sexual assault victims experience?

The development of a posttraumatic stress disorder, manifested by sleep disturbances, feelings of guilt, memory impairment, and detachment from the world and others may occur in the days to weeks following the assault. Long-term psychological sequelae in the form of rape trauma syndrome also may occur. Many communities have rape crisis centers with social workers and volunteers who are trained to provide counseling for sexual assault survivors. Sexual assault response teams have been organized in other areas to provide a coordinated approach to the sexual assault victim, including emotional support after the event. Physicians should be aware of the availability of such services so that they can recommend them to their patients.

CONTROVERSY

17. My patient is terrified of contracting HIV after her sexual assault. What do I do now?

Although not routinely recommended, postexposure prophylaxis (PEP) for HIV infection may be appropriate after sexual assault. The true risk of contracting HIV after a single sexual encounter is unknown but believed to be small. Risk of contracting HIV is believed to be highest for unprotected, receptive anal intercourse; trauma, bleeding, and inflammation can increase the risk. Physicians should consider the likelihood of exposure to HIV based on the assailant's HIV status (if known), any high-risk HIV behaviors exhibited by the assailant, the nature of the assault, the interval between the exposure and therapy, and the risks and benefits of PEP. Other complicating factors include the potential inability to test the assailant for HIV, the expense of PEP, the side effects of the medications, and the need for close follow-up. If PEP is offered, the guidelines for mucous membrane exposure should be followed.

BIBLIOGRAPHY

1. DeLahunta EA, Baram DA: Sexual assault. Clin Obstet Gynecol 40:648–660, 1997.
2. Feldhaus KM: Female and male sexual assault. In Tintinalli JE, et al (eds): Emergency Medicine: A Comprehensive Study Guide, 5th ed. New York, McGraw-Hill, 2000, pp 1952–1956.
3. Feldhaus KM, Houry D, Kaminsky R: Lifetime sexual assault prevalence rates and reporting practices in an emergency department population. Ann Emerg Med 36:23–27, 2000.
4. Fong C: Post-exposure prophylaxis for HIV infection after sexual assault: When is it indicated. Emerg Med J 18:242–245, 2001.
5. Linden JA: Sexual assault. Emerg Med Clin North Am 17:685–697, 1999.
6. Moran GJ: Pharmacologic management of HIV/STD exposure. Emerg Med Clin North Am 18:829–842 2000.
7. Patel M, Minshall L: Management of sexual assault. Emerg Med Clin North Am 19:817–831, 2001.

8. Riggs N, Houry D, Long G, et al: Analysis of 1,076 cases of sexual assault. Ann Emerg Med 35:358–362, 2000.
9. U.S. Department of Health and Human Services: Guidelines for treatment of sexually transmitted diseases. MMWR Morb Mortal Wkly Rep 47(RR-1):1–111, 1998.
10. U.S. Department of Justice, National Institute of Justice: Full report of the prevalence, incidence, and consequences of violence against women. NCJ 183781, November 2000.

98. SPONTANEOUS ABORTION

Kim M. Feldhaus, M.D.

1. What is abortion?

Termination of pregnancy before achieving fetal weight or maturity compatible with survival—less than 20 weeks' gestation or less than 500 g fetal weight. Abortions may be spontaneous, therapeutic, or elective.

2. State the incidence of spontaneous abortion.

Approximately 20% to 25% of pregnant patients experience some bleeding during the first 4 to 20 weeks of their pregnancy. Of these, approximately 50% miscarry.

3. What is the most common cause of spontaneous abortion?

Abnormal development of the zygote. Chromosomal abnormalities are seen in 50% to 60% of early spontaneous abortions occurring in the first 4 to 8 weeks of gestation. Spontaneous abortions occurring later in the first trimester often are due to isolated chromosomal abnormalities, maternal factors (insufficient progesterone support, alcohol use, cocaine use, or tobacco use), or structural uterine abnormalities.

4. When do most spontaneous abortions occur?

Most commonly between 8 and 12 weeks' gestation. Fetal demise procedes clinical symptoms in most cases by several weeks.

5. Describe the pathology of spontaneous abortion.

There is hemorrhage into the decidua basalis with subsequent necrotic changes in the area of implantation. The ovum becomes partially or completely detached, acts as a foreign body in the uterus, stimulates contractions, and results in expulsion of uterine contents.

6. What are the stages of miscarriage?

Any pregnant patient with vaginal bleeding in the first half of pregnancy and a closed internal os is said to have a **threatened abortion**. Crampy abdominal pain or back pain may be present. If the internal os is open on examination, this is an **inevitable abortion**. Patients with products of conception present in the cervical os or the vaginal canal are described as having an **incomplete abortion**, whereas **complete abortions** occur after all products of conception have been passed. Pain and bleeding cease after a complete abortion.

7. Besides a threatened abortion, what else causes vaginal bleeding in the first half of pregnancy?

The primary diagnosis to be excluded is an **ectopic pregnancy**. Other causes of early vaginal bleeding include vaginal ulcers, trophoblastic disease, cervical erosion, cervical polyps, cancer, and decidual reactions of the cervix.

8. What is a blighted ovum?

An ovum with no visible fetus in the sac because the embryo has degenerated or is absent.

9. Describe the sonographic findings in a healthy pregnancy.

There is a distinct, well-formed gestational ring, with central echoes indicating a fetal pole. A sac with no central echoes from an embryo or fetus implies, but does not prove, death of the conceptus. Serial sonograms are important to follow the progression or lack of fetal growth.

10. Summarize the treatment for threatened abortion.

1. **Examination**. Is the patient hemodynamically stable? Is there abdominal tenderness or rebound (indicating a possible ectopic pregnancy)? Are there products of conception visible in the cervical os or vaginal canal (an incomplete abortion)? Is the cervical os open (an inevitable abortion) or closed?

2. Identify an interuterine pregnancy, by ultrasound, if not previously documented to rule out an ectopic pregnancy.

3. Restrict sexual intercourse and strenuous physical exercise.

4. Follow serial quantitative β-human chorionic gonadotropin tests. If levels decrease, prognosis is poor.

5. If bleeding persists, obtain hematocrit and hemoglobin tests.

6. If bleeding is perfuse, causing hypotension, evacuation is necessary.

11. What are the earliest symptoms of a miscarriage?

Bleeding or spotting is usually first, followed by crampy abdominal pain.

12. What is the prognosis for patients with threatened abortion?

Patients with bleeding and a closed internal os have a risk of miscarriage estimated at 35% to 50%, although the fetal loss rate is probably higher in ED populations. If fetal cardiac activity is shown on ultrasound, risk of subsequent miscarriage is much lower. There is no treatment regimen that influences the course of a threatened abortion.

13. What is the treatment for an incomplete abortion?

Dilation and and evacuation or dilation and curettage with local cervical anesthesia and procedural sedation. If there is tissue protruding from the os on pelvic examination, removal can be attempted by gentle traction with ring forceps, which in most instances decreases the amount of uterine hemorrhage.

14. What is a missed abortion?

In a missed abortion, the conceptus dies but is not passed, with retention of products of conception in utero for 4 to 8 weeks or more. Uterine size decreases and symptoms of pregnancy regress. Most usually abort spontaneously.

15. What is the danger of prolonged retention of products of conception?

The occurrence of disseminated intravascular coagulation. Laboratory studies for coagulation defects, including prothrombin time, partial thromboplastin time, fibrinogen, and fibrin split products, need to be obtained.

16. Do diagnostic radiographs cause spontaneous abortion?

No. Diagnostic radiographs (< 10 rads) place a pregnant woman at little or no increased risk for miscarriage, although there is a risk for the development of fetal chromosomal abnormalities. Therapeutic radiation and antineoplastic agents *do* increase the incidence of spontaneous abortion.

17. What is a septic abortion?

A spontaneous abortion complicated by endometritis, parametritis, or peritonitis.

18. List the symptoms of a septic abortion.
1. Malodorous discharge from the cervix or vagina
2. Pelvic and abdominal pain
3. Fever
4. Uterine tenderness
5. Hyperthermia, which may be an indication of endotoxic shock

19. List the causes of spontaneous abortion.
1. Chromosomal abnormalities: most common is autosomal trisomy (52%).
2. Risk increases with increased maternal parity and increased maternal and paternal age. The frequency increases from 12% in women younger than age 20 to 26% in women older than age 40.
3. Conception within 3 months after a live birth.
4. Systemic disease of the mother (e.g., diabetes mellitus, cancer, hypothyroidism or hyperthyroidism).
5. Autoimmune mechanisms: antiphospholipid autoantibodies.
6. Laparotomy: The closer the surgery to the pelvic organs, the greater the risk of spontaneous abortion.
7. Uterine defects:
   • **Acquired**
   Leiomyomas: The location is more important than the size. Submucous fibroids are more dangerous.
   Intrauterine adhesions: synechiae or Asherman's syndrome secondary to curettage.
   • **Developmental**
   Abnormal müllerian duct formation or fusion. May be secondary to diethylstilbestrol use. Septate, bicornate, or unicornate uterus.

20. Is the drug isotretinoin (Accutane) safe for use in pregnancy?
No. It has been associated with spontaneous abortion and fetal abnormalities. Do *not* use in pregnant women or in women planning to become pregnant.

21. Has the use of oral contraceptives been associated with spontaneous abortion?
No. Oral contraceptives taken either before or during pregnancy have not been associated with spontaneous abortion.

22. Is trauma a major factor associated with spontaneous abortion?
No. Fetuses are well protected by maternal structures and amniotic fluid from minor falls or blows, but penetrating trauma such as a gunshot wound or stab wound is dangerous to the fetus.

23. Name drugs, chemicals, or noxious agents associated with spontaneous abortion.
1. Cigarettes
2. Alcohol (at high-exposure range)
3. Contraceptive agents (conception with an intrauterine device in place increases the risk of spontaneous abortion)
4. Environmental chemicals (anesthetic agents, arsenic, aniline, benzene, ethylene oxide, formaldehyde, lead)

24. Is exposure to spermicide before or after conception deleterious to a pregnancy?
No.

25. Is life event stress associated with spontaneous abortions?
Increased life stess has been reported to increase the risk of spontaneous abortions in women greater than 11 weeks' gestation, implying an increased risk of miscarriage of chromosomally normal fetuses. This association has not been clearly proved.

26. Define cervical incompetence.

Cervical incompetence is the painless dilation of the cervix during the second trimester, followed by spontaneous rupture of membranes, with subsequent expulsion of uterine contents.

27. Name the drug used to prevent Rh immunization.

Rh immunoglobulin or RhoGAM. Any pregnant woman who is experiencing vaginal bleeding must have an Rh (rhesus) type checked; if she is Rh negative and less than 12 weeks' gestation, she should receive a mini-dose of RhoGAM, 50 μg. If she is greater than 12 weeks' gestation, the full dose of RhoGAM, 300 μg, should be given.

28. What follow-up instructions should be given to a patient with a threatened abortion?

Careful instructions are given to return if she has a significant increase in pain, bleeding, or signs of hemodynamic instability, such as sycopal episodes. The patient should be instructed to bring any tissue she passes in with her to the ED or her primary care physician. Arrangements to repeat quantitative β-human chorionic gonadotropin measurements should be made. Patients with a history of recurrent miscarriages should be referred to a specialist for further testing.

29. What about the emotional aspects of an early miscarriage?

Miscarriage is associated with a significant amount of psychological stress and grieving. Important therapeutic messages include informing the patient that early miscarriages are common and that miscarriages are usually due to chromosomal abnormalities and not to the patient's own actions.

BIBLIOGRAPHY

1. Boyles SH, Ness RB, Grisso JA, et al: Life event stress and the association with spontaneous abortion in gravid women at an urban emergency department. Health Psychol 19:510–514, 2000.
2. Grant J, Hysolp M: Underutilization of Rh prophylaxis in the emergency department: A retrospective survey. Ann Emerg Med 21:181–183, 1992.
3. Nadukhovskaya L, Dart R: Emergency management of the nonviable intrauterine pregnancy. Am J Emerg Med 19:495–500, 2001.
4. Nybo Andersen AM, Wohlfahrt J, Christens P, et al: Maternal age and fetal loss population based register linkage study. BMJ 320:1708–1712, 2000.
5. Rosenberg L, Palmer JR, Kaufman DW, et al: Breast cancer in relation to the occurrence and time of induced and spontaneous abortion. Am J Epidemiol 127:981–989, 1988.
6. Scott JR, Disaia PJ, Hammond CB, et al (eds): Danforth's Obstetrics and Gynecology, 7th ed. Philadelphia, J.B. Lippincott, 1994.
7. Wichit Srisuphan PH, Bracken MB: Caffeine consumption during pregnancy and association with late spontaneous abortion. Am J Obstet Gynecol 154:14–20, 1986.
8. Zaccardi R, Abbott J, Koziol-McLain J: Loss and grief reactions after spontaneous miscarriage in the emergency department. Ann Emerg Med 22:799–804, 1992.

99. ECTOPIC PREGNANCY

Jean T. Abbott, M.D.

1. What is an ectopic pregnancy (EP)?

A pregnancy in which implantation of the gestational sac occurs outside of the uterus. In most cases, the pregnancy is located in the fallopian tubes, but EPs can occur in the interstitial or cornual portion of the uterus (2%), intraabdominally (1.5%), on the ovary (0.1%), or within the cervix (0.1%). EP occurs in approximately 1 in 60 pregnancies in the United States; the risk is higher in older women and minorities. Most ED series report that about 7% of first-trimester patients presenting to EDs have EP diagnosed.

2. What are the risk factors for EP?

Common risk factors are pelvic inflammatory disease, prior ectopic pregnancy, tubal ligation, intrauterine device use, prior pelvic surgery, infertility, and fertilization procedures. These are present in 50% of ED patients presenting with EP. The risk of EP has increased markedly primarily because of an increased incidence of pelvic inflammatory disease, which can be seen histologically in 50% of patients with EP. Other structural abnormalities of the fallopian tubes and host abnormalities that discourage implantation in the endometrium may cause some cases of ectopic implantation. New technology, such as artificial fertilization, ovulation stimulation, and surgical procedures that result in salvage of potentially abnormal fallopian tubes, also may contribute to the increased incidence.

3. What is the risk of heterotopic (combined intrauterine and ectopic) pregnancy?

The classic risk has been cited as 1 in 30,000 pregnancies. More recent estimates put the risk at closer to 1 in 4,000, and the risk in infertility patients with pregnancy stimulation or embryo transfer procedures may be much higher.

4. How reliable are routine serum and urine pregnancy tests in a patient with EP?

Sensitive serum or urine pregnancy tests are almost always positive in EP. β-Human chorionic gonadotropin (hCG) is secreted from the time of implantation, about 7 to 8 days after implantation of the fertilized ovum. Qualitative pregnancy tests positive at a level of 10 to 50 mIU/mL are positive in almost 99% of patients with EP. Home pregnancy tests and less sensitive tests with higher thresholds may be falsely negative. Serum and urine tests provide similar accuracy for qualitative testing if their thresholds are similar.

5. What clinical signs and symptoms are useful to increase suspicion of an EP?

The classic picture of EP is of vaginal bleeding, pelvic or abdominal pain, prior missed menses, and an adnexal mass. This picture is neither sensitive nor specific. Missed menses occur in only 85% of EP patients. Vaginal bleeding and pain may occur only later, when the growing EP begins to fail or overstretch its abnormal implantation site. Adnexal masses are palpated in only 50% of patients, even under anesthesia; they may represent the corpus luteum of the pregnancy rather than the ectopic gestation itself. Patients at high risk for EP are those with first-trimester pregnancy and either pelvic pain or risk factors for EP. Peritoneal signs, severe pain on pelvic examination, and cervical motion tenderness also increase suspicion of EP. There is, however, no constellation of historical factors or findings that confirms or excludes EP with sufficient reliability to avoid ancillary studies discussed subsequently.

6. Why are corpus luteum cysts frequently confused with EPs?

The corpus luteum of the ovary, originating from the graafian follicle, supports the pregnancy with secretion of hCG and progesterone during the first 6 to 7 weeks of gestation and may become cystic, growing to 5 cm in diameter or more. Cyst rupture can occur in the first trimester, presenting as a patient in early pregnancy with sudden pain, unilateral peritoneal findings, adnexal tenderness, and perhaps a mass.

7. What is the risk of EP in a patient with painless vaginal bleeding?

Although the risk of EP is low in patients with painless bleeding in the first trimester, occasionally women with EP present this way initially. Although use of ultrasound to locate all pregnancies in the first trimester in the ED is not feasible or necessary, instructions should be given to all women as if they could have an EP until an intrauterine pregnancy (IUP) is proved by ultrasound, auscultation of fetal heart sounds, or tissue diagnosis of an abortion.

8. What is the most efficient way to diagnose or exclude EP in the ED?

Ultrasound evaluation of early pregnancy is the best first ancillary study. Of patients, 50% to 75% have a definitive diagnosis of either IUP or EP (less commonly) from imaging. Normal

IUPs can be seen by transvaginal sonography by about 5.5 weeks' gestation. EPs occasionally can be seen, but the more common finding is an empty uterus. In 25% to 50% of patients seen in the first trimester for vaginal bleeding or pain, ultrasound is indeterminant. The risk of EP can be defined further by obtaining a quantitative hCG level if the ultrasound is inconclusive.

9. What is the role of quantitative hCG? Should it be a *stat* test in every patient with possible EP?

hCG levels double every 2 to 3 days during the first 7 to 8 weeks of normal pregnancies. Because many women do not know the date of their last menstrual period, quantitative levels may be useful to estimate gestational age and correlate with expected sonographic findings (see earlier). With hCG greater than 2,000 mIU/mL, a healthy IUP should be visible by transvaginal sonography. Failure to double normally during the first 7 weeks indicates the pregnancy is failing—either within the uterus or at an ectopic site. EP is likely if the ultrasound is indeterminant and the quantitative hCG is greater than 2,000 mIU/mL or is rising on serial measurements (usually done at 48-hour intervals). A rapidly falling hCG level (less than half of the original in 48 hours) is unlikely to be an EP, but slowly falling levels also are consistent with EP. A failed pregnancy is likely to be ectopic if dilation and curettage fails to detect villi or if no products of conception are found at the time of miscarriage. The most efficient method of diagnosing EP is to measure the hCG level only if the ultrasound is indeterminant. An alternative algorithm that is almost as efficient employs an initial hCG level and an ultrasound when the hCG level is greater than 2,000 mIU/mL.

10. What is the role of culdocentesis?

Sonography has obviated the need for culdocentesis in most instances. Culdocentesis is indicated in patients who are unstable and need rapid confirmation of intraperitoneal bleeding or in EDs where sonography is not readily available but diagnosis needs to be made urgently. Although 20% of aspirations from culdocentesis may be dry and give no information, greater than 90% of the remainder are positive in EP, even in women with subacute presentations and without signs of peritonitis.

11. Does every patient with bleeding or pain in the first trimester require ultrasound before discharge from the ED?

The unstable patient probably should have a rapid culdocentesis and be taken to the operating room. Urgent sonography should be reserved for patients with acute pain, significant risk factors, or unreliable follow-up. Most patients can be managed with the possibility that they could be harboring an EP. They should get an urgent ultrasound within 1 to 2 days; daytime sonographic studies frequently are more complete and accurate. All first-trimester complaints are treated as *rule out EP* until an IUP is shown on ultrasound. These patients should receive careful instructions to return if they develop pain and can be scheduled safely for a later ultrasound.

12. Sumarize the ultrasound findings in patients with suspected EP.

Ultrasound Findings in Patients with Suspected EP

Diagnostic of IUP	Indeterminate
Double gestational sac	Empty uterus
Intrauterine fetal pole or yolk sac	Nonspecific fluid collections
Intrauterine fetal heart activity	Echogenic material
Diagnostic of EP	Abnormal sac
Ectopic fetal heart activity or	Single gestational sac
Ectopic fetal pole	
Suggestive of EP	
Moderate or large cul-de-sac fluid without IUP	
Adnexal mass* without IUP	

* Complex mass most suggestive of EP but cyst also can be seen with EP.
Modified from Dart RG: Role of pelvic ultrasonography in evaluation of symptomatic first trimester pregnancy. Ann Emerg Med 33:310–320, 1999.

13. What patients with EPs can be discharged from the ED?

Women who are unstable with significant pain or signs of significant blood loss require admission. ED or inpatient observation may be useful in stable patients with worrisome symptoms, risk factors, or expected poor compliance to facilitate rapid sonography, quantitative hCG interpretation, or specialist consultation. Stable patients with indeterminant ultrasound results (*rule out EP*) or known but relatively asymptomatic EPs may be followed on an outpatient basis. Conservative outpatient treatment modalities for EP are becoming more common. Expectant management or chemotherapy for women with few symptoms and low hormonal levels should be directed by the patient's obstetrician/gynecologist. The role of the ED physician is to consider the diagnosis, make every effort to exclude or make the diagnosis of EP expeditiously, make the patient aware of the differential diagnosis and signs that should be of concern to her, and ensure access to close follow-up care for this potentially serious problem.

14. Summarize the management of possible EP.

Clinical Suspicion of Ectopic Pregnancy

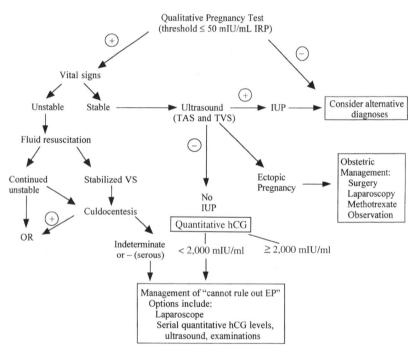

Management of possible ectopic pregnancy. *Note*: All patients at high risk for EP should receive a gynecologic consultation. TAS = transabdominal sonography; TVS = transvaginal ultrasonography.

15. Why is methotrexate used for EP?

Methotrexate, which is a chemical poison for the rapidly growing cells of pregnancy, has replaced surgery for many patients with small EPs (usually without fetal heart tones, < 4 cm diameter, or hCG level < 10,000 mIU/mL IRP [International Reference Preparation]) without signs of significant peritoneal bleeding. Failure rates of about 10% are seen, so the patient still must be followed closely. Patients commonly have significant pain and may have peritoneal findings several days after treatment with methotrexate. Abnormal vital signs, a decreasing hematocrit, or diffuse peritoneal signs are indications that rupture of the EP may have occurred. The gynecologist administering methotrexate should be involved in assessment of these patients.

BIBLIOGRAPHY

1. Abbott JT, Emmans L, Lowenstein SR: Ectopic pregnancy: Ten common pitfalls in diagnosis. Am J Emerg Med 8:515–522, 1990.
2. Barnhart K, Mennuti MT, Benjamin I, et al: Prompt diagnosis of ectopic pregnancy in an emergency department setting. Obstet Gynecol 84:1010–1015, 1994.
3. Dart RG, Kaplan B, Varaklis K: Predictive value of history and physical examination in patients with suspected ectopic pregnancy. Ann Emerg Med 33:283–290, 1999.
4. Garcia CR, Barnhart KT: Diagnosing ectopic pregnancy: Decision analysis comparing six strategies. Obstet Gynecol 97:464–470, 2001.
5. Houry D, Abbott JT: Acute complications of pregnancy. In Marx JA, et al (eds): Rosen's Emergency Medicine: Concepts and Clinical Practice, 5th ed. St. Louis, Mosby, 1998, pp 2413–2433.
6. Kaplan BC, Dart RG, Moskos M, et al: Ectopic pregnancy: Prospective study with improved diagnostic accuracy. Ann Emerg Med 28:10–17, 1996.
7. Mol BWJ, Hajenius PJ, Engelsbel S, et al: Serum human chorionic gonadotropin measurement in the diagnosis of ectopic pregnancy when transvaginal sonography is inconclusive. Fertil Steril 70:972–981, 1998.

100. THIRD-TRIMESTER VAGINAL BLEEDING

John M. Howell, M.D.

1. Name the sources of third-trimester vaginal bleeding.
The vagina, cervix, and uterus.

2. List the causes.
Placenta previa
Placental abruption
Marginal sinus rupture
Bloody show
Local trauma
Cervical polyps and lesions

3. Name the life-threatening causes.
Placenta previa, placental abruption, and uterine rupture.

4. What is the frequency of placenta previa?
0.3% to 0.5% of live births.

5. What is placenta previa?
Placenta previa occurs when the placenta implants on or near the cervical os. Total coverage of the cervical os by placenta is called **complete placenta previa**, whereas subtotal coverage is called **partial placenta previa**. Marginal placenta previa occurs when the margin of the placenta approaches but does not cover any of the cervical os.

6. Why is placenta previa dangerous?
Vaginal penetration or manipulation of the placenta during a pelvic examination may rupture blood vessels and cause massive hemorrhage, which in turn may cause maternal or fetal demise.

7. How is placenta previa diagnosed?
Color flow Doppler ultrasound is 82% sensitive and 91% to 96% specific in diagnosing placenta previa. Placenta previa frequently is diagnosed early in pregnancy and followed with serial

ultrasound studies until delivery. Occasionally, gravid women present with vaginal bleeding and an undiagnosed placental abnormality.

8. What is the clinical presentation?

If vaginal bleeding occurs, it is generally painless and bright red in color. Palpation of the fetus is not difficult. Fetal heart tones are heard, and there is no coagulopathy.

9. How is placenta previa treated?

If the diagnosis is considered, call for an immediate obstetric consultation. Do not perform a pelvic examination unless you are in the operating room or delivery suite with an experienced obstetrician; life-threatening bleeding may occur if the placenta is manipulated inadvertently. Place the patient on her left side in the recumbent position. In patients who are hemodynamically stable with small amounts of bleeding, start an intravenous line, and admit the patient for ultrasound, serial maternal vital signs, and fetal monitoring. In selected cases, delivery is delayed to optimize fetal development. If serious vaginal bleeding occurs, start two large-bore intravenous lines, administer oxygen, monitor fetal heart tones, and admit the patient for delivery.

10. What is placental abruption (abruptio placentae)?

The premature separation of the placenta from its insertion on the uterine wall.

11. What is the incidence of placental abruption?

0.8% to 1.2% of pregnancies.

12. Why is placental abruption dangerous?

A large amount of blood may collect between the placenta and the uterine wall, causing maternal shock and fetal demise.

13. What is the clinical presentation?

Abruption occurs spontaneously or after mild, moderate, or severe trauma. The uterus is firm or hard, and the patient reports severe abdominal pain. Hypotension may occur, and vaginal bleeding occurs in about 80% of patients. If vaginal bleeding does occur, the blood is dark red. This presentation is in contrast to the painless, bright red bleeding of placenta previa. The presence of additional blood in the uterus makes palpating the fetus and measuring fetal heart tones difficult. Coagulopathy may occur.

14. What percentage of patients with placental abruption have no vaginal bleeding?

15% to 20%.

15. How is placental abruption diagnosed?

Ultrasound. A clinical diagnosis is made when the mother or fetus is in danger, and the signs and symptoms suggest placental abruption.

16. Describe the treatment of placental abruption.

Start two large-bore intravenous lines, and administer oxygen. Monitor fetal heart tones and the mother's vital signs frequently. If possible, place on a fetal monitor. Obtain coagulation studies to diagnose coagulopathy. If the mother and fetus are stable, arrange an immediate ultrasound. Take unstable patients directly to the operating room or delivery suite for delivery.

17. What is uterine rupture?

A grave complication of late pregnancy in which the uterus ruptures, usually during contractions.

18. What is the frequency of uterine rupture?

0.05% of pregnancies.

19. Why is uterine rupture dangerous?

It can produce massive, life-threatening intraabdominal hemorrhage. Maternal mortality is 8%, and fetal mortality is about 50%.

20. List the causes of uterine rupture.

- Excessive intrauterine pressures during oxytocin stimulation or a difficult labor with cephalopelvic disproportion
- Weakening of the uterine wall owing to multiparity
- Placenta percreta (extension of villi through the uterine myometrium)

21. What is the clinical presentation of uterine rupture?

Sudden abdominal pain and shock late in pregnancy associated with uterine contractions. There is scant vaginal bleeding, and the abdomen is extremely tender.

22. What is the treatment?

Start two large-bore intravenous lines, and administer oxygen with immediate transfer to the operating room or delivery suite for laparotomy and hysterectomy. Ultrasound may be necessary in selected cases to distinguish uterine rupture from placental abruption.

23. Describe the non-life-threatening causes of third-trimester vaginal bleeding.

Bloody show is a pink mucous discharge caused by cervical changes that precedes labor by several hours to a week. The cervix is prone to hemorrhage during late pregnancy, and local trauma from vaginal penetration, including intercourse, may cause bleeding. Cervical erosions or preexisting polyps produce limited bleeding. Marginal sinus rupture is a premature separation of the placenta limited to the placental margin.

BIBLIOGRAPHY

1. Catanzarite V, Maida C, Thomas W, et al: Prenatal sonographic diagnosis of vasa previa: Ultrasound findings and obstetric outcome in ten cases. Ultrasound Obstet Gynecol 18:109–115, 2001.
2. Chou MM, Ho ES, Lee YH: Prenatal diagnosis of placenta previa accreta by transabdominal color Doppler ultrasound. Ultrasound Obstet Gynecol 15:28–35, 2000.
3. Crane S, Chun B, Acker D: Treatment of obstetrical hemorrhagic emergencies. Curr Opin Obstet Gynecol 5:675–682, 1993.
4. Cunningham FG, MacDonald PC, Gant NF, et al: Williams Obstetrics, 20th ed. Stamford CT, Appleton & Lange, 1997, pp 745–782.
5. Lavery JP: Placenta previa. Clin Obstet Gynecol 33:414–431, 1990.
6. McKennett M, Fullerton JT: Vaginal bleeding in pregnancy. Am Fam Physician 51:639–646, 1995.
7. Mishell DR, Brenner PF (eds): Management of Common Problems in Obstetrics and Gynecology, 3rd ed. Boston, Blackwell Scientific, 1994, pp 211–215.
8. Scott JR, Disaia PJ, Hammond CB, et al (eds): Danforth's Obstetrics and Gynecology, 7th ed. Philadelphia, J.B. Lippincott, 1994.

101. PREECLAMPSIA AND ECLAMPSIA

Robert S. Van Hare, M.D.

1. Is every pregnant patient with hypertension considered preeclamptic or eclamptic?

No. Hypertension during gestation can be divided into four categories:

1. Preeclampsia/eclampsia
2. Chronic hypertension
3. Chronic hypertension with superimposed preeclampsia
4. Late or transient hypertension

Preeclampsia/eclampsia and chronic hypertension with superimposed preeclampsia pose the greatest threat to fetal and maternal well-being. Chronic hypertension is hypertension of whatever cause that predates the pregnancy; it accounts for one third of all cases of hypertension in pregnancy. Late or transient hypertension consists of mild or at most moderate elevation of blood pressure near term but may herald the development of essential hypertension later in life.

2. How does toxemia of pregnancy fit into this categorization?

It is an older term that refers to the specific entities of preeclampsia and eclampsia and is defined as the onset of hypertension and proteinuria or edema after the 20th gestational week.

3. Define preeclampsia.

Acute elevation of blood pressure (> 140/90 mmHg, > 30 mmHg elevation in systolic blood pressure, or > 15 mmHg elevation in diastolic blood pressure above baseline levels) accompanied by proteinuria (1 g/L in random specimens at least 6 hours apart or > 3 g/L in a 24-hour collection). The third traditional requirement is generalized edema (no longer recognized by many authorities).

4. What is the cause of preeclampsia/eclampsia?

This is an easy question to answer correctly because if you do not know the answer, you are right! Despite decades of research, the exact pathogenesis of preeclampsia is not fully understood. It generally is accepted that there is a problem in the early development of the placental blood supply. This hypoperfused placenta releases toxic mediators that result in end-organ hypoperfusion and damage.

5. State the incidence of preeclampsia/eclampsia.

5% to 10% of all pregnancies.

6. Who is predisposed to preeclampsia/eclampsia?

Preeclampsia/eclampsia occurs most commonly in young primiparous women, older multiparous women, and women with a positive family history. Diabetes, obesity, multiple gestation, preexisting hypertension, hydatidiform mole, and fetal hydrops are predisposing factors. It is also more prevalent in lower socioeconomic groups.

7. What laboratory tests predict who will develop preeclampsia/eclampsia?

No test has emerged as an early indicator of preeclampsia/eclampsia. Rising uric acid levels and declining platelet counts are the earliest signs, but these usually appear late in the disease process and may precede a symptomatic crisis by less than 1 week.

8. Are there any proven treatments to prevent preeclampsia?

No. There is no proven way to prevent preeclampsia. Initial trials of aspirin were favorable but now seem only to benefit high-risk patients. Calcium supplementation is more effective in patients with transient hypertension than patients with preeclampsia. Good prenatal care and regular obstetric visits focusing on early detection are essential.

9. Is there a role for outpatient management of preeclampsia?

Not usually. Clinical evaluation of the preeclamptic patient is inaccurate in predicting which patients may develop eclamptic seizures. The blood pressure of the preeclamptic patient can escalate quickly to dangerous levels. A patient with mild preeclampsia who can be relied on to follow the physician's instructions can be managed closely on an outpatient basis. Obstetric consultation is essential, however, and admission usually is indicated because of the potential maternal and fetal risks.

10. List some of the signs of severe preeclampsia.

Rising blood pressure (> 160/110 mmHg)	Right upper quadrant pain
Heavy proteinuria (> 5 g/L in 24 hours)	Hemolytic anemia
Oliguria	Elevated liver enzymes
Headache	Elevated serum creatinine
Visual disturbances	Fetal growth retardation
Apprehension	Thrombocytopenia
Pulmonary edema	Hyperreflexia

11. Name the most frequent cause of maternal death in preeclampsia/eclampsia.

Central nervous system disorders, including cortical and subcortical hemorrhages, microinfarctions, cerebral edema, subarachnoid hemorrhage, and large intracerebral hematomas.

12. What are the fetal risks in a preeclamptic/eclamptic pregnancy?

The fetus experiences complications from the mother's toxemic state, including severe growth retardation, hypoxemia, acidosis, prematurity, and death.

13. Define eclampsia.

The development of seizures (generalized motor type) or coma in a patient with preeclampsia. It carries a grave prognosis. With proper management, maternal mortality is less than 1%; fetal mortality is greater than 10%.

14. Does a patient have to be pregnant to become eclamptic?

No, but this is a trick question. A preeclamptic patient may worsen after delivery (technically no longer pregnant) and develop late postpartum eclampsia, which usually occurs in the first 24 to 48 hours postpartum but which may not present until several weeks after delivery.

15. Describe the treatment for a preeclamptic/eclamptic patient.

If preeclampsia develops after 34 weeks' gestation and the fetus has adequate pulmonary maturity, delivery is the definitive treatment. Before 34 weeks, delivery may be postponed if the blood pressure can be controlled adequately and there are no signs of impending eclampsia. Depending on ethical considerations, delivery also is indicated at any gestational age if the patient has severe preeclampsia or impending eclampsia. Before delivery, blood pressure must be controlled and seizure prophylaxis initiated.

16. What is the current prophylaxis and treatment of eclamptic seizures?

Prophylaxis should be considered in all preeclamptic patients during risk periods: labor, delivery, and 24 hours postpartum. Although controversy continues, magnesium sulfate still is the drug of choice of obstetricians in the United States. The loading dose is 4 to 6 g of magnesium sulfate in a 10% solution infused slowly over 5 to 10 minutes. The maintenance dose is 1 to 2 g/h intravenously.

17. Is magnesium sulfate the standard of care worldwide?

No. In Europe, Great Britain, and Australia, phenytoin and benzodiazepines are used much more frequently than magnesium in the treatment of eclamptic seizures. This is changing, however. More recent studies have shown the superiority of magnesium sulfate over phenytoin and benzodiazepines in controlling and preventing recurrent seizures in eclamptic patients. ED physicians need to establish a therapeutic management plan that is acceptable to consulting obstetricians and neurologists.

18. What are the risks of magnesium therapy?

Excessive magnesium sulfate can lead to loss of reflexes (> 8 mEq/L), double vision, flushing, somnolence, slurred speech, and, eventually cardiac and respiratory arrest (> 12 mEq/L).

Monitor reflexes; when they disappear, stop the infusion. If magnesium toxicity ensues, it should be treated with 10 mL of 10% calcium gluconate slow intravenous push.

19. How is the elevated blood pressure of preeclampsia/eclampsia emergently controlled?

Antihypertensive agents usually are reserved until the blood pressure is 160/110 mmHg. Treatment goals are a blood pressure range of 140 to 150/90 to 100 mmHg. Hydralazine is the most frequent drug of choice. Labetalol is also an acceptable choice. Diazoxide is popular in Australia but is not used as widely in the United States. In a life-threatening situation unresponsive to prior measures, nitroprusside may be used but only for a short duration because of the risk of fetal cyanide toxicity. Nifedipine is advocated by some authors; diuretics and angiotensin-converting enzyme inhibitors are contraindicated.

20. What is the HELLP syndrome?

Hemolysis, elevated liver enzymes, and low platelet count. Described in 1982, it is controversial whether HELLP syndrome is a variant of preeclampsia/eclampsia or a separate complication of pregnancy. It is present in about 5% to 10% of patients with severe preeclampsia. The HELLP syndrome should be managed in the same manner as severe preeclampsia.

21. What are the clinical manifestations of the HELLP syndrome?

Most patients usually present before term complaining of epigastric and right upper quadrant pain, nausea or vomiting, and nonspecific viral illness-like symptoms. Headache is a frequent complaint. Hypertension and proteinuria may be absent or minimal.

22. What are the primary differential diagnoses of the HELLP syndrome?

The differential diagnosis includes many entities ranging from gastroenteritis and hyperemesis gravidarum to gallbladder and peptic ulcer disease. A more specific differential includes acute fatty liver of pregnancy, hepatitis, thrombotic thrombocytopenic purpura, idiopathic thrombocytopenic purpura, disseminated intravascular coagulation (caused by sepsis, hypovolemia, hemorrhage), and hemolytic-uremic syndrome.

23. What is an acute life-threatening complication of the HELLP syndrome?

Any patient who presents with shoulder pain, shock, evidence of massive ascites, or a pleural effusion may have a ruptured or unruptured subcapsular liver hematoma. Even appropriate management results in greater than 60% fetal mortality and 50% maternal mortality.

BIBLIOGRAPHY

1. Abbot J: Complications related to pregnancy. In Rosen P, Barkin RM (eds): Emergency Medicine: Concepts and Clinical Practice, 4th ed. St. Louis, Mosby, 1998, pp 2353–2355.
2. Ellison J, Sattar N, Greer I: HELLP syndrome: Mechanisms and management. Hosp Med 60:243–249, 1999.
3. Mabie WC, Sibai BM: Hypertensive states of pregnancy. In DeCherney AH, Pernoll ML (eds): Current Obstetric and Gynecologic Diagnosis and Treatment, 8th ed. East Norwalk, CT, Appleton & Lange, 1994.
4. Mathews J: Hypertension. In Rosen P, Barkin RM (eds): Emergency Medicine: Concepts and Clinical Practice, 4th ed. St. Louis, Mosby, 1998, pp1761–1762.
5. Mushambi MC, Halligan AW, Williamson K: Recent developments in the pathophysiology and management of pre-eclampsia. Br J Anaesth 76:133–148, 1996.
6. Patrick T, Roberts J: Current concepts in preeclampsia. MCN Am J Matern Child Nurs 24:193–201, 1999.
7. Sibai B, Ramadan M: Preeclampsia and exlampsia. In Sciarra J (ed): Gynecology and Obstetrics, 3rd ed. Philadelphia, Lippincott Williams & Wilkins, 2000, pp 1–15.
8. Usta IM, Sibai BM: Emergent management of puerperal eclampsia. Obstet Gynecol Clin North Am 22:315–335, 1995.

9. VanWijk M, Kublickiene K, Boer K, VanBavel E: Vascular function in preeclampsia. Cardiovasc Res 47:38–48, 2000.
10. Witlin AG, Sibai BM: Hypertension in pregnancy: Current concepts of preeclampsia. Ann Rev Med 48:115–127, 1997.
11. Zamorski MA, Green LA: Preeclampsia and hypertensive disorders of pregnancy. Am Fam Physician 53:1595–1604, 1996.

102. CHILDBIRTH

Richard O. Jones, M.D.

1. I'm an ED physician. Why should I learn about childbirth?
The delivery of newborn infants in the ED is a fact of life. The main objective should be a healthy infant and mother. Help should be sought from Obstetrics and Pediatrics as soon as it is evident that the delivery of an infant is going to occur in the ED. Most mistakes in the care of the newborn are made as the result of panic, which can be avoided if the guidelines presented here are followed.

2. What is the most important thing to learn from this chapter?
Labor and delivery is a natural process, which usually proceeds to its conclusion without difficulty. Little intervention is required on the part of the health care provider.

3. When a pregnant patient is brought to the ED, what factors should direct treatment?
The welfare of the mother must come first. After the mother is evaluated and stabilized, the pregnancy and fetus can be evaluated. If your hospital has obstetric coverage, the obstetrician should be notified as soon as possible.

4. What information do I need to care properly for the pregnant patient?
If the patient is conscious, she can give the due date and relate if the fetus is moving. She can also tell you if she is contracting, bleeding, or leaking fluid. Problems with the pregnancy and what medications she is taking and why can be discussed.

5. How are the fetus and pregnancy evaluated?
Indirect evaluation of the fetus can provide a great deal of information. Fetal heart tones should be obtained as soon as the mother is stabilized. Next, the fundal height (the distance in centimeters from the symphysis pubis to the top of the pregnant uterus) should be measured to give a rough estimate of gestational age. A fundal height of 32 cm would give a rough estimate of a pregnancy between 30 and 34 weeks. Ultrasound can confirm the gestational age, weight, and position of the fetus. Ultrasound also can locate the placenta and evaluate amniotic fluid. External fetal monitoring can identify the pattern of the fetal heart rate and the mother's contraction pattern.

6. What is false labor?
Contractions without cervical change. This is a common occurrence.

7. When can the diagnosis of true labor be made?
When the patient is having effacement and dilation of the cervix with contractions.

8. If the evaluation shows the patient is in labor but is not very dilated, can she be taken to labor and delivery?
If delivery is not imminent, taking the patient to labor and delivery is the best option. If the patient is well along in labor, and delivery is imminent, you should prepare for delivery in the ED.

9. How can I determine if a delivery is imminent?

This can be difficult. If examination of the patient reveals the cervix is ≥ 7 cm dilated, and the patient has the urge to push with (or especially between) contractions, delivery may occur before or during transport to Labor and Delivery.

10. How long does labor usually last?

In a first-time mother (**primigravida**), labor lasts an average of 10 hours but can last 26 hours (5th percentile). If the mother has had a baby previously (**multipara**), this time is shortened to less than 7 hours on average to 20 hours (5th percentile).

11. What is the most important sign of the progress of labor?

Cervical dilation.

12. How do you check cervical dilation?

Under sterile conditions, a digital pelvic examination is performed. The diameter of the cervical opening in front of the fetus's head is estimated in centimeters. The measurements vary from *closed* up to 10 cm. Practice is required for accuracy.

13. Describe the sequence of a normal labor.

First stage: The cervix thins out and dilates in response to contractions. This is divided into latent phase, active phase, and deceleration phase. The **latent phase** can last 20 hours (average 6.5 hours) in a primigravida and 14 hours (average 5 hours) in a multigravida. During the **active phase**, the most rapid dilation of the cervix takes place. The contractions are much stronger and more painful than in the latent phase. This phase usually lasts no longer than 5 hours in a primigravida and 3 hours in a multigravida. The **deceleration phase** takes place in the last hour or so before the cervix is completely dilated at 10 cm. During this phase, dilation slows, and the head begins to descend down the birth canal.

Second stage: The patient is completely dilated. This stage ends when the infant is delivered. The patient is allowed to push when the cervix is completely dilated. This shortens the second stage. Even if the patient did not push, the uterine contractions would cause delivery. The second stage can last 2 hours in a primigravida and usually is much shorter in a multigravida.

Third stage: The third stage begins after the infant is delivered and ends when the placenta is delivered; 30 minutes may be reasonably allowed for the third stage.

14. I have a pregnant patient in the ED and the infant's head can be seen distending the perineum. The obstetrician is on the way but will not make it in time. How do I deliver the baby?

Wearing sterile gloves, apply gentle pressure against the infant's head to prevent sudden expulsion and to allow gradual stretching of the perineum. It may be necessary to rupture the membranes with a clamp before the head is delivered.

15. If the umbilical cord is wrapped around the neck during a delivery, what should I do?

If the cord is wrapped around the neck, it should be pulled gently over the head if possible so that it does not tighten as the infant is being born. If the cord is too tight to lift over the head, apply two clamps to the cord and cut the cord between the clamps. Then the cord can be unwound from around the neck.

16. Okay, the head is out. What do I do next?

With the mother pushing and with your hands on the sides of the infant's head, apply gentle downward pressure to allow the infant's anterior shoulder to slip underneath the mother's pubic bone. Then apply gentle upward pressure to deliver the infant's posterior shoulder. The rest of the infant's body should follow quickly, so keep a good grip. Be sure to note the time of delivery.

17. What do I do now that the infant is delivered?

Holding the infant head down, suction the nose and mouth with a bulb syringe. Most infants cough out the amniotic fluid without help as long as they are held head down. Then apply two clamps to the umbilical cord (at least several centimeters from the infant's abdomen), and cut the cord between the clamps. To prevent the infant from becoming too cold from evaporation, the infant should be dried and kept warm. After drying, the infant can be placed on the mother's abdomen for skin-to-skin contact, which provides warmth.

18. Do I need to deliver the placenta?

There is no hurry to deliver the placenta until the obstetrician arrives, unless there is heavy bleeding. If there is heavy bleeding, have the mother push out the placenta. Do not pull on the cord. Massaging the uterus through the mother's abdominal wall helps control blood loss.

19. The placenta is out, but there was a tear at the bottom of the perineum that is bleeding. What do I do?

As with any laceration, applying pressure usually stems the bleeding until the obstetrician arrives. If necessary, local anesthetic can be given to allow suturing of the laceration.

20. What is premature labor?

Labor that takes place when the patient is between 20 and 37 weeks' gestation.

21. Why is premature labor important?

Premature delivery is the number one cause of damage and death of infants worldwide; 10% to 12% of pregnancies deliver prematurely. The earlier in pregnancy the infant is born, the more likely the infant is to suffer permanent damage or die. At 24 weeks, only 30% to 60% of infants survive. Of the 24-week infants that survive, 19 out of 20 suffer permanent damage. It is estimated that 50% of permanent neurologic damage suffered by newborns is due to premature delivery.

22. If a premature baby is going to deliver in the ED, do I do anything differently?

No, the delivery technique is the same. Keep the baby warm and dry and be ready to help with breathing problems. Turn the baby over to the pediatrician as soon as possible. (See Chapter 80, Neonatal Resuscitation.)

BIBLIOGRAPHY

1. American Academy of Pediatrics and the American College of Obstetricians and Gynecologists: Guidelines for Perinatal Care, 4th ed. Washington, DC, AAP and ACOG, 1997.
2. American College of Obstetricians and Gynecologists: Ultrasonography in Pregnancy. ACOG Technical Bulletin 187. Washington, DC, ACOG, 1993.
3. Eason E, Labrecque M, Wells G, Feldman P: Preventing perineal trauma during childbirth: A systematic review. Obstet Gynecol 95:464, 2000.
4. Gabbe SG, Niebyl JR, Simpson JL, et al (eds): Obstetrics, 4th ed. Philadelphia, Churchill Livingstone, 2002.

XVI. Trauma

103. INJURY PREVENTION

Kerry B. Broderick, M.D.

1. What is injury?
A harmful event that occurs from the transfer of energy to a living organism that results in tissue damage. The injury triangle **agent**, **host**, and **environment** was subdivided further in the 1960s by Haddon, who divided each factor into three phases: preinjury, injury, and postinjury. This phase matrix has become the mainstay of injury prevention work.

2. List the factors involved in injury prevention.
- **Epidemiology**—understanding patterns of disease and outcomes of prevention interventions
- **Biomechanics**—understanding how the agent interacts with the host and improving factors to decrease possible injury
- **Public and patient education**
- **Public policy and law enforcement**

3. Why should I care?
Of all ED visits, 33% are the result of injury. Each year, 1 in 4 Americans seeks medical care because of an injury. An estimated 23 to 28 million people are treated by emergency physicians for injury, with 10% being admitted to the hospital. Of injured people, 90% are seen only in the ED. The ED encounter may be the only opportunity for a health care provider to intervene and have an impact on decreasing future injury risk behavior in patients.

4. Name the agents involved in causing injury.
Vehicles, motorized and nonmotorized; guns; falls; blunt force; and knives and other sharp penetrating objects.

5. What is the most common cause of injury?
Motor vehicle crashes (MVCs). Estimates are greater than 3 million injuries a year and 40,000 fatalities from motorized vehicles. On average, 115 people die each day as a result of MVCs.

6. What is the estimated cost of MVC injuries?
Greater than $150 billion a year, or 2.2% of the gross domestic product. This is more than the entire 1998 Medicaid budget.

7. Are there any high-risk groups in MVCs?
- In 1998, more 18-year-olds died in MVCs than any other single age.
- The ages of 15 to 20 account for more than one fifth of all passenger fatalities (22%).
- More 21-year-olds died in alcohol-related crashes than any other age.

8. Is there a high-risk time of year for MVCs?
The greatest number of fatalities occur in June, July, and August.

9. Is there any good news regarding MVC injury prevention?

Since 1982, there has been a 63% reduction of alcohol-related motor vehicle injuries and fatalities. The National Highway Traffic Safety Administration (NHTSA) estimated that raising the minimal drinking age and zero tolerance laws have saved about 20,000 lives since 1975.

10. Do motor vehicle restraint devices really prevent injury?

Overall, it is estimated that safety belts, air bags, and child restraint seats save about 11,000 lives annually.

Seat belts reduce the risk of death by 60% and the risk of serious injury by 65%. If everyone buckled up every time, almost 10,000 lives would be saved every year.

Air bags reduce the risk of injury to drivers by 36% and car passengers by 32%. The NHTSA estimates that 7,585 people are alive today because of air bags.

Child restraint seats reduce deaths by almost 70%.

The average hospital cost for MVC victims is 55% higher for those who did not use a restraint device compared with those who did.

11. Can air bags be dangerous?

Air bags deploy in $\frac{1}{25}$ of a second at speeds reaching 150 to 200 mph, with deflation occurring within 2 seconds. Since 1990, there have been a total of 202 confirmed air-bag deaths (68 drivers, 8 adult passengers, and 126 children) with proximity to the air bag being the issue in nearly every death. Children are more likely to suffer injuries because of their short stature: The head and neck are likely to be impacted, and they cannot brace themselves against the floor. Most injuries are the result of severe closed head injury or cervical spine injuries with associated spinal cord transection. Children younger than 12 years old should be appropriately restrained and in the back seat.

Almost all adults, including adults of small stature and older adults, can be protected best from air-bag injury by buckling their seat belt and keeping at least a 10-inch distance between the air bag cover and their breastbone. There is a serious risk to injury only if one is close to the air bag cover when it deploys (within 2 to 3 inches). If a person is unable, because of health or physical stature reasons, to keep 10 inches away from the air bag cover, automobile manufacturers as of 1998 installed on-off switches. People should visit NHTSA's web site for a request and information brochure at http://www.nhtsa.dot.gov or call the NHTSA's toll-free auto safety hotline at 1-800-424-9393.

12. Do helmets really work?

Motorcycle helmets: The NHTSA estimated that motorcycle helmets reduce the likelihood of dying in a crash by about 29% and the risk of fatal head injury by 40%. Studies of individual states documented sharp declines in death rates after enactment of comprehensive helmet laws and corresponding increases after repeal of these laws. Texas and Arkansas weakened their helmet laws in 1997, and the following year helmet use decreased dramatically in both states (Arkansas 97% to 55%, Texas 97% to 62%), and fatalities increased by 21% in Arkansas and 31% in Texas.

Bicycle helmets: National Electronic Injury Surveillance System data indicate that about half a million nonfatal bicycle-related injuries and 1,000 deaths are treated in EDs each year with a cost of $8 billion. Approximately one third of the total injuries involve the head or face; however, 62% of the fatalities involved a head injury. Children younger than 10 years old have a higher rate of head injury (50%) than children aged 10 and older (19%). Although studies showed that helmets reduce the risk of head injury by 50% to 60%, only about 18% (11.8 million) of bicycle riders wear helmets all or most of the time, and 6% (4 million) wear helmets less than half the time.

Snowboarding and skiing: Head injuries represent about 14% of all skiing and snowboarding injuries. In the age group less than 15 years old, head injuries account for about 22% of all injuries. In 1998, the Consumer Product Safety Commission estimated that 44% of head injuries (7,700) could have been attenuated by helmet use.

13. Do all states now have comprehensive motorcycle helmet laws?

In 1996, 25 states and Washington, D.C., had comprehensive helmet laws in effect, and another 22 states had underage helmet laws. The only 3 states with no helmet laws were Colorado, Illinois, and Iowa.

14. Do firearms really cause much injury?

Yes. Overall, including adults, in 1998 there were 30,708 firearm fatalities. In 1998, on average, one child or adolescent died from firearm-related injuries every 2 hours, resulting in 3,800 youth deaths. According to a 1994 report, the homicide rate for children in the United States was five times higher than for children in 25 other countries combined (2.57 per 100,000 compared with 0.51). For unintentional injury, the United States was nine times higher than 25 other countries (0.36 per 100,000 compared with 0.04). Handguns account for more than 50% of gun deaths, and suicides account for nearly 70% of gun deaths in urban and rural areas.

15. What about suicide and guns and teenagers?

In 1988, 1,372 adolescents intentionally killed themselves with firearms. The odds of death increase 75-fold when a suicidal teenager has access to a gun in the home.

16. Can education have an impact on firearm safety?

It is unclear if education has an improved outcome with firearm safety. Firearm safety counseling has been shown to increase the rate of safer firearm storage, particularly among parents. Studies showed that in homes with guns, the non-gun owner reported significantly lower rates of loaded guns and higher rates of locked guns than the gun owner. These data support other studies that show many married women are unaware that a gun is in the home. These data also suggest that a gun often is stored in a manner that experts believe is unsafe.

17. Summarize the facts on poisonings.

In 2000, there were 2 million reported poison exposures in the United States. On average, U.S. poison centers handled one poison exposure every 15 minutes.

Site of exposure:	92% occurred in the home, 2.5% in the workplace, 1.6% in schools, 0.5% in restaurants or food services, and 0.3% in health care facilities.
Age:	Children less than 3 years old accounted for 40% and children less than 6 years old accounted for 53% of exposures reported to national poison centers.
Gender:	Boys younger than 13 years old predominated; this trend reversed in teenage and adult years, with women predominating.
Substance:	Exposures were single substance in 92% and multiple substances in 2.4%.
Intention:	Exposures were unintentional in 86%, suicidal intent in 7.5%, and therapeutic error in 7.0%.
Site of care:	78% of patients were treated at a non-health care facility, and 22% were treated at a health care facility.
Fatalities:	Fatalities were 2.2% in children younger than 6 years old and 59% in adults 20 to 49 years old. 94% of adolescent deaths and 79% of adult deaths were intentional exposures.

18. What legislative initiatives have been effective in injury prevention?

Helmet laws, seatbelt laws, air-bag installation laws, and alcohol and motor vehicle use laws all have been proved to be effective. Since 1991, there have been seven published studies and one multistate study recently completed regarding the effectiveness of 0.08 g/dL blood alcohol level laws in reducing alcohol-related fatal crashes. These studies examined the experiences of 14 states that have enacted 0.08 g/dL blood alcohol level laws and provided consistent and persuasive evidence that these laws, particularly in combination with administrative license revocation laws, are associated with reductions in alcohol-related fatal crashes and fatalities. Multistate studies reported reductions ranging from 6% to 16%.

19. How can the ED best assist with injury prevention?
Patients present to the ED with various injuries and are vulnerable at that time to education and intervention regarding the events that may have affected their degree of injury. The ED staff can discuss this with the patient and give the patient educational materials to read at a later time. Multiple studies have looked at brief interventions in the ED and decreasing risk behavior. In one study, Bernstein et al showed that brief ED assessment and intervention for drugs and alcohol can reduce drug severity problems by 45%, reduce alcohol use by 56%, and reduce the frequency of 6 or more drinks at one sitting by 64%. This and other studies show that ED physicians can directly affect patient behavior through education in the ED.

BIBLIOGRAPHY

1. Branas CC, Knudson MM: State helmet laws and motorcycle rider death rates. Accid Anal Prev 33:641–648, 2001.
2. CDC: Rates of homicide, suicide, and firearm-related death among children—26 industrialized countries. JAMA 277:704–705, 1997.
3. Litovitz TL, Klein-Scwhartz W, White S, et al: 2000 Annual report of the American Association of Poison Control Centers Toxic Exposure Surveillance System. Am J Emerg Med 19:337–347, 2001.
4. Marx JA, Hockberger RS, Walls RM (eds): Rosen's Emergency Medicine: Concepts and Clinical Practice, 5th ed. St. Louis, Mosby, 2002.
5. NHTSA: Evaluation of motorcycle helmet law repeal in Arkansas and Texas. Available at www.nhtsa.dot. gov, pp 1–47.
6. NHTSA: 1998 Youth fatal crash and alcohol facts. Available at www.nhtsa.dot.gov, pp 1–13.
7. Rodgers G: Part I: An overview of the Bicycle Study. Consumer Product Safety Commission. 1988, pp 1–18.
8. Rodgers G: Part II. Bicycle and bicycle helmet use patterns in the United States: A description and analysis of national survey data. 1988, pp 19–54.
9. www.nhtsa.dot.gov/airbags/factsheets/numbers.html.
10. www.cdc.gov/ncipc/factsheets/fafacts.htm.

104. MULTIPLE TRAUMA

Peter Rosen, M.D.

1. What is multiple trauma?
Significant injury to more than one major body system or organ.

2. Can severity of injury be determined at the scene?
Not accurately because many younger patients have great reserves and do not show injuries that may be serious until they are ready to decompensate. A variety of different trauma scales and scoring devices have been developed to quantify the extent of injury. These devices are imperfect, however, and to maintain an acceptable safety margin, systems need to **overtriage** potential multiple-trauma victims. Transport to a trauma center should be based on the mechanism of injury, underlying disease, physiologic parameters such as alterations in vital signs and neurologic status, and the presence of obvious multiple organ system injury.

3. Define mechanism of injury.
Mechanism of injury refers to the events and conditions that lead to known and unknown traumatic injuries. Significant mechanism of injury is associated with a higher likelihood of multiple trauma. Less obvious mechanism is of greater concern with increasing age or preexisting disease. A 70-year-old patient with ankylosing spondylitis is much less able to tolerate blunt trauma to the spinal column and pelvis than is a healthy younger person.

4. Give examples of significant mechanisms of injury.

BLUNT TRAUMA		PENETRATING TRAUMA
Automobile accidents	Automobile-pedestrian accidents	Gunshot wounds to
Fatality at the scene	High speed	head, neck, torso
Passenger ejection	Damage to exterior of vehicle	
Vehicle rollover		Stab wounds to neck,
Significant interior	Falls	torso
damage	Greater than 1 story	
	(12–15 feet)	

5. List the first steps in managing multiple trauma in the ED.
- Activate the trauma resuscitation team.
- Designate a trauma captain and call for O-negative blood if indicated by prehospital course.
- Transfer the patient from the ambulance stretcher or other conveyance to the ED resuscitation bed.
- Quickly obtain a history, including the mechanism of injury, field treatment, and response to this field treatment.
- Obtain vital signs while the patient is being undressed.
- Assess the ABCs and intervene as necessary.
- Draw blood for type, crossmatching, and baseline laboratory testing.

6. How should the patient be undressed?
Because immobilization is necessary until the spine can be cleared, all movement should be avoided. To obtain complete visualization rapidly while protecting the spine, simply cut the clothes away. Keep in mind that one of the purposes of clothing removal is to rid the patient of objects that can cause further damage to the patient or injury to the health care providers, such as shards of broken glass, bits of metal, or weapons.

7. What are the ABCs (and D) of trauma?
Airway
Airway patency is evaluated by listening for vocalizations, asking for the patient's name, and looking in the patient's mouth for signs of obstruction (blood, emesis, or foreign debris). The trauma captain must determine if the patient needs active airway management and verify that supplemental oxygen is being administered continuously to all patients who do not require immediate intubation.

Mandatory indications for airway management in trauma:
- Massive facial injuries
- Head injury with Glasgow Coma Scale (GCS) less than 8
- Penetrating injury to the cranial vault
- Missile penetrating injury to the neck
- Blunt injury to the neck with expanding hematoma or alteration of the voice
- Multisystem trauma with persistent shock

Relative indications for airway management in trauma:
- Upper airway obstruction from any cause
- Any patient with injuries impairing ventilation
- Flail chest with increasing respiratory rate or deteriorating oxygenation
- Any patient with one or more rib fractures who is going to need a ventilator or a general anesthetic
- Patients with bilateral pneumothorax
- Bilateral missile penetrating injuries of the thorax
- Patients with continuing hemothorax that recurs or does not respond to tube thoracostomy
- Patients with severe hypovolemic shock

Breathing

Ventilation is assessed by observing for symmetric rise and fall of the chest and by listening for bilateral breath sounds over the anterior chest and axillae. The chest should be palpated gently for subcutaneous air and bony crepitus. Oxygen saturation should be monitored continuously. The trauma captain determines whether or not tube thoracostomies or ventilatory support is needed immediately.

Circulation

Circulatory function is assessed by noting the patient's mental status; skin color and character (cool and clammy versus warm and dry); vital signs; and presence or absence of radial, femoral, and carotid pulses. Continuous cardiac monitoring should be started. Prehospital vascular access and type and amount of volume infused are assessed. The trauma captain determines whether additional vascular access or volume of crystalloid is needed and if blood should be administered.

Disability

The patient's neurologic status should be assessed (level of consciousness and gross motor function). An initial ED GCS rating should be ascertained, and this should be compared with the prehospital GCS. With any alteration of consciousness, it is useful to perform a rectal examination to determine anal sphincter tone.

8. **What type of intravenous access should be established in a patient with major trauma?**

At least two large-bore ($\geq$ 16G) intravenous catheters should be placed. Forearm or antecubital veins are the preferred sites for initial access. Although subclavian and internal jugular catheters allow central venous pressure monitoring, they rarely provide access for high-volume intravenous infusions unless a Cordis introducer is left in place. These routes should be used only if no other access exists, and catheters should be placed on the ipsilateral side of the chest trauma unless a subclavian vascular injury is suspected. Femoral lines and cutdowns are indicated in patients with a dropping blood pressure because large-volume infusions will be needed quickly.

9. **Where should cutdowns be performed?**

The ankle. The distal saphenous vein can be found between the anterior tibialis tendon and the medial malleolus. Bedside ultrasound can increase the ability to insert a central line successfully.

10. **What parameters should be monitored in multiple trauma victims?**

Vital signs, neurologic status, cardiac rhythm, oxygen saturation, and, if possible, central venous pressure and urinary output. Hypothermia adversely affects outcome, and core temperature can drop rapidly when the patient is disrobed and receives large quantities of cold intravenous fluid. Tachypnea is a sensitive sign of hypoxia and acidosis and should be measured accurately rather than estimated. Neurologic status, skin color and character, and urinary output over time should be monitored.

11. **When should blood be administered?**

O-negative (universal donor) blood should be reserved for patients who are in arrest from hypovolemic shock. If 40 mL/kg of crystalloid is infused rapidly and there is no significant improvement in the patient's circulatory status, type-specific noncrossmatched blood should be administered if available. Otherwise, use type O initially. (For more details, see Chapter 4, Shock.)

12. **Are laboratory tests useful?**

No, although all major trauma victims should have a clot sent for type and crossmatch. Baseline values of hematocrit and serum amylase (or preferably lipase) may be useful in detecting occult injuries and preexisting anemia. Urinalysis should be done to detect hematuria. Many trauma centers obtain an extensive trauma panel, which may be useful if the patient requires surgery or has underlying disease. No laboratory test defines injury, however, and the trauma panel is of little use in determining initial management, disposition, or need for surgery.

Initial Laboratory Tests in Multiple Trauma

Complete blood cell count	Clot for type and crossmatch
Electrolytes	Urinalysis
Blood urea nitrogen, creatinine	Blood alcohol as indicated
Glucose	Toxicology screen as indicated
Prothrombin and partial thromboplastin times	Amylase lipase

13. What is the secondary survey?

The complete physical examination performed after the ABCs have been assessed and stabilized. This survey includes assessment of the chest, abdomen, pelvis, back, and extremities. A repeat neurologic examination and rectal examination also should be done. The purpose of the rectal examination is to determine if there is gross blood in the rectum, if there is adequate sphincter tone and sensation, and if the prostate gland is in a normal position.

14. Which radiologic studies need to be obtained immediately?

When the patient is stabilized, portable radiographs of the lateral cervical spine, chest, and pelvis should be obtained. In gunshot wounds, portable films in two planes may be needed to determine the location of the bullet. If the mechanism of injury is an ejection or a fall, a cross-table lumbar spine film should be added to the initial series.

15. How do I prioritize diagnostic tests?

Prioritization is based on potential life threats. After external hemorrhage is controlled, diagnosing intraperitoneal hemorrhage takes precedence. Unless an indication for immediate laparatomy is present, the patient should undergo diagnostic peritoneal lavage, abdominal CT scan, or abdominal ultrasound to assess the intraperitoneal cavity. After these procedures, attention should be focused on ruling out correctable intracranial hemorrhage, such as a subdural or an epidural hematoma. Based on the mechanism of injury and the initial course, other specialized studies to evaluate the aorta and the retroperitoneum should be done. If the patient has a bleeding diathesis (e.g., hemophilia) or is on an anticoagulant, even minor head injury mandates a CT scan.

BIBLIOGRAPHY

1. Feliciano DV, Moore EE, Mattox KL (eds): Trauma, 3rd ed. Stamford, CT, Appleton & Lange, 1996.
2. Gin-Shaw S, Jorden RC: Approach to the multiple trauma patient. In Marx JA, Hockberger RS, Walls RM (eds): Rosen's Emergency Medicine: Concepts and Clinical Practice, 5th ed. St. Louis, Mosby, 2002, pp 242–256.
3. Greenfield LJ, Mulholland MW, Oldham KT, et al (eds): Surgery: Scientific Principles and Practice, 2nd ed. Philadelphia, Lippincott-Raven, 1997.
4. Rosen P: General principles of trauma. In Harwood-Nuss AL, Linden CH, Luten RC, et al (eds): The Clinical Practice of Emergency Medicine, 3rd ed. Philadelphia, Lippincott-Raven, 2001, pp 410–416.

105. MAXILLOFACIAL TRAUMA

Carlo L. Rosen. M.D.

1. What is maxillofacial trauma?

Injury to the anatomic area bounded inferiorly by the mandible, superiorly by the scalp, and laterally from ear to ear. Trauma ranges from simple abrasion, contusion, laceration, fracture, or burn (contact or inhalation) to any combination of the above. The facial bones that may be injured are the frontal, temporal, nasal, ethmoid, lacrimal, palatine, sphenoid, zygoma, maxilla, and mandible.

2. What is the primary concern in a patient with maxillofacial trauma?

The initial management of patients with facial trauma should follow the **ABCs** (airway, breathing, circulation) of trauma resuscitation. The airway is the primary concern and can be challenging in these patients. Significant facial trauma may cause swelling or distortion of the airway as a result of bleeding, loose teeth, or fractures. In patients with mandibular fractures, the tongue loses its support and can occlude the airway. Early endotracheal intubation should be considered in patients with significant midface or mandibular trauma, especially if they exhibit any signs of airway distress. Stridor is the classic sign of an upper airway obstruction caused by a foreign body; hematoma; or edema of the tongue, oropharynx, hypopharynx, or larynx. Edema of the soft tissues progresses rapidly, compromising the patient's airway and the physician's ability to visualize the vocal cords. Standard methods of intubation, such as rapid-sequence intubation, should be attempted first; however, airway distortion resulting from facial trauma sometimes necessitates a cricothyrotomy. All patients with facial and head trauma should be assumed to have a cervical spine injury. In-line cervical spine stabilization should be used during the intubation. More recent data suggest that the incidence of cervical spine trauma in patients with facial fractures is 1% to 4%.

3. Which procedure is contraindicated in patients with maxillofacial trauma?

Nasogastric tube placement because of the risk of intracranial placement through a fracture in the cribriform plate. The small size and flexibility of the nasogastric tube allow it to be misdirected through a fracture into the brain. There is also a theoretical concern about placing a nasotracheal tube through the cribriform plate into the brain, even though an endotracheal tube is larger and more rigid than a nasogastric tube. Some authors showed that the risk of intracranial placement of a nasotracheal tube is low.

4. What is a blow-out fracture, and what is the entrapment syndrome?

A **blow-out fracture** is a fracture of the orbital floor that results from a direct blow to the orbit. Increased intraorbital pressure causes rupture of the floor of the orbit. The **entrapment syndrome** is binocular diplopia and paralysis of upward gaze that results from entrapment of the inferior rectus muscle in the orbital wall defect. Diplopia is noted by having the patient follow and count fingers on upward gaze. Other physical findings include infraorbital anesthesia and enophthalmos (posterior displacement of the globe into the orbit). Patients may have tenderness or step-offs at the infraorbital rim or subcutaneous emphysema secondary to a fracture into the maxillary sinus. Ophthalmologic evaluation for associated orbital trauma (hyphema, retinal tear or detachment, closed-angle glaucoma, blindness) despite an initially normal visual acuity and funduscopic examination should be considered.

5. What are Le Fort fractures?

Midface fractures diagnosed by grasping the upper alveolar ridge and noting which part of the midface moves. **Le Fort 1**, a transverse fracture just above the teeth at the level of the nasal fossa, allows movement of the alveolar ridge and hard palate. **Le Fort 2**, a pyramid fracture with its apex just above the bridge of the nose and extending laterally and inferiorly through the infraorbital rims, allows movement of the maxilla, nose, and infraorbital rims. **Le Fort 3**, the most serious of the Le Fort fractures, represents complete craniofacial disruption and involves fractures of the zygoma, infraorbital rims, and maxilla. It is rare for these fracture types to occur in isolation; they usually occur in combination (one type on one side of the face and another on the other side).

Cerebrospinal fluid leaks, although occult in presentation, may result in significant morbidity if unrecognized and should be assessed by checking for glucose with a Dextrostix or by observing for a halo ring on the gurney linen. Cervical spine injury should be suspected, given the force necessary to produce a midfacial fracture. Plain radiographs are a useful screening examination, but CT is the diagnostic modality of choice.

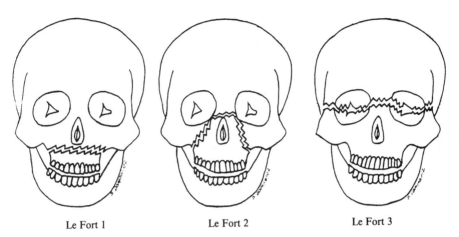

| Le Fort 1 | Le Fort 2 | Le Fort 3 |

Classification of true Le Fort fractures. Typically patients with Le Fort fractures present with a combination of the above.

6. When are nasal radiographs indicated?

Almost never. Nasal fractures typically are a clinical diagnosis without the need for routine radiographs. Physical examination may reveal swelling, angulation, bony crepitus, deformity, pain on palpation, epistaxis, and periorbital ecchymosis. Nasal radiographs are neither sensitive nor specific for fractures. The results do not alter management.

7. What is a septal hematoma, and why is it important?

All patients with nasal trauma and suspicion of a nasal fracture require inspection of the nasal septum for a septal hematoma. This is a collection of blood between the mucoperichondrium and the cartilage of the septum. It appears as a grapelike swelling over the nasal septum. If left undrained, it may result in septal abscess, necrosis of the nasal cartilage, and permanent deformity. If a septal hematoma is identified, incision and drainage is indicated in the ED, followed by nasal packing, antistaphylococcal antibiotics (prophylaxis for toxic shock syndrome), and prompt referral.

8. When should a consultation be obtained for a nasal fracture?

Most nasal fractures do not require immediate reduction unless there is significant deformity and malalignment. After anesthetizing the nose with cocaine-soaked or tetracaine-soaked gauze or pledgets, early reduction of an angulated fracture is done by exerting firm, quick pressure toward the midline with both thumbs. Patients should be referred to a maxillofacial surgeon for follow-up in 4 to 7 days after resolution of edema. Immediate consultation is suggested for nasal fractures with associated facial fractures, cerebrospinal fluid rhinorrhea, and sustained epistaxis.

9. How is a frontal sinus fracture diagnosed?

Frontal sinus fracture should be suspected in any patient with a severe blow to the forehead. The clinical signs include supraorbital nerve anesthesia, anosmia, cerebrospinal fluid rhinorrhea, subconjunctival hematoma, crepitus, and tenderness to palpation. The preferred diagnostic modality is CT to determine if there is involvement of the anterior or posterior walls of the sinus. Because of the proximity to the brain, cranial CT should be obtained to rule out intracranial hemorrhage.

10. How are frontal sinus fractures treated?

After surgical consultation, patients with nondisplaced anterior wall fractures may be discharged on prophylactic antibiotics, with instructions to avoid Valsalva maneuvers and to follow-up in 1 week with the surgical consultant. Patients with displaced anterior wall and sinus floor fractures require surgical consultation, admission, and antibiotic therapy. Patients with posterior wall fractures require antibiotics and immediate neurosurgical consultation.

11. What are the classic zygoma fractures?

The zygoma is the third most commonly fractured facial bone (after the nose and mandible). Zygoma fractures are classified into three basic types:

1. **Arch:** The bone may be fractured in one or two places and may be nondisplaced or displaced medially. Pain and trismus are caused by bony arch fragments abutting the coronoid process of the mandible. Because the masseter muscle originates on the zygoma, any movement causes further arch disruption. The fracture is diagnosed by the plain radiograph bucket-handle view (submentovertex).

2. **Tripod:** This is the most serious type of zygoma fracture, which involves the infraorbital rim, the zygomaticofrontal suture, and the zygomaticotemporal suture. Clinical signs include deformity (flatness of the cheek), infraorbital nerve hypesthesia, inferior rectus muscle entrapment, and diplopia on upward gaze. Although these fractures may be detected on plain radiographs (Waters and Caldwell views), CT is necessary to define better the extent of the fracture. For these fractures, admission and consultation with a maxillofacial surgeon are required.

3. **Body:** Fracture of the body of the zygoma, which involves the clinical signs and symptoms of the tripod fracture, results from severe force and leads to exaggerated malar depression.

12. What is the tongue blade test?

Patients with mandible fractures have mandibular tenderness and deformity and sublingual hematoma and malocclusion on physical examination. The jaw appears asymmetric, with deviation toward the side of the fracture. The tongue blade test is done by asking the patient to bite down on a tongue depressor. The tongue blade should be twisted by the examiner. If there is no fracture, the patient should be able to break the blade. In the presence of a mandible fracture, the patient opens his or her mouth and the tongue blade remains intact.

13. Which imaging studies should be ordered to diagnose a mandible fracture?

Mandible fractures are the second most common facial fracture. Multiple fractures are common (> 50%) because of the ring structure of the bone. Always check for a second fracture. The standard mandible series includes the posteroanterior view (for detecting fractures of the angle and body of the mandible), lateral oblique views (for detection of rami fractures), and the Towne view (anteroposterior view that projects the rami and condyles). The Panorex view is the most useful view for detecting mandible fractures. It provides a 180° view of the mandible and can detect fractures in all regions of the mandible, including symphyseal fractures that can be missed with the other views. A condylar fracture may be missed by plain radiographs. If this fracture is suspected and the plain radiographs are negative, facial CT is indicated.

14. What is the mechanism for a temporomandibular joint dislocation, and how is it treated?

Temporomandibular joint dislocation can result from blunt trauma to the mandible, but it also can occur after a seizure or with yawning. Patients with a temporomandibular joint dislocation present with jaw deviation away from the side of the dislocation if it is a unilateral dislocation or with the mandible pushed forward if it is a bilateral dislocation. After conscious sedation with a benzodiazepine for masseter muscle relaxation and a narcotic for pain relief, the emergency physician should place gauze-wrapped thumbs on the posterior molars. The mandible is then pushed downward and posterior.

15. When is a CT scan indicated in the evaluation of maxillofacial trauma?

In patients with a history of facial trauma but with minimal physical findings consistent with fractures or an equivocal examination, plain radiography can be used as a screening test. The standard plain film series of the face includes a Waters view (occipitomental) view, Caldwell (occipitofrontal) view, submentovertex view, and lateral view. The Waters view visualizes the orbital rim, infraorbital floor, maxilla, and maxillary sinuses and is useful as an initial examination in patients with suspected orbital floor fractures. Performance of this view requires that the cervical spine is clear because the patient is in the prone position. Fluid in the maxillary sinus is indirect evidence of fracture. The Caldwell view allows visualization of the superior orbital rim and the frontal sinuses. The lateral view shows the anterior wall of the frontal sinus and the anterior and posterior walls of the maxillary sinus.

In patients with physical findings that are highly suggestive of facial fractures (tenderness, step-offs, crepitus, or evidence of entrapment), some authors recommend proceeding directly to CT. This allows appropriate surgical planning. High-resolution, thin-cut CT scanning is the preferred modality for the elucidation of bony and soft tissue destruction inherent in maxillofacial trauma. This is the preferred test in any patient with suspected tripod, orbital, or midface fractures. In patients with suspected orbital fractures, CT scan with coronal and axial sections should be ordered (2- to 3-mm cuts).

16. How do I recognize an injury to Stenson's duct?

Stenson's (parotid) duct arises from the parotid gland and courses from the level of the external auditory canal (superficial) through the buccinator muscle to open at the level of the upper second molar. Any laceration at this level may involve the parotid gland, parotid duct, or buccal branch of the facial nerve. Laceration of the parotid system is recognized by a flow of saliva from the wound or bloody drainage from the duct orifice. Careful exploration reveals whether the flow is from the parotid gland or duct. The buccal branch of the facial nerve travels in close proximity to Stenson's duct; injury leads to drooping of the upper lip, which indicates a possible parotid duct injury. To assess for parotid duct patency, the parotid gland should be milked to see if saliva is expressed from the intraoral opening of the parotid duct. Damage to the duct requires repair over a stent and plastic surgical consultation.

17. When should closure of a facial laceration be deferred?

Closure of facial lacerations in the ED depends on the severity of facial and systemic injuries. Complex lacerations in patients needing operative intervention should be cleansed with normal saline, covered with dampened gauze, and deferred for intraoperative closure. Closure of the highly vascular tissues of the face may be delayed routinely 24 hours. Wounds involving the facial nerve, lacrimal duct, parotid duct, and avulsions should be referred on presentation to the appropriate surgeon for definitive care.

18. How do I control persistent hemorrhage from a facial laceration?

First, inject with 1% lidocaine with epinephrine. If hemorrhage continues and discrete arterial or venous bleeders can be visualized, they can be ligated with absorbable suture. If hemorrhage is from muscle, insert gauze followed by external pressure.

19. How is the ear anesthetized?

By raising a wheal of anesthesia (lidocaine without epinephrine) around the entire base of the ear. The external canal and concha require direct infiltration if they are involved. Small lacerations can be anesthetized with topical 4% lidocaine.

20. What are the clinical signs of an inhalation injury in a facial burn?

Significant inhalation thermal injury should be suspected in patients with facial burns, stridor, a hoarse voice, singed nasal and facial hairs, carbonaceous sputum, oropharyngeal mucosa edema, and altered mental status. Aggressive intervention, including endotracheal intubation and transfer to a burn center, is recommended.

BIBLIOGRAPHY

1. Cantrill SV: Face. In Marx JA, Hockberger RS, Walls RM, et al (eds): Rosen's Emergency Medicine Concepts and Clinical Practice, 5th ed. St. Louis, Mosby, 2002, pp 314–329.
2. Druelinger L, Guenther M, Marchand EG: Radiographic evaluation of the facial complex. Emerg Med Clin North Am 18:393–410, 2000.
3. Ellis E, Kirk S: Assessment of patients with facial fractures. Emerg Med Clin North Am 18:411–448, 2000.
4. Isenhour JL, Colucciello SA: Maxillofacial trauma. In Ferrera PC, Colucciello SA, Marx JA, et al (eds): Trauma Management, An Emergency Medicine Approach. St. Louis, Mosby, 2001, pp 180–196.
5. Rosen CL, Wolfe RE, Chew S, et al: Blind nasotracheal intubation in the presence of facial trauma. J Emerg Med 15:141–145, 1997.
6. Shepherd SM, Reyes IM: Maxillofacial injuries. In Harwood-Nuss A, Wolfson AB, Linden CH, et al (eds): The Clinical Practice of Emergency Medicine, 3rd ed. Philadelphia, Lippincott Williams & Wilkins, 2001, pp 465–474.

106. SPINE AND SPINAL CORD TRAUMA

Robert M. McNamara, M.D., and Michael J. Klevens, M.D.

1. Name the most common causes of spinal injury.
Vehicular crashes (39%); violence, primarily gunshot wounds (26%); falls (22%); sporting injuries (7%).

2. How many cases of spinal cord injury are reported each year in the United States?
About 11,000.

3. What percentage of patients with a vertebral column fracture or dislocation present with neurologic impairment?
14% to 15%. Injury to the cervical spine has a higher rate of neurologic compromise than do lower spine injuries.

4. If most spinal injuries do not cause neurologic injury, why is their management so important?
Some patients sustain permanent neurologic injury caused by improper medical care resulting from inadequate suspicion of injury, improper patient immobilization and handling, errant radiographic interpretation, poor-quality radiographs, or misleading seemingly normal radiographs despite a definite injury.

5. Why do you not want your patient to contribute to the aforementioned statistics?
Spinal cord injury with resultant permanent paralysis is one of the most devastating catastrophes. It generally affects young healthy adults with an average age of 32.1 years. The financial, social, and psychological sequelae are enormous to the patient and the patient's family. The estimated yearly costs, not including the first year, range from $21,274 to $102,491 per year depending on the severity of the injury.

6. Who is at risk, and how should one approach the patient with potential spinal injury?
The most important issue to establish is whether the patient's mental status is normal. If pain perception is altered by alcohol, drugs, head injury, shock, or other causes, injury is assumed to be present. A helpful reminder in potential spine injury is that "a proper history is **A MUST**":

A = Altered mental state. Check for drugs or alcohol.

M = Mechanism. Does the potential for injury exist?

U = Underlying conditions. Are high-risk factors for fractures present?

S = Symptoms. Is pain or paresthesia part of the picture?

T = Timing. When did the symptoms begin in relation to the event?

7. What are the underlying conditions of concern?

Less force is required to cause fractures in elderly patients than in younger patients. Rheumatoid arthritis can lead to subluxation problems at C1 and C2, whereas patients with Down syndrome may lack normal development of the odontoid. A patient with osteopetrosis or metastatic bone cancer should raise concern about possible fracture. As the population ages, there has been an increased prevalence of injury among the elderly, especially women with osteoporosis.

8. What parameters should be assessed on physical examination?

The two key areas of focus are the spine itself and the neurologic examination. The spine is palpated to assess for tenderness, deformity, and muscle spasm. Because the examiner feels only the posterior elements of the vertebrae, a fracture may be present despite a lack of tenderness. The neurologic examination should include motor function, sensory function, some aspect of posterior column function (position, vibration), and a rectal examination. In the unconscious patient, the only clues may be poor rectal tone, priapism, absence of deep tendon reflexes, or diaphragmatic breathing.

9. If the history or physical examination suggests a potential spine injury, how do I immobilize the patient?

When any spinal injury is suspected, the entire spine should be immobilized initially with a long board. The cervical spine can be immobilized with either a hard collar or a Philadelphia collar and the forehead taped to the board to prevent further neck flexion and extension. Previous studies also advocated the tape and sandbag method of immobilization.

10. How do I determine which patients need spine radiographs?

Because spinal injuries can create such devasting consequences, there has been liberal use of radiography to diagnose spinal injury. Studies stated that approximately 800,000 cervical spine radiographs are ordered annually in the United States. If there are 11,000 new cases of spinal cord injury per year in the United States, it can be seen that many of these radiographs may not be needed. Two studies tried to identify stable, nonobtunded, blunt trauma patients at risk for cervical spine injury. The National Emergency X-Radiography Utilization Study (NEXUS) created a decision instrument to identify patients with a low probability of injury using the following five crtieria: (1) no midline cervical tenderness, (2) no focal neurologic deficit, (3) normal alertness, (4) no intoxication, and (5) no painful distracting injury. If patients meet the criteria, there is a high likelihood that they have a low probability of injury and that cervical spine radiography is not needed. In this large multicenter study, the overall rate of missed cervical spine injuries was less than 1 in 4,000 patients. Similar to the NEXUS study, the Canadian C-Spine Rule for Radiography in Alert and Stable Trauma Patients presented a decision rule that is sensitive for detecting cervical spine injury. The Canadian study asks three questions: (1) Is there any high-risk factor that mandates radiography (i.e., age, severe mechanism, or focal neurologic signs)? (2) Can the patient be assessed safely for range of motion (simple mechanism, sitting position in the ED, ambulatory at any time, delayed onset of neck pain, or absence of midline cervical spine tenderness)? (3) Can the patient actively rotate the neck 45° to the left and right? This study had a sensitivity of 100% and a specificity of 42.5% for identifying clinically important cervical spine injuries. Both of these studies suggest that there can be a reduction in the number of radiographs ordered, having savings in terms of cost and irradiation to the patient. Any decision to have spinal radiography done should be in light of the current clinical situation and degree of suspicion of spinal injury.

11. Can this decision rule be applied to children?

Although the NEXUS study did include patients who were younger than 18 years old and correctly identified spinal cord injury victims, there were only 4 children younger than age 9 years who had cervical spine injury. It is difficult to apply the decision rule to children at this time. Ssome of the critera are difficult to verify in toddlers and children because of their inherent immaturity and unpredictability.

12. Which radiographs should be obtained initially in potential spinal injuries?

Cross-table lateral radiographs because they can be taken without moving the patient. Depending on the stability of the patient, they are taken either in a portable fashion or in the radiology suite.

13. If the cross-table lateral radiograph of the cervical spine is normal, can the patient be mobilized?

The patient should not be mobilized because 18% of cervical spine injuries are missed with the sole cross-table lateral radiograph. Although the most commonly missed injuries are at the C1–C2 level, missed injuries also occur at the lower cervical spine. It is recommended that at least three views of the spine be obtained if films are taken. The additional radiographs are the open-mouth odointoid and anteroposterior views.

14. How is the lateral cervical spine radiograph interpreted?

The first rule is to count all seven cervical vertebrae and be sure that the top of T1 is visible on the film. Next, follow the **ABCS**:

A = **Alignment.** Check for a smooth line at the anterior and posterior aspect of the vertebral bodies and the spinolaminal line from C1 to T1.

B = **Bones.** Carefully check each vertebral body to ensure that the anterior and posterior heights are similar (> 3 mm difference suggests fracture); follow the vertebrae out to the laminae and spinous process. Pay particular attention to the upper and lower cervical segments, where many missed fractures occur. Check the ring of C2, which can show a fracture through the upper portion of the vertebral body of C2.

C = **Cartilage.** Check the intervertebral joint spaces and the facet joints

S = **Soft tissue spaces.** Look for prevertebral swelling, especially at C2 C3 (> 5 mm), and check the predental space, which should be less than 3 mm in adults and less than 5 mm in children.

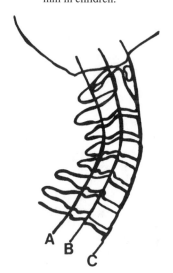

Curve of alignment. *A*, Spinolaminal line; *B*, posterior cerivcal bodies; *C*, anterior cervical bodies.

15. What are the indications for flexion-extension views of the cervical spine?

Flexion-extension views have been used if a ligamentous injury was suspected or if the physician was concerned about bony injury despite negative or nondiagnostic radiographs. Flexion-extension views are controversial because some believe they serve no purpose in the acute setting with the advent of newer modalities of testing such as CT and MRI. Reviews of the NEXUS data suggest that flexion-extension views add little in the acute setting. The preferential technique in the acute setting is MRI and, if necessary, a flexion-extension view 10 to 14 days after injury. This strategy can be employed only in settings where MRI is readily available without the transfer of the patient. In cases in which flexion-extension views are necessary, they should be obtained only in alert, cooperative patients and must be supervised by a physician.

16. When would more complex imaging of the cervical spine, such as CT or MRI, be considered?

Such studies are useful if plain radiographs are inconclusive or difficult to interpret. CT is useful to identify vertebral fractures and some correctable problems, such as hematomas or disc fragments within the spinal canal. MRI is useful to evaluate injury to the spinal cord itself or rupture of intervertebral discs. MRI shows areas of contusion and edema within the cord and areas of compression. It is less useful than CT for imaging vertebral fractures, however. Because multiple injuries are present in two thirds of patients with a cervical spine injury, these studies should be considered in all patients having at least one identified injury. Another reason to obtain a CT scan is for clearance of the cervical spine in obtunded or comatose patients. In a study of patients with traumatic brain injury, 5.4% of the patients had C1 or C2 fractures and 4% had occipital condyle fractures that were not visualized on the three-view radiograph series. If the lower cervical spine through T1 is inadequate through the normal lateral view and a further swimmer's view, CT is indicated.

17. Describe Jefferson's fracture, hangman's fracture, and clay-shoveler's fracture.

Jefferson's fracture is a burst fracture of the ring of C1 that occurs from axial loading.

A **hangman's fracture** is a disruption of the posterior arch of C2.

A **clay-shoveler's fracture** is a fracture of the spinous process that classically is caused by forceful cervical extension.

18. Describe the incomplete cord syndromes or injuries.

Anterior cord syndrome results in loss of function in the anterior two thirds of the spinal cord from damage to the corticospinal and spinothalamic pathways. Findings include loss of voluntary motor function and pain and temperature sensation below the level of injury, with preservation of the posterior column functions of position and vibration. The key issue is the potential reversibility of this lesion if a compressing hematoma or disc fragment can be removed. This condition requires immediate neurosurgical consultation.

Central cord syndrome results from injury to the central portion of the spinal cord. Because more proximal innervation is placed centrally within the cord, this lesion results in greater involvement of the upper extremities than of the lower extremities. Bowel or bladder control usually is preserved. The mechanism of injury is hyperextension of a cervical spine with a cord space narrowed by congenital variation, degenerative spurring, or hypertrophic ligaments. This syndrome can occur without actual fracture or ligamentous disruption.

Brown-Séquard syndrome is a hemisection of the spinal cord, usually from penetrating trauma. Contralateral sensation of pain and temperature is lost, and motor and posterior column functions are absent on the side of the injury.

Cauda equina syndrome is an injury to the lumbar, sacral, and coccygeal nerve roots causing a peripheral nerve injury. There can be motor and sensory loss in the lower extremities, bowel and bladder dysfunction, and loss of pain sensation at the perineum (saddle anesthesia).

19. What is the significance of sacral sparing and spinal shock?

Sacral sparing refers to the preservation of any function of the sacral roots, such as toe movement or perianal sensation. If sacral sparing is present, the chance of functional neurologic recovery is good. **Spinal shock** is a temporary concussive-like condition in which cord-mediated reflexes, such as the anal wink, are absent. Spinal shock also may result in bradycardia and hypotension. The extent of cord injury—and prognosis—cannot be determined until these reflexes return.

20. What are the general principles of emergency treatment in the patient with spinal injury?

The general principles of trauma resuscitation must be followed as necessary. Specific issues related to the cervical spine include preventing a worsening of the injury by proper immobilization and cautious patient handling. A higher level of cervical injury results in more devastation to the patient. Any patient with an injury above C5 probably should be intubated because the phrenic nerve roots, which supply the diaphragm, emerge from C3 to C5. The respiratory status must be monitored carefully. Gastric and bladder decompression are indicated early in the care of these patients. Overhydration is to be avoided. The absence of pain below the level of injured spinal cord can mask other injuries.

21. What is SCIWORA?

Spinal cord injury without radiographic abnormalities. Central cord syndrome can present in this manner, although this term is used most commonly regarding pediatric cervical spine injuries. Children are more susceptible to SCIWORA because of the greater elasticity of their cervical structures.

22. What is the status of steroids in acute spinal cord injury?

The first National Acute Spinal Cord Injury Study (NASCIS) was established in 1975 to evaluate pharmacologic therapy in the first hours after spinal cord injury. NASCIS 2 was completed in 1993 and followed by completion of NASCIS 3 in 1998. The *Cochrane Database Review* of pharmacologic therapies in acute spinal cord injuries was written by the lead author in the NASCIS studies. This review of all studies to date for pharmacologic therapy in acute spinal cord injuries concludes that methylprednisolone sodium succinate is the sole therapy shown to have sustained and improved neurologic outcome. The dosage is an initial bolus of 30 mg/kg intravenously over 15 minutes, followed 45 minutes later by a continuous infusion of 5.4 mg/kg/h for 24 hours. This should be given within 3 hours of injury. When the therapy is initiated 3 to 8 hours after injury, patients should be maintained on an infusion for 48 hours. This therapy is controversial because there have been questions raised about NASCIS's statistical analysis and lack of Food and Drug Administration approval for this still experimental therapy. Medicolegally the overwhelming desire for any improvement has made this therapy the *de facto* standard of care until other therapies are deemed more appropriate. Other therapies on the horizon include ganglioside G_{M1}, opiate receptor antagonists, calcium channel antagonists, glutamate receptor antagonists, and thyroid-releasing homone analogs.

23. What can physicians do to prevent spinal injuries?

Because motor vehicle accidents are the leading cause of spinal injuries, one can work to reduce problems such as driving under the influence of alcohol or drugs and to encourage the use of safety belts (ejected accident victims are at high risk for cervical spine injury). Diving and tackling injuries can be reduced by proper public education and coaching. Because handgun violence is increasing, physicians need to voice their opinions on this issue.

BIBLIOGRAPHY

1. Bracken MB: Pharmacological interventions for acute spinal cord injury. Cochrane Review. The Cochrane Library, Issue 4, 2001.
2. Bracken MB, Shepard MJ, Holford TR, et al: Administration of methylprednisolone for 24 or 48 hours or tirilazad mesylate for 48 hours in the treatment of acute spinal cord injury: Results of the third national acute spinal cord injury randomized controlled trial. JAMA 227:1597–1604, 1997.

3. Chandler DR, Nenej L, Adkins RH, et al: Emergency cervical-spine immobilization. Ann Emerg Med 21:1185–1188, 1992.
4. Davis JW, Phreaner DL, Hoyt DB, et al: The etiology of missed cervical spine injuries. J Trauma 34:342–346, 1993.
5. Hoffman JR, Mower WR, Wolfson AB, et al: Validity of a set of clinical criteria to rule out injury to the cervical spine in patients with blunt trauma. N Engl J Med 343:94–99, 2000.
6. Lowery DW, Wald MM, Browne BJ, et al: Epidemiology of cervical spine injury victims. Ann Emerg Med 38:12–16, 2001.
7. Marion DW, Domeier R, Dunham CM, et al: Practice Management Guidelines for Identifying Cervical Spine Injuries Following Trauma. Winston-Salem, NC, Eastern Association for the Surgery of Trauma, 1998–2000.
8. McNamara RM, Heine E, Espositio B: Cervical spine injury and radiography in alert, high-risk patients. J Emerg Med 8:177–182, 1990.
9. Nesathurai S: Steroids and spinal cord injury: revisiting the NASCIS 2 and NASCIS 3 trials. J Trauma 45:1088–1093, 1998.
10. Pollack CV, Hendley GW, Martin DR, et al: Use of flexion-extension radiographs of the cervical spine in blunt trauma. Ann Emerg Med 38:8–11, 2001.
11. Ruoff B, West OC: The cervical spine. In Schwartz DT, Reisdorff EJ (eds): Emergency Radiology. New York, McGraw-Hill, 2000, pp 269–318.
12. Spinal cord injury facts and figures at a glance. National Spinal Cord Injury Statistical Center, Birminham, AL, 2001.
13. Stiell IG, Wells GA, Vandemheen KL: The Canadian c-spine rule for radiography in alert and stable trauma patients. JAMA 286:1841–1848, 2001.
14. Sweeney TA, Marx JA: Blunt neck injury. Emerg Med Clin North Am 11:71–79, 1993.
15. Van Hare RS, Yaron M: The ring of C2 and evaluation of the cross-table lateral view of the cervical spine. Ann Emerg Med 21:733–735, 1992.
16. Viccellio P, Simon H, Pressman BD, et al: A prospective multicenter study of cervical spine injury in children. Pediatrics 108:E20, 2001.
17. Wales LR, Knopp RK, Morishima MS: Recommendations for evaluation of the acutely injured cervical spine: A clinical radiologic algorithm. Ann Emerg Med 9:422–428, 1980.

107. HEAD TRAUMA

Edward Newton, M.D.

1. What is the scope of head injury in the United States?

There are more 1.5 million ED visits and approximately 70,000 deaths as a result of head injury every year in the United States. Although the incidence of severe head injury is decreasing, most likely owing to the preventive benefits of helmets and seat belts and air bags in automobiles, head trauma remains the most lethal traumatic injury and accounts for a large proportion of patients with permanent disability. The peak incidence of head injury is in the 15- to 24-year-old age group with males affected twice as often as females. The spectrum of head injury includes relatively minor problems, such as lacerations and scalp contusions, and major, often lethal intracranial trauma. Distinguishing between minor and potentially lethal head injuries while using diagnostic resources appropriately is one of the most difficult tasks facing the emergency physician.

2. What groups of patients are at particular risk from head trauma?

Because assessment of mental status is such an integral part of the evaluation of head-injured patients, patients who are unable to communicate because they are preverbal (e.g., infants), are intoxicated, are mentally impaired, are aphasic, or have a language barrier pose a special challenge. When such communication barriers are present, there should be a lower threshold for obtaining a CT scan.

Certain age groups are at higher risk for intracranial injury. **Infants** are at higher risk because of their relatively large head size and compressibility of the skull. Infants also are at high risk for nonaccidental trauma (e.g., **shaken baby syndrome**), in which case an accurate history may be unavailable. If the cranial sutures and fontanelles are not closed, the cranium can expand as a result of intracranial bleeding. Infants can bleed sufficiently intracranially to produce hemorrhagic shock, whereas in older children and adults, another source of bleeding is inevitably responsible for shock. The **elderly** also are at higher risk of intracranial injury, particularly subdural hematoma. Cerebral atrophy results in stretching of bridging veins from the dura to the brain parenchyma, making these veins vulnerable to tearing from deceleration forces. **Chronic alcoholics** are at risk because of their greater frequency of head trauma, cerebral atrophy, and coagulopathy. Patients who are taking anticoagulants or have intrinsic **bleeding diastheses** bleed more actively than patients with normal coagulation.

3. What is a cerebral concussion?

Sudden, transient loss of central neurologic function secondary to trauma. It is characterized by loss of consciousness, transient amnesia, confusion, disorientation, or visual changes, without any gross cerebral abnormalities.

4. What is the postconcussive syndrome?

Although the patient may have a completely normal neurologic examination after a concussion, there are common sequelae from this type of injury. Patients frequently report migraine-type headaches, dizziness, inability to concentrate, and irritability. Although in 90% of cases these symptoms resolve within 2 weeks, they may persist for 1 year. Treatment is supportive, and the long-term prognosis is good. A phenomenon known as the **second impact syndrome** is recognized in which a second head trauma during a vulnerable period after a concussion results in severe and often fatal diffuse cerebral edema. Consequently, athletes should be held out of contact sports until all postconcussive symptoms have resolved.

5. How do you detect cerebrospinal fluid (CSF) leaks caused by basilar skull fractures?

A patient with signs of basilar skull fracture (raccoon eyes, hemotympanum, or Battle's sign) with clear drainage from the nose or ear canal should be suspected of having a CSF leak. Analysis of the glucose content of the drainage by glucometer or laboratory analysis may distinguish CSF (containing 60% of serum glucose levels) from nasal mucus (glucose not present). In cases in which blood is mixed with CSF, applying a drop of the fluid to filter paper reveals CSF in a target shape with blood at the center and pink-tinged CSF forming an outer ring. Bedside tests are neither specific nor sensitive for detecting CSF leaks.

6. How are CSF leaks treated?

CSF leaks through tears in the dura generally are managed conservatively. The use of prophylactic antibiotics is controversial because they have not been shown to reduce significantly the incidence of meningitis and may select for antibiotic-resistant bacteria. Patients must be followed closely until the dural tear heals because of the risk of meningitis. Dural tears that fail to close spontaneously over 2 to 3 weeks usually require operative repair.

7. How does a patient with epidural hematoma present?

Epidural hematoma occurs in 5% to 10% of severe head injuries. The classic pattern is a patient loses consciousness from the initial concussion, gradually recovers over a few minutes, and enters a lucid interval wherein he or she is relatively asymptomatic and has a normal neurologic examination. During this interval, accumulation of arterial blood in the epidural space, usually from a lacerated middle meningeal artery, eventually causes compression and shift of brain across the midline. This process is accompanied by a second reduction in the level of consciousness and the pupillary and motor signs of herniation. This classic pattern occurs in only about 30% of cases, however. Many patients remain unconscious after the initial impact or in minor hemorrhages may not develop increased intracranial pressure (ICP) at all. The characteristic CT scan appearance of an epidural hematoma is a hyperdense lenticular collection of blood that indents adjacent brain parenchyma and does not extend beyond cranial sutures where the dura is attached.

8. How does a subdural hematoma (SDH) present?

SDH may be acute, subacute (6 to 14 days), or chronic (> 14 days after trauma). **Acute SDH** is associated with a high incidence of underlying brain injury. The presentation varies with the severity of the underlying injury, but patients commonly present with a diminished level of consciousness, headache, and focal neurologic deficits corresponding to the area of brain injury. If sufficient bleeding occurs, ICP increases, and herniation may occur. The characteristic appearance of an acute SDH on CT scan is a collection of hyperdense blood in a crescent-shaped pattern conforming to the convexity of the hemisphere and often extending past cranial sutures. At times, the injury causes a minimal amount of bleeding, and the patient does not immediately seek medical care. The SDH undergoes lysis over a period of several days and eventually organizes into an encapsulated mass. **Subacute** or **chronic SDH** is a difficult clinical diagnosis because the symptoms are vague and common (e.g., persistent headache, difficulty concentrating, lethargy), and the trauma may have been forgotten. Even the CT scan diagnosis is difficult because subacute SDH becomes isodense and indistinguishable from surrounding brain unless special CT techniques are used. Chronic SDH appears as an encapsulated lucent collection of fluid in the same position as the acute type.

9. What is axonal shear injury?

Axonal shear injury occurs during abrupt deceleration because white and gray matter have different densities and different rates of deceleration. This produces a shearing force that may tear axons at the white-gray interface, resulting in coma or other severe neurologic derangements. The CT scan may appear completely normal or show only small petechial hemorrhages. MRI of the brain is a more sensitive tool in detecting these injuries but is currently impractical in the acute phase.

10. What is brain herniation?

Herniation is caused by increased ICP. Because the cranium is a rigid structure, pressure varies with the volume of its contents. Approximately 10% of intracranial volume is blood, another 10% is CSF, and the remainder is brain parenchyma and intracellular fluid. An increase in any of these compartments by blood, tumor, or edema causes a predictable response. Initially, CSF is forced into the spinal canal, and the ventricles and cisterns collapse. When this has occurred, ICP rises steeply, and the brain parenchyma shifts away from the accumulating blood and herniates through one of several spaces, eventually causing death by compressing the brainstem.

11. Describe the four types of herniation syndrome.

1. **Uncal herniation.** The uncus is the most medial portion of the hemisphere and is often the first structure to shift below the tentorium that separates the hemispheres from the midbrain. As the uncus is forced medially and downward, the ipsilateral third cranial nerve is compressed, producing pupillary dilation, ptosis, and oculomotor paresis. As herniation progresses, the ipsilateral cerebral peduncle and pyramidal tract are compressed, resulting in contralateral hemiplegia. In approximately 10% of cases, the hemiparesis occurs on the same side as the brain lesion, making this a less reliable finding for localizing the injury. Further progression results in brainstem compression with respiratory and cardiac arrest. Transtentorial herniation of this type is the most common variety.

2. **Central herniation.** Occasionally, hematomas located at the vertex or frontal lobes cause simultaneous downward herniation of both hemispheres through the tentorium. Clinical findings are similar to uncal herniation except that bilateral motor weakness occurs.

3. **Cingulate herniation.** Rarely the cingulate gyrus is forced medically beneath the falx by an expanding lateral hematoma, causing compression of the ventricles and impairing cerebral blood flow.

4. **Posterior fossa herniation.** Bleeding or edema in the posterior fossa can result in herniation of the cerebellar tonsils either upward through the tentorium or downward through the foramen magnum. In the latter case, coma and fatal brainstem dysfunction may occur rapidly and with little warning.

12. What is the ED treatment for increased ICP?

1. **Maintain adequate cerebral perfusion pressure**. Although there is often misguided reluctance to hydrate vigorously patients with concomitant head and systemic injuries, cerebral perfusion must be maintained for resuscitation to be successful. Hypotension must be avoided, and often laparotomy to correct intraabdominal bleeding must take precedence over neurosurgical intervention to maintain cerebral perfusion.

2. **Avoid secondary injuries to the central nervous system**. After brain trauma, there is a cascade of secondary neuronal metabolic injuries that are detrimental to recovery of neurologic function. At present, few interventions have proved effective in limiting these changes. Certain other treatable conditions either increase the metabolic demands of the brain or decrease cerebral perfusion and worsen the prognosis unless they are corrected. The **5 Hs** (**hypotension**, **hypoxia**, **hypercarbia**, **hypoglycemia**, **hyperthermia** and **seizures**) are conditions that should be avoided or corrected in the ED. Anticonvulsant prophylaxis with diphenylhydantoin is indicated particularly for penetrating injuries and depressed skull fractures. Raising the head of the bed while maintaining spinal precautions may decrease ICP slightly.

3. **Hyperventilation**: Carbon dioxide is one of the main determinants of cerebrovascular tone. High levels produce cerebral vasodilation; low levels cause vasoconstriction. Hyperventilation to a PCO_2 level of 25 mmHg decreases blood flow to the brain by 50%, which decreases the vascular compartment of the brain, "buying some time" for definitive surgical interventions. When blood flow to the brain decreases, delivery of oxygen and glucose also decreases, resulting in ischemic injury and worse edema. The optimal level of hypocarbia is uncertain at present, but most clinicians use mild hyperventilation, with a PCO_2 level of 30 to 35 mmHg as the goal. To accomplish this degree of hypocarbia, it is necessary to intubate the patient with rapid-sequence intubation and mechanically ventilate with settings determined by arterial blood gases to maintain the PCO_2 between 30 and 35 mmHg. The indication for implementing hyperventilation is increased ICP resulting in clinical signs of focal neurologic deficit (i.e., herniation).

4. **Diuresis**. The use of an osmotic diuretic, such as mannitol, 0.5 to 1.0 g/kg intravenously over 15 minutes, or a loop diuretic, such as furosemide, 0.5 to 1.0 mg/kg intravenously, is effective in reducing brain edema. Infusion of mannitol creates an osmotic gradient between the intravascular space and the extracellular fluid, drawing fluid from the extracellular fluid and reducing brain water content and ICP. Mannitol is filtered by the kidneys, producing systemic dehydration. Clinical experience and animal studies seem to support the concomitant administration of osmotic diuretics and volume resuscitation in patients with hypovolemic shock.

5. **Barbiturates**. Conscious patients who are paralyzed for intubation also must be sedated. A short-acting barbiturate is the ideal agent for this purpose because it lowers ICP, prevents seizures, and decreases cerebral metabolism. Such agents cannot be used in a hypotensive patient, however. In these cases, a reversible agent, such as morphine, 0.1 mg/kg; lorazepam, 0.01 mg/kg; or midazolam, 1 mg/kg/h, is preferred because adverse effects on blood pressure and cardiac output can be reversed by specific antagonists. Etomidate, 0.3 mg/kg, is a short-acting agent that decreases ICP without adversely affecting cardiac output, cerebral perfusion pressure, and systemic blood pressure. Fentanyl, 3 to 5 µg/kg, causes a slight increase in ICP and is not the preferred agent for sedation of a head-injured patient.

13. If a patient has a normal CT scan after head trauma, is it completely safe to discharge him or her home?

Nothing is completely safe. There are well-documented instances of delayed epidural and subdural bleeding many hours after injury. Consequently, although it is generally safe to discharge such patients, head injury instructions should be given to responsible family members, and the patient should be instructed to return immediately if symptoms worsen. If the patient is socially isolated or unreliable, a judgment has to be made regarding the seriousness of the mechanism of injury and the risk of discharge. Intoxicated patients should be kept under observation until their mental status can be evaluated properly.

14. Since CT scan is available, is there any role for plain skull films?
The usefulness of plain radiographs of the skull has been far outstripped by more informative imaging modalities such as CT and MRI. Skull films still have certain indications in evaluation of the following:

- Penetrating trauma (gunshot wounds)
- Suspected depressed skull fracture
- Suspected basilar skull fracture
- As part of the skeletal survey for suspected child abuse
- In patients with prior craniotomies or shunts

BIBLIOGRAPHY

1. Borczuk P: Mild head trauma. Emerg Med Clin North Am 15:563–579, 1997.
2. Cheung DS, Kharasch M: Evaluation of the patient with closed head trauma: An evidence based approach. Emerg Med Clin North Am 17:9–23, 1999.
3. Eisenberg HM, Aldrich EF (eds): Management of Head Injury. Neurosurg Clin North Am 2:1–501, 1991.
4. Evans RW: Postconcussive syndrome and the sequelae of mild head injury. Neurol Clin 10:815–847, 1992.
5. Lehman LB: Intracranial pressure monitoring: A contemporary view. Ann Emerg Med 19:295–303, 1990.
6. Livingston DH, Loder PA, Koziol J, et al: The use of CT scanning to triage patients requiring admission following minor head injury. J Trauma 31:483–489, 1991.
7. Redan JA, Livingston DH, Tortella NJ, et al: Value of intubating and paralyzing patients with suspected head injury in the emergency department. J Trauma 31:371–375, 1991.
8. Rosner MJ, Rosner SD, Johnson AH: Cerebral perfusion pressure: Management protocol and clinical results. J Neurosurg 83:949–961, 1995.
9. Stein CS, Young GS, Talucci RC, et al: Delayed brain injury after head trauma: Significance of coagulopathy. Neurosurgery 30:160–165, 1992.
10. Walls RM: Rapid sequence intubation in head trauma. Ann Emerg Med 22:1008–1013, 1993.

108. TRAUMATIC OPHTHALMOLOGIC EMERGENCIES

Harold Thomas, M.D.

1. Name the two most time-critical emergencies in ophthalmology.
Central retinal artery occlusion and chemical burns to the eyes.

2. What is the treatment for a chemical burn of the eye?
Immediate copious irrigation of the eyes (for at least 20 minutes). If you receive a phone call from a patient at home or from the paramedics, irrigation should be initiated before transport to the ED.

3. How do you know when you have irrigated the eye enough?
Nitrazine paper can be used to ensure that the pH has been corrected to normal. This usually requires at least 3 L of normal saline in each eye and continuous irrigation for 20 minutes. Alkalis, which cause the most damaging burns, tend to adhere to the tissue of the eye and are difficult to remove completely with irrigation. After irrigation, emergent ophthalmologic consultation is indicated.

4. What is the significance of pain from an eye injury that is not relieved with topical anesthesia?
Complete symptomatic relief with topical anesthesia indicates a superficial injury involving only the cornea. If a patient still has significant pain after application of anesthetic drops, a

deeper injury (often traumatic iritis) must be suspected, even in the presence of an obvious superficial injury.

5. List nine potential injuries that must be considered in a patient sustaining a blunt injury to the eye.

1. Blow-out fracture of the floor of the orbit	4. Lens dislocation	8. Traumatic iritis
2. Corneal abrasion	5. Traumatic mydriasis	9. Ruptured globe (rare after blunt injuries)
3. Anterior hyphema	6. Vitreous hemorrhage	
	7. Retinal detachment	

6. What is the most common eye injury seen in the ED?
Corneal abrasion with or without a superficial foreign body.

7. How is corneal abrasion diagnosed?
The anesthetized eye can be stained with fluorescein and illuminated by an ultraviolet or Wood's lamp; corneal defects fluoresce bright yellow-orange. Visual acuity should be checked, and the eye should be inspected, with particular emphasis on the anterior chamber to look for an anterior hyphema. A funduscopic examination for evidence of vitreous hemorrhage or retinal detachment, a visual field examination (also for evidence of retinal detachment), and testing of extraocular movement should be done.

8. What is the treatment for a corneal abrasion?
Because this injury is extremely painful, narcotic analgesics are indicated. **Never dispense topical anesthesia from the ED**. One frequently overlooked aspect of therapy is the instillation of a cycloplegic, usually cyclopentolate (Cyclogyl), to relieve the ciliary spasm that commonly accompanies this injury. Patients also need evaluation for tetanus prophylaxis. Most should receive topical antibiotics, drops, or ointment.

9. What is the role of an eye patch in treatment of corneal abrasions?
A pressure patch previously was considered the most important aspect of management of a corneal abrasion. Patches were thought to increase comfort and hasten healing. It is now known that not only are eye patches uncomfortable, but also they do not increase healing and may promote infection. They do *not* prevent the involved eye from moving and should not be used for most superficial corneal abrasions. If you do use a patch, be sure to instruct the patient not to drive because depth perception depends on binocular vision.

10. How does a corneal abrasion from a contact lens differ from other causes of corneal trauma?
Corneal abrasions secondary to overuse of contact lenses are much more likely to have a bacterial process involved, often *Pseudomonas*. These patients should receive topical antibiotics effective against *Pseudomonas* organisms (tobramycin or gentamicin) and should never be given an eye patch. If the emergency physician is unable to do a slit-lamp examination, early ophthalmologic referral to rule out ulcerative keratitis (corneal ulcer) is indicated.

11. What is the most common location of an ocular foreign body?
Foreign bodies often are lodged just beneath the upper eyelid along the palpebral conjunctiva. The eyelid needs to be everted with a cotton swab to examine this area adequately. Conjunctival foreign bodies should be suspected when many vertical linear streaks are noted on the cornea with fluorescein examination.

12. What is the proper treatment for a corneal foreign body?
First, topical anesthesia is applied, usually proparacaine. Nonembedded foreign bodies should be removed with a sterile, moist cotton swab. Embedded foreign bodies are removed with

a 27G needle or an eye spud. Most metallic foreign bodies leave a residual rust ring that should be removed in approximately 24 hours, after the cornea has softened.

13. What is an anterior hyphema?

A collection of blood in the anterior chamber of the eye; it is seen as a layering of cells that pool along the bottom of the eye when the patient is sitting upright. When the patient is lying down, a hyphema is not recognized easily; it may appear as a diffuse haziness of the anterior chamber. Small hyphemas, termed **microhyphemas**, may be identified only with a slit-lamp.

14. How is an anterior hyphema treated?

The standard in the past was to admit all patients for bed rest; today the dominant tendency is toward outpatient management. The patient should be kept upright, the eye patched, and ophthalmologic consultation initiated, at least by phone. Complications include rebleeding, glaucoma formation (particularly in black patients with sickle-cell trait), and corneal staining.

15. What physical findings lead to the suspicion of a blow-out fracture?

Classic findings with a blow-out fracture (fracture of the inferior orbital wall with herniation of the eye contents into the maxillary sinus) are (1) decreased sensation over the inferior orbital rim, extending to the edge of the nose and ipsilateral upper lip, secondary to compromise of the inferior orbital nerve; (2) enophthalmos, or a sunken appearance of the eye, which may be masked by edema; and (3) paralysis or limitation of upward gaze (manifested as diplopia), resulting from entrapment of the inferior rectus muscle.

16. What is traumatic mydriasis?

An efferent pupillary defect manifested by a dilated (in most instances irregular) pupil that does not react to direct or consensual light, usually as a result of minor trauma to the eye. Because such a patient is at risk for other more serious eye injuries, a careful eye examination is mandatory. The possibility of uncal herniation secondary to intracranial injury should be considered if level of consciousness is decreased in the presence of a perfectly round, nonreactive, unilateral, dilated pupil. If level of consciousness is unaltered, this is most likely an isolated ocular injury.

17. Why is a history of hammering metal on metal important in a patient presenting with an eye complaint?

Often a small, high-velocity fragment penetrates the globe with minimal or no physical findings. This injury, which can cause inflammation weeks later, is diagnosed with soft tissue radiographs of the orbit or a CT scan of the globe.

18. Which eyelid lacerations should be repaired by an ophthalmologist or plastic surgeon?

- Those involving the lid margin or gray line
- Those involving the tear duct mechanism along the lower eyelid
- Those involving the tarsal plate or levator muscle

19. When should penetration of the globe be suspected?

The pupil is usually misshapen, pointing in the direction of the penetration. The globe may appear soft because of decreased intraocular pressure. Intraocular pressure should not be tested if a penetrating injury is suspected because the test promotes extrusion of aqueous humor.

20. What is the significance of a subscleral (subconjunctival) hemorrhage?

Subscleral hemorrhages are usually benign and often occur spontaneously with complete resolution over 2 to 3 weeks. When associated with trauma, other potentially more serious eye injuries should be suspected and ruled out.

21. List traumatic ophthalmologic injuries that require immediate ophthalmologic consultation.

- Chemical burns of the eye, particularly with corneal opacification
- Perforation of the globe or cornea
- Lens dislocation
- Orbital hemorrhage with increased intraocular pressure
- Lacerations involving the lid margin, tarsal plate, or tear duct

22. Name ophthalmologic injuries that require urgent ophthalmologic consultation (within 12 to 24 hours).
Anterior hyphema, blow-out fracture, and retinal injuries.

23. What is solar keratitis?
Also known as **flash burns** or **snow blindness**, solar keratitis is a corneal injury secondary to overexposure to ultraviolet light. Diagnosis is made with fluorescein staining, which shows multiple punctate lesions of the cornea. Treatment consists of resting the eyes with adequate narcotic analgesia. Spontaneous resolution can be expected in 12 to 24 hours.

24. What is the cause of a dilated pupil that fails to constrict with topical pilocarpine?
A dilated pupil that fails to constrict with topical miotic agents is due to topical application of a mydriatic agent often because of rubbing the eye after application of a scopolamine patch (for motion sickness).

25. What is rose bengal stain used for?
Suspected herpetic keratitis.

BIBLIOGRAPHY

1. Bartfield JM, Holmes TJ, Raccio-Robak N: A comparison of proparacaine and tetracaine eye anesthetics. Acad Emerg Med 1:364–367, 1994.
2. Kirkpatrick JN, Hoh HB, Cook SD: No eye pad for corneal abrasion. Eye 7:468–471, 1993.
3. Lawrence T, Wilison D, Harvey J: The incidence of secondary hemorrhage after traumatic hyphema. Ann Ophthalmol 22:276–278, 1990.
4. Schein OD: Contact lens abrasions and the nonophthalmologist. Ann J Emerg Med 11:606–608, 1993.
5. Snyder RW, Glasser DB: Antibiotic therapy for ocular infection. West J Med 161:579–584, 1994.

109. NECK TRAUMA

Jeffrey J. Schaider, M.D.

1. Is neck trauma a complicated topic?
Yes. The lack of bony protection makes the anterior neck especially vulnerable to severe, life-threatening injuries. The exposed anatomic structure of the neck, which contains many vital parts of the vascular, airway, and gastrointestinal systems, provides a fertile ground for debate and myriad opinions about modality of treatment.

2. What are the most urgent concerns in the initial management of neck trauma?
Airway and **hemorrhage control**. Airway management comes before anything else discussed in this chapter. Early endotracheal intubation is indicated for any patient with existing or potential airway compromise. Delay in airway management increases the difficulty of intubation because of swelling and compression of the anatomic structures. If severe damage to the larynx and cricoid cartilage makes endotracheal intubation impossible, tracheostomy is preferred over

cricothyrotomy for airway management. Bleeding should be controlled with pressure rather than with blind clamping. The wound should be examined to determine whether it has violated the platysma. Injudicious probing of the wound may be dangerous, however, because a vascular structure that has ceased to bleed may resume when its tamponade is released with disastrous consequences.

3. What common findings indicate significant neck injury?

Injuries involving the **vascular system** result in hematomas, bleeding, pulse deficit, shock, and neurologic deficit secondary to arterial interruption. **Laryngeal trauma** causes voice alteration, airway compromise, subcutaneous emphysema, crepitus, and hemoptysis. Signs and symptoms of **esophageal disruption** include pain and tenderness in the neck, resistance of the neck to passive motion, crepitation, dysphagia, and bleeding from the mouth or nasogastric tube. The diagnosis of esophageal disruption is difficult because of injuries to other overlying structures. Ancillary testing must be used to assist in the diagnosis of these injuries.

4. What are the signs and symptoms of blunt carotid artery trauma?

Of patients with blunt carotid trauma, 25% to 50% have no external signs of trauma. Delayed neurologic signs are the rule rather than the exception; only 10% of patients have symptoms of transient ischemic attacks or strokes within 1 hour of injury. Most patients develop symptoms within the first 24 hours, but 17% develop symptoms days or weeks after injury. Carotid artery injuries may present with a hematoma of the lateral neck, bruit over carotid circulation, Horner's syndrome, transient ischemic attack, aphasia, or hemiparesis. The clinical manifestations of vertebral artery injury include, ataxia, vertigo, nystagmus, hemiparesis, dysarthria, and diplopia.

5. Name the main controversy regarding management of penetrating neck trauma.

The management of penetrating neck trauma that violates the platysma. In the 1990s, physicians and surgeons changed from a mandatory exploration policy for penetrating neck wound to a selective management approach.

6. What is mandatory exploration for penetrating neck wounds?

All patients who have wounds that penetrate the platysma muscle in the neck are explored surgically to determine the presence or absence of injury to the deeper structures in the neck. Some ancillary diagnostic testing (angiography, esophagography, esophagoscopy, laryngoscopy) may be done preoperatively, depending on the location of the wound and the stability of the patient.

7. What are the advantages of mandatory exploration for penetrating neck wounds?

During the 1940s, mandatory exploration was instituted for all penetrating wounds that violate the platysma. This policy reduced mortality significantly and remained the only mode of therapy until the mid-1970s. Proponents of mandatory exploration warn of the catastrophic complications from delayed treatment and missed injuries. Neck exploration is relatively simple, and a negative exploration has low morbidity and mortality.

8. State the disadvantages of mandatory exploration for penetrating neck wounds.

Because the negative exploration rate (no injuries found at surgery) is 50%, the cost of the operation and the added length of hospital stay are unwarranted. Many of these operations could be avoided with the selective approach to neck exploration.

9. Describe the theory behind the selective surgical management of penetrating neck wounds.

With the improved sensitivity and specificity of ancillary diagnostic testing (angiography, carotid duplex scanning, CT, esophagography, esophagoscopy, laryngoscopy), a nonoperative approach to a select group of patients, based on physical examination and results of ancillary tests, is safe. The selective approach has reduced the negative exploration rate significantly from 50% to 30%.

10. What are the three anatomic zones of the neck?

Zone I is the area below the cricoid cartilage.

Zone II extends from the cricoid cartilage to the angle of the mandible.

Zone III extends from the angle of the mandible to the base of the skull (see Figure).

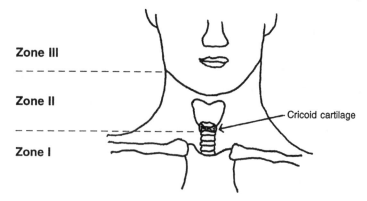

11. Why is the neck divided into three zones?

The location of the injury plays a major role in assessing the need for angiography. All **zone I** injuries require angiography to determine the integrity of the thoracic outlet vessels. In stable but symptomatic patients needing surgery, angiography should be done preoperatively because positive findings necessitate a thoracotomy before neck exploration.

The familiar anatomy of **zone II**, coupled with relative ease of surgical exposure, minimizes the need for angiography in symptomatic patients undergoing surgery. Some clinicians observe asymptomatic patients with penetrating injuries without angiography. Others perform angiography, carotid duplex scanning, or helical CT on asymptomatic patients to detect occult injuries and involvement of vertebral vessels before observation.

The management of **zone III** injuries is controversial because of the complex anatomy of the area and the difficulty in obtaining adequate exposure. Most clinicians agree that for asymptomatic patients not undergoing surgery, angiography is necessary to assess the status of the internal carotid artery and the intracerebral circulation. For symptomatic patients, preoperative angiography is helpful because high internal carotid artery injuries are difficult to visualize at operation and may require carotid artery ligation and concomitant extracranial-intracranial bypass.

12. Can carotid duplex scanning or helical CT replace angiography for detection of vascular injuries in penetrating neck injuries?

With experienced operators, carotid duplex scanning approaches 100% sensitivity for excluding zone II and III injuries in stable, asymptomatic patients with penetrating neck injuries. Because carotid duplex scanning has a lower specificity (85% to 95%), positive carotid duplex scanning should be followed by carotid angiography before making a decision regarding surgical intervention. In two small studies, helical CT had a sensitivity of 90% and 80% in detecting carotid artery injuries. In the latter study, using direct signs of injury (wall irregularity, contrast extravasation, lack of vascular enhancement, caliber changes) and indirect signs of injury (bone and bullet fragment < 5 mm from major vessel, path of injury through major vessel, hematoma in carotid sheath) increase sensitivity from 80% to 100%.

13. What diagnostic testing is preferred in detection of blunt vascular injuries?

Blunt vascular injuries were found in 27% of high-risk patients screened for blunt vascular injury (combination of injury mechanism [cervical hyperextension or hyperflexion, direct cervical blow, near-hanging] and injury pattern [carotid canal, midface, and cervical spine fracture]). **Angiography** is the study of choice in acutely injured and symptomatic patients. Of lesions, 90%

occur at the bifurcation of carotids or higher. Four-vessel angiography is recommended because multiple vessel injuries occur in 40% to 80%. The diagnostic accuracy of helical **CT angiography** has not been studied extensively in blunt trauma. In a small study comparing CT angiography with conventional angiography, CT angiography had a sensitivity of 85% and specificity of 71%. CT angiography has been shown to decrease significantly the time to diagnose the injury. **Color flow Doppler ultrasound** provides rapid identification and quantification of arterial dissection, but it is unable to assess distal upper extracranial and intracranial internal carotid artery and is operator dependent. With an experienced operator, ultrasound can be used as a screening test in lower risk patients. **MR angiography** accurately detects carotid and vertebral artery injuries with a sensitivity and specificity greater than 95% for carotid artery dissection. It is ideal for follow-up or for stable patients; MR angiography is difficult to perform in acutely injured unstable patient.

14. Which diagnostic studies are important in suspected laryngeal injuries?

Soft tissue cervical **radiographs** may show a fractured larynx, subcutaneous air, or prevertebral air. **CT** accurately identifies the location and extent of laryngeal fractures. Flexible **laryngoscopy** provides valuable information regarding the integrity of the cartilaginous framework and the function of the vocal cords. CT should be done when the diagnosis of a laryngeal fracture is still suspected despite a negative examination of the endolarynx or when flexible laryngoscopy cannot be done (e.g., intubated patient).

15. Are diagnostic studies necessary in suspected esophageal injuries?

Yes. Soft tissue cervical radiographs may show subcutaneous emphysema or an increased prevertebral shadow. Chest radiograph findings include pleural effusion, pneumothorax, mediastinal air, and mediastinal widening. Esophageal contrast studies should be done initially with radiopaque contract medium (Gastrografin); if negative, studies should be repeated with barium to increase diagnostic yield. Radiographic imaging is difficult because of the high false-negative rate. Esophagography has a 30% to 50% false-negative rate and should be followed by esophagoscopy in patients with suspected esophageal injury. Rigid endoscopy is more sensitive than flexible endoscopy. No one study can exclude esophageal perforation; a combination of physical signs, plain and contrast radiographs, and esophagoscopy should be used to make the diagnosis.

BIBLIOGRAPHY

1. Asensio JA, Valenziano CP, Falcone RE, Grosh JD: Management of penetrating neck injuries: The controversy surrounding zone II injuries. Surg Clin North Am 71:267–296, 1991.
2. Biffl WL, Moore EE: Identifying the asymptomatic patient with blunt carotid arterial injury. J Trauma 47:1163–1164, 1999.
3. Demetriades D, Theodorou D, Cornwell E, et al: Evaluation of penetrating injuries of the neck: Prospective study of 223 patients. World J Surg 21:47–48, 1997.
4. Fry WR, Dort JA, Smith RS, et al: Duplex scanning replaces arteriography and operative exploration in the diagnosis of potential cervical vascular injury. Am J Surg 168:693–695, 1994.
5. Ginzburg E, Montalvo B, LeBlang S, et al: The use of duplex ultrasonography in penetrating neck trauma. Arch Surg 131:691–693, 1996.
6. LeBlang SD, Nunez DB, Rivas LA, et al: Helical computed tomographic angiography in penetrating neck trauma. Emerg Radiol 4:200–206, 1997.
7. LeBlang SD, Nunez DB: Noninvasive imaging of cervical vascular injuries. AJR Am J Roentgenol 175:1269–1278, 2002.
8. Montalvo BM, LeBlang SD, Nunez DB Jr, et al: Color Doppler sonography in penetrating injuries of the neck. AJNR Am J Neuroradiol 17:943–951, 1996.
9. Munera F, Soto JA, Palacio D, et al: Diagnosis of arterial injuries caused by penetrating trauma to the neck: Comparison of helical CT angiography and conventional angiography. Radiology 216:356–362, 2000.

110. CHEST TRAUMA

Justin C. Chang, M.D., and Robert C. Jorden, M.D.

1. How should the patient with chest trauma be approached?

One must immediately identify actual or potential life threats based on the clinical evaluation. This evaluation consists of the standard inspection, auscultation, and palpation.

Inspection. Completely undress the patient and visually inspect the entire chest, which necessitates rolling over a supine patient. Look for a flail chest (paradoxical movement of the chest wall) and sucking chest wounds. Identify the exact location, number, and type (i.e., penetrating or blunt) of wounds.

Auscultation. Listen for diminished or absent breath sounds and bowel sounds in the chest. The former indicates a pneumothorax if the subcutaneous emphysema is located over the ribs or a pneumomediastinum if the location is supraclavicular. Bony crepitus indicates a rib or sternal fracture with the potential for intrathoracic injury.

Palpation. It is important to palpate the chest wall gently at first to detect subcutaneous emphysema and bony crepitus. The former indicates a major blow to the chest with rib fractures and the potential for underlying organ damage, and the latter, depending on location, indicates pneumothorax or pneumomediastinum.

2. What is a flail chest?

A flail chest occurs when a segment of the chest wall becomes unattached from the rest of the chest. It occurs in one of three settings: (1) two or more ribs are broken in two or more places; (2) more than one rib is fractured in association with costal cartilage disarticulation; or (3) the costal cartilages on both sides of the sternum are disarticulated, resulting in a sternal or central flail segment. The significance of a flail chest lies in the tremendous force that caused it and the near certainty of associated intrathoracic injuries.

3. What is the treatment for flail chest?

The condition of the underlying lung generally dictates the treatment. Underlying pulmonary contusion and resultant hypoxemia indicate the need for intervention. In general, a flail chest should be treated supportively; if the patient is doing well and tolerating the flail (i.e., blood gases do not show hypoxemia or hypercarbia), only supplemental oxygen is indicated. If the patient is in respiratory distress either clinically or as indicated by blood gas analysis or oxygen saturation measurements, intubation and positive-pressure ventilation should be initiated. Positive-pressure ventilation results in uniform expansion of the chest from within and stabilizes the flail segment.

4. What significant history should be obtained from the victim of a motor vehicle accident?

1. What was the nature of the accident (rollover, head-on collision)?
2. Was the patient wearing a seat belt?
3. Did the air bag deploy?
4. Was the steering wheel or windshield broken?
5. Was there substantial vehicular damage?
6. Was there intrusion into the passenger space?

When a frontal deceleration mechanism is operative, one should consider not only chest wall injuries and pulmonary contusion, but also two other specific entities—myocardial contusion and aortic rupture.

5. How is myocardial contusion diagnosed and treated?

There is no gold standard for the diagnosis of myocardial contusion. Many modalities have been used in the attempt, including ECG, radionuclide scanning, cardiac enzyme analysis, and echocardiography. Because a contusion rarely causes serious arrhythmias or compromises cardiac output, there is a trend away from aggressive monitoring of patients based on mechanism only. Instead, most recommend using ECG and clinical assessment as a screening device. A normal ECG in the absence of hemodynamic instability precludes the need for extended monitoring and probably effectively rules out a clinically significant contusion. An abnormal ECG or unexplained hypotension may merit further diagnostic evaluation, such as echocardiogram or radionuclide scan. Treatment is symptomatic, with arrhythmia control and measures to optimize cardiac output.

6. How can anyone survive a ruptured aorta?

Approximately 85% to 90% of patients with aortic rupture die, and they do so before medical aid reaches them. The 10% to 15% who survive do so because not all three layers of the aorta are ruptured; the adventitia remains intact and temporarily contains the hemorrhage. Left untreated, this injury usually results in complete rupture and exsanguination, usually in hours to days, but this may be delayed for years in the form of a pseudoaneurysm rupture.

7. What is the mechanism of a traumatic aortic tear?

The thoracic aorta is particularly susceptible to acceleration-deceleration shearing forces because the arch is less mobile than the heart and the aorta distal to the ligamentum arteriosum. Frontal or transverse deceleration causes shearing forces at the points of fixation, with the most common site for disruption being just distal to the left subclavian artery. Vertical acceleration-deceleration injuries such as falls may result in a tear of the ascending aorta with coronary artery compromise or acute pericardial tamponade.

8. Describe the first steps in diagnosing aortic rupture.

Traditionally the initial screening for aortic rupture includes obtaining the mechanism of injury and a standard upright **chest radiograph**. The finding of an abnormal-appearing or widened mediastinal silhouette usually triggers additional workup for these patients. Other suggestive radiographic findings include deviation of the nasogastric tube to the right, an apical cap, left pleural effusion, loss of the aortic window or the left pleural stripe, and depression of the left main stem bronchus. A supine chest radiograph can have a falsely widened mediastinum, and aortic rupture can be present even with a normal-appearing chest radiograph. If clinical suspicion is strong enough based on mechanism or clinical findings, further evaluation of the aorta by helical chest CT or aortography is warranted.

9. Should aortography or helical CT be used in diagnosing aortic rupture?

Classically, aortography has been considered the gold standard for diagnosing this condition. It is a relatively safe procedure with high sensitivity and specificity (both generally regarded as being > 90%). It is also an invasive, costly, and time-consuming procedure, however, which may not be available at all institutions or during off hours.

The introduction of helical CT technology has resulted in CT becoming an increasingly used alternative method of diagnosis. It is more widely available, quicker, and usually accessible 24 hours a day. Also, many trauma patients often require a trip to the CT scanner for other reasons. Large, prospective studies showed helical CT to have 100% sensitivity and 100% negative predictive value for diagnosing traumatic aortic injury. Patients with negative scans effectively require no further evaluation. Helical CT also can diagnose subtle intimal injuries sometimes missed by aortography. The major drawback with helical CT is its lower specificity (83% to 98%) compared with aortography. Nevertheless, when used as a screening test, helical CT can reduce dramatically the number of unnecessary aortograms performed. A dynamic helical CT scan of the chest is accepted as an initial screening test to rule out traumatic aortic dissection because a completely normal CT scan effectively rules out aortic injury.

10. How is penetrating chest trauma managed?

Multiple diagnostic and therapeutic approaches exist depending on the location of the chest wound and the nature of the wounding implement.

11. What is the significance of the location of the wound?

Wound location dictates the clinical approach by virtue of the organs at risk. From a functional standpoint, wounds are categorized as central, peripheral, thoracoabdominal, and those in adjacent areas (abdomen and neck). Anatomically speaking, central wounds are located anteriorly (bordered by the midclavicular lines, the clavicles superiorly, and the costal margins inferiorly). All other wounds are considered peripheral; they are either lateral (bordered by the midclavicular lines, the posterior axillary lines, the axilla, and the costal margins) or posterior (bordered by the posterior axillary lines, the shoulders, and the costal margins). Thoracoabdominal wounds are those in the inferior positions of all three anatomic areas. The inferior portions are defined by the nipple line anteriorly, the sixth rib laterally, and the tip of the scapulas posteriorly. Any wound below these landmarks is considered thoracoabdominal.

12. How are penetrating wounds of the central region managed?

Patients who are grossly unstable require an emergent thoracotomy with no ED workup. Stable patients should be monitored closely while a diagnostic workup (consisting of aortography, an esophagogram with or without esophagoscopy, and possibly bronchoscopy) is done. If the workup is negative, observation for 24 to 48 hours is appropriate; if positive, surgical intervention is needed. A helical CT scan of the chest can be extremely useful to determine the presence and location of mediastinal hemorrhage. If the hemorrhage is periaortic or direct signs of aortic injury are seen, the patient should proceed to aortography or possibly directly to the operating room.

13. What are the indications for ED thoracotomy?

Victims of penetrating trauma who arrest after arrival to the hospital or who arrest in the field and do not require prolonged cardiopulmonary resuscitation (CPR). If more than 10 minutes of CPR are performed, ED thoracotomy is futile. Similarly, victims of blunt trauma who arrest should not undergo thoracotomy because survival is essentially 0%. The only exception may be patients with suspected cardiac rupture, who might be salvaged by prompt thoracotomy.

14. What are the radiographic findings of a tension pneumothorax?

There should not be any because this diagnosis should be made on clinical grounds, and treatment should be undertaken before a radiograph is obtained. If a radiograph is obtained, a hyperlucent, overexpanded hemithorax with an evident pneumothorax and a mediastinal shift to the opposite side would be observed.

15. What are the clinical signs of a tension pneumothorax?

Respiratory distress, an overexpanded hemithorax, hyperresonance to percussion, absent or markedly diminished breath sounds, tracheal shift away from the pneumothorax (the trachea must be palpated above the sternal notch; it is not appreciated on inspection), tachycardia, jugular venous distention, subcutaneous emphysema, and hypotension. In addition, in patients who are intubated and are being bag ventilated, increasing resistance to ventilation (requiring more manual pressure to insufflate air into the lungs) is often the earliest sign of tension pneumothorax.

16. Why does tension pneumothorax cause hypotension?

The mediastinal shift compromises vena caval blood return to the heart. The severely altered preload results in reduced stroke volume, reduced cardiac output, and hypotension.

17. What is the treatment for a tension pneumothorax?

Immediate reduction in the intrapleural pressure on the affected side is appropriate therapy. For patients in extremis, the best way to accomplish this is also the quickest: placement of a 14G over-the-needle catheter over the fourth or fifth rib in the midaxillary line, followed by aspiration with a 50-mL syringe. After vital signs improve, the procedure should be followed immediately by **tube thoracostomy**, which is the definitive treatment. For patients who are stable, aspiration need not precede insertion of a chest tube.

18. When should pericardial tamponade be suspected?

Acute pericardial tamponade is a clinical condition that results from the accumulation of blood and clots in the pericardial space. When pericardial pressure exceeds cardiac filling pressure, shock and ultimately death rapidly ensue. It should be suspected in any patient with a penetrating wound of the chest (particularly in the central area) who develops hypotension, tachycardia, and elevated central venous pressure after tension pneumothorax has been treated or ruled out. The most accurate means of diagnosing a pericardial effusion is bedside ultrasonography.

19. How is acute pericardial tamponade treated?

The proper course of action in an unstable patient is **pericardiocentesis** followed by immediate transfer to the operating room for definitive therapy. If vital signs are lost in the ED, an immediate thoracotomy is indicated. In stable patients with impending tamponade, the presence of pericardial blood can be confirmed by bedside ultrasonography. In unstable patients, diagnosis is confirmed by response to therapeutic interventions.

20. Should all patients with a stab wound of the chest be admitted to the hospital?

Patients with peripheral wounds not in the thoracoabdominal area who are stable and have an initial chest radiograph that is normal usually do not require admission. They should be observed in the ED and have a repeat radiograph and hematocrit done in 4 to 6 hours. If repeat studies are normal, the patient may be discharged.

21. Are peripheral gunshot wounds that cross the mediastinum handled differently?

Determining missile trajectory based on entry wound and final resting position or exit wound is not always accurate. Nevertheless, if the estimated trajectory does traverse the mediastinum, these patients require a more thorough diagnostic evaluation while they are observed as inpatients. They should undergo the same workup as patients who have sustained a penetrating injury of the central chest.

22. How are thoracoabdominal wounds managed?

By virtue of their low chest location, such wounds risk injury to the infradiaphragmatic, intraperitoneal, and retroperitoneal organs. There is no clear consensus on how to manage these patients. Some recommend observation alone, basing surgical intervention on positive physical findings. Others use diagnostic peritoneal lavage with lowered red blood cell criteria (> 5,000 or 10,000 red cells as opposed to the usual 50,000 to 100,000). Others use laparoscopy as a more definitive but more difficult and time-consuming means of evaluation. Posterior thoracoabdominal wounds are particularly difficult to evaluate because retroperitoneal injuries are predominant, and they are undetected by peritoneal lavage. Observation with a variable diagnostic workup is recommended. Some merely observe, whereas others recommend adding an intravenous pyelogram, diagnostic peritoneal lavage, abdominal CT scan, contrast-enhanced CT enema, or varying combinations of these alternatives. Contrast-enhanced CT enema adds rectally instilled contrast material to the usual intravenous and oral contrast agents given during abdominal scanning. The goal is early diagnosis of an occult colon injury.

BIBLIOGRAPHY

 1. Borlase BC, Moore EE, Moore FA: Penetrating wounds to the posterior chest: Analysis of exigent thoracotomy and laparotomy. J Emerg Med 7:445–447, 1989.
 2. Durham LA, Richardson RJ, Wall MJ, et al: Emergency center thoracotomy: Impact of prehospital resuscitation. J Trauma 32:775–779, 1992.
 3. Dyer DS, Moore EE, Ilke DN, et al: Thoracic aortic injury: How predictive is mechanism and is chest computed tomography a reliable screening tool? A prospective study of 1,561 patients. J Trauma 48:673–683, 2000.
 4. Fabian TC, Davis KA, Gavant ML, et al: Prospective study of blunt aortic injury: Helical CT is diagnostic and antihypertensive therapy reduces rupture. Ann Surg 227:666–677, 1998.

5. Fabian TC, Richardson JD, Croce MA, et al: Prospective study of blunt aortic injury: Multicenter trial of the American Association for the Surgery of Trauma. J Trauma Inj Inf Crit Care 47:374–383, 1997.
6. Fildes JJ, Betlej TM, Manglano R, et al: Limiting cardiac evaluation in patients with suspected myocardial contusion. Am Surg 61:832–835, 1995.
7. Ivatory RR, Simon RJ, Weksler B, et al: Laparoscopy in the evaluation of the intrathoracic abdomen after penetrating injury. J Trauma 33:101–109, 1992.
8. Merlotti GJ, Dillon BC, Lange DA: Peritoneal lavage in penetrating thoraco-abdominal trauma. J Trauma 28:17–23, 1988.
9. Phillips T, Sclafani SJ, Goldstein A: Use of the contrast-enhanced CT enema in the management of penetrating trauma to the flank and back. J Trauma 26:593–601, 1986.
10. Plummer D, Brunette D, Asinger R, et al: Emergency department echocardiography improves outcome in penetrating cardiac injury. Ann Emerg Med 21:709–712, 1992.

111. ABDOMINAL TRAUMA

Reginald J. Franciose, M.D., and Ernest E. Moore, M.D.

1. What is the difference in pathophysiology between blunt and penetrating trauma?

Blunt trauma results from a combination of crushing, stretching, and shearing forces. The magnitude of these forces is proportional to the mass of the objects, rate of change in velocity (acceleration and deceleration), direction of impact, and elasticity of the tissues. Injury results when the sum of these forces exceeds the cohesive strength and mobility of the tissues and organs involved. High-energy transfer to the abdomen induces a pronounced rise in intraabdominal pressure that can produce hollow viscus rupture or solid-organ burst injuries. Compression of abdominal contents against the thoracic cage or spinal column may result in visceral crush injuries, and abrupt shearing forces may avulse organs from their vascular pedicles. The injuries produce a constellation of tissue contusions, abrasions, fractures, or organ ruptures. **Penetrating injuries** result from the dissipation of energy and tissue disruption along the path of the offending projectile. Typically, injuries result in localized tears or contusions of involved organs. The magnitude of injury depends on the penetrating object (i.e., knife versus bullet) and the trajectory.

2. What is the difference in pathophysiology between stab wounds and gunshot wounds?

Stab wounds typically produce clean lacerations of contiguous structures along the path of penetration. Although crucial structures may be involved, the physical damage is limited and generally requires only débridement and hemostasis or primary repair. **Gunshot wounds** are more extensive and are defined by the weapon and trajectory and the tissues traversed. The wounding potential of a projectile is determined largely by the kinetic energy (KE) imparted to the tissue. The KE of a missile is proportional to its mass (M) and the square of its velocity (V):

$$KE = \frac{MV^2}{2}$$

An increase in the mass of a given missile by a factor of 2 doubles its KE, whereas the same increment in velocity quadruples the KE. The efficiency of energy dissipation in tissue for a given projectile is determined by its physical characteristics and pattern of flight. Soft lead or hollow-tip projectiles are prone to mushrooming, fragmentation, and tumbling, which make them more destructive than fully jacketed spiraling projectiles. Low-velocity weapons produce injury predominantly by direct crushing and tearing, whereas high-velocity missiles induce variable tissue cavitation as well. The extent of cavitation is governed by the rate of energy dissipation and physical characteristics of the tissues involved. Solid, inelastic organs, such as the liver, spleen, and brain, are more susceptible than relatively pliant lung and skeletal muscle. A shotgun fires a group of pellets that disperse as a function of distance and length or taper of the gun barrel.

Shotgun loads vary in the number and size of pellets per load; at close range (< 7 m), the predominant determinant of wounding potential is the aggregate KE of the pellets. Because of the spherical shape of the pellets, velocity dissipates rapidly at greater distance.

3. What are the common injury patterns produced by blunt abdominal trauma?

Blunt injuries usually represent energy transfer to underlying visceral and vascular structures in the anatomic region sustaining the direct impact and can be compounded by crushing against the rigid vertebral column. Specific examples of these patterns are as follows:

DIRECT IMPACT	RESULTANT INJURIES
Right lower rib fractures	Liver, gallbladder
Left lower rib fractures	Spleen, left kidney
Mid epigastric contusion	Duodenum, pancreas, small bowel mesentery
Lumbar transverse process fracture	Kidney, ureter
Anterior pelvic fracture	Bladder, urethra

4. List the common patterns of injury associated with penetrating abdominal wounds.

REGION	LIKELY INJURY	FREQUENTLY ASSOCIATED INJURIES
Right upper quadrant	Liver	Diaphragm, gallbladder, right colon
Left upper quadrant	Spleen	Stomach, pancreas (tail), left kidney diaphragm
Midepigastric	Stomach	Pancreas (body), abdominal aorta
	Duodenum	Inferior vena cava
	Portal vein	Hepatic artery, common bile duct
	Superior mesenteric artery	Pancreas (neck), left renal vein, abdominal aorta
Pelvis	Iliac artery	Iliac vein, bladder, rectum

5. Discuss the key aspects of the history and physical examination in the initial evaluation of abdominal trauma.

The history is important in establishing the tempo, sequence, and extent of early diagnostic efforts. After blunt trauma caused by a motor vehicle accident, the size of the motor vehicle, its velocity and direction of impact, the use of lap and shoulder restraints, air bag deployment, associated steering wheel and windshield damage, and patient ejection are crucial facts to glean from prehospital providers. The initial physical examination is divided conceptually into the primary and secondary survey. The primary survey is a rapid search for immediate life-threatening injuries, whereas the second survey is a comprehensive examination that includes a systematic review for signs of potential occult injury. Upper abdominal and lower thoracic trauma should be considered as a unit because the dome of the diaphragm rises to the fourth intercostal space during full expiration, rendering the upper abdominal contents at risk for injury after impact to the lower chest. Gentle pressure over the lower ribs helps to establish the presence of fractures; fractures of the left and right lower ribs result in a 20% chance of splenic injury and a 10% chance of hepatic injury. The physical findings most often associated with internal injury are abdominal tenderness and guarding; rebound tenderness and rigidity are relatively infrequent. Most importantly, 20% to 40% of patients with serious intraabdominal injury in the context of multisystem trauma may be asymptomatic.

6. Which diagnostic tools are most helpful for the initial evaluation of blunt abdominal trauma?

1. **Ultrasound**: Ultrasound is currently the initial test of choice in the evaluation of multisystem trauma patients with blunt abdominal trauma. It is noninvasive and portable and can be

performed rapidly at the patient's bedside while resuscitation is in progress. A major advantage of ultrasound is that it is easily repeatable, allowing for serial examinations. It is most sensitive (86% to 98%) for the detection of free intraperitoneal fluid. Ultrasound also readily visualizes the heart and pericardial space, providing additional information. The major disadvantage of ultrasound is that it does not show specific organ injury well or identify the precise site of bleeding. It does not evaluate for retroperitoneum or hollow viscous injuries or distinguish blood from other fluids (i.e., ascites), and it is operator dependent.

2. **Diagnostic peritoneal lavage (DPL)**: DPL is a safe, rapid method to identify life-threatening intraperitoneal hemorrhage. Introduced in 1965, DPL was the gold standard for evaluation of the critically injured for more than 2 decades. It is an extremely sensitive (98% to 100%) technique for detecting intraperitoneal hemorrhage and is relatively effective in evaluating for hollow viscus injuries. With current standards for nonoperative management of hepatic and spleen injuries, DPL has become an overly sensitive means to detect intraperitoneal hemorrhage. Results must be interpreted cautiously in hemodynamically stable patients to prevent nontherapeutic laparotomies. Disadvantages of DPL include lack of organ specificity, inability to evaluate the retroperitoneum, and the morbidity of an invasive procedure. Reported complication rates of DPL range from 0.5% to 5% and include perforations of the small bowel, mesentery, bladder, and retroperitoneal vascular structures and wound infection. Relative contraindications to DPL include morbid obesity, multiple previous abdominal surgeries, and portal hypertension (risk of variceal perforation).

3. **CT**: CT has an important role as a noninvasive diagnostic adjunct in the early evaluation of abdominal and pelvic injuries. In addition to excellent sensitivity (93% to 98%) for intraperitoneal hemorrhage, CT adds injury specificity and shows the magnitude of solid-organ injury. This is an essential component of managing patients expectantly who are hemodynamically stable with liver, spleen, or kidney injuries. It is imperative that patients never be sent to the CT scanner until they have shown hemodynamic stability. Four additional groups of patients are particularly suitable for CT scanning: (1) patients with delayed (> 6 hours) presentation who are hemodynamically stable and do not have overt signs of peritonitis; (2) patients in whom ultrasound or DPL results are equivocal, and repeated physical examination is unreliable or untenable (e.g., patients who require prolonged general anesthesia for neurosurgical or orthopedic procedures, patients with altered mental status, patients with spinal cord injury); (3) patients in whom ultrasound or DPL is difficult to perform or is unreliable (e.g., morbid obesity, portal hypertension, previous laparotomies); and (4) patients at high risk for retroperitoneal injuries in whom the ultrasound or DPL is unrevealing (e.g., an unrestrained, intoxicated driver who strikes the steering column; a patient with postinjury hyperamylasemia). CT is valuable in defining the geometry of complex pelvic fractures, and with the addition of intravenous and bladder contrast material (CT cystogram), CT can be used to evaluate hematuria. Disadvantages of CT include necessity for oral and intravenous contrast agents, issues involving timely completion and transport from the ED, lack of availability of experienced radiologists, and expense. CT scanning may not show blunt pancreatic fractures in the first 6 hours after injury and may not be reliable for early detection of hollow viscous injuries. CT signs suggestive of hollow viscous injuries include free fluid without solid-organ injury, free air, or mesentric streaking. Contrast extravasation is pathognomonic for hollow viscous injury.

7. How are DPL results interpreted after blunt abdominal trauma?

DPL is considered positive if greater than 10 mL of free blood is aspirated. Otherwise, 1 L of warmed 0.9% sodium chloride is infused (15 mL/kg in children). If the clinical condition permits, the patient is rolled from side to side to enhance intraperitoneal sampling. The saline bag is lowered to the floor for the return of lavage fluid by siphonage. A minimal recovery of 75% of lavage effluent is required for the test to be considered valid. The fluid is sent for laboratory analysis of red blood cell (RBC) and white blood cell (WBC) counts, levels of lavage amylase and lavage alkaline phosphatase, and bilirubin. The criteria for positive DPL are outlined in the table. In the context of blunt abdominal trauma, significant visceral damage is encountered in greater than 90% of patients in whom the RBC count exceeds 100,000/mm³ but in less than 2% of patients in whom the count is less than 20,000 mm³. RBC counts between 20,000 and 100,000/mm³ may reflect serious injury in 15% to 35% of cases and merit further diagnostic evaluation. Occasionally an elevated WBC count (> 500/mm³) signals an otherwise occult intestinal injury. The contents of a perforated viscus evoke migration of leukocytes into the peritoneal cavity, but this response may be delayed for several hours after injury. Conversely an isolated WBC count exceeding 500/mm³ in a DPL done promptly after injury is often nonspecific. If the initial WBC count is elevated, repeat the DPL in 12 hours and do a laparotomy only if the count remains elevated. A lavage amylase level is more accurate in the detection of hollow visceral injury; a lavage amylase level greater than 20 IU/L combined with a lavage alkaline phosphatase level greater than 3 IU/L has a specificity greater than 95% for small bowel perforation.

Criteria for Positive DPL after Abdominal Trauma

INDEX	POSITIVE	EQUIVOCAL
Aspirate		
Blood	> 10 mL	
Fluid	Enteric contents	
Lavage		
RBCs	> 100,000/mm³	> 20,000/mm³
WBCs		> 500/mm³
Enzyme	Amylase > 20 IU/L and alkaline phosphatase > 3 IU	Amylase > 20 or alkaline phosphatase > 3 IU
Bilirubin	Greater than serum level	

8. Which diagnostic tests are most useful for the initial evaluation for penetrating abdominal wounds?

The management of penetrating abdominal wounds is dichotomous. Gunshot wounds that violate the peritoneum warrant mandatory laparotomy, whereas stab wounds can be managed selectively. Only two thirds of stab wounds to the anterior abdomen penetrate the peritoneal cavity, and only one half of those entering the peritoneum produce injuries requiring laparotomy. Consequently the first diagnostic question is whether the stab wound traverses the peritoneum. Local wound exploration, done under local anesthesia in the ED, answers this question reliably. Patients with an unequivocally negative wound exploration can be discharged. If peritoneal violation has occurred, the next question is whether significant intraabdominal injury is involved. DPL has proved to be exceedingly useful in the decision for laparotomy is this scenario. In a hemodynamically stable patient in whom peritoneal integrity is indeterminate, laparoscopy may be used to ascertain violation of the peritoneum.

9. What are the indications and interpretation of DPL after penetrating trauma?

The DPL indications for laparotomy are controversial, but most authorities recommend the same criteria employed for blunt trauma. Because of a proportionally high number of isolated intestinal perforations after stab wound, DPL has a 5% false-negative rate. All patients with a negative lavage are admitted for at least 24 hours of observation and undergo prompt exploration if signs of peritoneal irritation ensue. Most injuries missed by the initial DPL are isolated small bowel perforations, which usually are recognized within 12 hours and, if managed promptly, yield minimal additional morbidity. Lower chest stab wounds are associated with a 15% risk of abdominal injury because the diaphragm rises to the midchest during deep expiration. Unrecognized diaphragmatic rents pose a lifelong threat because the continuous negative pleuroperitoneal pressure gradient encourages visceral herniation into the pleural cavity, which results in strangulated intestine. The physical examination of patients with thoracoabdominal trauma is notoriously inaccurate. Consequently, DPL is recommended for all lower thoracic wounds. Blood loss may be minimal after perforation of the diaphragm; the RBC threshold for laparotomy is lowered to 10,000/mm³. Laparoscopy and thoracoscopy may prove to have a role in the evaluation of lower thoracic stab wounds with associated RBC counts between 1,000 and 10,000/mm³. Occasionally, patients who are hemodynamically stable with superficial tangential gunshot wounds that do not seem to traverse the peritoneum can be evaluated by DPL. In this scenario, a RBC count greater than 5,000/mm³ should be considered diagnostic for peritoneal violation.

10. How are management priorities different for penetrating versus blunt abdominal trauma?

In general, initial management of **penetrating trauma** comprises three elements: (1) aggressive resuscitation for any sign of hypovolemia, (2) directed physical examination, and (3) quick diagnostic studies with appropriate interventions. Gunshot wounds that traverse the peritoneum mandate immediate laparotomy. When the wound is in proximity to the thorax, a chest radiograph should be obtained to ensure that a bullet has not entered the chest. In hemodynamically stable patients, anteroposterior and lateral abdominal films with radiopaque markers on the entrance wounds are valuable in determining the bullet path during exploration. For stab wounds, hemodynamic instability, obvious evisceration, peritoneal signs, and intraperitoneal fluid shown by ultrasound (the exception with ultrasound being a question of ascites secondary to cirrhosis) are indications for immediate laparotomy. Otherwise the management of stab wounds is local wound exploration followed by DPL when indicated (see question 8).

The initial management of **blunt abdominal trauma** (see figure) consists of (1) gathering pertinent information from the patient, paramedics, flight nurses, and family; (2) aggressive resuscitation for any sign of hypovolemia; (3) systematic physical examination; and (4) directed laboratory and diagnostic studies, performed in a fashion dictated by the patient's physiologic status. The initial screening test is bedside ultrasound. If intraperitoneal fluid is identified, the patient's hemodynamic status determines whether to proceed to laparotomy or to CT scan for stable patients who are not operative candidates. For patients with an equivocal ultrasound or signs of peritoneal irritation, proceed to DPL. Patients who are hemodynamically stable with a negative ultrasound are followed with serial examination and ultrasound.

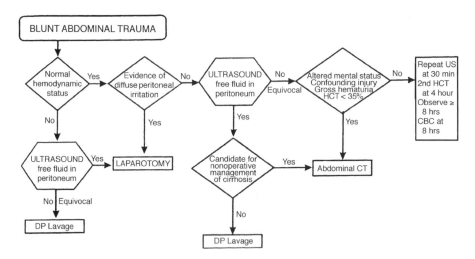

Algorithm for blunt abdominal trauma. US = ultrasound; HCT = hematocrit; CBC = complete blood cell count; CT = computed tomography; DP = diagnostic peritoneal. (From Branney SW, Moore EE, Cantrill SV, et al: Ultrasound based key clinical pathway reduces the use of hospital resources for the evaluation of blunt abdominal trauma. J Trauma 42:1086–1090, 1997; with permission.)

11. What are the concerns in a pregnant patient with abdominal trauma?

The prevailing rule when managing a pregnant trauma patient is that optimal care of the mother ensures the best outcome for the fetus. Pregnancy alters the susceptibility to blunt injury and the physiologic response to injury. The gravid uterus occupies the pelvis and lower abdomen and is vulnerable to a variety of insults from direct blows or seat belt injuries. These insults result in a spectrum of injuries from minor soft tissue contusions to uterine wall disruption, placental abruption, potential exsanguination, and fetal loss. The significance of relatively minor injuries mandates an aggressive posture in the early evaluation of pregnant patients. Ultrasound and DPL (open technique) are used routinely; the gravid uterus is evaluated simultaneously with ultrasound and noninvasive fetal monitoring. Hemodynamic instability, uterine rupture, placental abruption, or fetal distress indicates the need for emergent abdominal exploration and uterine evacuation with the rare possibility of hysterectomy. (See Chapter 115, Trauma in Pregnancy.)

12. What about the pediatric patient?

Pediatric trauma provides unique challenges because of patient size and different injury patterns. The elasticity of the child's lower rib cage and the relative large size of the abdominal cavity increase susceptibility to intraabdominal injury. Blunt injuries commonly are minor, with modest liver or splenic fractures that are self-limited. Pancreatic fractures and intestinal perforations are infrequent in children. Despite the enthusiasm for nonoperative management, an aggressive operative policy is warranted in the context of pediatric multisystem trauma because of the child's limited physiologic reserve. Although grossly positive DPLs in hemodynamically stable children can be elucidated further by CT scan to verify solid-organ injury amenable to expectant care, abdominal exploration is undertaken promptly for hemodynamic instability, need for ongoing blood transfusions, or DPLs positive by enzymes. (See Chapter 116, Pediatric Trauma.)

BIBLIOGRAPHY

1. American College of Surgeons Committee on Trauma: Advanced Trauma Life Support Course. Chicago, American College of Surgeons, 1997.
2. Branney SW, Moore EE, Cantrill SV, et al: Ultrasound based key clinical pathway reduces the use of hospital resources for the evaluation of blunt abdominal trauma. J Trauma 42:1086–1090, 1997.
3. Burch JM, Franciose RJ, Moore EE: Trauma. In Schwartz SI (ed): Principles of Surgery, 7th ed. New York, McGraw-Hill, 1998, pp 155–221.
4. Demetriades D: Indications for laparotomy. In Moore EE, Feliciano DV, Mattox KL (eds): Trauma, 5th ed. New York, McGraw-Hill, 2002.
5. Henneman PL, Marx JA, Moore EE, et al: Diagnostic peritoneal lavage: Accuracy in predicting necessary laparotomy following blunt and penetrating trauma. J Trauma 30:1345–1355, 1990.
6. Tso P, Rodriquez A, Cooper C, et al: Sonography in blunt abdominal trauma: A preliminary progress report. J Trauma 33:39–43, 1992.
7. Livingston D, Lavery R, Passannate M, et al: Free fluid on abdominal computed tomography without solid organ injury after blunt abdominal injury does not mandate celitomy. Am J Surg 182:6, 2001.
8. Omert L, Salyer D, Dunham M, et al: Implications of the "contrast blush" finding on computed tomographic scan of the spleen in trauma. J Trauma 51:272, 2001.
9. McCarter FD, Luchette FA, Malloy M, et al: Institutional and individual learning curves for focused abdominal ultrasound for trauma. Ann Surg 231:689, 2000.
10. Ochsner MG, Knudson MM, Pachter HL, et al: Significance of minimal or no intraperitoneal fluid visible on CT scan associated with blunt liver and splenic injuries. J Trauma 49:505, 2000.
11. Malhotra AK, Fabian TC, Katsis SB, et al: Blunt bowel and mesenteric injuries: The role of screening computed tomography. J Trauma 48:991, 2000.
12. Peitzman AB, Heil B, Rivera L, et al: Blunt splenic injury in adults: Multi-institutional study. J Trauma 49:177, 2000.

112. HEMORRHAGE FROM PELVIC FRACTURES

Walter L. Biffl, M.D., and Ernest E. Moore, M.D.

1. Why are pelvic fractures so deadly?

Fractured pelvic bones bleed briskly and can lacerate surrounding soft tissues and disrupt their extensive arterial and venous networks. The resultant hemorrhage and secondary coagulopathy can be lethal; to confound matters, the considerable force required to fracture the pelvis typically results in significant associated injuries. Collectively, these factors account for high rates of morbidity and mortality.

2. What is the approach to the patient with a pelvic fracture?

The evaluation of patients with pelvic fractures begins with the primary trauma survey (the **ABCs**) and resuscitation. Unstable patients with pelvic fractures require a multispecialty approach, with the fundamental objectives being: (1) control of hemorrhage, (2) restoration of hemodynamic stability, (3) identification of associated injuries, and (4) prioritization of treatment based on threat to life. Life-threatening associated injuries are evaluated and treated simultaneously with systematic assessment of the pelvic fractures. The physical examination directed at the pelvis includes **gentle** manual compression of the bony pelvis and inspection of the perineum, rectum, and vagina for ecchymosis, ongoing bleeding, and open wounds. Plain anteroposterior radiography of the pelvis is a priority in patients with suspected fracture. Hemodynamically stable patients may be evaluated further with additional views (e.g., inlet/outlet) or CT, but this should not interfere with resuscitation or necessary interventions. Because these patients may require coordinated interventions by multiple specialties, the recognition of a hemodynamically unstable patient with a potentially mechanically unstable pelvic fracture warrants the immediate presence of the attending trauma surgeon, attending orthopedic surgeon, and interventional radiologist in the ED.

3. How are pelvic fractures classified?

Multiple classification systems have been developed based on a variety of perspectives, including injury mechanism, fracture geography, and fracture stability. Currently the most useful classification system is Young's modification of the Pennel and Sutherland classification. This scheme is based on **injury mechanism** (i.e., anteroposterior compression, lateral compression, vertical shear); further grading (I, II, or III) suggests a likelihood of fracture-related bleeding, hemorrhagic shock, associated injuries, morbidity, and mortality. Anteroposterior compression fractures are associated with pubic symphyseal diastasis and sacroiliac (SI) disruption. Similarly, vertical shear injuries consist of displaced fractures of the anterior rami and posterior columns, including SI dislocation. Lateral compression fractures result in compression of posterior ligaments.

4. What are the sources and sites of bleeding from major pelvic fractures?

Uncontrolled hemorrhage is the leading cause of early death in patients with complex pelvic fractures. Massive bleeding is associated most frequently with vertical shear or anteroposterior compression fractures. SI disruption leads to bleeding from the internal iliac system, particularly the superior gluteal artery, bridging the anterior surface of the SI joint. Pubic diastasis and anterior fractures may result in significant blood loss, notably from vesicular branches of the pudendal artery. The most frequent source of bleeding is venous. Branches of the veins in the superior gluteal and pudendal distributions and the lumbosacral venous plexus contribute significantly to retroperitoneal and pelvic hemorrhage. Because lateral compression fractures result in compression of local vasculature, they are not usually associated with major pelvic blood loss.

5. What is the role of mechanical pelvic stabilization?

To reduce the pelvic volume, promote tamponade of bleeding bone and vessels, and prevent further fracture motion.

6. Name four ways to stabilize the pelvis.

1. Wrapping the pelvis with sheets or large straps
2. Resuscitation (C-) clamps
3. External fixation frames
4. Pneumatic antishock garments (PASG)

7. Discuss the role of the four methods of pelvic stabilization.

1. Wrapping the pelvis with sheets and binding the knees and ankles with tape is a simple maneuver that can be performed by virtually anybody in the ED or in the prehospital setting. This intervention is effective and should be performed immediately on discovery of an unstable pelvic fracture, particularly before patient transport. It can be used only temporarily, however, because prolonged periods of tight immobilization may result in extremity or abdominal compartment syndrome.

2. The C-clamp has the advantage of rapid application, without the need for fluoroscopy. It can be placed in any setting and can be rotated cephalad or caudad to allow virtually any required intervention. It is more effective than a standard anterior frame in stabilizing the posterior pelvis but requires the expertise of an orthopedic surgeon.

3. External fixation of complex pelvic fractures in the ED is becoming standard. Compression of the fractured pelvis decreases fracture mobility and limits expansion of the pelvic ring; it may contribute to tamponade of ongoing hemorrhage. The most favorable situation is the anteroposterior **open-book fracture** (i.e., disruption of the anterior ligaments of the SI joint with symphyseal diastasis). In this setting, the external frame can close the book, reducing the overall pelvic volume. More complex fractures, including complete SI disruption (i.e., vertical shear injury) also may benefit from early fracture stabilization, but fixation is not as complete because of the instability of the posterior column.

4. The use of PASG is controversial, particularly in prehospital trauma care in urban areas with short transport times. There is general support that PASG has a role in the acute management of pelvic fractures in hemodynamically unstable patients, to provide temporary splinting and tamponade of ongoing venous and small arterial hemorrhage. Given the efficacy of pelvic wrapping, there is little role for the PASG today.

8. Which abdominal injuries are associated with pelvic trauma?

Nearly 90% of patients with significant pelvic fractures have associated injuries. Associated abdominal injuries occur in approximately 15% to 20% of patients and increase with the magnitude and direction of force on impact (i.e., fracture classification).

Relative Frequency of Intraabdominal Injuries Associated with Major Pelvic Fractures (%)

	ANTERO-POSTERIOR	LATERAL COMPRESSION	VERTICAL SHEAR	COMBINED MECHANICAL
Spleen	20	0	25	12
Liver	10	0	7	5
Bowel	15	15	5	5
Kidney	1	1	4	4
Bladder	5	0	1	10
Vascular	25	25	5	5
Retroperitoneal hematoma	60	60	50	25

9. Which physical findings suggest injuries associated with major pelvic fractures?

Anterior pelvic instability, perineal hematomas, or blood at the urethral meatus are suggestive of urethral lacerations and bladder disruptions. These physical signs mandate complete urologic examination, including a retrograde cystourethrogram and commensurate therapy. Similarly, vaginal or rectal blood is strong evidence for laceration of these structures. Although the treatment for vaginal lacerations is unclear, open pelvic fractures with rectal tears portend profound septic complications and consequently require prompt interventions (see questions 14 and 15).

10. What is the role of abdominal ultrasound in the early evaluation of pelvic fractures?

With significant blood loss, early recognition of an extrapelvic source is imperative; the risk of active intraperitoneal visceral bleeding is 20% to 30%. Ultrasound is an integral part of the initial evaluation. If ultrasound is not available, diagnostic peritoneal lavage is done at the infraumbilical ring to avoid the dissecting pelvic hematoma; if results are negative, the catheter can be left in place to facilitate serial lavages as other diagnostic procedures are completed.

11. When should patients with pelvic trauma undergo laparotomy?

An ultrasound showing overt intraperitoneal fluid should prompt immediate laparotomy. Similarly a grossly positive diagnostic peritoneal lavage aspirate in a hemodynamically unstable patient mandates emergent abdominal exploration because aspiration of greater than 20 mL of gross blood is associated with a 95% chance of active splenic, hepatic, or mesenteric hemorrhage. A grossly negative tap but cell count-positive lavage must be interpreted cautiously because 20% are falsely positive from a ruptured pelvic hematoma or trivial hepatic or splenic injury. In the stable patient, CT should be used to clarify the source of bleeding after the immediate life-threatening problems have been addressed.

12. How is continued pelvic bleeding managed in these patients?

The patient with ongoing hemorrhage demands a critical triage decision. The unstable individual with a positive abdominal ultrasound or a grossly positive diagnostic peritoneal lavage should undergo laparotomy because of the high probability of solid visceral or major vascular injury. In the patient with a negative ultrasound or a positive lavage by red blood cell count, the pelvic bleeding should be managed first. The key decision is whether to employ skeletal fixation or selective pelvic arterial embolization; prompt consultation of orthopedic and interventional radiology specialists is imperative. (See figure, top of next page.)

13. How frequently are rectal injuries associated with pelvic injuries, and how are they managed?

Approximately 5% of major pelvic fractures are associated with rectal injuries. These complex injuries result in a high mortality rate secondary to septic complications. Current management principles are based on accumulated wartime experience, which has proved the efficacy of fracture stabilization, hemorrhage control, and fecal diversion with rectal washout, perineal débridement, and pelvic drainage via the presacral space.

14. What is rectal washout?

With the identification of a rectal injury in association with a pelvic fracture, the patient undergoes a diverting colostomy (usually sigmoid) with exclusion of the distal colon and rectum. The anal sphincters are gently dilated, and the excluded distal colon and rectum are copiously irrigated until gross fecal material has been removed. This technique has been shown to reduce morbidity and mortality significantly in critically injured patients.

15. What are the common urologic injuries associated with pelvic fractures?

Pelvic fractures usually cause posterior (above the urogenital diaphragm) urethral tears, as opposed to anterior lesions, which typically are associated with perineal straddle trauma (see Chapter 113, Genitourinary and Pelvic Trauma). If urethral disruption is suspected, Foley catheterization should be deferred until a retrograde urethrogram can be obtained. The ED management of complete urethral disruption is transcutaneous suprapubic cystostomy. Displaced pelvic rami fractures also may perforate the extraperitoneal bladder. Hematuria is absent in more than 10% of such patients, and the ability to void does not exclude the injury. Gravity flow

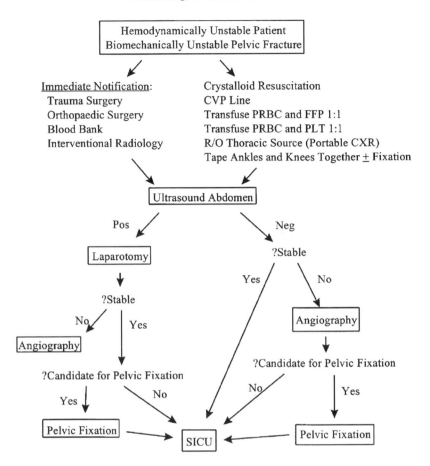

cystography with 250 mL of contrast material and postvoiding views should be done in patients with displaced anterior pelvic fractures.

16. What are the major causes of death following pelvic trauma?
The overall mortality from pelvic trauma is 30%. **Early mortality** results from uncontrolled hemorrhage, refractory shock, or associated multisystem injuries. **Delayed mortality** is most frequently the result of septic complications or multiple organ failure and may be 50% in the subset of patients with open pelvic fractures.

BIBLIOGRAPHY

1. Agolini SF, Shah K, Jaffe J, et al: Arterial embolization is a rapid and effective technique for controlling pelvic fracture hemorrhage. J Trauma 43:395–399, 1997.
2. Biffl WL, Smith WR, Moore EE, et al: Evolution of a multidisciplinary clinical pathway for the management of unstable patients with pelvic fractures. Ann Surg 233:843–850, 2001.
3. Buckle R, Browner BD, Morandi M: Emergency reduction for pelvic ring disruptions and control of associated hemorrhage using the pelvic stabilizer. Tech Orthop 9:258–266, 1995.
4. Burgess AR, Eastridge BJ, Young JWR, et al: Pelvic ring disruptions: Effective classification system and treatment protocols. J Trauma 30:848–856, 1990.
5. Parreira JG, Coimbra R, Rasslan S, et al: The role of associated injuries on outcome of blunt trauma patients sustaining pelvic fractures. Injury 31:677–682, 2000.
6. Routt MLC, Simonian PT, Swiontkowski MF: Stabilization of pelvic ring disruptions. Orthop Clin North Am 28:369–388, 1997.

7. Scalea TM, Burgess AR: Pelvic fractures. In Mattox KL, Feliciano DV, Moore EE (eds): Trauma, 4th ed. New York, McGraw-Hill, 2000, pp 807–837.
8. Shannon FL, Moore EE, Moore FA, McCroskey BL: Value of distal colon washout in civilian rectal trauma—reducing gut bacterial translocation. J Trauma 28:989–994, 1988.
9. Woods RK, O'Keefe G, Rhee P, et al: Open pelvic fracture and fecal diversion. Arch Surg 133:281–286, 1998.

113. GENITOURINARY AND PELVIC TRAUMA

Joanne M. Edney, M.D.

1. What are the primary mechanisms of renal trauma?

Blunt traumatic injuries caused by direct impact or severe deceleration (> 80%) and penetrating injuries generally from gunshot or stab wounds (20%). Renal injury should be suspected in the presence of lower posterior rib fractures, transverse process fractures of the upper lumbar spine, acute scoliosis, flank tenderness or ecchymoses, or hematuria.

2. Name the two true genitourinary emergencies.

Uncontrolled hemorrhage and renal pedicle injuries resulting in ischemia. The kidneys move to a limited degree on the vascular pedicle. Victims with a complete severance of the renal pedicle usually exsanguinate at the scene. Deceleration injuries may cause shearing of the major renal vessels, leading to thrombosis and subsequent ischemia. Early diagnosis and surgical intervention are crucial for salvage of the affected kidney. In the multiple-trauma patient, the guidelines of the Advanced Trauma Life Support program should be followed, focusing initially on the airway, breathing, and circulation (ABCs) and on life-threatening thoracic and abdominal injuries.

3. Describe the general classifications of renal injury.

American Association for the Surgery of Trauma Organ Injury Severity Scale for the Kidney

GRADE*	TYPE	DESCRIPTION
I	Contusion	Microscopic or gross hematuria, urologic studies normal
	Hematoma	Subcapsular, nonexpanding without parenchymal laceration
II	Hematoma	Nonexpanding perirenal hematoma confined to renal retroperitoneum
	Laceration	< 1.0 cm parenchymal depth of renal cortex without urinary extravasation
III	Laceration	> 1.0 cm parenchymal depth of renal cortex without collecting system rupture or urinary extravasation
IV	Laceration	Parenchymal laceration extending through renal cortex, medulla, and collecting system
	Vascular	Main renal artery or vein injury with contained hemorrhage
V	Laceration	Completely shattered kidney
	Vascular	Avulsion of renal hilum, devascularizing the kidney

* Advance one grade for bilateral injuries up to grade III.

4. What is the clinical course of these injuries?

Almost all renal contusions and minor lacerations heal spontaneously with bed rest and observation. Treatment of major lacerations should be left to the urologist. There has been an increasing trend to treat all stable renal trauma patients (with the exception of grade V injuries) expectantly. Renal pedicle injuries and shattered kidneys often require early surgical intervention.

5. What are the roles of CT, intravenous pyelography (IVP), selective angiography, and MRI in the evaluation of renal trauma?

CT is superior to IVP in defining the severity and extent of injury and has become the modality of choice for definitive evaluation of the renal parenchyma. Contrast-enhanced CT is also an accurate method of diagnosing renal artery injuries, decreasing the need for arteriography. Helical CT has improved the sensitivity of CT in identifying ureteral trauma. **IVP** may be used as a screening test to rule out significant blunt renal trauma and isolated ureteral injury if CT is not available or the patient is unstable. Abnormal or indeterminate IVP studies require additional studies to define the injury. IVP does not assess associated intraabdominal injuries. IVP may be useful in an unstable patient requiring immediate operative intervention because it can be done outside the radiology department (i.e., in the ED or operating room). Renal **angiography** may be indicated in the presence of a suspected vascular injury, although it has largely been replaced by CT. **MRI** shows anatomic detail similar to CT. It is limited, however, by the increased imaging time, cost, and monitoring difficulties. MRI may be useful in stable patients with dye allergies.

6. When should ureteral trauma be suspected?

In the presence of penetrating injuries in proximity to the ureter. Hematuria may be absent. IVP or CT identifies the injury. Blunt ureteral trauma usually is associated with other intraabdominal injuries and often is diagnosed intraoperatively.

7. What are the contraindications to urethral catheterization in the traumatized patient?

Catheterization should not be done in a patient with suspected urethral injury because a partial tear may be converted into a complete tear, and the risks of infection and further damage are increased. Of patients with urethral injury, 80% to 90% have blood at the urethral meatus. Scrotal and perineal hematomas or a high-riding prostate on rectal examination are other signs of urethral rupture. Patients with these findings should not be catheterized until a retrograde urethrogram is done to rule out urethral injury.

8. How is a retrograde urethrogram performed?

The urethrogram is obtained using a 12F urinary catheter secured in the meatal fossa by inflating the balloon to approximately 3 mL. Alternatively a catheter-tipped syringe may be used. Standard water-soluble contrast material (25 to 30 mL) is injected under gentle pressure as the anteroposterior and oblique views are taken.

9. Describe the methods used to diagnose bladder injuries.

Conventional **retrograde cystography** has long been considered the gold standard for diagnosing traumatic bladder injuries. Proper technique is important. The bladder should be filled under gravity with 300 to 400 mL of contrast material through the indwelling catheter. A flat anteroposterior abdominal radiograph is obtained after instillation of contrast material and after drainage. The postdrainage radiograph identifies small ruptures not apparent on the initial distended view.

CT cystography has emerged as a reliable and accurate method of identifying bladder injuries and has replaced conventional cystography in many centers. The accuracy of either method depends on adequate distention of the bladder. Initial studies evaluating CT cystography reported decreased sensitivity owing to inadequate filling of the bladder. Retrograde filling of the bladder ensures adequate distention and is less time-consuming. When indicated, CT cystography may be done as an adjunct to routine abdominopelvic CT in the trauma setting, which saves time and eliminates the need to move further a patient with a potentially unstable spine or pelvic fracture. CT cystography also may identify small amounts of intraperitoneal or extraperitoneal fluid with the density of water, suggesting extravasated urine. Disadvantages of CT cystography are increased radiation exposure and cost.

10. What are the indications for retrograde cystography?

Conventional retrograde cystography or CT cystography is indicated if **bladder rupture** is suspected. The recommendations for bladder imaging in blunt trauma are controversial. The combination of gross hematuria and pelvic fracture is an absolute indication for cystography. Relative indications include gross hematuria without pelvic fractures and pelvic fracture with microhematuria. Penetrating trauma with any degree of microscopic hematuria should be evaluated for genitourinary injury. If the wound is in the vicinity of the bladder, regardless of the presence of hematuria, a cystogram should be obtained.

11. What are the associated clinical findings in bladder injury?

Approximately 10% of all pelvic fractures are associated with bladder or urethral rupture. Lower abdominal compression, as seen with lap belt and steering wheel injuries, may rupture the distended bladder without injuring the pelvic girdle. Gross hematuria is present in more than 95% of patients with bladder rupture after blunt trauma.

12. What is a penile fracture?

A sudden tear in the tunica albuginea with subsequent rupture of the corpora cavernosum. It occurs only in the erect penis and usually is associated with falls or sudden unexpected moves during sexual intercourse. It has also been reported with direct blunt trauma. A sudden intense pain associated with a snapping noise and immediate detumescence usually occurs. Most authors support surgical intervention in an attempt to restore normal function and prevent angulation. Inability to urinate, bleeding from the urethral meatus, or extravasation of urine may indicate injury to the corpora spongiosum and urethra, which occurs in approximately 20% of cases.

13. Describe the approach to the amputated penis.

Penile amputation may result from accidental trauma or deliberate mutilation. Survival of penile skin is unlikely after 2 hours of warm ischemia time. Overall, graft survival is approximately 18 hours. The amputated part should be immersed in cold Ringer's lactate containing heparin and antibiotics, which may extend survival time while immediate urology consultation is obtained. Psychiatric evaluation is indicated in cases of intentional mutilation.

14. What is the role of ultrasound in the evaluation of testicular trauma?

Ultrasound is a valuable tool in assessing the integrity of the testicles. Adequate palpation may be prevented by hematoma formation. Ultrasound can distinguish between simple hematoma and disruption of the parenchyma. Failure to suspect and diagnose testicular rupture may result in subsequent loss of the testicle.

15. What is the diagnostic approach to asymptomatic microhematuria in the patient with blunt trauma?

Any trauma patient with gross hematuria, microhematuria and shock, or penetrating injuries and any degree of hematuria requires further radiographic evaluation. Studies of adult and pediatric blunt trauma patients showed, however, that asymptomatic microscopic hematuria is not a good predictor of genitourinary tract injury. The amount of blood in the urine does not correlate with severity of injury. The relatively low incidence of positive studies requiring surgery does not justify an extensive radiographic evaluation. Close follow-up of these patients and repeat urinalyses are recommended, with additional studies only if the hematuria persists. Controversy still exists regarding the evaluation of pediatric patients with asymptomatic microhematuria. Pediatric patients are more susceptible to significant renal injury with relatively benign mechanisms, and consequently many advocate imaging studies with any degree of hematuria regardless of symptoms.

BIBLIOGRAPHY

1. Brown S, Elder J, Spirnak J: Are pediatric patients more susceptible to major renal injury from blunt trauma? A comparative study. J Urol 160:138–140, 1998.
2. Dreitlein D, Suner S, Basler J: Genitourinary Trauma. Emerg Med Clin North Am 19, 2001.
3. Fergany A, Angermeier K, Montague D: Review of Cleveland Clinic experience with penile fracture. Urology 54:352–355, 1999.

4. Mattox K, Feliciano D, Moore E: Trauma, 4th ed. New York, McGraw-Hill, 1999.
5. Moore E, Shackford S, Pachter H, et al: Organ injury scaling: Spleen, liver, and kidney. J Trauma 29:1664–1666, 1989.
6. Morey A, Iverson A, Swan A, et al: Bladder rupture after blunt trauma: Guidelines for diagnostic imaging. J Trauma 51:683–686, 2001.
7. Peng M, Parisky Y, Cornwell E, et al: CT cystography versus conventional cystography in evaluation of bladder injury. AJR Am J Roentgenol 173:1269–1272, 1999.
8. Rosen P, Barkin RM (eds): Emergency Medicine: Concepts and Clinical Practice, 4th ed. St. Louis, Mosby, 1998.
9. Santucci R, McAninch J: Diagnosis and management of renal trauma: Past, present, and future. J Am Coll Surg 191:443–451, 2000.
10. Tintinelli J, Gabor D, Stapczynski S: Emergency Medicine: A Comprehensive Study Guide, 5th ed. New York, McGraw-Hill, 1999.
11. Vaccaro J, Brody J: CT cystography in the evaluation of major bladder trauma. Radiographics 20:1373–1381.

114. FOREIGN BODIES

W. Peter Vellman, M.D.

1. State the generic, three-step initial approach to a patient with a foreign body.

1. Attempt to visualize it.
2. Palpate for it.
3. If it is not visible or palpable, order appropriate diagnostic studies to determine its presence and location.

2. What is the best approach for evaluating and removing superficial foreign bodies from the eye?

Patients generally report a foreign-body sensation associated with tearing and conjunctival injection. Meticulous examination of the eye is done under magnification (i.e., loupe or slit-lamp), including eversion of both lids to look for foreign bodies in the conjunctival sacs. If a foreign body is not visualized, the inner aspects of the lids are swept with a moist cotton swab, or the eye is irrigated gently with normal saline. Fluorescein staining and examination under blue light should reveal corneal abrasions, which may present with the same symptoms as a foreign body. The safest way to remove corneal or conjunctival foreign bodies is with an eye spud or moist cotton swab under direct magnification. Rust rings may require removal with a hand-held burr.

3. How can you avoid missing an ocular foreign body?

The physician always must have a high index of suspicion for an ocular foreign body, particularly with orbital trauma, sudden eye pain with or without a history of trauma, or visual loss. A hyphema may be the only clue to a penetrating ocular foreign body. The physical examination must include visual acuity testing and meticulous inspection of the eyelids and globe. Careful funduscopic examination should be done but may be difficult in the presence of hemorrhage or cataract formation. External pressure on the globe should be avoided. Small, high-velocity missiles that penetrate the orbital soft tissue or globe may leave no obvious sign of entry. If there is any suspicion, plain films, ultrasonography, or CT scan should be performed. Missed ocular foreign bodies with subsequent loss of visual acuity are a leading source of malpractice losses.

4. What is the best way to remove a foreign body from the ear canal?

There is no one correct answer. The physician must use his or her knowledge and experience to optimize patient comfort and to limit injury to the ear structures when extracting the foreign body. Techniques vary from simple irrigation or suction to forceps extraction under direct visualization. Conscious sedation may be required, especially in children. Fine right-angle forceps, a right-angle hook, or small suction cups may be particularly useful. If extraction cannot be accomplished readily, referral to an otolaryngologist for removal under anesthesia, with or without an operating microscope, may be required. After removal of the foreign body, the canal and the tympanic membrane should be inspected. Any evidence of injury to the tympanic membrane should prompt acuity testing and referral to a specialist.

5. How is an insect removed from the external ear?

A 2% lidocaine solution is effective in immediately paralyzing live insects and facilitates their removal.

6. When should a nasal foreign body be suspected?

Always suspect a retained nasal foreign body when there is a history of persistent unilateral nasal discharge. Nasal foreign body is a common ED presentation, particularly in small children and the mentally retarded. Careful examination of the nasal cavity requires patience and the proper equipment.

7. How is a nasal foreign body removed?

Techniques of removal are based on the physician's experience and ability; safe removal occasionally requires general anesthesia. There is always a risk of airway compromise if the foreign body dislodges posteriorly during attempted extraction or with forced inhalation. Administration of a topical vasoconstrictor to shrink the nasal mucosa may facilitate removal of the foreign body by any method, including the use of forceps, magnets, suction cup, wire ear loops, hooked probes, wall suction, and balloon catheters.

8. What is the positive-pressure technique?

After the installation of a local vasoconstrictor, a caregiver (usually a parent) gently occludes the unobstructed nares with his or her thumb, being careful not to deviate the septum. The parent tells the child that he or she is going to give the child "a big kiss." With the child in a supine position with his or her mouth open, the parent delivers, mouth-to-mouth, a short, sharp puff of air. The foreign body is usually delivered to the parent's cheek, along with other intranasal material.

9. How do you handle the adult with an esophageal foreign body?

A careful history is crucial to the management of such patients. More than 80% of swallowed foreign bodies pass through the gastrointestinal (GI) tract without incident. Sharp objects (e.g., bones, needles, wire) may impale the wall of the esophagus, whereas soft objects, such as meat, may obstruct the anatomic points of constriction of the esophagus: the postcricoid area, the aortic arch, and the gastroesophageal junction. Flexible esophagoscopy is the accepted method of removal for sharp, inert, radiopaque, or recently impacted foreign objects and should be performed on patients with foreign body symptoms for more than 12 hours. Balloon catheter retrieval may be effective for removal of nonsharp objects, such as coins, but is controversial. Intravenous glucagon or sublingual nitroglycerin or nifedipine results in smooth muscle relaxation of the distal esophagus and may be useful in relieving obstructions at that level. Gas-forming agents have been used to propel a food-bolus impaction into the stomach from the distal esophagus. This method should not be used in patients with pain suggestive of perforation or prolonged impaction.

10. What about the swallowed foreign body without esophageal symptoms?

The general rule regarding management is conservative observation. A careful history should eliminate sharp versus blunt swallowed objects. Plain radiographs of the neck, chest, and upper abdomen and serial radiographs when indicated to follow the progress through the GI tract should be obtained. Sharp objects should be removed by flexible esophagoscopy. Early retrieval should be considered for any object larger than 2 cm wide × 6 cm long because of the potential for obstruction at the pylorus or duodenal sweep.

11. What about the body packer?
Patients who conceal prepared illicit drug packets in the GI tract pose a challenging problem. First, any patient showing signs of obstruction or toxicity must have therapy directed at the specific signs and symptoms and immediate attempts at packet removal by endoscopy or surgery. In stable patients, the number and location of packets should be ascertained. History is frequently unreliable, and plain radiographs and CT scan may not detect all packets. Asymptomatic body packers should be treated with activated charcoal and whole-body irrigation with polyethylene glycol. If cocaine is suspected, alkalinizing the gastric contents may neutralize the drug to its inactive metabolite (benzoylecgonine). Endoscopic removal of packets carries a risk of packet rupture.

12. Do children with possible coin ingestion and no symptoms need a radiograph?
Yes. Many children with an esophageal coin are asymptomatic. Delayed diagnosis may lead to mistreatment and complications resulting from esophageal erosion, such as bleeding, perforation, and obstruction. In general, if the coin passes the gastroesophageal junction, it traverses the remainder of the GI tract without complication. Subtle symptoms, such as failure to thrive, eating complications, and wheezing secondary to tracheal compression, may be the result of unsuspected esophageal coins.

13. How do you evaluate the patient with a fish bone in the throat?
The dilemma of a fish bone in the throat is whether the symptoms are caused by a retained foreign body or mucosal abrasion. Tenderness on palpation of the neck is an unreliable sign, whereas pooled secretions on laryngoscopy almost always are associated with a retained foreign body. Careful physician examination with visualization and removal of the bone obviates the need for radiologic studies or specialty referral. Plain radiography is rarely helpful; however, barium swallow or CT scan may detect retained foreign bodies or show a perforation. Removal can be achieved by direct laryngoscopy with Magill forceps or may require subspecialty referral.

14. How do you remove a rectal foreign body?
The preferred route of removal is through the same orifice into which it was originally inserted. This may not always be feasible, however, because of the size or shape of the foreign body or because of fragmentation or possible breakage. Laparotomy is rarely required. Mucosal edema also may preclude easy extraction. Direct visualization with a vaginal speculum and extraction with a ring forceps or tenaculum, sometimes with the tip of a Foley catheter passed proximal to the foreign body to overcome suction, is a common technique. If this is unsuccessful, removal in the operating room under general anesthesia may be required.

15. What are the common foreign bodies found in the rectum?
Glass or ceramic objects, sexual devices, and foods, primarily fruits and vegetables. The type of foreign body dictates the best approach for removal. Large-bowel injuries should be suspected with all rectal foreign bodies and appropriate evaluation should be done after removal of the foreign body.

16. Why are button batteries a cause of concern?
Most button batteries contain an alkaline electrolyte and a heavy metal, such as lithium or mercury. Impaction in a mucosa-lined cavity (i.e., the nose, GI tract, respiratory tract) may result in corrosive inflammation that leads to perforation. Injury may occur by one of the following four mechanisms: (1) electrolyte leakage, (2) alkali produced from external current, (3) mercury toxicity, and (4) pressure necrosis. Early diagnosis and removal are crucial to prevent complications, such as perforation of the nasal septum or GI tract. Button batteries lodged in the external auditory canal can result in caustic injury to the canal and erosive perforation of the tympanic membrane.

17. How do you determine whether a foreign body has been aspirated into the tracheobronchial tree?

Patients may give a history of aspiration; peak incidences for aspiration occur before the age of 3 and after the age of 50 and in patients with altered mentation. The **penetration syndrome** is a sudden onset of choking and intractable cough with or without vomiting. It may occur in half of patients with tracheobronchial foreign bodies and should prompt further investigation. Half of young children with aspirated foreign bodies are asymptomatic. Hoarseness or stridor indicates a tracheal or laryngeal obstruction, whereas unilateral wheezing and decreased breath sounds imply a bronchial obstruction. Delayed presentation is the rule in children, with only one third of patients presenting within 24 hours. If plain radiographs are unrevealing, fluoroscopy should be done. Positive findings include a mediastinal shift away from the side of the foreign body and obstructive emphysema. MRI T1-weighted images, which are extremely sensitive to fat compounds, have been used to identify and locate aspirated peanuts and other such foreign bodies in the airway. Foreign bodies are rarely expulsed spontaneously and generally require removal with a rigid bronchoscope. Bronchoscopy is indicated if the index of suspicion is high despite the absence of symptoms and x-ray findings.

18. Which radiologic studies are helpful in elucidating subcutaneous foreign bodies?

Plain radiographs should be used as an initial screening device. Although some foreign bodies are radiopaque (e.g., metal, glass with and without lead), many, including wood, are not. If plain films are unrevealing, ultrasound is clinically useful in detecting wood foreign bodies. Glass foreign bodies are more likely to result in a foreign body sensation on palpation, and glass foreign bodies 2 mm or larger can be detected by radiographs nearly 100% of the time. Xeroradiography does not seem to offer any advantage over standard radiography and requires much larger doses of radiation. For deep foreign bodies not detected by plain films or ultrasound or for studying the complications of retained foreign bodies, CT or MRI should be used.

19. How is a subcutaneous foreign body removed?

After localization, local anesthesia, and sterile preparation, the foreign body may be removed directly with forceps or with a hemostat. This may require extending the entrance wound with a scalpel. The ED physician should feel comfortable with simple foreign body removal under fluoroscopy. Complicated or difficult-to-remove foreign bodies may require surgical consultation.

20. What if the foreign body is metallic?

These may be removed using a sterile eye magnet. A magnet is inserted through an extended entrance wound, then probed until a click is appreciated.

BIBLIOGRAPHY

1. Backlin SA: Positive-pressure technique for nasal foreign body removal in children. Ann Emerg Med 25:554–555, 1995.
2. Baharloo F, Veyckemans F, Francis C, et al: Tracheobronchial foreign bodies: Presentation and management in children and adults. Chest 115:1357–1362, 1999.
3. Busch DB, Starling JR: Rectal foreign bodies: Case reports and a comprehensive review of the world's literature. Surgery 100:512–519, 1986.
4. Courter BJ: Radiographic screening for glass foreign bodies: What does a "negative" foreign body series really mean? Ann Emerg Med 19:997–1000, 1990.
5. Flom LL, Ellis GL: Radiologic evaluation of foreign bodies. Emerg Med Clin North Am 10:163–177, 1992.
6. Fritz S, Kelen GD, Sivertson K: Foreign bodies of the external auditory canal. Emerg Med Clin North Am 5:183–192, 1987.
7. Graham DD: Ultrasound in the emergency department: Detection of wooden foreign bodies in the soft tissues. J Emerg Med 22:75–79, 2001.
8. Imaizumi H, Kaneko M, Nara S, et al: Definitive diagnosis and location of peanuts in the airways using magnetic resonance imaging techniques. Ann Emerg Med 23:1379–1382, 1994.

9. Lam HCK, Woo JKS, Van Hasslect CA: Management of ingested foreign bodies: A retrospective review of 5240 patients. J Laryngol Otol 115:954–957, 2001.
10. Olmedo R, Nelson L, Chu J, Hoffman R: Is surgical decontamination definitive treatment of "body-packers"? Am J Emerg Med 19:593–596, 2001.
11. Steele MT, Tran LV, Watson WA, Muelleman RL: Retained glass foreign bodies in wounds: Predictive value of wound characteristics, patient perception and wound exploration. Am J Emerg Med 16:627–630, 1998.

115. TRAUMA IN PREGNANCY

Jedd Roe, M.D., M.B.A.

1. What is the most important concept I need to remember from this chapter?

Fetal outcome is largely related to maternal morbidity. The best fetal resuscitation is aggressive maternal resuscitation.

2. How common is trauma in pregnancy?

An estimated 6% to 7% of pregnancies are complicated by trauma. In blunt abdominal trauma, the usual causes are motor vehicle accidents (MVAs) (67%), falls, and direct blows to the abdomen. One study showed the serious MVAs accounted for a 7% maternal mortality rate, whereas the fetal mortality rate was 15%. Of falls, 80% occur after 32 weeks of gestation.

3. Is physical or sexual abuse seen frequently in pregnant patients?

Yes. One large study reported a prevalence of abuse in pregnant women in urban settings of 32%. Of physically abused women, 60% reported two or more episodes of assault. Injury was more common to the head, neck, and extremities; a fourfold increase in the incidence of genital trauma was noted in this population. When pregnant patients are physically abused, there is a higher incidence of low-birth-weight infants, low maternal weight gain, maternal anemia, and drug and alcohol abuse. Homicides account for one third of maternal trauma deaths.

4. How do physiologic changes in pregnancy affect the evaluation of the trauma victim?

First, decreasing blood pressure and rising heart rate might indicate hypovolemic shock in a nonpregnant woman, but in pregnancy this may merely reflect physiologic changes or supine positioning. Because of increased blood volume, signs of shock may not be clinically apparent until 35% of maternal blood volume is lost. Given the markedly increased blood flow to the uterus, there is a new potential source of blood loss that requires aggressive investigation. Because physiologic changes result in a decreased maternal oxygen reserve, tissue hypoxia develops more rapidly in response to a traumatic insult.

5. How do physiologic changes of pregnancy affect laboratory values?

A physiologic anemia is seen as the plasma volume rises by more than twice the amount of red blood cells. It is not unusual for one to see hematocrits of 32% to 34% by the third trimester. Fibrinogen levels are double those seen in other trauma patients. Disseminated intravascular coagulation may be seen with normal fibrinogen levels. Because of hormonal stimulation of the central respiratory drive, PCO_2 falls to approximately 30 mmHg, and injury sufficient to cause a respiratory acidosis might be manifested by what ordinarily would be considered a normal PCO_2 of 40 mmHg.

6. Are serious maternal injuries required for fetal injury to be present?

Not always. Although in utero damage is often associated with maternal pelvic fractures, 7% of maternal cases of minor trauma have been associated with poor fetal outcome. Direct injuries to the fetus in utero are unusual, but given the size of the fetal head, when direct trauma occurs, fetal head injury is the most common injury.

7. Name the most common causes of fetal death.
Maternal death, maternal shock, and placental abruption.

8. How does placental abruption occur?
Abruption results from the separation of a relatively inelastic placenta from an elastic uterus secondary to a shearing, deceleration force. There may be little or no external evidence of such a mechanism. Although abruption may be present in 50% of patients with life-threatening injuries, it also exists in 1% to 3% of minor mechanisms. Classically the clinical findings of abruption have included vaginal bleeding and abdominal and uterine tenderness. In many cases, fetal distress may be the only presenting sign because the reduction in placental blood flow to the fetus causes hypoxia and acidosis. A consumptive coagulopathy may occur with placental injury, and evaluation for disseminated intravascular coagulation should be done in all instances of suspected abruption.

9. How often does ultrasound detect cases of placental abruption?
Because a large separation must be present for ultrasound to be diagnostic, it detects only about half of cases. In many instances, fetal distress is present before the clear visualization of an abruption by ultrasound. Fetal mortality from abruption is reported to be 30% to 68%. Usually an abruption large enough to place the fetus at risk becomes apparent within 48 hours. Detection of fetal distress mandates prompt delivery of the fetus.

10. Are radiologic investigations harmful to the fetus?
Fetal organs are maximally sensitive to radiation when younger than 8 weeks of gestational age. Most authorities agree that a radiation dose of less than 5 to 10 rad carries no significant fetal risk. In general, all radiographic studies should be undertaken with appropriate fetal shielding. All **clinically indicated** studies should be done regardless of any radiation concerns. Consideration also should be given to nonradiographic alternative evaluation with ultrasound. The following table lists doses received from exposure during production of commonly ordered investigations.

EXAMINATION	ESTIMATED DOSE TO UTERUS/FETUS (MRAD)
Cervical spine series	0.0–1.0
Extremity (one view)	0.0–1.0
Chest posteroanterior radiograph	0.0–5.0
Head or chest CT	< 50
Pelvis radiograph	200–300
Lumbar spine anteroposterior/lateral	200–1300
Abdominal CT	3,000–10,300

11. How should these patients be managed in the field?
Given the reduced maternal oxygen reserve, oxygen therapy is crucial. Intravenous volume resuscitation with crystalloid and blood should proceed as with other trauma patients. Avoid compression of the inferior vena cava by transporting the patient on her left side, or if the patient is immobilized, elevate the right side of the backboard to 15° or 20°. Aside from early transport, the most important aspect of prehospital management is to notify the ED so that the appropriate obstetric consultants may participate on the trauma team.

12. How do I begin to evaluate the fetus?
First, determine the size of the uterus and the presence of abdominal and uterine tenderness. Uterine size, measured in centimeters from the pubic symphysis to fundus, provides a rough estimate

of gestational age and potential viability. Carefully inspect the vaginal introitus for evidence of vaginal bleeding. Next, assess for fetal distress, which may be the earliest indication of maternal hypovolemia. Abnormal fetal heart rates are greater than 160 beats/min and less than 120 beats/min. Continuous cardiotocographic monitoring should be performed to ascertain early signs of fetal distress (e.g., decreased variability of heart rate or fetal decelerations after contractions). Ultrasound should be done as soon as possible to confirm gestational age, fetal viability, and the integrity of the placenta.

13. Is diagnostic peritoneal lavage (DPL) safe and accurate in pregnant women?

DPL has been reported to be safe and accurate when using an open, supraumbilical technique. Although the cell count thresholds and clinical indications for DPL are the same, ED ultrasound has become the more prevalent investigation. The physiologic changes that take place with pregnancy and the elimination of radiation exposure from abdominal CT provide persuasive arguments for aggressive use of ED ultrasound as a diagnostic tool. With the exception of concern for diaphragmatic injury secondary to penetrating trauma, the need for DPL as an evaluation modality has largely been supplanted by the use of ED ultrasound to determine rapidly the presence of intraperitoneal hemorrhage.

14. What is fetomaternal hemorrhage (FMH)?

Hemorrhage of fetal blood into the usually distinct maternal circulation. The incidence of FMH in trauma patients has been reported to be 30% (four to five times the incidence of noninjured controls). With FMH, the complications of maternal Rh sensitization, fetal anemia, and fetal death can occur. Laboratory techniques are not sensitive enough to diagnose FMH accurately. The prudent course is to give Rh immunoglobulin to all Rh-negative patients who present with the suspicion of abdominal trauma because a 300-μg dose of Rh immunoglobulin given within 72 hours of antigenic exposure prevents Rh isoimmunization. Massive transfusion (> 30 mL) into the maternal circulation sometimes is seen with severe abdominal trauma. When such mechanisms are present, the Kleihauer-Betke test should be ordered to identify patients in whom massive transfusion has occurred and who require additional administration of Rh immunoglobulin.

15. When is cesarean section indicated?

The first factor to be considered is the stability of the mother. If the mother has sustained serious injuries elsewhere and is critically ill, she may not be able to tolerate an additional procedure and the blood loss it would entail. Next, fetuses whose gestational age is 24 weeks or whose weight is estimated to be greater than 750 g are predicted to have a 50% survival rate in the neonatal ICU setting and are considered viable. The most common indication for cesarean section is fetal distress. Other indications are uterine rupture and malpresentation of the fetus. Perimortem cesarean section should be done when ultrasound or uterine size suggests viability (i.e., above the umbilicus) and maternal decompensation is acute. Resuscitation should be instituted within 6 minutes, but fetal survival has occurred 15 minutes after maternal decompensation.

16. Which pregnant patients with abdominal trauma require admission for fetal monitoring?

Any viable (> 24 weeks) fetus requires monitoring. Monitoring is recommended even for patients without external evidence of trauma because it has been well documented that these patients are at risk from placental abruption. Current guidelines suggest that these patients be observed for a minimum of 4 hours with a cardiotocograph. If any abnormalities are discovered, the observation should be extended 24 hours.

BIBLIOGRAPHY

1. Drost TF, Rosemurgy AS, Sherman HF, et al: Major trauma in pregnant women: Maternal/fetal outcome. J Trauma 30:574–578, 1990.
2. Henderson SO, Mallon WK: Trauma in pregnancy. Emerg Med Clin North Am 16:209–228, 1998.
3. McFarlane J, Parker B, Soeken K, Bullock L: Assessing for abuse during pregnancy: Severity and frequency of injuries and associated entry into prenatal care. JAMA 267:3176–3178, 1992.

4. Pearlman MD, Tintinalli JE, Lorenz RP: Blunt trauma during pregnancy. N Engl J Med 323:1609–1613, 1990.
5. Pearlman MD, Tintinalli JE, Lorenz RP: A prospective, controlled study of outcome after trauma during pregnancy. Am J Obstet Gynecol 162:1502–1507, 1990.
6. Poole GV, Martin JN, Penny KG, et al: Trauma in pregnancy: The role of interpersonal violence. Am J Obstet Gynecol 174:1873–1877, 1996.
7. Scorpio RJ, Esposito TJ, Smith LG, Gens DR: Blunt trauma during pregnancy: Factors affecting fetal outcome. J Trauma 32:213–216, 1992.
8. Sherman HF, Scott LM, Rosemurgy AS: Changes affecting the initial evaluation and care of the pregnant trauma victim. J Emerg Med 8:575–582, 1990.
9. Williams JK, McClain L, Rosemurgy AS: Evaluation of blunt abdominal trauma in the third trimester of pregnancy. Obstet Gynecol 75:33–37, 1990.
10. Kass LE, Abbot JT: Trauma in pregnancy. In Ferrara PC, Colucciello SA, Marx JA, et al (eds): Trauma Management: An Emergency Medicine Approach. St. Louis, Mosby, 2001, pp 489–503.

116. PEDIATRIC TRAUMA

Walter L. Biffl, M.D., and Holly U. Biffl, M.D.

1. What kids get injured, and how do they do it?

Every year, nearly one in three children is injured, and trauma is the leading cause of child-hood mortality. Motor vehicle crashes account for most deaths, but the next most common site of lethal pediatric trauma is the home. Boys are injured twice as often as girls. Falls are the most common cause of severe injury in infants and toddlers; bicycle accidents are the most common cause in children and adolescents.

2. Aren't children just small little adults?

No. Anatomically, three unique characteristics in children require special consideration:

1. A smaller body mass results in more force applied per unit area, with a propensity toward multiple injuries in a child.

2. A child's incompletely calcified skeleton allows internal organ damage without overlying fractures.

3. A high body surface area-to-volume ratio results in significant thermal energy loss and early hypothermia in a child.

3. How do the ABCs differ between children and adults?

They don't. Airway, Breathing, and Circulation always take priority.

4. What factors affect the patency of a child's airway?

Craniofacial disproportion (the child's occiput is relatively large compared with the midface) results in cervical flexion when the child is lying supine. Compared with an adult, a child has a large tongue, floppy epiglottis, and increased lymphoid tissue; these factors may contribute to airway obstruction. The **sniffing position** (slight superior and anterior positioning of the mid-face) is employed to maintain a patent airway. Infants are obligate nasal breathers, so their nos-trils should not be occluded. Oral airways should be inserted only in unconscious children because they may induce vomiting. The airway should be inserted directly, rather than the adult practice of rotating it in the oropharynx.

5. What factors affect endotracheal intubation of a child?

A child's larynx lies higher and more anterior in the neck, and the vocal cords have a more anterocaudal angle; the cords may be more difficult to visualize for intubation. The most narrow part of a child's airway is the cricoid ring, which forms a natural seal with the endotracheal tube. Uncuffed tubes generally are used in children younger than 12 years old. The size of the tube is estimated by the diameter of the child's external nares or little finger. The trachea is short, so the tube should be placed just 2 to 3 cm distal to the vocal cords. Nasotracheal intubation should not be attempted in children younger than 12 years old.

6. Describe rapid-sequence intubation in a child.

The airway should be opened by placing the child in the sniffing position (or chin left/jaw thrust). The airway is cleared of debris, and the patient is preoxygenated. Atropine sulfate is given to ensure a high heart rate. The child should be sedated with thiopental (if normovolemic) or midazolam (if hypovolemic). Cricoid pressure is maintained with the Sellick maneuver. Neuromuscular blockade is administered (succinylcholine or vecuronium).

7. What do I do if I cannot endotracheally intubate the patient?

A surgical airway should be performed. Tracheostomy is the procedure of choice because there is a high risk of subglottic stenosis in children younger than age 11 who undergo cricothyroidotomy. As a temporizing measure, needle cricothyroidotomy with a 14-G or 16-G catheter allows jet insufflation of oxygen. It does not provide adequate ventilation, however.

8. How do I recognize shock in a pediatric patient?

Tachycardia is the primary response to hypovolemia. Other, more subtle signs include decreased pulse pressure, mottling of the skin, cool extremities, capillary refill greater than 2 seconds, and a depressed level of consciousness. The systolic blood pressure is normally greater than 80 mmHg + (2 × age in years). Hypotension indicates a loss of 45% of blood volume and often is accompanied by bradycardia.

9. Name the preferred sites for venous access.

In order, peripheral, intraosseus, saphenous vein cutdown at the ankle, and percutaneous femoral–subclavian–external jugular–internal jugular.

10. What are some considerations regarding an intraosseus line?

It is most appropriate in children younger than 6 years old and allows administration of virtually any fluid or drug and blood draws. The preferred site is the proximal tibia below the tibial tuberosity. It should not be placed distal to a fracture and should be removed when peripheral intravenous access is secured. It may be complicated by cellulitis or osteomyelitis.

11. What is a child's normal blood volume?

80 mL/kg.

12. How should I resuscitate a pediatric trauma patient?

A 25% reduction in blood volume (20 mL/kg) generally is required to manifest signs of shock. The 3:1 rule (crystalloid resuscitation-to-blood loss) applies as it does in adults. For a 20-mL/kg blood loss, 60 mL/kg should be given. Either warmed normal saline or lactated Ringer's solution can be given in boluses of 20 mL/kg. After 60 mL/kg, consideration should be given to transfusing packed red blood cells (10 mL/kg). At this point, a surgeon should be involved.

13. Why are children prone to head trauma?

They lead with their head because it is larger in proportion to their body than that of an adult.

14. What kinds of head injuries do children get?

Compared with adults, mass lesions are less common, but cerebral edema and postinjury seizures are more common. Hemorrhagic shock may occur secondary to blood loss in the subgaleal or epidural space, owing to open cranial sutures and fontanelle. Bulging sutures or fontanelle suggests a significant brain injury and warrants aggressive management and neurosurgical consultation before decompensation occurs.

15. What children need cranial imaging after head trauma?

Symptomatic (history of loss of consciousness, vomiting, drowsiness, irritability, headache, amnesia) or neurologically abnormal (depressed mental status, seizures, focal deficits) **children less than 1 year old** should have head CT. If the child is asymptomatic and neurologically normal and has no scalp hematoma, no studies are required. If there is a scalp hematoma, skull radiographs should be obtained; if normal, no CT is required, but if abnormal, CT scan should be performed. **Children older than 1 year** who are neurologically normal and asymptomatic require no studies. If neurologically normal but symptomatic, CT may be done; alternatively a child may be sent home with a reliable parent (or admitted) with CT scan performed for deterioration. Neurologic abnormalities, skull depression, or signs of basilar skull fracture warrant CT scanning.

16. What is SCIWORA?

Spinal cord injury without radiographic abnormality. Normal spine radiographs are found in two thirds of children with spinal cord injury. Normal films do not exclude injury. Continued immobilization and appropriate consultation are warranted if there is suspicion of spinal cord injury, particularly in the presence of neurologic deficits.

17. How common are rib fractures in children?

Not very. The compliant chest wall allows transmission of a great deal of force to the underlying lung or heart, potentially resulting in life-threatening contusions. Two thirds of children have associated organ system injuries. A mobile mediastinum allows tension pneumothorax to develop more readily than in adults.

18. How reliable is physical examination to exclude abdominal trauma?

You might as well flip a coin. Decompression of the stomach, which almost invariably is distended in children who have been crying, and bladder may facilitate the examination, but some diagnostic test generally is warranted.

19. Compare and contrast the primary diagnostic modalities for evaluating children for abdominal trauma.

CT, diagnostic peritoneal lavage, and ultrasonography, are the primary diagnostic tests. **CT** is appropriate in stable patients. It is the most specific of the tests, identifying solid organ and hollow viscus injuries. It also evaluates the retroperitoneum. **Diagnostic peritoneal lavage** is greater than 95% accurate in identifying injuries, but it is invasive and leads to nontherapeutic laparotomy in many children because of its sensitivity for hemoperitoneum. It is most useful in patients who are hemodynamically unstable with an equivocal ultrasound examination or patients undergoing an operative procedure whose abdomen cannot be serially evaluated. **Ultrasound** is simple, rapid, repeatable, and accurate in identifying hemoperitoneum. It may be used to triage unstable patients to the operating room or to exclude rapidly the abdomen as a source of significant blood loss.

20. What is a handlebar injury?

An injury (typically a duodenal hematoma or pancreatic injury) resulting from a bicycle handlebar—or elbow—striking the child in the right upper quadrant or epigastrium.

21. What is the seat belt complex?

Ecchymosis of the abdominal wall, a flexion-distraction injury of the lumbar spine. (Chance fracture), and intestinal or mesenteric injury.

22. How much of a problem is nonaccidental trauma?

It is the most common cause of traumatic death in the first year of life. Of abused children, 50% who are released to those who abuse them ultimately sustain fatal nonaccidental trauma injuries. (See Chapter 78, Emergency Department Evaluation of Child Abuse.)

23. List some situations that should arouse suspicion of child abuse.
- Trauma in a child < 1 year old
- A discrepancy between the history and the degree of injury
- A prolonged interval between injury and seeking medical care
- A history of multiple traumatic injuries treated in different EDs
- Inappropriate responses or noncompliance by parents
- Different accounts of the event given by different caregivers

24. List physical findings that should arouse suspicion of child abuse.
- Multiple subdural hematomas
- Retinal hemorrhage
- Perioral or perineal injuries
- Evidence of frequent injuries (old scars, healed fractures)
- Long bone fractures in children < 3 years old
- Bizarre injuries (cigarette burns, bites, rope burns)
- Sharply demarcated burns in unusual areas

The suspicion of abuse mandates reporting by physicians.

BIBLIOGRAPHY

1. American College of Surgeons Committee on Trauma: Advanced Trauma Life Support for Doctors. Chicago, American College of Surgeons, 1997.
2. Arkovitz MD, Johnson N, Garcia VF: Pancreatic trauma in children: Mechanisms of injury. J Trauma 42:49–53, 1997.
3. Bensard DD, Beaver BL, Besner GE, Cooney DR: Small bowel injury in children after blunt abdominal trauma: Is diagnostic delay important? J Trauma 41:476–483, 1996.
4. Manary MJ, Jaffe DM: Cervical spine injuries in children. Pediatr Ann 25:423–428, 1996.
5. McAllister JD, Gnauck KA: Rapid sequence intubation of the pediatric patient. Pediatr Clin North Am 46:1249–1280, 1999.
6. Partrick DA, Bensard DD, Moore EE, et al: Ultrasound is an effective triage tool to evaluate blunt abdominal trauma in the pediatric population. J Trauma 45:57–63, 1998.
7. Quayle KS: Minor head injury in the pediatric patient. Pediatr Clin North Am 46:1189–1199, 1999.
8. Tepas JJ III: Pediatric trauma. In Mattox KL, Feliciano DV, Moore EE (eds): Trauma, 4th ed. New York, McGraw-Hill, 2000.

117. MUSCULOSKELETAL TRAUMA AND CONDITIONS OF THE EXTREMITY

Steven J. Morgan, M.D., and Wade R. Smith, M.D.

GENERAL PRINCIPLES

1. What are the immediate treatment priorities in an open fracture?

As in any trauma patient, the immediate priorities are the **ABCs**. Any break in the skin near a fracture site should be assumed to communicate with the fracture until proved otherwise. After careful examination with neurologic and vascular assessment, the wound should be cleaned of gross contamination, and a sterile dressing impregnated with a 1% povidone-iodine (Betadine) solution should be applied. Direct pressure can be used for hemorrhage control. Axial realignment and splinting immobilizes the bone, decreasing blood loss and protecting the soft tissue from further damage. Probing of the wound, wound cultures, extensive irrigation, and multiple examinations of the wound should be avoided, owing to the increased potential for secondary contamination and soft tissue damage. Tetanus prophylaxis and intravenous antibiotics are usually administered. A first-generation cephalosporin, with or without an aminoglycoside, is used most commonly for antibiotic prophylaxis. When open fractures occur in grossly contaminated environments, such as barnyards, penicillin is added, secondary to the increased risk of anaerobic organisms. Consult an orthopedic surgeon immediately. Open fractures are **orthopedic emergencies**.

2. What percentage of polytrauma patients have unrecognized fractures at the time of admission?

Of patients with multiple system injuries, 20% have unrecognized fractures at the time of initial assessment. In general, these do not typically involve the axial skeleton or long bones. These unrecognized injuries are located most commonly in the hands and feet. This important fact shows the need for repetitive examination of the multiply injured patient and discussions with the family of the injured party regarding the potential of unrecognized fractures.

3. What is compartment syndrome?

A condition that develops when the pressure in the confined space of the muscle compartment exceeds the filling pressure of the venules and the arterioles supplying the muscle, resulting in muscle ischemia and the eventual necrosis of muscle and nerve tissue. Conditions or situations that cause an increase in the compartment contents or decrease the expansive nature of the compartment can result in compartment syndrome. Common causes include fracture, crush injuries, hemorrhage, postischemic swelling after repair of vascular injury, tight-fitting casts or dressings, MAST (Military Anti-Shock Trousers), and burns.

4. What are the signs and symptoms of compartment syndrome?

The classic diagnosis of compartment syndrome is indicated by the **5 Ps**: **pain**, **pallor**, **paresthesias**, **pulselessness**, and **paralysis**. **Pain** is the earliest and most common symptom associated with compartment syndrome. The pain is typically more severe than what is normally expected, based on the associated cause. The pain often is exacerbated when the muscles of the involved compartment are put on stretch. The pain is typically ischemic in nature and often not relieved by narcotics. **Paresthesia** is another common finding but indicates a prolonged period of increased compartment pressures. **Pallor**, **lack of pulse**, and **paralysis** are late findings, and the condition is often not reversible at that point. There are various methods of measuring intracompartmental pressure to obtain objective evidence of compartment syndrome. The gold standard of diagnosis is a positive clinical examination combined with a plausible history. Missed or delayed diagnosis of compartment syndrome is catastrophic, warranting a high index of suspicion and early specialist consultation.

5. What are the most common sites of compartment syndrome?

The volar compartment of the forearm and the anterior compartment of the leg. The deep posterior compartment of the leg is the site most often missed for this event. Supracondylar fractures of the humerus in children and both-bone forearm fractures are the injuries most commonly associated with this process in the upper extremity. Proximal tibial fractures are the most common cause of compartment syndrome in the leg. Compartment syndrome also is known to occur in the feet, thighs, and upper arm. Fractures may or may not be present.

6. What is the treatment of compartment syndrome?

Surgical release of the investing fascia of the compartment is the only effective treatment for this condition. Temporary measures that may be used to prevent compartment syndrome include elevation of the extremity to heart level and maintenance of a normal arteriole filling pressure by maintaining a normotensive blood pressure.

7. Describe the trauma patient who can have their cervical spine clinically cleared.

Clinical clearance of the trauma patient without radiographs requires a patient who is awake, is alert, and has not been involved with mind-altering substances. The patient should not have a distracting injury, such as major long bone fractures; pelvic fractures; or fractures involving the proximal humerus, clavicle, or scapula. If the patient has no complaints of pain, has no tenderness on examination, and can move through an unrestricted range of motion without pain, the cervical spine immobilization can be discontinued. If these requirements are not met, radiographs are required to complete the evaluation.

8. Describe the joint fluid analysis consistent with septic arthritis.

On visual inspection, the fluid is cloudy. Gram stain of the fluid often shows the presence of polymorphonuclear cells and may or may not indicate the presence of bacteria. A cell count is probably the most important aspect of joint fluid analysis. The total white blood cell count is generally greater than 75,000 cells with more than 80% of them being polymorphonuclear cells. The glucose level in the joint fluid is low when compared with the serum level.

9. Describe the microscopic findings consistent with gout during joint fluid analysis.

Joint aspiration is required to make the diagnosis of gout. Monosodium urate crystals are long and thin or needle-shaped and show strong negative birefringence when viewed under polarized light.

10. Name the associated radiologic finding consistent with pseudogout or calcium pyrophosphate deposition disease of the knee.

Calcification of the meniscus.

11. Can gout and septic arthritis coexist?

Yes.

12. What is the most common infecting bacterium associated with septic arthritis?

Staphylococcus aureus.

13. What organism must be considered in the patient with septic arthritis and risk factors for sexually transmitted disease?

Neisseria gonorrhoeae.

14. How do I diagnose a traumatic open joint?

Probing of a wound in proximity to a joint is insufficient, may increase the risk of infection, and generally should be avoided. Radiographs of the involved joint may reveal the presence of air in the joint, indicating joint violation. The definitive diagnosis is made by performing an arthrogram. Sterile saline combined with a small amount of methylene blue should be injected in the joint. A significant amount of fluid needs to be injected to distend the joint. The traumatic wound is inspected for egress of the injected fluid. The fluid should be withdrawn from the joint.

15. When should I order radiographs, and how many should I order?

Radiographs should be ordered based on the physical examination findings. Radiographs should include the joints above and below the perceived area of injury. Two orthogonal views always should be obtained. Obtaining radiographs should not obstruct the resuscitation process in the multiply-injured patient. In situations in which significant deformity of the limb results in vascular compromise or devitalization of the overlying skin, radiographs should be delayed, pending emergent realignment and splinting of the involved extremity.

HAND AND UPPER EXTREMITY

16. What is the best method to control bleeding in a hand or forearm laceration?

Direct pressure. Tourniquets are rarely necessary. The practice of blindly placing clamps into the wound is dangerous and often can damage structures in close proximity to the offending vessel, such as the median or ulnar nerve.

17. What metacarpophalangeal joint most commonly sustains a laceration when an individual engages in "fist diplomacy"?

The third metacarpophalangeal joint because it is the most prominent knuckle when making a fist.

18. How much deformity can be tolerated in a metacarpal fracture?

Rotational deformity is not tolerated well and should be corrected. Rotation in a metacarpal neck or shaft fracture causes the fingers to cross when the individual makes a fist. Flexion deformity of the fracture is the most common and best tolerated. You can accept 10°, 20°, 30°, and 40° of flexion in the index through small fingers. A greater degree of deformity is tolerated at the small finger, secondary to the increased motion at the carpometacarpal joint. The same is true for a thumb metacarpal fracture, in which 40° of angular deformity can be accepted.

19. What bacterium is often associated with cat bites, and what is the antibiotic treatment?

Pasteurella multocida. Penicillin G.

20. What should be done with an amputated part that may be replanted?

1. Remove gross contamination by irrigating with saline.
2. Wrap the part in a saline-moistened (not soaked) sterile gauze.
3. Place the wrapped part into a sealed plastic bag or container.
4. Place the bag or container into an ice water bath.

21. List traumatic amputations that should be considered for replantation.

1. Children
2. Multiple finger amputations
3. Thumb
4. Hand
5. Arm

The ultimate decision always should be deferred to a hand surgery specialist. It is usually best to defer detailed discussion of replantation with the patient or family to the consulting microvascular specialist.

22. What is the appropriate treatment for a patient with pain in the snuffbox of the wrist and normal radiographs after a traumatic event to the wrist?

The scaphoid is easily palpable in the anatomic snuffbox of the wrist. The snuffbox is the space between the extensor pollicis longus and the extensor pollicis brevis. Tenderness in this area is suggestive of a scaphoid fracture. The absence of fracture on the initial radiographs is not unusual. As the necrotic bone at the fracture site is resorbed, the fracture line often becomes apparent on radiographs approximately 14 days after injury. Individuals with this condition should be immobilized in a thumb spica splint or cast and referred to an orthopedist for evaluation. For this reason, bone scans and MRI are not indicated in the acute evaluation.

23. State the incidence and common causes of posterior shoulder dislocations.

Incidence is 5% of shoulder dislocations. Tonic-clonic seizures, electrical shock, and direct anterior shoulder trauma are causes.

24. What percent of patients with first-time anterior shoulder dislocations experience a recurrent dislocation?

Of patients aged 30 years old or younger, 90% experience a recurrent dislocation. For older patients, the percentage is lower and more variable, depending on the mechanism of injury.

25. What are the potential complications of anterior shoulder dislocation?

The axillary nerve is at risk for injury at the time of dislocation. Careful examination of the deltoid muscle should be done to assess motor function. The axillary nerve also provides sensation to the lateral aspect of the shoulder, and sensation should be checked in this area. In addition to axillary nerve injury, a rotator cuff tear can occur at the time of dislocation.

26. How is a rotator cuff tear diagnosed?
The patient often complains of pain with overhead activity, night pain, and pain with abduction of the arm. The patient has difficulty abducting the arm and often is unable to lift the arm above the level of the shoulder. With the shoulder in 90° abduction, 30° forward flexion, and maximal internal rotation, the patient cannot resist against downward pressure on the extremity (supraspinatus strength test). A drop test is done in the same manner with the arm simply at 90° abduction. The patient is not able to lower the arm **slowly** from 90° abduction. When these conditions exist, it is important to differentiate a rotator cuff tear from subacromial impingement (condition that irritates the rotator cuff). Inject 10 mL 1% lidocaine in the subacromial space. If the patient obtains pain relief and still cannot initiate abduction, the diagnosis of rotator cuff tear is confirmed.

27. How is a posterior sternoclavicular dislocation diagnosed?
Radiographs are generally unsuccessfuls. CT scan is the most sensitive diagnostic modality.

28. Describe the significance of anterior versus posterior dislocation of a sternoclavicular joint.
Anterior dislocations are not associated with major complications and are treated easily with a sling. Of **posterior** sternoclavicular dislocations, 25% are associated with complications, including rupture or compression of the trachea; esophageal occlusion or rupture; lung contusion; and laceration or occlusion of the superior vena cava, subclavian vein, or artery. Reduction of posterior sternoclavicular dislocation should be done only in the operating room, with a cardiothoracic surgeon immediately available.

29. What is the most common neurologic deficit seen with a humeral shaft fracture?
The radial nerve may be stretched (**neurapraxia**) or rarely lacerated (**neurotmesis**). This condition typically occurs with fractures involving the distal one third of the humerus. Disability includes inability to extend the wrist and fingers at the metacarpophalangeal joints and numbness on the dorsum of the radial side of the hand. Interphalangeal extension, representing ulnar and median nerve function, is preserved.

30. What is the difference between a nightstick fracture and a Monteggia fracture?
A fracture of the ulna (typically the proximal one third) with a radial head dislocation is a **Monteggia fracture**. This fracture occurs as a result of a fall on an outstretched hand with associated valgus force on the extremity. The treatment requires internal fixation of the ulna fracture. A nightstick fracture is a fracture of the ulna resulting from a direct blow to the shaft of the ulna. There is no associated injury to the proximal radial ulnar humeral joint. In most cases, these injuries can be treated by closed means and early range of motion. Nightstick fractures with significant comminution, 10° to 15° of angulation, or greater than 50% displacement may be considered for operative fixation.

31. What nerve is commonly injured in a Monteggia fracture?
The posterior interosseous nerve lies in close proximity to the neck of the radius. When the radial head is dislocated, this nerve is often stretched, resulting in a neurapraxia and inability to extend the thumb or wrist.

LOWER EXTREMITY AND PELVIC FRACTURES

32. Name the major complications that are directly related to pelvic fracture.
Hemorrhage and urologic injuries, including bladder rupture and urethral tear.

33. What is the mortality rate in patients with open pelvic fracture?
50%.

34. Discuss the major management considerations of hemorrhage in patients with pelvic fracture.
A thorough evaluation for other life-threatening injuries must be done. Patients with major pelvic fractures often have associated injuries. Closed head injuries or visceral bleeding are the most common causes of death in patients with major pelvic fracture. Immediate surgical consultation should be obtained. A pelvic fracture itself can result in significant, even fatal hemorrhage, especially with biomechanically unstable fractures. Aggressive administration of crystalloid, blood, platelets, and fresh frozen plasma is required. Transfusion with 6 U or more of packed red blood cells is not unusual. In open book injury patterns, stabilization of the fracture with pelvic external fixation or pelvic clamps can reduce pelvic volume, promoting tamponade of venous hemorrhage (the cause of pelvic fracture bleeding in approximately 85% of cases). On initial presentation, the pelvis can be stabilized easily and quickly by a sheet or binder wrapping. If bleeding persists, angiography with embolization should be considered to control the arterial bleeding that is present in about 15% of pelvic fractures. Multidisciplinary protocols involving emergency physicians, trauma surgeons, orthopedic surgeons, and interventional radiologists have been shown to reduce mortality significantly.

35. What is the incidence and mechanism of injury in posterior hip dislocation?
Greater than 80% are posterior and result from a force directed posteriorly to a flexed knee, as occurs when the knee strikes the dashboard in a motor vehicle accident.

36. What are the complications of posterior hip dislocation?
Sciatic nerve deficit is found in about 10% of patients, resulting in weakness or loss of hamstring function in the thigh and all of the muscles of the leg. **Avascular necrosis** occurs in 10% to 15% of patients, but increases almost to 50% if reduction is delayed beyond 12 hours. With prompt reduction, 20% of patients develop **osteoarthritis**.

37. How is posterior hip dislocation differentiated clinically from a femoral neck fracture or intertrochanteric femoral fracture?
Both result in lower extremity shortening. In posterior hip dislocation, the hip is flexed, adducted, and internally rotated. This is often referred to as the position of modesty. With a femoral neck or intertrochanteric fracture, the lower extremity is not flexed but is shortened, abducted, and externally rotated.

38. How much blood loss can be expected with a fracture of the femoral shaft?
500 to 1,500 mL.

39. How are femoral shaft fractures best stabilized in the ED?
Hare longitudinal traction, involving a self-contained traction unit. Most emergency providers carry these and can place them in the field or ambulance. Hare traction should not be left in place for more than 2 hours without frequent neurovascular checks because of the potential for compartment syndrome and vascular compromise. A second option is placement of a distal femoral traction pin and in-line traction connected to the bed or gurney. Conventional splinting is ineffective.

40. Why do patients with hip pathology present with knee pain?
A patient with a hip problem may complain only of pain to the anterior distal thigh and medial aspect of the knee. The knee and the hip share a common innervation through the obturator nerve. Always suspect a hip problem in a patient who complains of knee pain without corresponding findings on physical examination. Careful examination of the knee and hip, with appropriate radiographs of the hip, is necessary to complete the evaluation.

41. Name the most common injury associated with traumatic hemarthrosis of the knee joint.

Anterior cruciate ligament rupture. If fat globules are noted in the joint aspiration fluid, the possibility of an associated intraarticular fracture should be pursued.

42. Name the ligament most commonly associated with an inversion ankle sprain.

Anterior talofibular ligament. The calcaneofibular ligament also can be injured in more severe sprains.

43. Describe the treatment for ankle sprains.

Ankle sprains are treated by the **RICE** protocol:

R = Rest
I = Ice
C = Compression
E = Elevation

Early protected weight bearing with crutches and an early range-of-motion program should be instituted. More severe sprains may require a short period of immobilization.

44. Discuss the Ottawa Rules regarding radiographs of the ankle.

The Ottawa Rules were developed from a large study done in Ottawa, Canada, which examined the necessity of routine ankle radiography in the assessment of patients with ankle injuries. It was determined that radiographs are not required when the following conditions are met:

1. The examiner is experienced.
2. The patient does not have significant deformity of the ankle.
3. The examination is consistent with an ankle sprain.
4. There is no tenderness on examination over the medial or lateral malleolus.

45. What is a locked knee, and what are the most common causes?

The patient is unable to extend the knee actively or passively beyond 10° to 45° flexion. True locking and unlocking occur suddenly. The most common causes are a tear of the medial meniscus, a loose body or **joint mouse** (osteochondral fragment) in the knee, or a dislocated patella.

46. What injuries are associated with a calcaneal fracture?

Depending on the exact mechanism of injury and the type of calcaneal fracture, 10% to 50% of patients have an associated compression fracture of the lumbar or lower thoracic spine. Of calcaneal injuries, 10% are bilateral, and about 25% are associated with other lower extremity injuries; 10% can result in a compartment syndrome of the foot, requiring fasciotomy.

47. What vascular injury must be considered with a tibiofemoral knee dislocation?

Injury or compression of the popliteal artery. Cadaver studies showed that anterior dislocations tend to cause intimal flaps and occlusion, whereas posterior dislocations are more likely to cause a rupture of the popliteal artery. Injuries also occur at the trifurcation just distal to the popliteal fossa. Postreduction angiography should be considered for all patients with abnormal pulse examination or antebrachial index.

PEDIATRIC ORTHOPEDICS

48. What is a torus or buckle fracture?

This fracture is typically seen in the metaphysis of the radius but is not limited to this bone. **Torus** means a round swelling or protuberance. In children, the cortical bone and metaphyseal bone fail in compression (**buckling**), while the opposite cortex remains intact. The area of bone that fails in compression forms a torus. Because the opposite cortex remains intact, these fractures are stable and require splint or cast immobilization for 4 weeks.

49. What is a greenstick fracture?

Children's bones have increased elasticity. An angular force applied to a long bone of a child causes a greenstick fracture. One cortex fails in tension, while the opposite cortex bows but does not fail or fracture in compression. The fracture is similar to what occurs when one attempts to break a green branch of a tree. This fracture pattern is common in the radius and ulna. These fractures require reduction, and often the fracture must be completed to achieve an adequate reduction. Immobilization in a cast is required for 6 weeks.

50. What is the Salter-Harris classification, and what is its clinical significance?

A method of classifying epiphyseal injuries. Fractures involving the epiphysis may result in growth disturbance, and parents must be informed of this potential. About 80% of these injuries are Salter-Harris types I and II, both of which have a low complication rate. Salter-Harris types III, IV, and V injuries have a more variable prognosis. Displaced Salter-Harris types III and IV fractures may require open reduction to restore the normal relationship of the epiphysis and articular surface.

Salter-Harris Classification

	DESCRIPTION	DIAGRAM
Type I	Fracture extends through the epiphyseal plate, resulting in displacement of the epiphysis (this may appear merely as widening of the radiolucent area representing the growth plate)	
Type II	As above, with an additional fracture of a triangular segment of metaphysis	
Type III	Fracture line runs from the joint surface through the epiphyseal plate and epiphysis	
Type IV	Fracture line also occurs in type III but also passes through adjacent metaphysis	
Type V	This is a crush injury of the epiphysis, which may be difficult to determine by x-ray examination	

51. Describe the vascular complications associated with pediatric supracondylar humerus fractures.

Displaced supracondylar humerus fractures in children have a 5% incidence of vascular compromise. The brachial artery typically is compressed or lacerated by the anteriorly displaced humeral shaft. Posterior lateral displacement of the supracondylar fracture is the fracture pattern most likely to result in vascular injury. The child with a viable hand and absent pulse should undergo prompt reduction and fracture fixation in the operating room, with reevaluation of the vascular status after the procedure. In the patient with an absent pulse and a devascularized hand, longitudinal traction and splinting should be done in the ED in an attempt to reconstitute flow to the distal extremity. Prompt consultation with orthopedic and vascular surgeons is required.

52. Describe the neurologic complications associated with pediatric supracondylar humerus fractures.

The anterior interosseous nerve (branch of the median nerve) is potentially the most commonly injured nerve. This nerve innervates the deep compartment of the forearm, which consists of the flexor digitorum profundus to the index, the pronator quadratus, and the flexor pollicis longus. The nerve can be checked by evaluating flexor pollicis longus function at the interphalangeal joint of the thumb. The radial nerve is the next most commonly injured nerve, followed by the ulnar nerve. A thorough physical examination must be done to identify these injuries, a difficult task in the small child.

53. What is a nursemaid's elbow? What is its management?

A longitudinal pull on the outstretched arm of a 1- to 5-year-old child may result in a subluxation of the annular ligament over cartilaginous radial head. The child typically presents with pseudoparalysis of the injured extremity. Radiographs are negative for fracture or radial head dislocation. Reduction involves simultaneous supination of the forearm and flexion of the elbow. A distinct click over the radial head signifies reduction. The child often begins to use the extremity within minutes of reduction. The parent or caregiver should be educated to avoid longitudinal traction on the arm to prevent this from occurring in the future.

54. Describe the potential implications of a humeral or femoral fracture in a small child.

In the nonambulating child with these fractures, the suspicion of child abuse should be high. An unwitnessed event or a history that does not correspond to the injuries is another potential sign of abuse. Careful examination of the child should be done, looking specifically for skin bruises or burns, retinal hemorrhage, and evidence of previous fracture. A skeletal survey should be considered because the presence of fractures at different stages of healing is a sign of abuse. All cases of suspected abuse need to be reported to the local authority. (See Chapter 78, Child Abuse.)

55. What is Waddell's triad?

The constellation of injuries in a child struck by a car:
1. Femoral fracture
2. Thoracic injury
3. Head injury

56. Which nontraumatic hip disorders cause a limp in a child?

Septic arthritis, transient synovitis (ages 2 to 12 years), idiopathic avascular necrosis (boys, ages 5 to 9 years), slipped capital femoral epiphysis (boys, ages 10 to 16 years), Perthes' disease, and juvenile rheumatoid arthritis; all of these are uncommon. Transient synovitis is probably the most common cause of nontraumatic limp in a child but is a diagnosis of exclusion. Symptomatic treatment is prescribed for transient synovitis, including nonsteroidal antiinflammatory drugs and non-weight bearing or bed rest. Untreated or delayed treatment of septic arthritis can lead to irreversible and catastrophic sequelae from permanent damage and deformation of the articular cartilage. Infection in a child presenting with atraumatic hip pain must be convincingly ruled out. The white blood cell count, erythrocyte sedimentation rate, and body temperature frequently are elevated in cases of infection. If doubt persists, the gold standard is hip aspiration, usually done in the operating room. Standard anteroposterior and lateral radiographs of the hip differentiate between Perthes' disease and a slipped capital femoral epiphysis.

57. What are the early radiographic findings of a slipped capital femoral epiphysis (SCFE)?

Any asymmetry of the relationship of the femoral head to the femoral neck should raise the suspicion of SCFE, even if evident on only one x-ray view. If anteroposterior and lateral radiographs are normal, frog-leg views should be obtained. Comparison of the two hips may not be helpful in discerning subtle changes because SCFE is bilateral in 20% of cases.

58. What is the ED management of a child with injury and tenderness over an open epiphysis but a normal radiograph?

It is best to assume the child has sustained an undeterminable fracture of the physis (Salter-Harris type I or V). Immobilize the joint in a posterior splint and keep the child non-weight bearing if the lower extremity is involved. Parents should be notified of the possibility of this type of injury and the potential for growth disturbance. The need for prompt follow-up must be emphasized and is best arranged before discharging the child from the ED. A nondisplaced physeal fracture that becomes displaced because of lack of immobilization can have significant long-term consequences. Short-term extremity immobilization in an appropriately applied splint or cast is well tolerated. When in doubt, immobilize.

BIBLIOGRAPHY

1. Browner BD, et al (eds): Skeletal Trauma: Basic Science, Management, and Reconstruction, 3rd ed. Philadelphia, W.B. Saunders, 2002.
2. Green DP, Hotchkiss RN, Pederson WC: Green's Operative Hand Surgery, 4th ed. New York, Churchill Livingstone, 1999.
3. Lovell WW, Winter RB, Morrissy RT, Weinstein SL: Lovell and Winter's Pediatric Orthopaedics, 5th ed. Philadelphia, Lippincott Williams & Wilkins, 2001.
4. Rockwood CA, Green DP, Bucholz RW, Heckman JD: Rockwood and Green's Fractures in Adults, 5th ed. Philadelphia, Lippincott Williams & Wilkins, 2001.
5. Rockwood CA, Green DP, Bucholz RW, Heckman JD: Rockwood and Green's Fractures in Children, 5th ed. Philadelphia, Lippincott Williams & Wilkins, 2001.

118. HAND INJURIES AND INFECTIONS

Michael A. Kohn, M.D., M.P.P.

1. Are hand problems important in emergency medicine?

Yes. More than 16 million hand injuries occur annually in the United States, most of which initially present to EDs. More than 30% of all industrial accidents involve the hand. Hand injuries account for 75% of all partially disabling injuries.

2. Name the essential elements of the history.

Age; dominant hand; occupation; how, where, and when injury occurred; posture of hand when injured; tetanus status; and prior injury or disability of the hand.

3. Name the elements of a complete hand examination.

Initial inspection of skin and soft tissue, vascular examination, evaluation of tendon function, nerve examination (motor and sensory), determination of joint capsule integrity, and skeletal examination.

4. What is topographical anticipation?

Looking at the skin wound and thinking about which underlying structure (vessel, tendon, nerve, bone, ligament, or joint) could be injured. Know the anatomy. Do not hesitate to consult an atlas.

5. What is the normal posture of the hand at rest?

With the wrist in slight extension, the resting fingers normally assume a "cascade," progressively more flexed from index to small. (See this by relaxing your own hand with the wrist in slight extension.) An alteration in the normal posture can lead to immediate diagnosis of major tendon and joint injuries.

6. Does dorsal swelling signify an injury or infection in the dorsum of the hand?

No. Most of the palmar lymphatics drain to lymph channels and lacunae located in the loose areolar layer on the dorsum of the hand. Always check for a palmar wound when a patient presents with dorsal swelling.

7. What is the Allen test, and how is it performed?

The Allen test verifies patency of the radial and ulnar arteries as follows: Occlude radial and ulnar arteries. Have patient open and close hand five or six times. Hand should blanch. Release ulnar artery; blanching should resolve within 3 to 5 seconds. Repeat test, releasing radial artery instead of ulnar artery. Blanching should resolve within 3 to 5 seconds. The most accurate form of the Allen test uses digital blood pressures rather than return of color to monitor reperfusion.

8. How is function of the flexor digitorum superficialis (FDS) tendon tested?

The FDS inserts on the middle phalanx and flexes the proximal interphalangeal (PIP) joint. The flexor digitorum profundus (FDP) inserts on the distal phalanx and flexes the PIP and the distal interphalangeal (DIP) joints. The FDS muscle-tendon units should be independent of one another, whereas the FDP tendons arise from a common muscle belly. Testing the FDS of a finger entails flexing it at the PIP joint, while stabilizing the other three fingers in full extension, thereby taking the FDP out of action as a potential flexor of the PIP joint.

9. In which finger is the test of FDS function unreliable?

Because the FDP to the index finger can be independent of the other profundi, the FDS test is unreliable in the index finger. Flexion at the PIP joint may be due to the FDP, even with the other fingers stabilized in extension. Suspected index finger FDS injuries must be explored.

10. Why is the flexor or palmar aspect of the hand called the "OR side," whereas the extensor or dorsal aspect is the "ED side"?

In contrast to the extensors, the flexor tendons run through delicate sheaths. Because of these sheaths, repairing flexor tendons requires more expertise and a more controlled environment in the operating room than repairing extensor tendons.

11. How is a partial tendon laceration diagnosed?

If the location of the skin laceration is suspicious, rule out an underlying partial tendon laceration by exploration and direct visualization under tourniquet hemostasis. Because a flexor tendon runs through its sheath like a piston through a cylinder, a sheath laceration implies a partial tendon laceration, which is visible only when the hand is in the same posture as when injured. Direct visualization of the tendon during full range of motion must occur to rule out a partial tendon laceration.

12. How do I test the extrinsic extensor tendons?

The extrinsic extensors alone extend the metacarpophalangeal (MCP) joints, whereas they combine with tendons from the interossei and lumbricals to form the extensor mechanism that extends the interphalangeal joints. To test the extrinsic extensor, lay the hand, palm down, on a flat surface and ask the patient to elevate the digit.

13. Can extensor function to a finger be intact despite complete laceration of the extensor digitorum communis (EDC) to that finger?

Yes. The juncturae tendinum interlink the EDC tendons at the midmetacarpal level. Even if the EDC to a finger is completely lacerated in the dorsum of the hand, extension at the MCP still may be possible because of the junctura.

14. How do I test sensory nerve function?

Assess nerve function before the use of anesthesia. Test digital nerves by checking two-point discrimination on the volar pad. The two points should be 5 mm apart and aligned longitudinally.

15. What are the sensory distributions of the median, ulnar, and radial nerves?

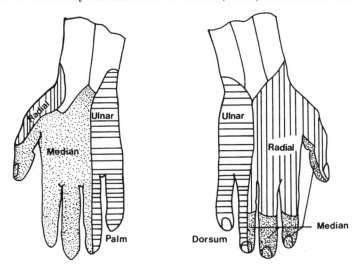

Sensory distribution of the median, ulnar, and radial nerves.

16. How is motor function of the median, ulnar, and radial nerves tested?

Median: Abductor pollicis brevis (APB)—abduct the thumb against resistance while palpating the APB muscle belly.

Ulnar: First dorsal interosseous—abduct the index finger against resistance.

Radial: (No intrinsics) Extensor pollicis longus (EPL)—extend the thumb interphalangeal joint against resistance.

17. Which is the most frequently dislocated carpal bone?

The carpal bones are as follows:

    Proximal row—scaphoid, lunate, triquetrum, pisiform
    Distal row—trapezium, trapezoid, capitate, hamate

The **lunate** is most frequently dislocated. Its blood supply comes through the volar and dorsal ligaments from the radius. If both ligaments are ruptured, avascular necrosis results.

18. Which is the most frequently fractured carpal bone?

The scaphoid. Its distal blood supply increases the likelihood of avascular necrosis in the proximal segment after fracture.

19. What is the classic sign of a scaphoid fracture?

Snuffbox tenderness. Even without radiographic evidence of a fracture, the patient with tenderness to palpation of the anatomic snuffbox gets a thumb spica splint and must have a repeat radiograph in 2 weeks.

20. How do I control hemorrhage from a hand injury?

Direct pressure and elevation. Rarely an incomplete arterial laceration requires a proximal tourniquet for temporary control, followed by sensory examination, anesthesia, scrub, and exploration under good light and magnification to tie off the bleeder. **Never blindly clamp a bleeder**.

21. Why the rule, "no blind clamping of bleeders"?

In the hand, the arteries run in close approximation to the nerves. Blindly clamping an artery may irreparably damage the associated nerve. Also, the clamp may damage a section of vessel vital to successful reanastomosis.

22. What should be done with an amputated digit?

Gently clean the digit with sterile saline, wrap it in moist gauze, place it in a sterile container, and float the container in ice water. (Avoid direct contact between ice and tissue to prevent freezing.)

23. What should be done with a devascularized but still partially attached digit?

Leave part attached (preserves veins for reimplantation), gently wrap in moist gauze, and apply a bulky dressing.

24. What are the indications and contraindications for reimplantation?

Indications: Multiple finger injury, thumb amputations (especially proximal to interphalangeal joint), single finger injury in children, clean amputation at hand, wrist, or distal forearm. (A clean amputation at the wrist is easier to reimplant than multiple-digit amputations.)

Contraindications: Severe crush or avulsion, heavy contamination, single-finger amputations in adults, severe associated medical problems or injuries, severe multilevel injury of amputated part, willful self-amputation.

Bottom line: Give the hand surgeon the opportunity to decide.

25. Which are the most deceptive of all serious hand injuries?

High-pressure injection injuries (from paint guns, grease guns, or hydraulic lines) initially may seem innocuous, often involving just the fingertip. In some reported series, 70% of such injuries resulted in some form of amputation and an average of 7 months' lost work time, even with early radical treatment.

26. List Kanavel's four cardinal signs of flexor tenosynovitis?

1. Slightly flexed posture of the digit.
2. Fusiform swelling of the digit.
3. Pain on passive extension.
4. Tenderness along the flexor tendon sheath.

Flexor tenosynovitis requires admission and surgery.

27. What is a paronychia, and how is it treated?

A common bacterial infection involving the folds of skin that hold the fingernail in place. In the absence of visible pus, treatment should consist of warm moist compresses, elevation, and antistaphylococcal antibiotics. If pus is present, do the minimum necessary to drain and maintain drainage. This usually consists of simply elevating the eponychial fold or making a small incision. Bilateral paronychia indicates subungual pus and necessitates removal of the proximal part of the nail plate.

28. How is whitlow different from a paronychia?

Whitlow is infection of the tissue around the nail plate with herpes simplex virus (rather than bacteria). The discharge is serous and crusting rather than purulent. The patient also may have perioral cold sores. Do **not** incise and drain herpetic whitlow.

29. What is a felon, and how is it treated?

A painful and potentially disabling infection of the fingertip pulp. Treatment is controversial. Some clinicians argue for immediate drainage of the tensely swollen and painful fingertip pad. Others argue that early treatment with antibiotics, elevation, and immobilization may prevent the need for surgical drainage. Even if drainage is necessary, the best method is also a matter of controversy. The full fishmouth incision has fallen out of favor, but the three quarters fishmouth incision and the simple lateral incision are both acceptable.

30. What is a football jersey finger, and how is it treated?

Rupture of the FDP occurs commonly when a football player catches his or her finger in an opponent's jersey. The tendon is avulsed from its insertion at the palmar base of the distal phalanx, often taking a bone fragment along. Surgical repair within the next several days is indicated.

31. What is a mallet finger, and how is it treated?

A mallet finger is the opposite of a football jersey finger; the insertion of the extensor tendon, rather than the flexor tendon, is avulsed from the dorsum of the distal phalanx, often pulling off a bone fragment. Appropriate treatment is to splint the DIP joint in extension (not hyperextension) for 6 weeks.

32. Describe a subungual hematoma. How is it treated?

A collection of blood under the nail plate can be painful. Classically, this occurs when a weekend carpenter strikes his or her thumb with a hammer. Relieving the pressure by nail trephinization (poking a hole in the nail) will make you a hero to the patient. Use electrocautery, a red hot paperclip, or an 18G needle (twisting it between your fingers like a drill bit). Removal of an intact nail plate is almost never indicated.

33. What is a gamekeeper's thumb?

A torn ulnar collateral ligament of the thumb MCP joint. In 1955, the injury was reported in 24 Scottish game wardens, arising from their technique for breaking the necks of wounded rabbits. The injury is more properly called **skier's thumb** because it most commonly occurs when a skier either catches the thumb on a planted ski pole or falls while holding a pole in the outstretched hand. The injury is potentially severely disabling. Complete rupture of the ligament always requires surgery. ED treatment consists of a thumb spica splint and referral.

34. What is a boxer's fracture?

Fracture of the fifth (small finger) metacarpal is common in barefisted pugilists. Because the small finger metacarpal is second only to the thumb metacarpal in mobility, large angles of angulation are tolerated without functional deficit. Nevertheless, attempts to correct significant angulation of an acute boxer's fracture are warranted. Any rotational deformity must be corrected. A laceration accompanying a boxer's fracture is assumed to be a fight bite.

CONTROVERSIES

35. What is a fight bite?

The most notorious of all nonvenomous bite wounds is the fight bite. As the name implies, the injury occurs when the soon-to-be-patient punches his or her adversary in the teeth, lacerating the dorsum of one or more MCP joints. Other names for this injury such as **morsus humanus** or **closed fist injury** have been proposed. **Fight bite** is more compact, descriptive, and poetic. All such wounds require formal exploration, including extension of the skin laceration if necessary. They should be débrided, irrigated, dressed open (no sutures), and splinted.

36. Are human bites more dangerous than other animal bites?

No. The fight bite gave human bites their reputation for being more prone to infection than other animal bites. This probably has more to do with the location of the bite and the typical delay in treatment than with the mix of organisms in the human mouth. True human bites (occlusive bites rather than fight bites) have no higher infection rates than animal bites. If humans punched animals in the teeth, these animal fight bites would have high infection rates also.

37. Should persons with uninfected fight bites be treated on an outpatient basis?

For:

1. Admitting every person with a fight bite, without evidence of infection, is extremely expensive.

2. Two studies (Peeples [1980] and Zubowicz [1992]) support outpatient management with oral antibiotics of reliable patients who present within 12 hours (Peeples) or 24 hours (Zubowicz) of the injury.

Against:

1. Treating a septic joint is more expensive in terms of hospital costs and patient disability costs than admitting a person with an uninfected fight bite for intravenous antibiotics.

2. All studies on the subject include fight bites and true occlusive bites to the hand, confusing the issue.

3. Fight-bite patients are notoriously unreliable and poor candidates for outpatient management.

Addendum: No controversy exists regarding patients with **infected** fight bites. All such patients are admitted.

BIBLIOGRAPHY

1. American Society for Surgery of the Hand: The Hand: Examination and Diagnosis. "Blue Book," 3rd ed. New York, Churchill Livingstone, 1990.
2. American Society for Surgery of the Hand: The Hand: Primary Care of Common Problems. "Red Book," 2nd ed. New York, Churchill Livingstone, 1985.
3. Antosia RE, Lyn E: The hand. In Rosen P, Barkin RM (eds): Emergency Medicine: Concepts and Clinical Practice, 4th ed. St. Louis, Mosby, 1998, pp 625–668.
4. Cambell CS: Gamekeeper's thumb. J Bone Joint Surg 37B:148–149, 1955.
5. Carter PR: Common Hand Injuries and Infections: A Practical Approach to Early Treatment. Philadelphia, W.B. Saunders, 1983.
6. Kanavel AB: Infection of the Hand. Philadelphia, Lea & Febiger, 1925.
7. Lampe EW (with ill. by F Netter): Surgical Anatomy of the Hand. Clin Symp 40:3, 1988.
8. Peeples E, Boswick JA, Scott FA: Wounds of the hand contaminated by human and animal saliva. J Trauma 20:383–389, 1980.
9. Szabo RM (ed): Common Hand Problems. Orthop Clin North Am 23:1, 1992.
10. Welch C: Human bite infections of the hand. N Engl J Med 215:901, 1936.
11. Zubowicz VN, Gravier M: Management of early human bites of the hand: A prospective randomized study. Plast Reconstr Surg 88:111–114, 1991.

119. BURNS

Jeffrey S. Hill, M.D.

1. List types of burns commonly seen in the ED.
- Direct thermal injuries (most common)
- Solar (i.e., sunburn)
- Chemical
- Electrical
- Radiation

2. How should thermal burns be assessed initially in the ED?
Rapid assessment of the type and severity of burn injury is key. The most important factors to evaluate include severity (estimated depth of injury), body surface area (BSA), and location. Other important factors are associated injuries and coexisting or preexisting medical conditions.

3. So where do I start?
Do a physical examination. Severity is estimated most easily in this way. **First-degree** burns (involving only the superficial layers of the skin) are erythematous and painful. **Second-degree (partial-thickness)** burns extend to the deeper layers of the dermis and can have a varied appearance. Erythema or mottled skin, often with blistering or a wet shiny surface, is often present; however, deeper partial-thickness burns can be pale and colorless. These burns are extremely and

exquisitely painful. **Third-degree (full-thickness)** burn injuries look like what they are: dead tissue. Here the burn extends through all the dermal layers, and the skin may appear translucent to off-color to frankly charred. These areas are insensate. **Fourth-degree** burns are direct current electrical injuries to deep tissue such as muscle, blood vessels, and nerves.

4. What is BSA, and why is it important?

BSA is a rapid means of estimating the extent of injury in a relatively simple and commonly recognized format. It is a means of quantifying the injury and has important clinical and prognostic implications. The **rule of nines** is the most widely employed topographic measurement and divides the regions of the body into approximate percentages of total surface area. These percentages differ between adults and children, and the differences are noteworthy.

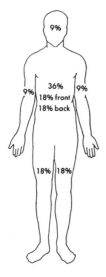

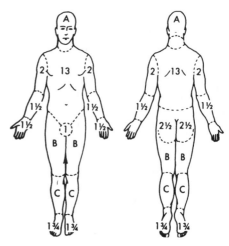

Relative Percentages of Areas Affected by Growth (Age in Years)

	0	1	5	10	15	ADULT
A: Half of head	9½	8½	6½	5½	4½	3½
B: Half of thigh	2¾	3¼	4	4¼	4½	4¾
C: Half of leg	2½	2¾	2	3	3¼	3½

Second degree_____ and Third degree _____ =
Total percent burned _____

Above left, Percentages used in determining extent of burn by "rule of nines" (From Miller RH: Textbook of Basic Emergency Medicine, 2nd ed. St. Louis, Mosby-Year Book, 1980, with permission.)

Above right, Classic Lund and Browder chart. The best method for determining percentage of body surface burn is to mark areas of injury on a chart and then compute total percentage according to patient's age. (From Artz CP, Yarbrough DR III: Burns: Including cold, chemical, and electrical injuries. In Sabiston DC Jr (ed): Textbook of Surgery, 11th ed. Philadelphia, W.B. Saunders, 1977, with permission.)

5. What are the indications for surgical consultation?

Any significant burn (second degree or greater) involving the face, neck, hands, feet, or perineum mandates surgical consultation and, at a minimum, surgical follow-up. These vital regions are important because significant burn injury may be complicated by swelling or edema, which can lead to neurovascular or airway compromise. Surgical consultation should be sought immediately for any patient with a potentially life-threatening burn injury, preferably a surgeon familiar with the care of burn patients. Particular burns may require immediate surgical intervention. Specifically, circumferential burns of the neck are a true emergency because rapid progression to airway compromise can develop. Aggressive airway management is mandatory. Circumferential burns of the extremities are also an emergency because the neurovascular supply to the areas distal to the burn site can be impaired and, as edema develops, tissue ischemia and frank compartment syndrome may develop. Early surgical intervention (escharotomy) may be limb-saving.

6. What are the criteria for admission?
Any infant or child with greater than 10% BSA burn or any adult with greater than 25% BSA burn must be hospitalized. These are loose guidelines at best and must be viewed in context with all other relevant clinical and social issues.

7. Are there special considerations in children?
Yes. The approach to the burned child must be as thorough and aggressive as for an adult, but the possibility of nonaccidental trauma, conditions surrounding the home and social situation, and reliability of the parents must be considered before releasing any child with a minor to moderate burn for outpatient care. Burn patients at the extremes of age are at greater risk for morbidity and mortality, and children and infants younger than 2 years of age should have more liberal admission criteria than older children.

8. Are there similar modifiers for adults?
Victims at the extremes of age with major burns have greater morbidity, and burn victims older than 60 years of age generally do poorly. Patients with alcoholism, HIV illness or other causes of immunocompromise, diabetes, malignancy, and cardiovascular or pulmonary impairment require more aggressive inpatient care.

9. How are superficial thermal burn injuries treated?
First-degree burns. Care is generally supportive; burns usually heal quickly without scarring. Application of cool water or saline, adequate analgesia, and follow-up with one's primary physician as needed are reasonable. For sunburn, addition of an antihistamine may be helpful for associated swelling or edema (as occurs on the face). A short course of oral steroids may be beneficial, although efficacy of this regimen has not been evaluated rigorously.

Second-degree burns. These burns are more complex and require more meticulous evaluation and care. After excluding any life-threatening or limb-threatening injury, the burn should be cleansed gently with a mild antiseptic solution. When intact blisters are encountered, it generally is recommended they be left intact. Ruptured blisters should be débrided. Outpatient care follows the usual tenets of basic wound care. Topical antibiotics should be applied liberally to the affected area. Silver sulfadiazine may affect pigmentation of healing tissue and should be used with caution on the face. One study from India showed raw, unrefined honey to be an excellent covering for such wounds. A nonadhesive dressing and bulky bandage are applied. If a joint surface is crossed, immobilization is appropriate. Aggressive pain control and follow-up in 24 to 48 hours for dressing change and reexamination are mandatory either in the ED or by a physician familiar with burn care.

10. Are there other burn dressing options?
Many. Topical antibiotics are the primary treatment for superficial burns. For partial-thickness burns, several alternatives are available. An occlusive hydrocolloid dressing (DuoDerm Hydroactive Burnpack) has been shown to be effective for second-degree burns. A polymyxin B sulfate/bacitracin/collagenase ointment regimen has been shown to be superior in improving healing times and decreasing eschar formation with these injuries. Skin substitutes (Biobrane) have been used successfully as an alternative covering for burned regions of the body. Such coverings have the advantage of greater comfort, decreased rates of infection, and cost-effectiveness.

11. How about a potentially life-threatening burn?
The approach to a seriously burned patient should be appropriately aggressive and thorough. The basic tenets of patient care (the **ABCs**) must be strictly followed. Attention to airway management and respiratory support is essential. Establishment of adequate intravenous access is required

(yes, you can place an angiocatheter through burned tissue if necessary). Because of the hemodynamic instability that may develop with major burns, central monitoring (including Swan-Ganz) is often used after the patient reaches the ICU. In the ED, central venous access is appropriate if indicated. Always consider conditions or circumstances that may have **contributed to or followed** the burn itself (e.g., toxic ingestion or exposure, alcohol, metabolic derangement, cardiovascular or central nervous system pathology). All patients who sustain a major burn in an enclosed space are assumed to have carbon monoxide poisoning until proved otherwise. All of these patients should be transferred to a burn unit.

12. What are the priorities in patients who have multisystem trauma and burns?

In **polytraumatized** patients with major burn injuries, the traumatic injuries are a major contributor to death. Any patient who sustains traumatic injuries concomitantly with the infliction of the burn needs prompt resuscitation, with attention to life-threatening traumatic injuries taking priority.

13. What about thermal injury to the airway?

The physiologic mechanisms of cooling inspired air are remarkably efficient. With the exception of steam inhalation injuries, direct thermal injury to the subglottic structures is uncommon. The glottic and supraglottic structures take the brunt of thermal inhalation injuries. There is little in the way of protection for the upper airway, and the most immediate life threat results from tissue edema in the hypopharynx. Aggressive airway management is the rule.

14. What other concerns must be kept in mind regarding smoke inhalation injuries?

Depending on the materials involved during combustion, additional toxic exposures may be sustained. These can be local (i.e., pulmonary) or systemic. The most toxic is cyanide. Aldehydes, hydrogen fluoride and chloride gases, and nitrogen oxides may be present. (See Chapter 93, Smoke Inhalation.)

15. What are the indications for active airway management?

Evidence of progressive airway obstruction (especially changes in voice, stridor) should be acted on immediately. Ongoing respiratory insufficiency despite 100% high-flow oxygen is an indication for support. For severe burns to the face and neck, early intubation is appropriate (early airway management under controlled conditions is preferable to the hurried and potentially hazardous circumstances that may develop later).

16. Which routes of intubation are appropriate?

If there is any concern about upper airway pathology or edema, blind nasotracheal intubation is contraindicated. Orotracheal intubation offers the clinician the ability to visualize the supraglottic structures directly and (it is hoped) allows placement of the endotracheal tube atraumatically. In a stable patient, fiberoptic intubation via the nasal or oral route may follow further visualization of the respiratory tract. This may be unacceptably time-consuming in an unstable patient unless the operator is highly proficient in the use of the scope. Emergency cricothyrotomy is indicated if glottic edema does not allow passage of the endotracheal tube.

17. Are any anesthetic or induction agents contraindicated in burn patients?

Several texts state that succinylcholine is contraindicated in the burn patient because of concerns about hyperkalemia. This is not relevant in the ED, however, because it is a delayed response. This phenomenon manifests 7 to 10 days after injury and is related to up-regulation of certain muscle receptors. It does **not** happen acutely, and succinylcholine and nondepolarizing muscle blocking agents are safe and may be used in any rapid-sequence intubation. The greater danger is the use of induction agents related to volume status. Depending on the amount of time between burn occurrence and emergency treatment, large intravascular fluid shifts occur, and the patient becomes effectively volume depleted. Hypotension and cardiovascular collapse are possible if fluid replacement has not been initiated. Judicious use of induction agents that can cause or exaggerate hypotension, such as barbiturates and narcotics, is essential.

18. What is burn shock?

After a major burn, vascular integrity in the affected region is lost, and significant amounts of fluid begin to leak from the intravascular to the extravascular spaces. These shifts are most pronounced in the first 8 hours after burn injury, and this **third spacing** of fluid can lead to profound intravascular volume depletion that results in hypovolemic shock.

19. How is fluid resuscitation carried out in the victim of a major burn?

Crystalloid (hypertonic and isotonic saline) and colloids have been examined with mixed results. Immediate fluid resuscitation using a balanced salt solution (i.e., lactated Ringer's solution or normal saline) is universally accepted.

20. How much and how fast?

Many formulas have been devised for fluid replacement, but the Parkland formula is widely used and easy to remember. It calculates the fluid requirements needed for the first 24 hours. One half of the calculated volume is to be replaced within the first 8 hours postburn (coinciding with the time when initial intravascular fluid shifts are more pronounced).

$$\text{Fluid required} = \text{Body weight (kg)} \times \text{BSA involved} \times 2\text{–}4 \text{ mL/kg}$$

This is a guideline. Clinical parameters, including vital signs, central venous pressure or pulmonary capillary wedge pressure, and urine output, should be monitored carefully. Urine output should be maintained at 30 to 60 mL/h in adults and 1 to 2 mL/kg/h in children.

21. Sounds simple enough. Anything else?

Yes. In most EMS systems, transported patients usually have had one or more intravenous lines established and some fluid administered before arrival to the ED. You must remember to include these fluids when calculating the fluid requirement to attempt to avoid early overhydration. The fluid shifts seen in the first hours after burn injury are dramatic, but causing acute pulmonary edema in your patient is not helpful. Other considerations (e.g., pulmonary or central nervous system injury) also complicate fluid management. Not so simple after all.

22. What about systemic pain control?

A common error is to undertreat pain. Appropriate and repeated use of narcotics, usually morphine, can be started in the field and should be withheld only if the patient is so hemodynamically unstable that these agents are life-threatening. It is difficult for paralyzed, intubated patients to let you know how they feel. Be humane.

23. What about application of ice water for pain?

Covering the affected area with sterile sheets or bandages, then wetting them down with cool saline is a reasonable first step. Burned areas do not have intact autonomic or vascular function, and application of iced solutions damages tissue further and can lead to global hyperthermia.

24. Is there a role for prophylactic parenteral antibiotics in the ED?

No.

BIBLIOGRAPHY

1. Barret JP, Dziewulski P, Ramzy PI, et al: Biobrane versus 1% silver sulfadianzine in second-degree pediatric burns. Plast Reconstr Surg 105:62–65, 2000.
2. Chung JY, Herbert ME: Myth: silver sulfadiazine is the best treatment for minor burns. West J Med 175:205–206, 2001.
3. Demling RH, DeSanti L: Management of partial thickness facial burns (comparison of topical antibiotics and bio-engineered skin substitutes). Burns 25:256–261, 1999.

4. Dougherty W, Waxman K: The complexities of managing severe burns with associated trauma. Surg Clin North Am 76:923–958, 1996.
5. Hedderich R, Ness TJ: Analgesia for trauma and burns. Crit Care Clin 15:167–184, 1999.
6. Leslie CL, Cushman M, McDonald GS, et al: Management of multiple burn casualties in a high volume ED without a verified burn unit. Am J Emerg Med 19:469–473, 2001.
7. Mlcak R, Cortiella J, Desai MH, Herndon DN: Emergency management of pediatric burn victims. Pediatr Emerg Care 14:51–54, 1998.
8. Monafo WW: Initial management of burns. N Engl J Med 335:1581–1586, 1996.
9. Nguyen TT, Gilpin DA, Meyer NA, Herndon DN: Current treatment of severely burned patients. Ann Surg 223:14–25, 1996.
10. Sheridan RL, Schnitzer JJ: Management of the high-risk pediatric burn patient. J Pediatr Surg 36:1308–1312, 2001.
11. Subrahmanyam M: A prospective randomised clinical and histological study of superficial burn wound healing with honey and silver sulfadiazine. Burns 24:157–161, 1998.

120. WOUND MANAGEMENT

Javier I. Escobar II, M.D., Bryce R. Tiller, M.D., and Ann L. Harwood-Nuss, M.D.

1. Why is wound healing important?

Approximately 12 million traumatic wounds are treated in EDs across the United States annually. This constitutes about 10% of all ED visits. Patients judge the competency of a physician based on their ultimate functional or cosmetic results and the development of complications.

2. What is the difference between functional and cosmetic closure?

Functional closure is closure of a wound in such a fashion as to return the patient to earliest full use of the injured part. A **cosmetic repair** is one that is done so as to result in the least visible scarring.

3. How do I remember what steps to take when repairing a wound?

Use the mnemonic **LACERATE**:

L = **Look.** Evaluate the wound to determine the most appropriate closure. Also be sure to examine thoroughly distal to the wound for movement, sensation, and pulsation.

A = **Anesthetize.**

C = **Clip and Clean.** Clipping hair leads to less infection than shaving. Methodical irrigation is one of the best ways to decrease infection risk.

E = **Equipment.** Be prepared. Have everything needed for repair at the bedside, including laceration kit, sterile gloves, suture, and dressing.

R = **Repair.** Perform the repair. Devitalized tissue may need to be débrided.

A = **Assess results.** Reevaluate the wound when the repair is near completion to determine the need for additional sutures.

T = **Tetanus.** Give tetanus prophylaxis for dirty or contaminated wounds when the patient has not had a booster in 5 years or for clean wounds when the patient has not had a booster in 10 years.

E = **Educate.** Educate the patient on how to care for the wound, signs of infection, and the timing of suture removal.

4. Which factors increase the visibility of scars and compromise wound healing? How are they minimized?

CONTRIBUTING FACTORS	METHODS TO MINIMIZE SCARRING
Direction of wound, e.g., perpendicular to lines of static and dynamic tension	Layered closure; proper direction in elective incisions of wound
Infection necessitating removal of sutures resulting in healing by secondary intention and a wide scar	Proper wound preparation; irrigation, débridement, and use of delayed closure in contaminated wounds
Wide scar secondary to tension	Layered closure; proper splinting and elevation
Suture marks	Remove all percutaneous sutures within 7 days
Uneven wound edges resulting in magnification of scar by shadows	Careful, even approximation of wound edges and top layer closure to prevent differential swelling of edges
Inversion of wound edges	Proper placement of simple sutures or use of horizontal mattress sutures
Tattooing secondary to retained dirt or foreign body	Proper wound preparation and débridement
Tissue necrosis	Use of corner sutures on flaps, splinting, and elevation of wounds with marginal circulation or venous return; excise nonviable wound edges before closure
Compromised healing secondary to hematoma	Use of properly conforming dressing and splints
Hyperpigmentation of scar or abraded skin	Use of #15 or greater SPF sunblock for 6 months
Superimposition of blood clots between healing wound edges	Proper hemostasis and closure; H_2O_2 frequent swabbing; proper application of compressive dressings
Failure to align anatomic structures properly such as vermilion border	Meticulous closure and alignment; marking or placement of alignment suture before distortion of wound edges with local anesthesia; use of field block

From Markovchick V: Suture materials and mechanical after care. Emerg Med Clin North Am 10:673–689, 1992, with permission.

5. What aspects of history should be obtained in a patient with a traumatic wound?

The time, setting, and mechanism of injury are essential because these features help determine whether the wound is contaminated, may contain a foreign body, or has the potential for infection. The patient's current medications and immune status (AIDS, diabetes, chemotherapy), the patient's occupation, and dominant hand if a hand injury has occurred are important. The patient's tetanus immunization history and allergies (specifically regarding anesthetics, antibiotics, or latex gloves) must be obtained.

6. What are the most important aspects of the physical examination?

To perform an adequate examination, it is important to be familiar with underlying anatomy, especially in the regions of the face, neck, hands, and feet. Examination of the injured site should begin with identification of any motor, sensory, and vascular deficits. With extremity injuries, examination can be conducted in the absence of hemorrhage by temporarily inflating a sphygomomanometer proximal to the injury. Palpation of the bones adjacent to the site of injury may detect instability or point tenderness of an underlying fracture. Direct inspection always should be performed when there is a suspicion of bone injury or deep penetration of a foreign body.

7. What is the most important step I can take to prevent infection?

For all traumatic wounds, irrigation with normal saline at 8 to 10 psi should be done with a 19G needle and a 30-mL syringe. The optimal volume of irrigant has not been determined; however, 60 mL per centimeter of wound length has been used as a guideline. In the presence of gross contamination, copious irrigation should be done and débridement considered. Although diluted 1% povidone-iodine (Betadine) solution is not likely to cause significant tissue injury, its use has not been shown to produce a significant benefit when compared with saline. Exploration; débridement when indicated; hemostasis; and proper repair, dressing, and immobilization are essential adjuncts for proper wound management. Antibiotics have no proven prophylactic benefit in the normal host. For contaminated or dirty extensive wounds, a mechanical irrigation device should be used.

8. Which anesthetic agent should be used for local anesthesia?

Selection of an appropriate anesthetic depends on many factors, including age of the patient, underlying health, prior drug reactions, wound size and location, and practice environment in the ED. Lidocaine traditionally has been the standard agent for local anesthesia in the ED; however, bupivacaine has advantages over lidocaine, related mainly to duration of anesthesia. Patients receiving bupivacaine experience significantly less discomfort during the 6-hour postinfiltration period. Also, in a busy ED, use of bupivacaine may prevent the need to reanesthetize a wound when repair has been interrupted by the arrival of a higher acuity patient. Contrary to popular belief, the onset of anesthesia is not significantly slower with bupivacaine; mixtures of lidocaine and bupivacaine are unnecessary.

9. What causes the pain of local anesthetic infiltration, and how can it be prevented?

Pain from the infiltration of lidocaine and bupivacaine is caused by distention of tissue from too-rapid injection with too large a needle directly into the dermis. Also, these agents are acidic, which causes pain. Pain from infiltration can be minimized by injecting slowly, with a small, 25G or 27G needle, directly through the wound margins. Pain from infiltration can be reduced by buffering the anesthetic agent with 1 mL of sodium bicarbonate for every 10 mL of lidocaine. Bupivacaine does not lend itself to buffering because it precipitates as its pH rises. Warming of lidocaine and bupivacaine is an efficacious and inexpensive method of decreasing the pain of infiltration.

10. What is the toxic dose of lidocaine and bupivacaine?

ANESTHETIC	CLASS	MAXIMUM DOSE	DURATION
Lidocaine	Amide	4.5 mg/kg	1–2 h
Lidocaine with epinephrine	Amide	7 mg/kg	2–4 h
Bupivacaine	Amide	2 mg/kg	4–8 h
Bupivacaine with epinephrine	Amide	3 mg/kg	8–16 h
Procaine	Ester	7 mg/kg	15–45 min
Procaine with epinephrine	Ester	9 mg/kg	30–60 min

When calculating the dose of milligrams infiltrated, 1 mL of 1% lidocaine = 10 mg of lidocaine, and 1 mL of 0.25% bupivacaine = 2.5 mg of bupivacaine. Lower maximal doses should be used for patients with chronic illness, for very young or very old patients, or when infiltrating highly vascular areas or mucous mucosa.

11. Describe the presentation of lidocaine toxicity.

In general, toxicity should not occur unless the recommended dosing is met or exceeded. The caveat to that statement is that toxicity may take place at lower than maximal doses when infiltrating highly vascular areas or mucous membranes or with patients at the extremes of age or chronically ill patients. The main effects are on the central nervous and cardiovascular systems. Central nervous system effects present as lightheadedness, nystagmus, and sensory disturbances, including visual aura or scotoma, tinnitus, perioral tingling, or a metallic taste in the mouth. Slurred speech, disorientation, muscle twitching, and finally seizures may follow. The cardiovascular effects are manifested by hypotension, bradycardia, and prolonged ECG intervals. In severe toxicity, the end result is coma and cardiorespiratory arrest.

12. What can I use to anesthetize a patient who is allergic to amide and ester anesthetics?
Subdermal diphenhydramine may be injected locally to obtain short-acting analgesia. Make a 0.5% to 1.0% solution by diluting 1 mL of 50 mg/mL diphenhydramine into 5 to 10 mL of saline. The anesthetic effect may take several minutes to become evident. Do not exceed a total dose of 50 mg in adults or 1 mg/kg in children. The patient may become drowsy after the injection.

13. What are the contraindications to epinephrine as an adjunct to lidocaine and bupivacaine?
Anesthetics with epinephrine should not be used on digits, on pinna, circumferentially around the penis, or in areas with poor or marginal blood supply, such as flap wounds of the anterior pretibial area. Epinephrine decreases resistance to infection because of its potent vasoconstrictor effect. In areas of the body such as the scalp and face, the vasoconstriction and resulting hemostasis aid in the exploration and repair of the wound and do not seem to increase wound infection.

14. What is TAC?
A commonly used topical anesthetic that consists of a mixture of **tetracaine, epinephrine (adrenaline)**, and **cocaine**. Cotton soaked with TAC and placed directly onto or into an open wound results in excellent local anesthesia. It is expensive, unreliable in areas below the head, and tissue toxic, however, and it can result in significant complications when used improperly. Its use has been associated with at least one death. TAC should no longer be used in wound care.

15. What is LET (LAT)?
A topical anesthetic that consists of a mixture of **lidocaine** (4%), **epinephrine (adrenaline)** 1:1000, and **tetracaine** (0.5%). LET has been shown to be as efficacious as TAC for wound anesthesia and at one tenth of the expense. It has a much greater margin of safety. For these reasons, it has replaced TAC as the topical agent of choice.

16. What are the contraindications to LET?
They are the same as for lidocaine-bupivacaine with epinephrine.

17. When do I use conscious or procedural sedation?
Conscious sedation is a pharmacologic means of lowering the level of consciousness for procedures to be performed easily. The goal is to maintain a patent airway and spontaneous respirations while providing enough sedation to perform the procedure. It is indicated when the wound cannot be explored thoroughly or closed properly using local or topical anesthetic. This method is particularly helpful in children. Risks include respiratory depression, aspiration, laryngospasm, and cardiac arrest depending on the particular agents used.

18. What is a contaminated wound?
Any wound that has a high inoculum of bacteria. Some examples are full-thickness bites; wounds of the perineum or axilla in which there is normally a high skin flora count; and wounds that are exposed to contaminated water, such as from ponds, lakes, or coral reefs.

19. List factors that contribute to wound infection.
- Wound age
- Presence of foreign material

- Amount of devitalized tissue
- Presence of bacterial contamination
- Advanced patient age
- Ability of the host to mount an adequate immune response

20. Is a dirty wound the same as a contaminated wound?

No. **Road rash**, resulting from road gravel, has a low bacterial count. In contrast, wounds that occur in a barnyard or are exposed to soil contaminated with fecal material have a high bacterial count and are contaminated.

21. What causes tattooing?

The retention of foreign material and incorporation of it in the dermis during the healing process. To prevent this cosmetic complication, all foreign material and dirt must be removed through proper débridement, scrubbing, and irrigation at the time of the initial patient encounter. A stiff brush, such as a toothbrush, is useful to remove dirt embedded in the dermis.

22. How do I treat road rash?

Anesthetize the area with viscous lidocaine and circumferential or field block anesthesia. Remove all foreign bodies with the methods described previously. Consider dressing with **silver sulfadiazine**, which greatly reduces the pain and may obviate the need the potent oral analgesics for deep, extensive, painful abrasions.

23. When do I get an x-ray?

Radiographs are useful to search for a foreign body or to look for an associated fracture. Obtain a radiograph if the history is suspicious for a foreign body. In the case of bite wounds, radiographs should be obtained to search for teeth. With severe pain or structural instability, radiographs may reveal an underlying open fracture, which necessitates an orthopedic consultation in most cases.

24. Which type of foreign bodies found in wounds are visible on radiographs?

Glass, metal, and gravel. In general, glass larger than 2 mm and gravel larger than 1 mm can be seen on radiographs. Foreign bodies that are radiolucent (not visible on radiographs) include wood, plastics, and some aluminum products.

25. What is the best method for hair removal?

Clipping or cutting hair with scissors as opposed to shaving has been shown to result in lower wound bacterial counts and decreased rates of infection.

26. Define the three different types of wound closure.

1. **Primary closure** is closure of wound margins with sutures, staples, glues, or adhesive tapes 24 hours after injury.

2. **Delayed primary closure** is closure of a wound 3 to 5 days after wounding to decrease the risk of infection.

3. **Secondary closure**, or healing by secondary intention, is allowing a wound to heal by granulation without mechanical approximation of the wound margins.

27. Which wounds should be closed primarily?

Any clean (not initially contaminated) wound if it is less than 6 to 8 hours old and is located anywhere on the body except for the face and scalp, which may be closed primarily up to 24 hours because of the rich vascular supply and resistance to infection.

28. When should secondary closure be used?

For contaminated wounds that penetrate deeply into tissue and cannot be irrigated adequately before closure. Examples of such wounds are puncture wounds of the sole of the foot or palm of the hand and stab wounds that penetrate into subcutaneous tissue and muscle.

29. When should delayed primary closure be used?

It should be strongly considered for all contaminated wounds that are gaping or have significant amounts of tension. It decreases the risk of infection, optimizes the cosmetic result, and accelerates the healing process.

30. How is a wound prepared for delayed primary closure?

The wound should be examined thoroughly, prepared, débrided, and irrigated. Hemorrhage should be controlled. A fine layer of mesh gauze should be laid in the wound; the wound should be packed open and followed closely. At 3 to 5 days, if there is no purulent drainage or wound-margin erythema, the wound may be closed in the same fashion as if it were being closed primarily.

31. What is the most important step when closing a lip laceration through the vermilion border?

Placement of the first stitch at the vermilion border. Use permanent suture to close the edges of the vermilion border. Be sure to line up the edges precisely. The remainder of the lip should be closed with absorbable suture. The skin should be closed with permanent suture.

32. When are surgical staples indicated?

To reapproximate linear lacerations that do not involve cosmetically sensitive areas, such as the face. Two approaches are commonly employed. One approach involves two operators with one everting both wound edges with forceps while the other staples the wound together. If only one operator is available, the wound edges should be aligned and one edge everted with forceps in one hand while stapling with the other.

33. What is surgical glue, and how is it used?

2-Octyl cyanoacrylate (Dermabond) is a polymer currently being used as an alternative for wound repair. Cyanoacrylate acts rapidly, polymerizing within 30 seconds at room air. It is best used for linear lacerations under low tension and may replace 5-0 or 6-0 sutures. The wound can be held together manually, and the cyanoacrylate can be painted over the wound in three to four coats to ensure adequate closure. Be careful not to apply any adhesive within the wound because this would impede healing. Tapes may be placed over the glued wound as a reinforcing dressing. The adhesive sloughs off in 7 to 10 days. Do not use antibiotic ointment or any other type of ointment on the wound because it destroys the adhesive bond.

34. What are the advantages and disadvantages of using 2-octyl cyanoacrylate (surgical glue)?

One major advantage is that it is essentially nontraumatic when compared with the infusion of local anesthesia and sutures or staples. Another advantage is that bacterial counts in wounds closed with cyanoacrylate have been shown to be significantly lower than those in sutured wounds. Presumably this is because suture material may be a nidus for infection and because cyanoacrylate has intrinsic antimicrobial properties. A disadvantage is that wounds closed with cyanoacrylate have been shown to have a lower tensile strength 3 to 4 days after repair than do wounds repaired with sutures. There is a risk of accidentally applying the tissue adhesive into an unintended area (eye or inside the wound), causing inadvertent damage or impedance of healing.

35. How do I remove tissue adhesive?

First, avoid getting tissue adhesive into undesirable areas by applying protective covering and petroleum jelly to areas surrounding the wound. Apply light coats of the adhesive and quickly wipe off excess fluid. You have about 15 seconds before the adhesive dries. If the adhesive dries on an undesirable area (e.g., eyelid glued shut), the bond may be loosened with petroleum jelly or antibiotic ointment.

36. Summarize the advantages and disadvantages of the available techniques for wound closure.

TECHNIQUE	ADVANTAGES	DISADVANTAGES
Sutures	Time-honored method Meticulous closure Greatest tensile strength Lowest dehiscence rate	Removal required Anesthesia required Greatest tissue reactivity Highest cost Slowness of application
Staples	Rapidity of application Low tissue reactivity Low cost Low risk of needle stick	Less meticulous closure than with sutures May interfere with CT and MRI
Tissue adhesives	Rapidity of application Patient comfort Resistance to bacterial growth No need for removal Low cost No risk of needle stick	Lower tensile strength than sutures Dehiscence over high-tension areas (joints)
Surgical tapes	Least tissue reactivity Lowest infection rates Rapidity of application Patient comfort Low cost No risk of needle stick	Lower tensile strength than sutures Highest rate of dehiscence Use of toxic adjuncts required Cannot be used in hairy areas Must remain dry

From Singer AJ, Hollander JE, Quinn JV: Evaluation and management of traumatic lacerations. N Engl J Med 337:1142–1148, 1997, with permission.

37. Which sutures are used, how is the wound repaired, and when do I remove the sutures?

LOCATION	SUTURE MATERIAL	TECHNIQUE OF CLOSURE AND DRESSING	SUTURE REMOVAL
Scalp	3-0 or 4-0 nylon or polypropylene	Interrupted in galea; single tight layer in scalp; horizontal mattress if bleeding not well controlled by simple sutures	7–12 d
Pinna (ear)	6-0 nylon or 5-0 SA in perichondrium	Close perichondrium with 5-0 SA interrupted; close skin with 6-0 nylon interrupted; stint dressing	4–6 d
Eyebrow	4-0 or 5-.0 SA and 6-0 nylon	Layered closure	4–5 d
Eyelid	6-0 nylon or silk	Single layer horizontal mattress	3–5 d
Lip	4-0 silk or SA (mucosa) 5-0 SA (Sq, muscle); 6-0 (skin); 4-0 SA	Three layers (mucosa, muscle, skin) if through and through, otherwise two layers	3–5 d
Oral cavity	4-0 SA	Simple interrupted or horizontal mattress: layered closure if the muscularis of the tongue is involved	7–8 d or allow to dissolve
Face	4-0 or 5-0 SA (Sq); 6-0 nylon (skin)	If full-thickness laceration, layered closure desirable	3–5 d
Neck	4-0 SA (Sq); 5-0 nylon (skin)	Two-layered closure for best cosmetic results	4–6 d

(Table continued on following page.)

LOCATION	SUTURE MATERIAL	TECHNIQUE OF CLOSURE AND DRESSING	SUTURE REMOVAL
Trunk	4-0 SA (Sq, fat); 4-0 or 5-0 nylon (skin)	Single or layered closure	7–12 d
Extremity	3-0 or 4-0 SA (Sq, fat, muscle); 4-0 or 5-0 nylon (skin)	Single or layered closure is adequate, although a layered or running Sq closure may give a better cosmetic result; apply a splint if the wound is over a joint	7–14 d
Hands and feet	4-0 or 5-0 nylon	Single-layer closure only with simple or interrupted horizontal mattress suture, at least 5 mm from cut wound edges; horizontal mattress sutures should be used if there is much tension on wound edges; apply splint if wound is over a joint	7–12 d
Nailbeds	5-0 SA	Gentle, meticulous placement to obtain even edges	Allow to dissolve

SA = synthetic absorbable sutures such as Vicryl and Dexon; Sq = subcutaneous.
From Markovchick V: Soft tissue injury and wound repair. In Reisdorff EJ, Roberts MR, Wiegenstein JG (eds): Pediatric Emergency Medicine. Philadelphia, W.B. Saunders, 1993, pp 899–908, with permission.

38. How are bites treated?

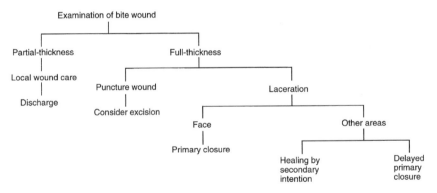

39. What should be included in all follow-up instructions?

Instructions on local wound care, signs of infection, and time of suture removal. Antimicrobial ointment may be applied to decrease the risk of infection; however, when tissue adhesives have been used, ointments dissolve the adhesive and may cause separation of the wound. Sunlight should be avoided, and sunscreen should be used to help minimize hyperpigmentation and scarring. Inform patients that all wounds will heal with a scar, all wounds may get infected, and all wounds may have retained foreign material.

CONTROVERSY

40. Are there any controversies in wound care?

1. The primary controversy relates to the use of **prophylactic antibiotics**. Their use is widespread and has developed with little scientific support. In general, the use of prophylactic antibiotics is not warranted in the normal host. Antibiotic therapy is indicated in patients with soft tissue wounds who are prone to infective endocarditis. Antibiotics may be indicated when the

risk for infection is high, including wounds of the distal foot; contaminated wounds; wounds in which there has been a delay in irrigation and débridement; and wounds that contain fecal material, pus, saliva, or vaginal secretions. Prophylactic antibiotic use should never replace proper wound decontamination.

2. With the rising cost of health care, economic concerns are at the forefront of many emergency medicine issues, including wound care. Numerous studies have shown that when used appropriately, tissue adhesives are an acceptable alternative to **traditional suturing**. Specifically, adhesives have been shown to decrease the duration of the ED visit and cut overall cost, while maintaining a similar result to suturing at 1 year postclosure. Stapling in selected patients can lower cost and increase time efficiency with end results close to those of traditional suturing. These alternatives should be kept in mind for suitable patients and situations.

BIBLIOGRAPHY

1. Hollander JE, Singer AJ: Wound management. In Harwood-Nuss AL, Wolfson AB (eds): The Clinical Practice of Emergency Medicine, 3rd ed. Philadelphia, Lippincott Williams & Wilkins, 2001, pp 449–459.
2. Hollander JE, Singer AJ, Valentine SM, Shofer FS: Risk factors for infection in patients with traumatic lacerations. Acad Emerg Med 8:716–720, 2001.
3. Howell JM, Chishholm CD: Wound care. Emerg Med Clin North Am 15:417–425, 1997.
4. Markovchick V: Soft tissue injury and wound repair. In Reisdorf EJ, Roberts MR, Wiegenstein JG (eds): Pediatric Emergency Medicine. Philadelphia, W.B. Saunders, 1993, pp 899–908.
5. Markovchick V: Suture materials and mechanical after care. Emerg Med Clin North Am 10:673–689, 1992.
6. Norris RL: Local anesthetics. Emerg Med Clin North Am 10:707–718, 1998.
7. Schilling CG, Bank DE, Borchert BA, Klatzko MD: Tetracaine, epinephrine (adrenaline), and cocaine (TAC) versus lidocaine, epinephrine, and tetracaine (LET) for anesthesia of lacerations in children. Ann Emerg Med 25:203–208, 1995.
8. Singer AJ, Hollander JE, Quinn JV: Evaluation and management of traumatic lacerations. N Engl J Med 337:1142–1148, 1997.
9. Wilson JL, Kocurek K, Doty BJ: A systematic approach to laceration repair: tricks to ensure the desired cosmetic result. Postgrad Med 107:77–88, 2000.

XVII. Behavioral Emergencies

121. ACUTE PSYCHOSIS
Eugene E. Kercher, M.D.

1. What is acute psychosis?

Psychosis is a dysfunction in the capacity for thought and information processing. The individual is unable coherently to perceive, retain, process, recall, or act on information in a consensually validated way. There is a decreased ability to willfully mobilize, shift, sustain, and direct attention. A major feature of the psychotic state is the failure in ranking the priority of stimuli. The ability to act on reality is unpredictable and diminished because the patient is unable to distinguish internal from external stimuli.

2. What is the difference between organic and functional psychosis?

Organic psychosis refers to a reversible or nonreversible dysfunctional mental condition that can be identified as a disturbance in the anatomy, physiology, or biochemistry of the brain.

Functional psychosis refers to a dysfunctional mental condition identified as schizophrenia, a major affective disorder, or other mental disorders with psychotic features.

3. What are the types of psychoses?

Classification of psychosis is found in the *Diagnostic and Statistical Manual of Mental Disorders* (DSM-IV), which is divided appropriately into functional and organic varieties. Most organically caused acute psychoses result from dementia, withdrawal states, and intoxications. Schizophrenia and the affective disorders are the major contributors to functionally caused acute psychoses.

4. List the possible causes of alcohol-related organic psychosis.

Chronic alcoholism
Thiamine deficiency (i.e., diet, starvation, and emesis)
Alcohol dependent withdrawal states
Comorbid substance abuse
Lack of psychosocial support system
Comorbid psychotic and mood disorder
Alcohol idiosyncratic intoxication (pathologic intoxication)

5. How does one differentiate amphetamine-induced psychosis from other forms of psychosis?

The absence of anger, avoidance behavior, lack of motivation, flat affect, and resolution of psychotic symptoms on discontinuance of the drug suggest the diagnosis of amphetamine-induced psychosis.

6. Is there a brief, self-limited, and nonorganic psychosis?

Yes. Some individuals may become acutely psychotic after exposure to an extremely traumatic experience. If such a psychosis lasts for fewer than 4 weeks, it is termed a **brief psychotic disorder**. Precipitants of the psychosis include the death of a loved one or a life-threatening situation, such as combat or a natural disaster, or other life stressors. Patients with hysterical, borderline, and narcissistic personalities are prone to brief psychotic disorder, and some studies support a genetic vulnerability. Emotional turmoil, confusion, and extremely bizarre behavior and speech are common symptoms on presentation.

7. How does a patient in a psychotic state typically present to the ED?

Patients who are in a psychotic state may act strangely (i.e., mannerisms, posturing), dress bizarrely, respond to hallucinations, harbor false and delusional beliefs, and consistently confuse the reality of events. They are frequently impulsive and in constant danger of acting on distorted perceptions or delusional ideas resulting in unintentional injury or death. Clarity of oneself and the environment is consistently blurred. The patient is unable to discriminate the stimuli that he or she perceives. Thinking is disorganized and incoherent, as evidenced from the patient's speech. Memory is impaired in registration, retention, and recall. Orientation may be impaired, especially for time. Psychomotor behavior may be hypoactive or hyperactive regarding movements and speech. Emotions can range from apathy and depression to fear and rage.

8. Why does the psychotic patient come to the ED?

Psychotic patients frequently are brought to the ED by relatives or friends who no longer can safely control the patient's behavior. Frequently a psychotic patient is brought in by police or paramedics because the psychotic condition is considered potentially dangerous to self or others. Some patients come to the ED seeking refuge from their overwhelming fears.

9. Why is it important to control psychotic behavior immediately?

Patients who present in a psychotic state are impulsive and unable to prioritize stimuli and their reactions to them. Because of this dysfunction, they always should be considered a danger to themselves or to others.

10. How can the potential for violent behavior be detected in the psychotic patient?

The best way to deal with violent behavior is to prevent it. Emergency physicians recognize patients who are obviously confused, irrational, paranoid, or excited. Emergency physicians also must develop an intuitive vigilance to detect the possibility of violence in patients who present more rationally and less floridly psychotic. Any history or comment that suggests violence should be taken seriously. The potential for violence in general is particularly high in patients who are psychotic secondary to psychostimulant drugs.

11. Are there behavioral controls that can be used immediately for the psychotic patient?

Yes. Recognizing the chance of violence and physical harm, definitive steps should be taken to avoid confrontation.

1. **Environmental**—keep the environment simple and stimuli-free, and minimize staff changes.

2. **Interpersonal**—assume the role of patient advocate, and engage the patient in a calm and self-assured voice.

12. What option can be exercised if the patient becomes increasingly disorganized and agitated?

Institute a formalized and rehearsed physical restraint plan. On summons by the physician, security guards should appear at the door, so the patient can see and feel their presence. This "show of force" indicates that any display of violence will not be tolerated and often helps the patient to organize and regain control of their thoughts and behavior. When the patient is physically restrained, he or she should be searched thoroughly for weapons or sharp objects.

13. Are there further methods of control if the patient continues to have psychotic turmoil?

Medication often complicates rather than accelerates the evaluation process of a patient in a psychotic state. The treatment goal in the ED is to decrease the patient's discomfort, anxiety, and disruptive behavior. The specific safety of the patient and the generalized safety of the staff are at stake. The standard medical treatment for acute psychosis is haloperidol.

14. How should priorities be set when I first encounter a psychotic patient?

1. Assess ABCs (airway, breathing, circulation) (if necessary).

2. Observe (quickly assess impulse control and tendency to physically act out).

3. Control and manage psychotic behavior (if necessary).

4. Obtain a history (gather from everyone who has been involved with the patient).

5. Differentiate between organic and functional causes through a formal mental status examination.

6. Do a physical examination, including complete vital signs.

7. Obtain laboratory (toxicologic and metabolic studies) tests and a head CT scan if clinically indicated.

8. Obtain psychiatric consultation and disposition.

15. What are other sources of information for psychotic patients, who are usually historically unreliable?

Because acutely psychotic patients may be unable to provide an adequate history, all avenues for obtaining information must be explored. This may include speaking to EMS personnel, family, friends, neighbors, and law enforcement officers and reviewing old medical records.

16. What historical information is important?

1. **Onset.** Did the behavior change suddenly or gradually?

2. **Longitudinal course.** Is this the first such event?

3. **Family history.** Do these symptoms or any other psychiatric disorders appear in the patient's family?

4. **Previous psychiatric disease.** Are organic brain disease, the use of medication, and any history of drug use present?

17. List pharmacologic agents that can cause acute psychosis.

Digitalis
Corticosteroids
Isoniazid (INH)
Disulfiram (Antabuse)
Tricyclics
Anticonvulsants
Cimetidine
Benzodiazepines
Amphetamines and related drugs
Antiarrhythmics
Narcotics
Barbiturates
Methyldopa
Nonsteroidal antiinflammatory drugs
Anticancer agents
Recreational drugs

18. How should my physical examination be tailored for a psychotic patient?

Always note the vital signs and pulse oximetry readings. Defer until last the rectal and pelvic examinations and other parts of the physical examination that require undressing. Start with the head, neck, and neurologic examination, which can be performed without undressing the patient. In most cases, emergency physicians will have built sufficient rapport with patients in time for the cooperation necessary for a more intimate examination. Tell the patient exactly what you are doing and what you are going to do during the examination. This helps to provide structure for the psychotic patient and avoids confusion or misunderstanding.

19. Is laboratory screening necessary in an appropriate workup of an acute psychotic patient?
Most laboratory investigations provide little help during the acute evaluation of a psychotic episode. The following tests are recommended if an organic cause is considered: complete blood count, electrolytes, toxicology screens, urinalysis, thyroid function tests, and liver function tests.

20. Summarize the key points to consider in the differentiation of organic from functional psychosis.

MADFOCS Mnemonic

		ORGANIC	FUNCTIONAL
M	**Memory deficit**	Recent impaired	Remote impaired
A	**Activity**	Hyperactivity and hypoactivity Tremor Ataxia	Repetitive activity Posturing Rocking
D	**Distortions**	Visual hallucinations	Auditory hallucinations
F	**Feelings**	Emotional lability	Flat affect
O	**Orientation**	Disoriented	Oriented
C	**Cognition**	Some lucid thoughts Perceives occasionally Attends occasionally Focuses occasionally	No lucid thoughts Unfiltered perceptions Unable to attend Unable to focus
S	**Some other findings**	Age > 40 Sudden onset Physical exam often abnormal Vital signs may be abnormal Social immodesty Aphasia Consciousness impaired Confabulation	Age < 40 Gradual onset Physical exam normal Vital signs usually normal Social modesty Intelligible speech Alert, awake Ambivalence

21. Name the life-threatening causes of acute psychosis.
WHHHIMP mnemonic:
Wernicke's encephalopathy
Hypoxia or hypoperfusion of the central nervous system
Hypoglycemia
Hypertensive encephalopathy
Intracerebral hemorrhage
Meningitis/encephalitis
Poisonings

22. Are there any other clinical "rules of thumb" in the workup of the acute psychotic patient?
1. Fever and psychosis = meningitis
2. Acute psychosis and alcoholism = Wernicke's encephalopathy
3. Headache and psychosis = tumor or intracranial hemorrhage
4. Abdominal pain and psychosis = porphyria
5. Sweating and psychosis = hypoglycemia or delirium tremens
6. Autonomic signs and psychosis = toxic or metabolic encephalopathy

23. Summarize the potentially reversible causes of psychosis.
DEMENTIA mnemonic:

Drug toxicity
Emotional disorders
Metabolic disorders
Endocrine disorders
Nutritional disorders
Tumors and trauma
Infection
Arteriosclerotic complications

24. What are the three basic questions to answer regarding the disposition of the psychotic patient?
 1. Is there risk of suicide or homicide?
 2. Is there realistic family support or supervision?
 3. What is the patient's initial response to medication?

25. When should hospitalization be recommended?
 1. If this is the patient's first psychotic episode
 2. If the patient is a danger to self or others
 3. If the patient is unable to care for self appropriately
 4. If the patient has no social support system
 5. If the functional psychotic patient is not sufficiently clear after initial ED tranquilization
 6. If an acute organic psychosis does not clear while the patient is in the ED

BIBLIOGRAPHY

1. American Psychiatric Association: Diagnostic and Statistical Manual of Mental Disorders, 4th ed, revised. Washington, DC, American Psychiatric Association, 1994, pp 273–315.
2. Anderson WH, Kuehanie JC: Diagnosis and early management of acute psychosis. N Engl J Med 305:1128, 1989.
3. Battaglia J, et al: Haloperidol, lorazepam, or both for psychotic agitation? A multicenter, prospective, double-blind, emergency department study, Am J Emerg Med 15:335, 1997.
4. Bresler RE, Klinger BI, Erickson BJ: Acute intoxication and substance abuse among patients presenting to a psychiatric emergency service. Gen Hospital Psychiatry 18:183, 1996.
5. Frame DS, Kercher EE: Acute psychosis: Functional vs. organic. Emerg Med Clin North Am 9:123–136, 1991.
6. Hillard JF: Emergency treatment of acute psychosis. J Clin Psychiatry 59:57, 1998.
7. Hockberger RS, Richards J: Thought disorders. In Marx JA, et al (eds): Rosen's Emergency Medicine: Concepts and Clinical Practice, 5th ed. Mosby, St. Louis, 2002, pp 1541–1548.
8. Kercher EE: Acute psychosis. In Rund DA, Barkin RM, Rosen P, Sternbach GL (eds): Essentials of Emergency Medicine, 2nd ed. Mosby, St. Louis, 1996, pp 647–655.
9. Richards JR, Derlet RW, Duncan DR: Chemical restraint for the agitated patient in the emergency department: Lorazepam versus droperido. J Emerg Med 16:567, 1998.

122. DEPRESSION AND SUICIDE

Douglas A. Rund, M.D., and Richard A. Nockowitz, M.D.

DEPRESSION

1. What are the symptoms of depression?
 The cardinal symptom of depression is a **dysphoric or sad mood**. To diagnose depression, a depressed mood must be present at least half of the time over a 2-week period. There must be at

least four of the following symptoms during this same period: sleep disturbance, loss of interest or pleasure in usual activities, feelings of guilt or worthlessness, lack of energy, decreased concentration or ability to make decisions, appetite disturbance (usually diminished), psychomotor changes (agitated or slowed), and suicidal thinking. The mnemonic **SIG E CAPS** can be remembered by thinking of what you want to do for depressed patients (figuratively): "prescribe energy capsules."

Depressed mood, plus four of the following:

S	Sleep disturbance	**C**	Concentration
I	Interests	**A**	Appetite disturbance
G	Guilt	**P**	Psychomotor changes
		S	Suicidal thinking
E	Energy		

2. Why is depression considered a mood disorder?

Mood refers to the subjective, internal state of a person, as reported by that person. *Affect* is a person's objective, outward appearance, as judged by another. The term *mood disorder* has replaced *affective disorder* in the current psychiatric literature. The main mood disorders are major depression (or unipolar disorder), which is exclusively depression, and manic-depression (or bipolar disorder), which is depression with a history of at least one manic episode.

3. What is the difference between primary and secondary depression?

Major depression is classified as **primary** if the symptom complex appears before or is unrelated to any other significant medical or psychiatric illness. It is considered **secondary** when it follows and is related to other medical or psychiatric illness.

4. List medical conditions that might cause secondary depression.

Endocrine disorders
Hypothyroidism
Diabetes mellitus
Cushing's syndrome

Neurologic disorders
Cerebrovascular accidents
Subdural hematoma
Multiple sclerosis
Brain neoplasm
Parkinson's disease
Seizure disorder
Dementia

Connective tissue diseases
Systemic lupus erythematosus

Neoplasms
Pancreatic cancer

5. List medications that might cause secondary depression.

Antihypertensives (reserpine, β-blockers, methyldopa)
Hypnotics and sedatives (benzodiazepines and barbiturates)
Corticosteroids
Cimetidine
Ranitidine

6. Why should the clinician always inquire about alcohol use when evaluating depression?

Alcohol use and abuse is an extremely common comorbid condition with depression and should be asked about routinely for several reasons. First, alcohol use can be disinhibiting with regard to behavior, putting a depressed and suicidal person at increased risk of impulsively acting on suicidal impulses. Second, depression cannot be treated effectively if there is ongoing alcohol abuse. Third, alcohol is a depressant and is a common cause for depression, a problem known as **alcohol-induced mood disorder**. It may be that the patient's depression is secondary to alcohol use and is treated best by abstaining from alcohol, rather than by administering an antidepressant. This situation is suggested when the onset of the mood disturbance is during an extended period of regular (usually daily) alcohol use, rather than before it.

7. When should I suspect depression when a patient presents with what seems to be a medical complaint?

Screen for depression when patients present with nonspecific complaints, such as "sick all over," "weak and dizzy," or "just feeling bad." Using the SIG E CAPS mnemonic (see question 1) aids in diagnosis. Often the depression is expressed in physical rather than emotional terms. Nonspecific physical complaints, such as fatigue, exhaustion, headache, gastrointestinal complaints, muscle aches, and nonspecific pain, are common. Anxiety is seen commonly with depression and can manifest as shortness of breath, nervousness, irritability, and difficulty swallowing, among other symptoms. Panic attacks, a severe form of anxiety that often occurs in the context of depression, are a common cause of ED presentations of atypical chest pain.

8. Are psychotic features ever a manifestation of depression?

Depression may be accompanied by psychotic symptoms, signifying a more severe and dangerous form of depression. When this is the case, psychiatric consultation and often psychiatric hospitalization are indicated. Patients with **psychotic depression** are at higher risk for suicide, especially when they have hallucinations commanding them to harm themselves. Other common psychotic symptoms are hearing guilt-provoking or self-critical voices, called *auditory hallucinations*, and fixed, false beliefs that can be persecutory or paranoid in nature, referred to as *delusions*.

9. Name therapies available for treatment of depression.

Antidepressant medications, psychotherapy, and electroconvulsive therapy.

10. What antidepressant medications are used to treat depression?

Tricyclic antidepressants (TCAs) and **monoamine oxidase inhibitors (MAOIs)** are the two original classes of antidepressants, both of which have fallen into relative disuse because of their side effects and dietary restrictions (in the case of MAOIs). The newer agents, **serotonin reuptake inhibitors**, are the most commonly prescribed class of antidepressants mainly because of comparable efficacy and greater ease of use. These are fluoxetine (Prozac), paroxetine (Paxil), sertraline (Zoloft), citalopram (Celexa), and fluvoxamine (Luvox). Newer (and more expensive) medications are available for treatment, which act on multiple neurotransmitter systems but with better side-effect profiles than the older TCAs or MAOIs. These include venlafaxine (Effexor), bupropion (Wellbutrin), nefazodone (Serzone), and mirtazapine (Remeron). Lithium, psychostimulants, and thyroid hormone are common adjunctive treatments.

11. What are some psychotropic-related emergencies or precautions?

MAOIs in combination with sympathomimetic agents can cause hyperadrenergic crisis, and their combination with meperidine (Demerol) or dextromethorphan can cause cardiovascular instability and central nervous system excitability. Neuroleptics can cause dystonias, including laryngeal spasm and neuroleptic malignant syndrome (delirium, rigidity, fever, and autonomic abnormalities), both medical emergencies. Anticholinergic toxicity may occur because many psychotropics have anticholinergic properties and often are used in combination; these include benztropine mesylate (Cogentin), trihexyphenidyl (Artane), diphenhydramine (Benadryl), TCAs, and low-potency and midpotency neuroleptics. Many other commonly used agents have frequent toxic side effects, particularly the *mood stabilizers*, which include lithium and the anticonvulsants valproic acid and carbamazepine.

12. When should the emergency physician begin antidepressant therapy?
Because antidepressants generally take weeks to begin working and often require monitoring of side effects and dose titration, prescribing them in the ED should be avoided whenever possible. Exceptions include a patient who is already on treatment and needs a refill or a patient who is initiating new treatment after an emergent consultative evaluation by a psychiatrist. Ideally, in both of these cases, a 2- to 4-day supply of medication can be prescribed, and the patient can follow-up with outpatient psychiatric care.

13. What is the most serious complication of depression?
Suicide. Major depression accounts for an estimated 50% of all suicides.

14. Which patients should be hospitalized for depression?
In most instances, depressed patients who express suicidal intent or have a plan for suicide and psychotic depressed patients. Also, patients who have just made a violent suicide attempt, have tried to avoid rescue, or are refusing help probably are best admitted for further observation. Do not forget to institute suicidal precautions while these patients are in the ED.

SUICIDE

15. What is the proper approach to a patient who has attempted suicide?
Medical management of any life-threatening condition precedes psychiatric evaluation. It is important, however, that as the treatment proceeds, the ED team maintain a nonjudgmental approach. Punishment or ridicule is neither therapeutic nor proper conduct for medical professionals. Nearly all patients who attempt suicide are at least ambivalent about the wish to live or die. Demeaning or harsh treatment of such patients, especially by health professionals who are symbols of medical authority, worsens the already low self-esteem and may make subsequent psychiatric care more difficult.

16. Describe suicide precautions.
Because some patients have been able to repeat a suicide attempt while in the ED, suicide precautions are necessary. Such precautions include searching the patient and recovering weapons, pills, or other potential causes of self-injury; keeping the patient under close observation; recovering any potential dangerous items from the immediate care area (e.g., needles, scalpels, glass, razors); and not allowing the patient to go anywhere (e.g., bathroom) unaccompanied. When constant staff observation is not possible, physical restraints may be necessary to protect the severely suicidal patient from further self-harm.

17. Are "accidents" ever suicide attempts?
It is important to remember that victims of trauma may have attempted suicide. Single-victim accidents, such as a car driven at high speed into a concrete structure, a pedestrian hit by a high-speed vehicle, or a fall, are classic examples of suicide attempts presenting as trauma. Medical management should be followed by an assessment of suicide intent, including a discussion with family members and perhaps psychiatric consultation.

18. What psychiatric disorders are associated with attempted suicide?
Major depression, alcohol and drug dependence, schizophrenia and other thought disorders, personality disorders, panic disorder, adjustment disorders, and organic brain syndromes.

19. How do I evaluate the risk of a subsequent suicide in a suicide attempter?
The following elements are part of an emergency assessment of suicide risks: age, gender, marital status, social supports, physical illness, previous attempts, family history of suicide, risk of the attempts versus likelihood of rescue, secondary gain, nature of any psychiatric illness, alcohol or drug abuse, attitude, affect, and future plans of the suicide attempter. If, after reviewing

these factors, the emergency physician is still unsure of the patient's risk, psychiatric consultation is often helpful.

20. How does age relate to suicide risk?
Older patients (especially > 45 years old) are statistically more likely to complete suicide than younger patients. Such patients may experience loss of spouse, loneliness, physical illness, or economic hardship in addition to depression. A worrisome increase in suicide among younger persons has emerged, however. Suicide is now the third leading cause of death in children 5 to 14 years old and the second leading cause of death in teenagers and young adults aged 14 to 24.

21. What role does gender play?
The rates of completed suicide in men are higher than those for women, whereas the rates of attempted suicide are higher for women than for men. This difference has to do with the lethality of the means. Men attempt suicide more often by violent means, such as shooting, stabbing, hanging, or jumping from a height, whereas women typically use less violent and less definitive methods, such as drug overdose.

22. What is the relationship of marital status to risk of successful suicide?
Never having been married carries the highest risk, followed in decreasing magnitude of risk by being widowed, separated, divorced, and married.

23. What about other social support?
Unemployment, loneliness, loss of home, and relative isolation increase the risks of suicide. Church, family, or community support helps to mitigate suicide risk.

24. Is there a relationship between physical illness and suicide risk?
Yes. Patients with a medical illness, especially a painful, incurable one, may seek a "way out" through suicide. The most common nonpsychiatric diagnoses associated with suicide are chronic medical conditions, such as cancer, chronic obstructive pulmonary disease, and chronic pain. Renal dialysis patients have a suicide rate 400 times higher than the general population, and HIV patients may have a higher than average rate.

25. Does a history of prior suicide attempts signify increased risk?
Yes, unless the previous attempts all have been minor and considered to be manipulative acts, especially if each subsequent attempt escalates in severity.

26. What is the relationship of family history to suicide risk?
Patients with a family history of suicide, alcoholism, or depression have a higher suicide risk than patients without such a family history. A family history of suicide in first-order relatives (e.g., parent or sibling) should cause particular concern.

27. How does the risk of the suicide attempt and the likelihood of rescue affect a suicide evaluation?
In general, a more serious or risky attempt is considered a more likely predictor of subsequent attempts than a minor attempt. An attempt carried out in such a way that rescue is likely is associated with a lower risk of subsequent successful suicide. The patient's belief about the lethality of the attempt is at least as important as the physician's assessment.

28. What is secondary gain as it applies to suicide attempt?
Sometimes a suicide attempt seems to have a goal other than death. This goal, which is termed *secondary gain*, may be increased attention from parents, friends, or lovers. In attempts with no expected gain other than death, the potential for subsequent successful suicide is great. With the increase in successful suicides among the young, the physician must be careful in ascribing

suicide attempts to the desire for attention or secondary gain until a reasonably thorough evaluation can be completed.

29. What is the value of assessing the suicidal patient's attitude and affect?

The patient who appears exhausted, helpless, hopeless, or lonely represents high risk. The patient who attempts suicide because of anger or in an effort to gain revenge has a much better prognosis than one who appears quiet, sad, fatigued, or apathetic.

30. Why is it important to inquire about a specific plan?

Never hesitate to ask the patient about any plans regarding suicide. The patient who continues to express suicidal ideation after one attempt is at risk for a subsequent attempt. The risk is highest if the plan is detailed, violent, or feasible.

31. What is the SAD PERSONS scale?

In 1983, Patterson et al used known high-risk characteristics to develop the mnemonic **SAD PERSONS** Scale. The scale was designed to be used by nonpsychiatrists to assess the need for hospitalization in suicidal patients. Hockberger and Rothstein modified the scale to facilitate use in the ED (see Table). A score of 5 or less indicates that a patient probably can be discharged safely. Scores of 6 or more require psychiatric consultation, and a score of 9 or more indicates the probable need for psychiatric hospitalization.

Modified SAD PERSONS Scale

MNEMONIC		CHARACTERISTIC	SCORE
S	Sex	Male	1
A	Age	< 19 or > 45	1
D	Depression or hopelessness	Admits to depression or decreased concentration, appetite, sleep, libido	2
P	Previous attempts or psychiatric care	Previous inpatient or outpatient psychiatric care	1
E	Excessive alcohol or drug use	Stigmata of chronic addiction or recent frequent use	1
R	Rational thinking loss	Organic brain syndrome or psychosis	2
S	Separated, widowed, or divorced		1
O	Organized or serious attempt	Well-thought-out plan or life-threatening presentation	2
N	No social supports	No close family, friends, job, or active religious affiliation	1
S	Stated future intent	Determined to repeat attempt or ambivalent	2

Scoring: A positive answer to the presence of depression or hopelessness, lack of rational thought processes, an organized plan or serious suicide attempt, and affirmative or ambivalent statement regarding future intent to commit suicide are each scored 2 points. Each other positive answer is scored 1 point.
(From Hockberger RS, Rothstein RJ: Assessment of suicide potential by non-psychiatrists using the SAD PERSONS score. J Emerg Med 99:6, 1988, with permission.)

32. In general, which suicidal patients should be hospitalized?

Absolute indications for hospitalization after suicide attempts (involuntarily, if necessary) usually include the following: presence of psychosis; a violent, nearly lethal preplanned attempt; and continued suicidal ideation with definite plans for a repeated attempt. **Relative indications** include age older than 45; high risk-to-rescue ratio; serious mental illness; alcoholism; drug addiction; living alone with poor social support; and hopelessness, helplessness, or exhaustion.

BIBLIOGRAPHY

1. Colucciello SA, Hockberger RS: Suicide. In Marx JA, Hockberger RS, Walls RM (eds): Emergency Medicine: Concepts and Clinical Practice, 5th ed. St. Louis, Mosby, 2002.
2. Kishi Y, Robinson RG, Kosier JT: Suicidal ideation among patients with acute life threatening physical illness in patients with stroke, traumatic brain injury, myocardial infarction and spinal cord injury. Psychosomatics 42:382–390, 2001.
3. Olfson M, Marcus SC, et al: National trends in the outpatient treatment of depression. JAMA 287:203–209, 2002.
4. Placidi GP, et al: Anxiety in major depression, relationship to suicide attempts. Am J Psychiatry 157:1614–1618, 2000.
5. Zametkin AJ, Alter MR, Yemini T: Suicide in teenagers: Assessment, management and prevention. JAMA 286:3120–3125, 2001.

123. MANAGEMENT OF THE VIOLENT PATIENT

Paul-André C. Abboud, M.D.

1. Is violence a problem in the ED?

Yes. Acts of violence resulting in death have occurred in 7% of major teaching hospitals.

2. What can hospitals do to decrease the risk of violence?

1. All unnecessary doors should be locked and access into the hospital limited to a few patrolled entrances.

2. Metal detectors should be used to screen patients and visitors for weapons.

3. Continuous-surveillance, closed-circuit television monitors help to ensure safety in the parking areas and the immediate grounds of the hospital.

4. Multiple methods of summoning police or security must be available to the ED without having to go through the hospital operator.

5. Responding police or security officers should be trained and equipped appropriately.

3. What can be done to preempt a violent episode?

1. Be aware of early signs of impending violent behavior, such as agitation, abusive language, and challenges to authority.

2. Completely undress major trauma victims as soon as possible, removing any weapons on their person.

3. Do not leave any instruments that can be used as weapons near a potentially violent patient.

4. What is the initial approach a physician can take to control an agitated or violent patient?

The first approach to any agitated patient should be verbal deescalation. When approaching the patient, the physician must appear calm and in control, use a tranquil and compassionate tone of voice, and convey his or her concern for the patient's well-being. The physician should remind the patient he or she is in a safe environment and that the ED staff is there to help. Improving the patient's comfort (perhaps with something to drink or a warm blanket) may go a long way toward soothing the patient's agitation. The patient needs to be told emphatically that the staff will maintain control to prevent any harm to the patient or others. Stationing security officers in the patient's presence may dissuade further inappropriate behavior. Most importantly, care providers must check their own emotions when dealing with agitated or violent patients. Yelling back at or exchanging threats with the patient only further escalates the situation.

5. What if that doesn't work?

In cases in which agitation continues to escalate and a patient becomes an increasing risk for violence or elopement, multiple different restraint techniques may be used. For patients who are disoriented and pulling at catheters and tubes, soft restraints may be used to tie the hands at the patient's sides. Two-point restraints, in which a single upper and lower extremity are placed in locking leather cuffs, may be more appropriate for nonviolent but disoriented or intoxicated patients who pose a high risk of falling out of bed or injuring themselves. In the case of the physically violent patient, four-point locking leather restraints should be used. These restraints should be placed by a team of at least five staff members: one for each limb plus an additional staff member to oversee the action and provide an ongoing explanation to the patient for what is happening and why. It is preferable for the physician not to be involved in this action because his or her therapeutic relationship with the patient may be jeopardized further.

6. What do I need to remember when I physically restrain a patient?

Some principles apply to all restrained patients regardless of the type used. The restraints must be snug enough only to maintain their grip but not impede circulation. Side rails always must be placed up for patients in restraints to minimize the risk of falling out of bed. Restrained patients must never be placed prone on a bed, owing to increased risk of mortality. Patients at increased risk for aspiration should be positioned on their side. When restraints are in place, they must be monitored for their continued need. Subsequent reevaluations may reveal that restraining measures can be downgraded or discontinued. The patient's behaviors, attempts at less restrictive measures, and reevaluations of the patient's mental status and vital signs after restraints are placed all must be documented.

7. Do I have any alternatives to restraining a patient?

Ideally, an ED should have an isolation room in which agitated patients can be placed to minimize stimulation. These rooms should be monitored easily (e.g., through windows or video camera) and emptied of any objects that can be used as weapons. Patients who need immediate medical attention are not candidates for this intervention.

8. How do I know when it's time to use chemicals to restrain a patient?

If continued efforts at verbal deescalation are unsuccessful, and the patient remains agitated or violent despite mechanical restraints, chemical sedation is indicated. Physical restraints often may increase patients' agitation despite decreasing their risk to themselves and others. Increasingly, chemical restraint is viewed as more humane and effective than physical restraint. Sometimes both are necessary.

9. What medications are recommended for chemical restraint?

It depends on what is causing the agitation. Two classes of drugs generally are used for chemical restraint: (1) butyrophenones, such as haloperidol and droperidol, and (2) benzodiazepines, such as lorazepam and diazepam.

Butyrophenones: Droperidol has been used extensively but no longer is recommended because of Food and Drug Administration warnings regarding it use. Haloperidol, 5 to 10 mg intravenously, is the preferred agent for chemical restraint.

Benzodiazepines: In sympathomimetic-induced (e.g., amphetamine, PCP, and cocaine) agitation and suspected anticholinergic toxicity, benzodiazepines are preferred because they reduce central nervous system production of catecholamines. Initial doses of 1 to 4 mg intramuscularly or intravenously of lorazepam may be given. Except in cases of liver disease, diazepam generally is preferred over lorazepam because it is cheaper and not as long acting, which allows for more frequent reassessment of the patient. Diazepam may be given as follows: 5 to 10 mg intravenously for an initial dose and repeated doses of 2 to 10 mg every 20 to 30 minutes as needed.

10. What do I do if two doses of haloperidol have not sedated the violent patient?
Don't give a third dose. To avoid toxicity from escalating doses of this drug, switch to a benzodiazepine such as diazepam in doses lower than if this agent were used alone. The combination of these two classes of drugs achieves optimal sedation in most haloperidol-refractory cases.

11. Summarize the main side effects to watch for with these drugs.
All benzodiazepines can cause hypotension and respiratory depression. The butyrophenones may cause hypotension and extrapyramidal or other dystonic reactions. Hypotension is rare, but dystonic reactions from haloperidol are relatively common. For this reason, consider prophylaxis with diphenhydramine or benztropine mesylate (Cogentin) for 2 to 3 days after haloperidol administration.

12. Why did the patient become violent in the first place?
When the patient is controlled, determine the underlying problem. Emphasis is on determining if the patient has one or more of the following:

Acute intoxication	Acute withdrawal
Metabolic disorder	Trauma
Infectious disease	Environmental injury
Cardiovascular disorder	Psychiatric disorders
Intracranial disorder	Hypoxia

13. What paperwork is required after physical or chemical restraint?
Clear documentation in the medical record should include justification for the application of restraints, administration of medication, patient monitoring, and a plan for removal of restraints. Ongoing observation of patients in restraints must be documented. All restraint documentation should comply with Joint Commission on Accreditation of Healthcare Organizationss (JCAHO) standards.

14. Does the ED staff need any treatment?
The effect of major unpredictable violence and mayhem on ED employees can be devastating. Physical and psychological trauma is only part of the long-lasting effects. Such episodes may affect future job performance. A comprehensive program patterned after the critical incident stress debriefing model should be established to provide immediate and long-term psychological support.

BIBLIOGRAPHY

1. Chambers R, Druss B: Droperidol: Efficacy and side effects in the psychiatric emergencies. J Clin Psychiatry 60:664–667, 1999.
2. Clinton JE, Sterner S, Stelmacher Z, Ruiz E: Haloperidol for sedation of disruptive emergency patients. Ann Emerg Med 16:319–322, 1987.
3. Dubin W, Feld J: Rapid tranquilization of the violent patient. Am J Emerg Med 7:313–320, 1989.
4. Ellenhorn MJ, Schonwald S, Ordog G, Wasserberger J: Ellenhorn's Medical Toxicology, Diagnosis, and Treatment of Human Poisoning, 2nd ed. Baltimore, Williams & Wilkins, 1997.
5. Hill S, Petit J: The violent patient. Emerg Med Clin North Am 18:301–315, 2001.
6. Lavoie FW, Carter GL, Danzl DF, Berg RL: Emergency department violence in United States teaching hospitals. Ann Emerg Med 17:1221–1233, 1988.
7. Wasserberger J, Ordog GJ, Hardin E, et al: Violence in the emergency department. Top Emerg Med 14:71–78, 1992.
8. Wasserberger J, Ordog GJ, Kolodny M, Allen K: Violence in a community emergency room. Arch Emerg Med 6:266–269, 1989.
9. Weisberg MP, Dwyer BJ (eds): Safe strategies for recognizing and managing violent patients. Emerg Med Rep 8:169–176, 1987.

124. DOMESTIC VIOLENCE

Kim M. Feldhaus, M.D.

1. Isn't domestic violence more of a law enforcement issue than it is a health issue?
No. Research shows that 50% of all women presenting to EDs for care have experienced abuse from an intimate partner or ex-partner at some point in her life and that 30% of women have experienced domestic violence within the past year. Injuries and illnesses caused by abuse affect their lives more frequently than diseases such as hypertension, cancer, or diabetes. Interpersonal violence has tremendous health implications in the United States.

2. Define domestic violence.
Domestic violence, in a broad sense, refers to all violence occurring within a family unit. By this definition, partner abuse, child abuse, and elder abuse are subsets of domestic violence. *Domestic violence* is the term most commonly used to refer to the victimization of one partner by his or her intimate partner or partners. *Intimate partner violence* (IPV) is a more specific term, and it is used in this chapter. IPV includes physical acts, such as battering and sexual assault, and nonphysical acts, such as emotional abuse, economic abuse, threats to harm children and property, and prevention of access to health care or prenatal care. Most battered women state that the nonphysical abuse is more humiliating and distressing to them than physical beatings.

3. Why is IPV a problem affecting all of society and not just women?
IPV affects men, women, and children. Nearly 50% of homeless women and children are fleeing from battering situations. In the United States, police spend one third of their time responding to partner violence calls, which result in 40,000 reported physician visits per year (although total visits are much higher). IPV costs society $5 to $10 billion per year for health care costs, property damage, investigation, protective services, lost time from work, and criminal justice proceedings.

4. Who has more shelters available to them—animals or battered women?
Animals have three times as many shelters as battered women.

5. What are the risk factors for IPV?
IPV occurs in all socioeconomic classes and in all races. Women at greatest risk include those with male partners who abuse alcohol or use drugs; are unemployed; have less than a high school education; or are the former husband, estranged husband, or former boyfriend of the woman. Women who are younger than 30 years; who are single, divorced, separated, or pregnant; or who abuse drugs or alcohol classically have been viewed as at increased risk for IPV. It is unclear, however, if some of these risk factors lead to the partner abuse or are a result of living in an abusive situation.

6. Are men *ever* victims of partner abuse?
Men certainly may be injured as a result of IPV. In any conflict that has escalated to the point of violence, the persons involved become mutual combatants, and injury may be inflicted on a man by his female partner. The woman is 13 times more likely to be injured than the man, however, and 30% more likely to be killed. Statistically, 95% of IPV victims are women, and women almost exclusively endure the pattern of recurrent nonphysical and physical abuse (the **battering syndrome**).

7. If IPV is so common, why have none of my patients experienced it?
Many of your patients may be experiencing partner abuse. Often, physicians do not know because they do not ask about it.

8. What is the result of a missed diagnosis of IPV?

Failure to diagnose IPV may return the woman to a dangerous situation. It also furthers the victim's sense of entrapment and helplessness. Inappropriate medications may be prescribed (tranquilizers and antidepressants) without a search for the underlying causes of these symptoms. Patients may be labeled as being hysterical, paranoid, and irrational.

9. State some of the reasons why physicians choose not to inquire about IPV.

The most commonly cited reason is **lack of time**. Health care providers believe that this issue is too time-consuming to deal with, especially in a busy ED. Other reasons include the belief that it is none of the physician's business, the belief that women would "tell" if they wanted to, the belief that there is nothing that can be done, the belief that the woman deserved the abuse, and the belief that a woman could just leave the situation if she wanted to.

10. State some of the reasons why victims of partner abuse might not disclose the abuse to health care providers, even if asked.

Women may be embarrassed and humiliated that it is happening to them. There may be cultural or religious beliefs that lead her to believe that this is normal or to be expected. She may have been told that she deserved the abuse. Her abuser might have threatened to harm her, her children, or other loved ones if she discloses to others, or she may believe that no one can help her.

11. What are some of the structural and system barriers that might prevent a woman from disclosing abuse?

Lack of privacy is a real concern in the ED. Women should be interviewed alone, without children or partners present. If necessary, hospital security may be recruited to ensure her safety. Also, family members or children should not be used as translators when inquiring about abuse.

12. How many women who present to an ED for care are there because of injuries or illness caused by IPV?

Studies indicate that approximately 10% to 14% of women who present to an ED are there because of illness or injuries related to partner abuse. Approximately 2% to 3% of all women seen in an ED have an acute injury caused by domestic assault.

13. What clues to IPV might be evident in a patient's history?

Most importantly, a history that is inconsistent with the physical examination findings should raise physician suspicion for IPV. Consider partner abuse in patients with threatened miscarriages (because of abdominal trauma), patients with suicidal intentions or attempts (frequently occur after a "fight" with a partner), patients who are depressed, patients who have evidence of drug and alcohol abuse, patients with frequent visits for chronic pain complaints, and patients who report no prenatal care (their partners may prevent them from accessing care).

14. What clues may be present on physical examination in a victim of IPV?

Common injury patterns include injuries to the face, neck and throat (especially signs or symptoms of strangulation), chest, breasts, abdomen, and genitals. Any injury that does not "fit" with the history obtained should create suspicion of abuse. Other physical examination findings of concern include evidence of sexual assault or frequent, recurrent sexually transmitted diseases.

15. How can I increase my recognition of partner abuse?

First, ask about IPV. Any woman who presents with an injury should be specifically asked who injured her. Second, raise your level of suspicion in women without injuries. Remember the clues that might be present in the history or physical examination. If you are considering partner abuse, ask about it.

16. What questions about partner violence can I ask a woman without injuries?

1. Have you ever been hurt or injured by a partner or expartner?
2. Are there situations in your relationship where you have felt afraid?
3. Has your partner ever abused you or your children?
4. Do you feel safe in your current relationship?
5. Is there a partner from a past relationship who is making you feel unsafe now?

17. What about screening all women for IPV?

Good idea! Because of the prevalence of this problem, many organizations have advocated screening all women for the presence of IPV. One screening tool that has been tested clinically is the Partner Violence Screen. This consists of these three questions: (1) Have you been hurt or injured in the past year by anyone? If so, by whom? (2) Do you feel safe in your current relationship? (3) Is there a partner from a previous relationship who is making you feel unsafe now? This tool is 71% sensitive for detecting IPV. Women who screen positive for IPV are 47 times more likely to experience severe physical violence and 11 times more likely to experience physical injury in the next 4 months than women who screen negative for IPV.

18. What comments or questions would be inappropriate when discussing IPV with women?

"What did you do to him?"
"What did you do that made him so mad?"
"This has happened before, and you are still married to him?"
"Why didn't you tell anyone?"
"You let him do that to you?"
"I wouldn't let anyone do that to me."
"Why don't you just leave?"

19. What do I do if my patient has an injury caused by her partner?

1. Treat her injuries.
2. Document her history and her injuries carefully in the medical records.
3. Provide support and empathy; women should be informed that IPV is a common problem, that no one deserves this abuse, and that help is available. Helping victims access community resources should be a primary goal of ED treatment.
4. Inquire about the woman's safety and that of her children. Not all women want or require shelter placement. Women who are experiencing increasingly severe physical injuries or whose batterers have access to firearms are at risk for severe or lethal injuries. Some of these interventions may be by a social worker or by a domestic violence advocate, depending on the clinical setting.

20. Summarize some important points to remember when documenting IPV.

Document what happened in the patient's own words, and document the relationship to her batterer. Record all areas of bruising or tenderness; a body map may be helpful. Photographs may be used, but care should be taken to follow local legal guidelines for photographing injuries. Be *sure* to obtain the patient's permission. Any treatment and intervention should be documented. In cases in which abuse is highly suspected and the patient is denying abuse, document the reason that you suspect abuse (e.g., the history does not match the physical examination findings). A well-documented medical record can mean the difference between convicting an abuser and allowing him to go free.

21. Don't I have any legal responsibilities?

You might. Some states mandate that all assaults be reported to the police, including IPV. If you are practicing in a state with mandated reporting, the police must be notified if you are treating an injury that has been inflicted on a person by another person.

22. I am practicing in a state that has mandated reporting of IPV, and my patient is begging me not to report her to the police. She says he will kill her if she tells anyone about what happened. What do I do?

By law, you are required to call the police; however, forcing an intervention on a patient without her consent violates her autonomy and furthers her sense of entrapment. Women need to be informed that the law requires that this be done, and some women are relieved that this decision has been taken out of their hands. The patient is not required to talk to the police when they arrive. States with mandated reporting should have a law enforcement response that provides for patient safety (e.g., strict restraining order policies, mandated arrest of the perpetrator, fast tracks to process domestic violence cases quickly, and adequate shelters to provide safe homes for victims). Knowledge of the typical law enforcement response to partner abuse calls helps you to reassure the victim when she does not want the police involved. Explain to the patient why you are involving the police, remind her that this is a crime, involve your social services agencies if possible, and ensure that she is going to a safe place. Use your best judgment with the goal of preventing further battering. There is a difference between doing something to a patient ("I am going to report you to the police"), and doing something *with* a patient ("We are going to make a police report together about this crime").

23. My patient just told me about an episode of battering that occurred several months ago. What do I do now?

If there is no recent assault, a police report is not required. You should let the patient know that this is a common problem, that help is available, and that she does not deserve the abuse. An inquiry into her safety is warranted. Women who are experiencing increasingly severe physical injuries or whose batterers have access to guns are considered to be at extreme risk for significant injuries and death.

24. Why is she going home to her batterer? Why doesn't she just leave him?

Why a woman does not leave her batterer is the wrong question to ask. It implies that the woman is to blame and that if she would just leave everything would be okay. Battered women are most likely to be killed during the act of leaving or after they have left their abuser. There are many other valid reasons why women stay in an abusive situation. She may have no money or job skills, she may have nowhere else to go, or she may feel she must stay to protect her children.

25. What can we do about IPV?

A more appropriate response to IPV is to ask ourselves why society tolerates this behavior and how we, as health care providers, might change those attitudes.

BIBLIOGRAPHY

1. Abbott J, Johnson R, Koziol-McLain J, et al: Domestic violence against women: Incidence and prevalence in an emergency department population. JAMA 273:1763–1767, 1995.
2. Abbott J: Assault-related injuries: What do we know, and what should we do about it? Ann Emerg Med 32:363–366, 1998.
3. Feldhaus KM, Koziol-McLain J, Amsbury HL, et al: Accuracy of 3 brief screening questions for detecting partner violence in the emergency department. JAMA 277:1357–1361, 1997.
4. Haywood YC, Haile-Mariam T: Violence against women. Emerg Med Clin North Am 17:603–615, 1999.
5. Koziol-McLain J, Coates CJ, Lowenstein SR: Predictive validity of a screen for partner violence against women. Am J Prev Med 21:93–100, 2001.
6. Kyriacou DN, Anglin D, Taliaferro E, et al: Risk factors for injury to women from domestic violence against women. N Engl J Med 341:1892–1898, 1999
7. McGrath ME, Bettacchi A, Duffy SJ, et al: Violence against women: Provider barriers to interventions in emergency departments. Acad Emerg Med 4:297–300, 1997.
8. Muelleman RL, Lenaghan PA, Pakieser RA: Battered women: Injury locations and types. Ann Emerg Med 28:486–492, 1996.
9. Rodriquez MA, McLoughlin E, Nah G, et al: Mandatory reporting of domestic violence to the police: What do emergency department patients think? JAMA 286:580–583, 2001.
10. Wilt S, Olson S: Prevalence of domestic violence in the United States. J Am Med Wom Assoc 51:77–82, 1996.

XVIII. Emergency Medicine Administration and Risk Management

125. COST CONTAINMENT AND RISK MANAGEMENT IN EMERGENCY MEDICINE

Stephen V. Cantrill, M.D.

COST CONTAINMENT

1. What is cost containment in emergency medicine?

An approach to limit medical care expenses without compromising quality of care.

2. Why is cost containment so important?

Medical care currently consumes nearly 14% of the gross national product (GNP), and health care costs traditionally have increased at a rate far above inflation. Because the federal government directly or indirectly pays for 42% of health care, they are quite concerned about this ongoing increase. One study concluded that one third of medical care may be unnecessary. If medicine continues to fail to deal with these issues, the federal government may step in and "help" us deal with them. The proliferation of health maintenance organizations (HMOs) and capitated-care contracts has placed additional pressure on physicians to curtail unnecessary health care costs, often with the health care provider sharing in the financial risk of providing patient care. Also, many practice environments are developing physician practice profiling systems to identify practitioners who order excessive numbers of tests and procedures.

3. In what area do emergency physicians have the most control in terms of containing costs?

Ancillary tests (clinical laboratory and radiology) constitute 44% of patient ED charges—the largest component. These tests are done at the request of the emergency physician and represent an area directly under our control.

4. List some reasons for excessive test ordering in emergency medicine.

Peer pressure (e.g., wanting to please a consultant)	Out-of-date hospital policies
	Intellectual curiosity
Ignorance of the costs of tests	Patient expectations
Defensive medicine	Reflex ordering/old habits

None of these reasons is adequate justification for ordering tests that are not medically indicated based on the patient's presentation.

5. What is the golden question to ask before ordering any test?

How useful will this test be in establishing a diagnosis or assisting in treatment?

6. List some additional strategies to reduce inappropriate test ordering?

1. Avoid ordering reflexively. Carefully consider the benefits before ordering a test.
2. Do not order a test because "it would be nice to know," unless you are willing to pay for the test.

3. Learn how much routine laboratory tests and radiographs cost. (Prepare yourself for a shock.)

4. Establish guidelines for the use of new technologies. Medicine is notorious for developing and using new tests without discontinuing tests that are old or outdated.

5. Avoid ordering studies for medicolegal reasons. Good medicine is good law. Order only studies that are medically indicated.

6. Use patient education to reshape patient expectations when possible.

7. Cancel studies that were ordered but later found to be unnecessary.

7. Shouldn't we order tests to "cover" ourselves?

No. Again, good medicine is good law. The criteria for ordering studies should be strictly medical, not based on the physician's notion of what would be helpful to have in a court of law. Laboratory or radiographic studies should not be used as a substitute for a proper history and physical examination.

8. Name some commonly overordered tests.

Extremity radiographs	Urine culture and sensitivity
Chest radiographs	Throat culture (excluding streptococcus screen)
Abdominal radiographs	Blood type and crossmatch
Rib radiographs	Blood ethanol level
Electrolyte panel	Arterial blood gases
Complete blood count	

9. How much can be saved with no compromise in patient care?

In a multicenter study of 20 hospital EDs, both teaching and nonteaching, a cost-containment educational program was used. Seventeen tests or groups of tests or studies (including those listed earlier) were targeted. A 12.5% decrease in targeted test charges was shown. No decrease in the perceived quality of care could be shown. The costs of medical testing in the ED can be contained by careful, thoughtful ordering without sacrificing patient care.

RISK MANAGEMENT

10. What is risk management?

Efforts to identify (and, when possible, improve or rectify) situations that place a service provider in jeopardy. This section addresses emergency physicians and how they are placed at risk. Good risk management not only deals with situations as they arise (e.g., dealing appropriately with a patient's complaint about care), but also anticipates health-delivery problems before they occur (e.g., establishing in advance the procedures for dealing with a patient who wishes to leave against medical advice).

11. Why are emergency physicians at high risk for malpractice lawsuits?

The primary reason is the lack of an established physician-patient relationship. The patient often feels little rapport with a physician unknown to the patient before the visit to the ED. The visit is usually not at the patient's wish, occurring at an unscheduled time and in a situation in which the patient is under stress and sometimes pain. All of these factors may contribute to feelings of anger and hostility, laying the groundwork for feelings of dissatisfaction about the provided care. A second major reason is that in emergency medicine, the decisions are often irrevocable. If a mistake or misjudgment is made on a patient who is admitted to the hospital, a second chance to correct the error usually exists because the patient is still accessible. In patients wrongly discharged from the ED, sometimes no such second chance exists.

12. What must be proved in a malpractice case?

1. **Duty to treat**. Was there an obligation for the physician in question to treat the patient? In emergency medicine, this answer is almost always yes. By working in an ED, an emergency

physician automatically assumes the duty to treat any patient presenting to the ED and requesting care.

2. **Actual negligence**. Was the care provided actually negligent? This often involves showing (to the jury's satisfaction) that the care provided fell below what is to be considered the *standard of care*. This point is the one most often contested by the opposing sides in a malpractice suit. Negligence may result from acts of commission or omission.

3. **Damages**. Did the patient suffer actual damages? This can include the nebulous *pain and suffering*.

4. **Proximate cause**. Did the negligence cause the damages? It must be shown to the jury's satisfaction that the alleged damages were truly the result of the alleged negligent care.

13. Give some examples of high-risk patients.

- **The hostile or belligerent patient**. These patients are difficult to deal with and sometimes get less than complete, careful evaluation. Intoxicated patients represent a significant subgroup of this class of patients. Demanding patients also fall into this class. When confronted with patients in this category, remember that "you don't have to love them to give them proper care."

- **The patient with a problem that may be a potential life threat**. With these patients, the challenge is to discover and address the life threat (see Chapter 1, Decision Making in Emergency Medicine). Inappropriately discharging these patients often results in a risk-management problem.

- **The returning patient**. The patient who returns unscheduled to the ED should raise a red flag. What problem is being missed? These patients deserve extra care in reevaluation. The threshold for admitting an unscheduled returning patient should be low.

- **The "private" patient**. Patients may be sent to the ED by a private physician for diagnostic studies or treatment but not to be seen and evaluated by the emergency physician. Any patient in the ED becomes the responsibility of the emergency physician. If something goes wrong with the care of these patients, the emergency physician also may be held liable. It is advisable to have an established policy that **every** patient who enters the ED will be seen and evaluated by the emergency physician.

14. What clinical problems tend to get emergency physicians into malpractice difficulty?

There is regional variation in clinical problems that tend to cause malpractice problems for emergency physicians, but the following entities are generally major causes: (1) FTD/FTT (failure to diagnose/failure to treat) myocardial infarction, (2) FTD/FTT meningitis/sepsis (especially in young children), (3) FTD fracture (including spine and pelvis), (4) FTD appendicitis, (5) FTD ectopic pregnancy, (6) FTD foreign bodies, (7) FTD tendon/nerve injuries associated with wounds, (8) FTD intracranial hemorrhage (subdural/epidural/subarachnoid hemorrhages), and (9) FTD wound infections.

15. What is the most common error emergency physicians make with regard to their malpractice insurance policy?

Failure to read carefully and understand the conditions of the policy (i.e., what is covered, what is not covered, what is required for a malpractice occurrence to be covered, what are the settlement options, and what are the "tail" requirements to provide coverage for past patient encounters when the current policy is no longer in force).

16. What common deficiencies in the medical record exacerbate malpractice problems for emergency physicians?

In a malpractice case, your record of a patient's visit can be your greatest friend or your worst foe. The following problems will place the record on the side of the opposing team:

- **An illegible record**. Think about how the record will look when it is enlarged to 4 feet by 4 feet by the plaintiff's attorney to show to the jury. Dictated or typed records avoid this problem.

• **Not addressing the chief complaint or nurses' and paramedics' notes**. Make sure your evaluation addresses why the patient came to the ED and what others observed and documented about the patient.

• **Not addressing abnormal vital signs**. As a rule, patients must not be discharged from the ED with abnormal vital signs. Whenever this *is* done, the record must contain a discussion of why the physician is taking this action.

• **An incomplete recorded history**. As with all other parts of the medical record, an attempt will be made to convince the jury that "not recorded equals not done." The history must include information concerning all potential serious problems consistent with the patient's presentation. Significant negatives should be recorded as well.

• **Labeling the patient with a diagnosis that cannot be substantiated by the rest of the record**. This not only may cause difficulty if the physician's "guess" is wrong, but also it leads to premature closure on the part of the next physician to treat the patient, removing the slim chance of correcting the diagnostic error if the patient returns to the ED because of no improvement.

• **Inadequate documentation of the patient's course in the ED** with inadequate attention to the patient's condition at discharge. Often the patient's condition may improve dramatically while in the ED justifying discharge, but this fact is not reflected in the record. If this case becomes a malpractice problem, it appears that the patient was discharged in the original (unimproved) condition.

• **Inadequate discharge (follow-up, aftercare) instructions**. The greatest risk in dealing with patients is being wrong in our judgment. The best insurance is careful and complete patient discharge instructions that include when and where to follow-up and under what conditions to return to the ED. It is striking how little effort is put into this component of the record. After completing your evaluation and treatment of a patient, ask yourself, "what if I am wrong, and what is the worst possible complication that can occur?" Address these possibilities completely in your discharge instructions and document them carefully in the record.

17. What "systems problems" often lead to lawsuits?

Systems problems are not under the emergency physician's control, but still can cause difficulty. Such problems include inadequate follow-up on radiology rereads of radiographs, inadequate follow-up of cardiology rereads of ECGs, inadequate follow-up of delayed clinical laboratory results (e.g., cultures), poor availability of previous medical records, inadequate handling of patient complaints (your chance possibly to head off a malpractice suit), and inadequate physician and ED staffing patterns (leading to prolonged patient waits and subsequent patient hostility).

18. When a patient refuses care, what are the two criteria that must be present?

If a patient desires to leave the ED against medical advice, the patient must (1) be competent to refuse care and (2) understand the possible untoward sequelae that could result from refusal of care. All patients have the right to refuse care if these two criteria are met. Common sense (and most risk managers) would tell you to err on the side of treating the patient if there is any doubt as to competence.

19. What clinical problem-solving approach is most helpful in avoiding lawsuits?

When dealing with any patient, make sure you address the life threats: major problems that could exist, given this presentation for this patient. The safe approach is to assume the presence of these life threats, then set about to disprove them (see Chapter 1, Decision Making in Emergency Medicine).

20. What physician behaviors may help avoid lawsuits?

1. Be courteous and kind to the patient and to the patient's family.

2. Take time to communicate with the patient. It takes only seconds to tell the patient what is going on, what the results of diagnostic studies are, and what you are thinking concerning his or her case. Make sure all patient questions and concerns are addressed.

3. Dress neatly.
4. Explain and apologize for inordinate delays in patient care.
5. Make sure the medical record accurately reflects the care provided and the thought processes behind the care.

This approach can be summarized in a simple statement: "Treat every patient as you would want your mother treated." This assumes you love your mother.

21. How can writing admission orders for admitted patients cause problems for the emergency physician?

In many situations, writing admission orders for patients has made the emergency physician liable for untoward events occurring to the patient in the hospital before he or she is seen by the private physician. There is often significant peer pressure for the emergency physician to write such orders. This practice is potentially dangerous and must be discouraged.

22. What are the criteria for reporting a physician to the National Practitioner Data Bank?

The National Practitioner Data Bank (NPDB) was established by the federal government in 1989 to track potential problem physicians. The criteria for reporting a physician to the NPDB are: (1) any payment made for a claim or judgment against a physician, (2) any action taken by a state medical licensing board against a physician, and (3) any disciplinary action lasting more than 30 days taken against a physician by a group or institution. A hospital must query the NPDB about any physician applying for staff privileges and at the time of reappointment of a physician to the medical staff.

23. How can clinical policies (standards of care) decrease malpractice risk for the emergency physician?

Many groups and organizations are developing standards of care—clinical policies, clinical guidelines, protocols, or standards. If it can be shown that a physician's care was consistent with an accepted standard, it may help to show the appropriateness of the care and the lack of negligence.

24. How can clinical policies potentially increase malpractice risk for emergency physicians?

Malpractice risk can be increased by applicable clinical policies or other standards of care if the emergency physician is not aware of those standards that apply to his or her practice or if he or she chooses not to follow a standard without carefully documenting the reasons for not doing so.

25. Does emergency medicine residency training decrease my malpractice risk?

One study revealed emergency medicine residency-trained physicians had significantly less malpractice indemnity than non-emergency medicine residency-trained physicians. This difference was not due to differences in the average indemnity but was due to significantly fewer closed claims against emergency medicine residency-trained physicians with indemnity paid. This resulted in a cost per physician-year of malpractice coverage for non-emergency medicine residency-trained physicians that was more than twice that of emergency medicine residency-trained physicians ($4905 versus $2212).

BIBLIOGRAPHY

1. Branney SW, Pons PT, Markovchick VJ, et al: Malpractice occurrence in emergency medicine: Does residency training make a difference? J Emerg Med 19:99–105, 2000.
2. Cantrill SV, Karas S (eds): Cost-Effective Diagnostic Testing in Emergency Medicine: Guidelines for Appropriate Utilization of Clinical Laboratory and Radiology Studies, 2nd ed. Dallas, American College of Emergency Physicians, 2000.
3. Cost Containment Task Force: Guidelines for Cost Containment in Emergency Medicine. Dallas, American College of Emergency Physicians, 1983.

4. Detsky AS, Naglie G: A clinician's guide to cost-effectiveness analysis. Ann Intern Med 113:147–154, 1990.
5. Henry GL: Emergency Medicine Risk Management: A Comprehensive Review. Dallas, American College of Emergency Physicians, 1991.
6. Karas S: Cost containment in emergency medicine. JAMA 243:1356–1359, 1980.

126. MANAGED CARE

John C. Moorhead, M.D., M.S.

1. What is managed care?

A contractual arrangement in which there is a health care funding mechanism that transfers health care risk by contracting selectively with health care providers to whom patients will be preferentially referred, in return for which the provider agrees to participate in less costly, more efficient patterns of care. It is health care that is *managed* by a health plan or a physician group to meet a predetermined financial budget or clinical service goal. Reimbursement from managed care plans varies from a discounted fee schedule for physicians and hospitals (i.e., a **preferred provider organization [PPO]**) to a fully capitated prepaid group health care plan, or **health maintenance organization** (**HMO**). In a capitated system, a single premium must cover all services provided with the plan. Providers are at risk financially if services exceed expectations. There are many models for reimbursing physicians in capitated plans. Often, emergency physicians are paid directly from pools controlled by primary care physicians.

In traditional fee-for-service health care, the financial incentives were always to provide *more* care, sometimes without regard to cost or clinical effectiveness. Early managed care entities, such as Kaiser or Group Health HMOs, attempted to provide the total realm of clinical services for a predetermined premium. These not-for-profit entities used *excess* revenues to provide additional benefits for their members and bonuses for the providers. So, in theory, managed care uses systematic, coordinated, evidence-based management of the health and health care needs of patients, their families, and communities.

2. Why has managed care become the dominant form of health care delivery?

With total health care expenditures in the United States raised to $1 trillion per year and the percentage of the gross national product projected to exceed 15%, business and the federal government chose to use managed care to bring health care costs under control.

3. How does managed care control cost?

The most easily implemented element is to contract selectively with physician groups and hospitals that agree to provide care at a discount in exchange for directed referrals. Another model involves transferring risk to providers and hospitals by providing a lump sum payment for a specific service (e.g., coronary artery bypass graft surgery) often adjusted for acuity. Individual resources (physician visits, hospital days, or supplies) are not reimbursed seperately. Managed care entities often control access to services by requiring prior authorization from their plan before agreeing to pay for a specific service. Prior authorization has been used extensively by managed care in an attempt to limit use of the ED as a site for delivering care. Managed care often requires providers to adhere to specific treatment protocols, which reduces variation in the care delivered.

4. Has managed care worked to solve these cost issues?

Managed care was effective in the 1990s by introducing significant cost efficiencies into the delivery of health care. Total health expenditures remained stable at 13.6% of the gross national product, and health care inflation, which was rising to 15% annually, has been stable at a level of approximately 4%. Most of the reduction in health care expenditures has come from discounted reimbursement to physicians and hospitals. Some of the efficiency has come from changes in use of health care services. One of the targets for decreasing patient use of health care services has been the ED, where care was perceived to be costly with suboptimal communication to primary care physicians. A key to controlling costs is limiting choice of providers and hospitals within a given plan. Public opinion surveys and reenrollment studies about patient preferences show strong support for maintaining choice of physicians, however. This limits the ability of managed care plans to differentiate their panel of providers and use this as a marketing tool.

5. Discuss problems with managed care.

In evaluating the delivery of health care services, health policy experts examine three issues: **cost**, **quality**, and **access**. It is believed that in controlling costs, there must be an effect on the quality of care or access to services. The financial incentives within the delivery of health care under managed care are viewed by many as a method to withhold or reduce the delivery of health care services to meet budgetary goals. Early discharge from the hospital, the need for second opinions, and the demand for preauthorization for many clinical services sometimes associated with poor clinical outcomes have led the public to question the need for this form of health care to exist without regulation. Many patients who sought emergency services for what they believed was a real emergency have had their reimbursement completely denied by managed health plans. Some plans educate their members to phone their health plan for preauthorization if they perceive the need for emergency care. This often leads to delays in the timeliness of receiving necessary care, however. Some case reports show death and disability arising from these practices. Managed care plans have been shown to benefit financially by delaying payments to providers for services rendered in good faith.

6. Are there different kinds of HMOs?

HMOs can be divided into for-profit and not-for-profit companies. The **not-for-profit** companies often organize their physicians into a *staff model* group of physicians who are primarily paid a salary. **For-profit** HMOs tend to place the physician much more at risk financially for their medical decision making. Physicians in these plans are often loosely organized. In many HMOs, emergency physicians are paid directly out of the capitated payment made to a primary care physician to provide and coordinate all of that member's health care. The plan or the primary care providers negotiate which services will be covered and predetermine reimbursement rates for those services.

7. Summarize the major concerns about managed care for emergency medicine.

Managed care has the potential to restrict access to emergency services to the public. The federal **Emergency Medical Treatment and Active Labor Act (EMTALA)** (see Chapter 127) legislation protects patients' access to EDs by mandating an evaluation for anyone who presents to an ED and requests care. By making patients responsible for charges the plan refuses to cover, managed care plans cause patients to think about financial coverage at times when they should be accessing emergent care immediately. Delay or avoiding necessary care may have serious medical consequences. Managed care also can mandate changes in the working conditions of emergency medicine specialists and decrease financial reimbursement for services. Additional paperwork and calls made to managed care plans for authorization of care can delay necessary care. The additional unreimbursed care can lead to a reduction in support services and make the delivery of care less efficient.

8. How is the public threatened by a reduction in access to emergency services?

By retrospectively denying reimbursement for emergency services, health plans may educate the individual to call the health plan for approval before seeking emergency services. For conditions such as heart attack and stroke, in which therapy and outcome are time dependent, these calls can mean less timely and less successful treatment when the patient presents to the ED.

Denial of reimbursement for services provided by emergency physicians in good faith adds to the high level of unreimbursed care in the ED. The economic downturn beginning in 1999 resulted in an increase in the uninsured population who access the ED for services that might have been provided in alternate settings. The shorter lengths of stays in hospitals have resulted in patients who have moderately acute conditions being managed in an outpatient setting. This situation results in an increased demand for unscheduled care. Combined with the aging of the population (elderly patients access the ED three times more frequently than younger patients), this has resulted in a tremendous increase in the numbers of patients presenting to EDs for care. In many EDs, declining reimbursement threatens the viability and function of their emergency services to provide emergent care for all patients.

9. What effect do HMOs have on ED staffing?

Cost efficiencies resulting from the delivery of health care by managed care entities have brought into question the mix of providers necessary in EDs. Many HMOs have indicated that much of the care can be provided by physician extenders who are reimbursed at a lower rate, which enables the HMO to decrease its care provider budget. Other changes in the staffing mix can leave an ED inadequately staffed by the number and mix of appropriate individuals. In many EDs, multiple phone calls between the physicians and health plans have been deemed mandatory to provide additional stabilizing services. This requirement has led to a significant increase in nonproductive time spent by emergency physicians advocating for their patients. Much of the delivery of services in a managed care plan is by protocol that may be perceived as a threat to physician autonomy in clinical decisions.

10. How has the emergency medicine community responded?

A legislative or regulatory approach was believed to be important to preserving access to emergency services. Legislative bills have been introduced federally and passed in many states to mandate the concept of a **prudent layperson** definition of an emergency. According to these bills and acts, health care provided to a *prudent layperson* who seeks emergency care because he or she believed an emergency existed is deemed legislatively appropriate and compensable by the health plan.

The American College of Emergency Physicians (ACEP) has worked successfully at the national and state levels with other specialty societies and state medical societies to pass **prompt payment legislation**, which mandates that plans are responsible for payment for services in a reasonable time frame or face financial or legal penalties.

ACEP, the Society for Academic Emergency Medicine, the Council of Residency Directors, and the Emergency Medicine Residents Association have undertaken two national studies to define the emergency medicine workforce. These data will help health policy experts determine the future need for residency-trained, board-certified emergency physicians. The American Board of Emergency Medicine has an ongoing longitudinal study of emergency physicians, which, among other things, delineates the attrition rate for emergency physicians.

11. How have EDs changed to provide services in the face of managed health care?

Many EDs have diversified their services to provide "one-stop shopping" for all unscheduled care. Emergency physicians have changed their charging pattern to align charges more closely with the level of services being provided. New products and technologies are being introduced in the ED to promote greater efficiency. Many departments have added observation services that encompass prolonged care provided in the ED or in an adjacent specialty unit as an alternative to inpatient care. These models have promoted further the concept of efficiently providing unscheduled care by emergency physicians. These changes have been received positively by the medical and insurance community and the public. Most emergency medicine groups have undertaken quality improvement efforts to increase timely communication between emergency medicine and primary care providers, which has resulted in increased efficiency in the delivery of care in the ED.

12. What lies in the future for managed care?

The health care delivery environment has changed from one that is predominately focused on controlling the cost of care to one in which controlling the cost of care is balanced by the need to maintain high quality. New "report cards" are being developed to look at the overall quality of care provided by HMOs, and some specifically address care provided in EDs. Emergency physicians are being challenged to provide high-quality care at a lower cost, while appropriately documenting that care and showing its value to the health plan and individual member. The public is demanding choice of providers in the delivery of health care and direct access to specialty providers, including the ED, without prior approval from their primary care provider. Health care costs are escalating again because of new technology and new pharmaceutical drug development. Direct marketing of prescription drugs to the public has increased demand for these products. Managed care is responding by consolidating to increase negotiating power and passing on cost increases directly to patients in the form of higher copayments and deductibles.

Managed care will continue to be used, as economist Reinhardt refers to it, as a *recession tool*. Some are predicting a multitiered system of care in the future in which the poor are restricted to a publicly financed delivery system, the rich have access 24 hours a day to their own physicians, and the rest some form of commercially insured care. It is likely that managed care will play a role in several of these delivery systems and continue to use some form of the various tools that have been successful in maintaining cost efficiency in the past. Plans also are turning to disease management programs to manage the 20% of the population with chronic diseases who account for 80% of the cost of care.

Outcome-oriented clinical research is being designed to meet the need to develop and validate evidence-based protocols. Managed care will continue to be used to maintain cost efficiencies in a new era of an explosion of health care costs (current insurance premiums are increasing 12% to 25% per year), while competition among plans, direct measurement of quality of service provided, political regulation, medical professionalism, and ethics will counterbalance these forces in an effort to maintain a high standard of emergency care. Emergency physicians will need to continue to be well educated in the financial and management aspects of the delivery of health care to evaluate appropriately potential contracts with medical groups or hospitals. It also will be important for emergency physicians to continue to advocate for patients to preserve the *safety net* role provided by emergency medicine.

BIBLIOGRAPHY

1. Carlson RP: The next generation of managed care? Physician Exec May/June:15–22, 2001.
2. Kohn L, Corrigan J, Donaldson M (eds), Committee on Quality of Health Care in America: To Err Is Human: Building a Safer Health System. Washington, DC, Institute of Medicine, 2000.
3. Krohn RW: Achieving the best-avoiding the worst-of capitation contracting. Group Pract J 44:18–24, 1995.
4. Mayer TA: Contracting with managed care. In Sulluzzo RF (ed): Emergency Department Management Principles and Applications. St. Louis, Mosby, 1997, pp 341–359.
5. Moorhead JC, Gallery ME, Mannle T, et al: A study of the workforce in emergency medicine. Ann Emerg Med 31:595–607, 1998.
6. Richardson LD, Hwang U. Access to care: A review of the emergency medicine literature. Acad Emerg Med 8:1030–1036, 2001.
7. Young GP, Ellis J, Becher J, et al: Managed care gatekeeping, emergency medicine coding, and insurance reimbursement outcomes for 980 emergency department visits from four states nationwide. Ann Emerg Med 39:24–30, 2002.
8. Young GP, Sklar D: Health care reform and emergency medicine. Ann Emerg Med 25:666–674, 1995.

127. EMTALA

Andrew L. Knaut , M.D., Ph.D., and Carolyn Sprinthall Knaut, J.D.

1. What is EMTALA?

Emergency Medical Treatment and Labor Act; not, as some would assert, Easy Method to Attract unwanted Legal Action. In 1986, Congress enacted EMTALA as part of the **Consolidated Omnibus Reconciliation Act (COBRA)**. Its intended purpose is to prevent the *dumping* of patients—that is, the inappropriate transfer or discharge of uninsured patients in an unstable condition solely for the economic benefit of the treating hospital. Put simply, EMTALA requires any hospital that participates in Medicare to do a medical screening examination (MSE) on each patient requesting medical evaluation at their facility to determine if an emergency medical condition exists without regard to the patient's ability to pay for services rendered. If such a condition is found to exist, the hospital and the treating physician must use all of the resources normally available to them in stabilizing the emergency medical condition before that patient can be discharged or transferred to another facility. Because more than 98% of hospitals in the United States participate in Medicare, the influence of EMTALA on emergency medical care is far-reaching. Failure to comply with its provisions can mean criminal sanctions, stiff financial penalties, and exclusion from participating in governmental programs such as Medicare and Medicaid.

2. Define emergency medical condition.

Any condition that without immediate medical attention might result in the patient's loss of life; a serious impairment of bodily function; severe pain; or, in the case of a woman in active labor, the death or disability of the unborn child.

3. Why does a statute such as EMTALA even exist?

Access to medical care in the United States has never been defined as a fundamental right. For much of the 20th century, private hospitals were under no obligation to offer emergency care to the uninsured. Consequently, indigent or *undesirable* patients often were denied such care and forced either to seek care elsewhere or to go without any assistance whatsoever. By the mid-20th century, a two-tiered emergency health care system existed in which the properly insured received better care than the poor. To mitigate the situation, Congress enacted the Hill Burton Act in 1946 that required any hospital receiving federal funds for construction or other expenses to open its doors to all persons residing within its territorial area. The statute lacked any real means of enforcement, however, and compliance was poor. Over the course of the 1960s and 1970s, the number of civil legal actions taken against hospitals that denied emergent medical treatment to indigent patients increased dramatically. As a result, important legal theories emerged as to how and why hospitals could be held liable for withholding medical care. Essentially, these theories held that any hospital holding itself out as a place that provides emergency care must provide that service competently and in a timely fashion to anyone in the public who relied on such advertisement in seeking emergent treatment during a time of need. Paralleling this development was the evolving concept that any hospital receiving public monies through such programs as Medicare and Medicaid reimbursement in turn held a duty to serve all sectors of the public equally. Ultimately, these concepts culminated in the 1986 enactment of EMTALA. Many amendments over the years have increased greatly the scope and the enforcement powers of the statute.

4. As a physician, can I personally be penalized for an EMTALA violation?

Yes. The hospital, the individual physician who provided care, or both can be penalized for an infraction of EMTALA. Formal sanctions include a $50,000 fine for each violation and termination of the Medicare provider agreement, which is in essence key to allowing hospitals and individual physicians to deliver medical care in the United States. The statute allows patients involved in an EMTALA violation to take private cause of action against the offending institution.

5. How is this any different from being sued for malpractice?

The most immediate difference to any physician implicated in an EMTALA violation is the fact that malpractice insurers generally do not cover monetary sanctions imposed for an infraction of the statute. As a result, the penalties amount to a major out-of-pocket expense for the practitioner. Another important difference is that EMTALA is not intended to police standards of medical care *per se* but rather to ensure that every patient is treated equally without regard to ability to pay. The patient does not have to suffer a poor outcome for a physician or a hospital to be cited for an EMTALA violation. If a patient suffers a poor outcome from treatment and alleges malpractice in the state courts, EMTALA is invoked only if it can be proved that the care was substantially different from what the hospital would provide uniformly to any other patient presenting with similar complaints and circumstances.

6. Does EMTALA apply only to patients presenting to the ED?

No. EMTALA's requirement of adequate medical screening for an emergency medical condition begins the moment a patient enters hospital property seeking care. An obstetric patient presenting to the obstetrics department or a psychiatric patient presenting to a psychiatric unit instead of the ED also is covered under the statute. *Hospital property* is defined broadly and has been found by the courts to include parking lots, sidewalks, and driveways that are part of a hospital's campus. It also includes any ambulance owned and operated by the hospital and any satellite clinic that operates under the same Medicare provider number as the hospital.

7. How does EMTALA define a proper MSE?

The simple answer: the adequate screening of a patient for an emergency medical condition using the resources normally available to the hospital's ED. The complex reality is that those resources are stated to include any laboratory studies; radiologic examinations such as CT, MRI, or angiography; and the services of any on-call consultant. Consequently an adequate MSE can range from a quick history and physical examination to confirm the presence of an upper respiratory tract infection to a complex workup involving multiple tests, diagnostic procedures, and hospital admission for further evaluation and treatment. When a physician or medical care provider designated by the hospital to provide an MSE can document in good faith that no emergency medical condition exists, EMTALA no longer applies.

8. Who can perform the MSE?

EMTALA states simply that "qualified medical personnel" must perform the MSE. The statute does not specify whether that means a physician, a nurse, or some other provider such as a physician's assistant or nurse-practitioner. Instead, EMTALA allows each hospital's governing body or the director of its ED to determine who is qualified to do screenings for the hospital. One person who clearly *cannot* perform an MSE is a triage nurse. The courts have held consistently that triage by a nurse is not adequate medical screening. Many hospitals have been cited for EMTALA violations because their triage nurses evaluated patients then referred them to an outside clinic or a private physician's office without a formal evaluation in the ED.

9. Is it an EMTALA violation if the patient decides to leave against medical advice before the MSE is complete?

That depends on when during the triage and evaluation process the patient decides to refuse care and on his or her competency to do so. If, during the course of the MSE, a patient refuses further evaluation and treatment after discussion of the potential risks of such a decision, the patient is considered to have withdrawn the initial request for evaluation, and EMTALA no longer applies. The burden of proof falls on the hospital and the treating physician, however, to show that no coercion was used to dissuade the patient from consenting to further treatment with suggestions or statements that the continued care could be prohibitively expensive. Proper chart-ing and documentation in such situations is essential. A more difficult situation arises when a pa-tient is triaged to the waiting room then decides to leave before being formally evaluated in the ED. On the surface, this situation can be interpreted as the patient withdrawing the initial request for medical evaluation. EMTALA and the courts have focused considerable attention on the po-tential for inequity in triage practices, with the uninsured or undesirable patient being subjected to long waiting times in the hopes that they simply will leave. In such situations, the hospital must be able to prove that no different standard of triage was used and that a reasonable effort was made to call the patient back to the ED to address the initial complaint.

10. What is meant by transfer under EMTALA?

EMTALA does not simply deal with patient transfers and the transferring facilities. EMTALA defines *transfer* as the movement of a patient away from the hospital, not simply as the act of transporting a patient to another hospital. By this definition, even a patient sent home from the ED is considered to have been transferred under the statute. If such a patient subsequently is found to have been discharged in unstable condition, claim of an EMTALA violation could be made.

11. When does EMTALA say it is okay to transfer a patient?

EMTALA applies only to the transfer of unstable patients. If a patient is deemed **stable** (i.e., an emergency medical condition is no longer present and no significant medical deterioration is likely during or after the transfer), a transfer can proceed without the statute being applicable. Unstable patients can be transferred under one of two conditions:

1. The patient requests the transfer. In that case, an informed request for the transfer must be signed by the patient, and it is important for the hospital and the treating physician to document that a discussion of cost did not enter into the patient's decision to ask for a transfer.

2. An unstable patient needs to be moved because the initial facility lacks the capability or the resources to treat the emergent condition adequately. This might occur when a multitrauma patient presents to a small rural ED and requires transfer to a level I trauma center for to receive proper care.

12. List the requirements for transferring an unstable patient.

1. A physician must certify that the benefits of the transfer outweigh the risks, and that when possible this has been discussed with the patient or responsible party.

2. Every effort shall be made to minimize the risk involved in the transfer in terms of proper treatment before the patient's departure.

3. The receiving facility has accepted the patient and has the capability to treat the emer-gency medical condition.

4. The receiving facility has been provided with all pertinent records of the patient's care to the point of transfer.

5. The transfer is conducted with proper equipment and personnel.

13. Can a hospital refuse to accept a transfer under EMTALA?

A receiving hospital cannot refuse an appropriate transfer as long as they have the capability to treat the patient.

14. If I receive an inappropriate transfer at my hospital, do I have an obligation to report an EMTALA violation?

EMTALA states that any hospital that receives an inappropriate transfer must report the sus-pected EMTALA violation within 72 hours or face penalties. This is an obligation of the hospital, however, not of an individual physician.

BIBLIOGRAPHY

1. Bitterman RA: Medicolegal and risk management. In Marx JA, et al (eds): Rosen's Emergency Medicine: Concepts and Clinical Practice, 5th ed. St. Louis, Mosby, 2002, pp 2747–2761.

2. *Bryan v. Rectors and Visitors of University of Virginia.* 95 F.3d 349 (4th Cir. 1996).
3. *Correa v. Hospital San Francisco.* 69 F.3d 1184 (1st Cir. 1995), *cert. denied*, 116 S. Ct. 1423, 517 U.S. 1136, 134 L.Ed. 2d 547.
4. Examination and treatment for emergency medical conditions and women in labor. 42 USC § 1395dd.
5. *Gerber v. Northwest Hosp. Center Inc.* 943 F. Supp. 571 (D. Md. 1996).
6. Guertler AT: The clinical practice of emergency medicine. Emerg Med Clin North Am 15:303–313, 1997.
7. Hubler JR: EMTALA update 2001: Guidelines, developments, and recent court opinions. ED Legal Letter 12:125–136, 2001.
8. *Summers v. Baptist Medical Center Arkadelphia.* 91 F.3d 1132 (8th Cir. 1996).
9. *Torres Nieves v. Hospital Metropolitano.* 998 F. Supp. 127 (D. Puerto Rico 1998).
10. Williams AR: Patient transfers: Legal issues. In Harwood-Nuss A (ed): The Clinical Practice of Emergency Medicine, 3rd ed. Philadelphia, Lippincott Williams & Wilkins, 2001, pp 1733–1740.

XIX. Medical Oversight and Disaster Management

128. MEDICAL OVERSIGHT AND DISASTER MANAGEMENT

Daniel W. Spaite, M.D., and Elizabeth A. Criss, R.N., C.E.N., M.A.Ed.

1. What is medical oversight?

The means by which physicians give direction and authority to nonphysicians to provide emergency medical care outside of the hospital and in the absence of a physician. The concept of medical oversight began with the development of organized EMS. Before 1970, ill and injured patients were transported by personnel who had little more than basic first aid training. There was essentially no physician input regarding the scope of practice or quality of care provided by prehospital personnel. Adoption of the first standardized EMS curriculum mandated more physician involvement. Medical oversight may be characterized as either on-line (direct) or off-line (indirect) medical direction.

2. Why is the medical oversight of prehospital care important?

The importance of medical oversight lies in the concept that nonphysicians can provide physician-level medical care safely and effectively when under the authority and in consultation with a physician.

3. Describe indirect medical direction.

Indirect, or off-line, medical direction is the process by which a physician develops and maintains the structure that ensures proper patient care, within an EMS system. This entails numerous responsibilities, such as training personnel; system design and evaluation; developing medical standards, protocols, and standing orders; reviewing prehospital care; and initiating a program of quality management. Maintaining high-quality patient care requires that the physician not only has the responsibility for indirect medical direction, but also the authority and organizational support to develop, alter, and maintain the medical care system.

4. What is direct medical direction?

Direct, or on-line, medical direction entails the direction, observation, and evaluation of prehospital medical care when care is being rendered. In many systems, direct medical oversight is carried out primarily by radio or cell phone communication between the prehospital personnel and a medical direction physician (or designee). The concept also includes the direct observation of prehospital personnel during physician "ride along" encounters. The percentage of EMS calls that have on-line medical direction varies widely among different systems. Some systems rely heavily on standing orders and little on direct communication during a patient encounter, whereas others require direct communication during all patient encounters.

5. Have there been any practical problems with the development of proper medical oversight?

Although the profound sense of need for medical direction is essentially universal among physicians, there has not always been unanimous interest in close physician supervision by system administrators. Much of the hesitation has been based on the fact that many physicians have little administrative, budgetary, public safety, or legislative expertise. A fire chief might be concerned that a medical director would mandate improvements in a system that require financial commitments beyond the agency's resources. This issue has led to the development, on a national scale, of specialized physician education and has spawned the development of postgraduate fellowships that provide subspecialization in prehospital care as an identifiable medical discipline.

6. Define the term *disaster*.

A disaster is best described as an imbalance between needs and resources. A disaster does not require a large-scale or globally catastrophic event (e.g., a train crash or hurricane). A disaster exists any time the available community resources are inadequate for either the number or the severity of casualties produced. The collapse of a section of bleachers at a public event that seriously injures 200 persons is a disaster. A one-vehicle rollover involving five seriously injured people in a rural or wilderness area that outstrips the local resources, although perhaps less apparent, may also constitute a disaster.

7. Why is there a need for disaster planning?

The quality of medical care in general is tied directly to the experience of the practitioner. Proficiency of a given medical intervention depends on the frequent performance of that intervention. Because in a disaster people are trying to do quickly what they do not ordinarily do, often in an unfamiliar environment, it makes sense to plan and exercise the plan regularly. No matter how experienced someone is, the level of care, resources, and framework for resource management undergo major alterations during a disaster. The development of a clear plan for the management of multiple casualties is imperative to ensure optimal outcome for the victims, given the available resources. Disaster planning must not be conducted in a vacuum, but rather must include the various pertinent agencies within a community, such as police and fire departments, EMS agencies, Red Cross, Salvation Army, hospitals, public works departments, utilities, and volunteers such as ham radio operators. Disaster plans and associated training must reflect the potential threats to a community.

8. How can prehospital care of disaster victims be optimized?

A concept that is believed to improve overall outcome during disasters is the **incident command system** (ICS). The principle behind an ICS is to direct, control, and coordinate emergency personnel and resources at a scene. The overarching role of the ICS is to oversee the situation and determine priorities. Through ICS, there are clear lines of authority and responsibility for such things as triage, communication, and transportation. ICS is especially helpful in disasters involving multiple agencies or multiple jurisdictions because prior agreements and planning have instituted command and control procedures.

9. Define *triage*.

Triage means "to sort." Although numerous systems exist for triaging victims of multicasualty incidents, the basic concept generally identifies four groups of patients: (1) minor illness or injury (walking wounded); (2) serious but not immediately life-threatening illness or injury (e.g., a patient with an intraabdominal injury who is currently not in shock); (3) critical or immediately life-threatening illness or injury (tension pneumothorax, hypovolemic shock); and (4) dead or resource-intensive victims. The actual categorization of specific patients is different in various types and magnitudes of disaster. A critically injured patient who might receive the benefit of a comprehensive life-saving effort in a three-patient incident might be deemed resource intensive in a disaster with several hundred victims.

10. When is it appropriate for a physician to respond to the scene of a multiple-casualty incident?

Although the answer to this question is unknown from a scientific perspective, most prehospital disaster plans include the potential request for a physician to respond to the scene. This is based on the concept that a well-trained and experienced physician can provide a higher level of patient assessment and care. This concept has several caveats. First, few physicians have substantial training and experience in prehospital patient management. A physician who is highly proficient in the care of critically ill and injured patients in the hospital may be a "duck out of water" in the field. A physician who does not have significant prehospital experience may make a scene less efficient. In general, personnel who deal with uncontrolled environments daily are best prepared to manage such situations efficiently. Second, a physician who is well known to prehospital personnel is likely to command significantly greater authority during a multicasualty incident than one who is unknown. In systems that do have a plan for physician response, it is appropriate to designate the system medical director or a small number of identified physicians who have participated in disaster drills to function as the on-scene medical authority.

BIBLIOGRAPHY

1. Augustine JJ: Medical direction and EMS. Emerg Med Serv 30:65–69, 2001.
2. Ayres Jr RJ: Legal considerations in prehospital care. Emerg Med Clin North Am 11:853–867, 1993.
3. Cuny FC: Principles of disaster management: Lesson 1: Introduction. Prehosp Disaster Med 13:88–92, 1998.
4. Cuny FC: Introduction to disaster management: Lesson 2: Program planning. Prehosp Disaster Med 13:63–79, 1998.
5. Davis EA, Billitier AJ: The utilization of quality assurance methods in emergency medical services. Prehosp Disaster Med 8:127–132, 1993.
6. Johnson GA, Calkins A: Prehospital triage and communication performance in small mass causality incidents: A gauge for disaster preparedness. Ann Emerg Med 17:148–150, 1999.
7. Kuehl AK (ed): National Association of EMS Physicians Prehospital Systems and Medical Oversight. St. Louis, Mosby, 1994.
8. Roush WR (ed): Principles of EMS Systems: A Comprehensive Text for Physicians. Dallas, American College of Emergency Physicians, 1989.
9. Stewart RD: Prehospital care: Education, evaluation, and medical control. Top Emerg Med 2:67–82, 1980.
10. Swor RA (ed): Quality Management in Prehospital Care. St. Louis, Mosby, 1993.

129. MEDICAL CARE AT MASS GATHERINGS

Peter T. Pons, M.D.

1. What constitutes a mass gathering?

Any event or occurrence that draws large numbers of spectators or participants.

2. Why is on-site medical care needed at mass gatherings?

Anytime a large number of people is gathered together in one place, it is likely that there will be some medical emergencies. One can expect the full gamut of potential problems from minor injuries to life-threatening emergencies such as cardiac arrest. A mass gathering is similar to a small community or city, all in one location for a short period of time, needing its own EMS system to handle medical emergencies while the event is occurring and everyone is gathered together. If no on-site medical care is provided, any medical emergency has to be handled by the local EMS system. Responding to calls for medical assistance at a special event or mass gathering can overburden the local EMS system and interfere with its handling of the normal daily EMS response.

3. What factors affect how much medical care needs to be provided at a mass gathering?

Many factors must be analyzed to determine the level of care to be provided, the type and number of medical personnel, and the amount of equipment and supplies: the type of event, the nature of the event venue, the location of the venue, and the number and characteristics of the attendees. Each of these factors influences the likelihood of and the potential for medical emergencies, affecting decisions about the level of medical staffing and services.

4. How does the type of event affect medical staffing?

Let's start by using a concert as an example. A classical music concert would attract a different audience than an event featuring a heavy metal hard rock group. There is a much greater potential for one or more medical emergencies to occur at the latter compared with the former. This is true for many types of events. At sporting events, a fan might be struck by a ball at a baseball game, possibly injured by an out-of-control vehicle at an automobile race, or potentially involved in a major riot at a soccer game.

5. Does the event venue have any impact on planning for medical staffing?

Indoor events usually are seated events occurring in a climate-controlled environment. **Outdoor events** often expose participants to temperature extremes, and some events such as fairs involve walking about over various types of terrain. There are usually more medical problems at an outdoor event than at an indoor event. Heat exposure is a particularly significant risk factor to bear in mind when planning medical coverage at an outdoor event. More persons require medical attention if the ambient temperature is increased.

Location is an important consideration. If the event is located at a site that is far from hospital facilities, planners might choose to provide for a more definitive and higher level of care, such as suturing and advanced life support, because prolonged transport and delayed care are likely. The event planner might add physicians and appropriate supplies and equipment to meet anticipated needs. Conversely, if the event is located in close proximity to a hospital, event planners may choose not to offer physician-level services but instead may rely on transport to a nearby medical facility.

6. Are there any other factors that affect the planned medical staffing?

It is important to ascertain whether alcoholic beverages will be served at the event or if there is a strong likelihood of drug or alcohol use by the event participants. Alcohol and drug use significantly increases the medical contact rate at an event.

7. After analyzing these factors, are there any guidelines or suggested staffing levels?

A good place to start is anticipated attendance. For every 25,000 attendees, 2 paramedics should be assigned. If physician staffing is included, 1 physician per 25,000 attendees should suffice. If the event is something like an outdoor, all-day rock music festival in August and drug or alcohol use is anticipated, the number of medical personnel is increased from this starting point. If the event is a classical music performance in a concert hall, the number of medical staffers may be decreased. Other issues that affect medical staffing include the number and location of medical aid stations and the need for on-site medical response capability. Medical aid stations should be centrally located and always should be staffed by medical providers during event hours. Provision of on-site EMS response personnel also has an impact on staffing and equipment requirements. Bicycles or stretcher-equipped golf carts can be used in many venues and for many events. Ambulance vehicles may be needed for events involving large geographic areas, such as marathons. The mix of personnel needed to staff a mass gathering can often reflect routine EMS—EMTs and paramedics for on-site EMS, nurses to staff aid stations, and physicians to provide on-site definitive care and medical control.

8. What should be done about on-site communications and medical system activation?

Because the planning effort should be creating a mini EMS system, communication is an integral component. A command post or communications center should be created with a representative from all appropriate venue services, such as police or security, fire control, and EMS. All on-site employees or ushers should be educated in how to access or request medical assistance.

Each on-site service should have a communications or radio system that is dedicated for that purpose and does not accommodate multiple purposes on the same frequency. The medical service should ensure a mechanism to obtain medical control and direction as warranted.

9. How is patient transport, when necessary, accomplished?

Ideally, there would be an ambulance and crew stationed at the venue with the primary purpose being patient transport. This increases the cost of providing on-site medical care. In some cases, the local EMS system is used to perform the transport after the on-site medical personnel have evaluated the patient and determined the need for transport to a hospital. If long distance transport is involved because the event venue is located some distance from a hospital, consideration for helicopter use is appropriate.

10. Okay, so who pays for all the medical services?

There is no one answer. In some cases, the cost of on-site medical care is built into a venue contract and is considered an event expense by the promoter. In some cases, medical care is part of the annual venue budget. Sometimes the cost is borne by the medical personnel provider, who then bills patients for medical services, and in some situations, the cost is covered entirely by the provider.

11. Are there any other important considerations?

One must also take into account security arrangements and the potential for a terrorist attack. Part of the overall analysis of an event is to determine the risk of the event being a terrorist target. A junior high school football game is likely not a target; however, a high-profile event with television coverage and participants from around the world might be an inviting target. In this case, additional contingency plans should be in place to ensure an appropriate medical response if something should occur.

BIBLIOGRAPHY

1. Bowdish GE, Cordell WH, Bock HC, et al: Using regression analysis to predict emergency patient volume at the Indianapolis 500 mile race. Ann Emerg Med 21:1200–1203, 1992.
2. Cohen DL, Montalvo MA, Turnbull GP: Medical support for a major military air show: The RAF Mildenhall Medical Emergency Support Plan. J Trauma 36:237–244, 1994.
3. DeLorenzo RA, Boyle MF, Garrison R: A proposed model for a residency experience in mass gathering medicine: The United States Air Show. Ann Emerg Med 22:1711–1714, 1993.
4. DeLorenzo RA, Gray BC, Bennett PC, et al: Effect of crowd size on patient volume at a large, multipurpose, indoor stadium. J Emerg Med 7:379–384, 1989.
5. Jasolow D, Drake M, Lewis J: Characteristics of state legislation governing medical care at mass gatherings. Prehosp Emerg Care 3:316–320, 1999.
6. Leonard RB, Petrilli R, Noji EK, et al: Provision of Emergency Medical Care for Crowds. Dallas, American College of Emergency Physicians, 1990.
7. Leonard RB: Medical support for mass gatherings. Emerg Med Clin North Am 14:383–397, 1996.
8. Parrillo SJ: Medical care at mass gatherings: Considerations for physician involvement. Prehosp Disaster Med 10:273–275, 1995.
9. Sanders AB, Criss E, Steckl P, et al: An analysis of medical care at mass gatherings. Ann Emerg Med 15:515–519, 1986.

XX. *Alternative Therapies and Tricks of the Trade*

130. COMPLEMENTARY AND ALTERNATIVE MEDICINE

Tracy R. McCubbin, M.D.

1. Does this chapter really belong in an emergency medicine text?

Well, that remains to be seen. Studies suggest that 50% of ED patients have used some form of **complementary and alternative medicine (CAM)**. Spontaneous disclosure rates are low—next to zero if health care providers do not inquire.

2. What is CAM?

According to the National Center for Complementary and Alternative Medicine (NCCAM) at the National Institutes of Health (NIH), CAM covers a broad range of healing philosophies, approaches, and therapies (e.g., acupuncture, herbal therapy, homeopathy) that mainstream allopathic medicine does not commonly use, accept, study, or understand.

3. List common CAM therapies.

Acupuncture	Homeopathy
Aromatherapy	Hypnotherapy
Ayurveda	Massage
Biofeedback	Naturopathy
Chiropractic	Reflexology
Craniosacral therapy	Relaxation therapy
Herbalism	Yoga

4. Aren't CAM therapies too expensive for the average person?

Some aspects of CAM are a bit costly. Many insurance companies (including some managed care organizations) provide discounts, however, on certain CAM therapies. Many patients do not seem to mind the cost. In 1997, consumers/patients spent an estimated $27 billion out-of-pocket for CAM.

5. Should I consider CAM use in pediatric patients?

Yes. It is estimated that 11% to 30% of parents explore CAM for their children. Although herbal medicine generally is considered safe in adults, little information is available regarding its use in children. There are numerous reports in the literature on the toxic effects of herbal medicines in children.

6. Name the most popular CAM therapy.

Herbal medicine. Consumers spend more than $5 billion annually on herbal therapies.

7. How safe is the use of medicinal herbs?

The primary problem with medicinal herbal products is the lack of regulation. These products do not fall under the purview of the Food and Drug Administration (FDA). Manufacturers of herbal preparations are not required to show safety or efficacy before marketing. The products are not regulated for quality, with respect to dosage, potency, or purity. Despite this, the FDA categorizes about 250 herbs as "generally recognized as safe" for consumption based on long-term or widespread use without significant side effects.

8. Which herbs are unsafe?

Borage, calamus, chaparral, comfrey, germander, licorice, life root, and sassafras. Kava (*Piper methysticum*) is currently under investigation by the FDA. There are approximately 25 case reports of hepatic toxicity associated with the use of products containing kava extract in Germany and Switzerland. These products have widespread use in the United States.

9. What about interactions with prescription medication?

We have relatively little information about interactions of traditional herbal medicine with prescription drugs. It is estimated that 15 million adults in the United States are at risk for such interactions, including altered bioavailability and efficacy of the prescribed medication. Documented herb-drug interactions, which might be useful to the emergency physician, are listed in the Table.

Common Herbal-Drug Interactions

HERBAL/ SUPPLEMENT	USE	DRUG	INTERACTION
Garlic	Elevated cholesterol, hypertension	ASA, anticoagulants	Prolonged blood clotting time
Ginkgo biloba	Vertigo, tinnitus, dementia	ASA, NSAIDs, anticoagulants	Increased risk of bleeding
Ginseng	Lethargy	Warfarin	Decreased INR
Ma Huang	Asthma, obesity	CNS stimulants	Increased herbal effect
St. John's wort	Depression	Amitriptyline, cyclosporin, digoxin, indinavir	Decreased effectiveness owing to reduced serum drug concentrations
		Paroxetine, sertraline	Additive serotonin effects
Valerian	Anxiety, insomnia	CNS depressants	Increased CNS depression

ASA, acetylsalicylic acid; NSAIDs, nonsteroidal antiinflammatory drugs; INR, international normalized ratio; CNS, central nervous system.

10. Is massage therapy efficacious, or does it just feel good?

For patients with chronic low back pain, the answer is yes to both. In a randomized trial of 262 patients, massage was superior to acupuncture and self-care/education at 10 weeks. At 52 weeks, massage remained superior to acupuncture and was the least expensive of the three in total costs of medical care.

11. How does acupuncture work?

According to Chinese philosophy, Qi is the life force. The basis of acupuncture lies in the assumption that Qi courses through channels in the body known as *meridians*. The acupuncture points represent *gates* where the channels come closest to the surface. Acupuncture is the practice of influencing the flow of Qi by stimulating these points. Most studies evaluating clinical outcomes are with the use of needling. The insertion of thin, stainless steel needles into these points establishes communication between the outer and inner body, correcting the flow of Qi and enhancing healing.

12. For what clinical conditions might acupuncture be considered useful?

The NIH Consensus Panel on Acupuncture cited clear evidence that acupuncture can treat effectively postoperative and chemotherapy-induced nausea and vomiting, hyperemesis gravidarum, and pain from dental procedures. This committee also concluded that acupuncture may be a useful adjunctive therapy for addictions, stroke rehabilitation, headache, menstrual cramps, fibromyalgia, low back pain, carpal tunnel syndrome, and asthma.

13. What is homeopathy?

The principle of "like cures like" is the basis of homeopathy. This theory originated with Hippocrates in the 4th century BC and was rediscovered by Hahnemann in 1790. Hahnemann spent much of his life extensively testing many common herbal and medicinal substances to determine what symptoms they might cause in healthy individuals. He began treating sick people with the medicine that most closely matched the symptoms of their illness. He discovered that the solutions became more effective with fewer side effects by serial dilutions in a water/alcohol solution. Gold and nitroglycerin are two homeopathic remedies used by conventional allopathic medicine.

14. Is homeopathy effective?

It depends on whom you ask. Homeopathic practitioners claim that the diluted substances work on the body's energy field, catalyzing natural healing responses; critics argue that homeopathic remedies are nothing but placebos. Some homeopathic remedies are so dilute that no single molecule of the original medicine theoretically can be found. According to a metaanalysis, there is some evidence that homeopathic treatments are more effective than placebo; however, the strength of the evidence is low because of the low methodologic quality of the trials.

15. What might CAM offer my patient or me?

For the true emergency, CAM probably has little to offer. Pneumonia resulting in respiratory distress requires intubation and antibiotics, not acupuncture and echinacea. True emergencies are only 20% to 30% of emergency practice, however. Emergency physicians evaluate many illnesses that traditional Western medicine has little to offer (low back pain, irritable bowel syndrome, migraine headache). CAM may increase the treatment modalities offered to these patients and provide additional referral sources at discharge. Consider suggesting echinacea for a patient with a viral upper respiratory infection instead of antibiotics. A patient with low back pain concerned about narcotic dependence may benefit from massage therapy or acupuncture. An open-minded approach regarding CAM may enhance your relationship with your patient.

16. What is my liability?

Some physicians do not inquire about the use of CAM for fear of being *at risk*; if they know about it, they may be deemed to endorse it. Others may be hesitant to refer patients to a CAM practitioner for fear of being sued in the case of a poor outcome. According to one study, you need not be overly concerned about the malpractice liability implications. Claims against CAM practitioners occur much less frequently and generally involve less severe injuries than claims against physicians. When referring a patient to a CAM practitioner, the same principles apply as in traditional allopathic medicine. Is there evidence in the medical literature to suggest that the patient may benefit from this treatment without unnecessary risk? Is this practitioner licensed in my state? The important issue is to open a professional dialogue between physicians and CAM practitioners to improve patient care.

17. Is there evidence in the medical literature to support CAM therapies?

Yes. The NIH created the Office of Alternative Medicine in 1992 with a $2 million budget. This was upgraded to the NCCAM in 1998. In fiscal year 2000, the NCCAM awarded $68 million to CAM researchers. The NIH is committed to investigating the utility of these therapies and exploring the integration of CAM and traditional allopathic medicine. There are randomized, double-blind, placebo-controlled trials published in the CAM arena. Some show benefit.

18. Which of these studies show benefit?

An extract of *Ginkgo biloba* (Egb) was used in a 52-week, randomized, double-blind, placebo-controlled, parallel-group multicenter study to assess efficacy and safety in the treatment of Alzheimer disease and multiinfarct dementia. It was concluded that Egb was capable of stabilizing and improving cognitive performance and social functioning of these patients.

A randomized, double-blind, placebo-controlled trial of 116 patients compared a Chinese herbal preparation with placebo in the treatment of irritable bowel syndrome. Patients receiving the Chinese herbal medicine had significant improvement in bowel symptom scores as rated by patients ($P = 0.03$) and by gastroenterologists ($P = 0.001$) and significant global improvement as rated by patients ($P = 0.007$) and gastroenterologists ($P = 0.002$).

A systematic quality assessment and metaanalysis was done of the clinical trials of glucosamine and chondroitin for the treatment the osteoarthritis. This therapy was determined to be effective, but quality issues and publication bias were believed to exaggerate these effects.

CONTROVERSY

This entire chapter is controversial. Need I say more?

BIBLIOGRAPHY

1. Benhousaan A, Talley NJ, Hing M: Treatment of irritable bowel syndrome with Chinese herbal medicine. JAMA 280:1585–1589, 1998.
2. Boullata JI, Nace AM: Safety issues with herbal medicine. Pharmacotherapy 20:257–269, 2000.
3. Cherkin DC, Eisenberg DM, Sherman KJ, et al: Randomized trial comparing traditional Chinese medical acupuncture, therapeutic massage, and self-care education for chronic low back pain. Arch Intern Med 161:1081–1088, 2001.
4. Cucherat M, Haugh MC, Gooch M, et al: Evidence of clinical efficacy of homeopathy: A meta-analysis of clinical trials. Eur J Clin Pharmacol 56:27–33, 2000.
5. Eisenberg DM, Davis RB, Ettner SL, et al: Trends in alternative medicine use in the United States, 1990–1997. JAMA 280:1569–1575, 1998.
6. Gulla J, Singer AJ: Use of alternative therapies among emergency department patients. Ann Emerg Med 35:226–228, 2000.
7. Klepser TB, Klepser ME: Unsafe and potentially safe herbal therapies. Am J Health Syst Pharm 56:125–138, 1999.
8. Le Bars PL, Katz MM, Berman N, et al: A placebo-controlled, double-blind, randomized trial of an extract of ginkgo biloba for dementia. JAMA 278:1327–1332, 1997.
9. McAlindon TE, LaValley MP, Gulin JP, et al: Glucosamine and chondroitin for treatment of osteoarthritis: A systematic quality assessment and meta-analysis. JAMA 283:1469–1475, 2000.
10. NIH consensus conference: Acupuncture. JAMA 280:1518–1524, 1998.
11. Studdert DM, Eisenberg DM, Miller FH, et al: Medical malpractice implications of alternative medicine. JAMA 280:1610–1615, 1998.
12. Weiss SJ, Takakuwa KM, Ernst AA: Use, understanding and beliefs about complementary and alternative medicine among emergency department patients. Acad Emerg Med 8:41–47, 2001.

131. TRICKS OF THE TRADE

Fred A. Severyn, M.D.

1. Why include a "tricks of the trade" chapter?

To have a chapter in which to associate freely and discuss various approaches to the *practice* of emergency medicine. In this way, we can learn some secrets in error reduction in emergency medicine and some procedural tips to practice safer, more effective emergency medicine.

2. As a good clinician, I never make a mistake (yeah, right). Why is error reduction important to me?

The truly gifted clinician recognizes his or her naiveté daily. The more you read, the more you learn and realize what you don't know. Overconfidence can result in careless workups, careless care, and poor patient outcome.

3. As an emergency medicine practitioner, what general steps can I follow to prevent errors?

The list is long; we can share, however, some basic secrets to providing careful, safe emergency care.

1. Read the nursing notes. You have the choice to read them now, concurrently, or later, at time of deposition. The nurses are truly your safety net and friends.

2. Vital signs are just that—vital to the longevity of the patient and your career. Look at them, critically interpret them, and formulate definitive answers to explain abnormalities.

3. A careful history and physical examination is essential and can lead you to a correct diagnosis in most patients. Confirmatory tests help to verify your suspicions, but *shotgun* testing is ineffective and costly.

4. Chart what you do and see, the pertinent positives and negatives. Common documentation of *WNL* (within normal limits) is just asking for trouble and is often interpreted as "we never looked."

5. Common things are common, but often the common disease has atypical presentations. So your diagnosis must match your patient. The diagnosis of gastroenteritis without vomiting or diarrhea is best left unsaid.

6. A major distinction between emergency medicine practice and that of other medical specialties is the lack of prior physician-patient relationship and of subsequent patient follow-up. Often the patient is seen at one point in the disease spectrum, and the disease process does not declare itself until a later time. Discharge instructions should be clear and explicit and contain some type of patient follow-up or return instructions.

4. I've noticed that there are a lot of *clinical rules* popping up, and I have a hard time remembering them. How do these fit in my practice of emergency medicine?

These rules are guidelines that are meant to give the clinician a suggested approach to a specific problem (usually a specific symptom) and consensus viewpoint on how best to approach this complaint or symptom. The clinician must balance clinical science, cost-effectiveness, local practice resources, and his or her risk management style in using clinical rules. The clinician may deviate from these guidelines if in his or her clinical judgment it is appropriate to do so.

5. Give an example of a clinical rule.

An example is a rule on deciding whether or not to order a cranial CT scan in the minor head injury patient, with a normal Glasgow Coma Scale score of 14 or 15. More recent literature shows that this patient population harbors an approximately 6% to 9% rate of intracranial pathology. Only about 0.5% needed neurosurgical intervention to alter their care, however. Cutting back on just 10% of cranial CT scan orders could save the U.S. health care system an estimated $20 million per year. Other clinical rules include ankle and knee radiographs, chest pain management, and the ordering of cervical spine films. Be cautious on whose rule you may be following because you may be following biased recommendations. Often studies give recommendations that support the side of a sponsored pharmaceutical or product, with its accompanying bias. As a clinician in any field of medicine, you must learn to read the literature critically, often between the lines, and formulate your own opinions.

6. I can never get an adequate cross-table lateral film on my trauma patient. How can I limit my frustration, added cost, and radiation exposure to my patient?

Give an adequate pull! But this comes with caveats as to how to improve visualization. A slow, gradual pull limits the "pullback reaction" of the patient with a fast motion. Talk to the patient, and have him or her relax (if possible) and try to touch their toes gently without lifting up their heads. Simple, gradual traction with internal rotation of the patient's arms during this process eliminates almost all muscle resistance, improving your efficiency of obtaining an adequate cross-table lateral film. In addition to getting a better film, make sure that you look into all four corners of the film and at areas that are not your prime interest. Look for air-fluid levels in the sphenoid, maxillary, and mastoid air spaces, and look for occult pneumothorax on anteroposterior neck films.

7. How can I improve my intubation skills?

Practice. Intubation requires not only the laryngoscopist, but also someone to hold cricoid pressure (Sellick's maneuver) after induction and paralysis. The BURP (backward, upward, rightward pressure) maneuver can be helpful during difficult laryngoscopy, and the assistant's guiding can bring the cords into view, rather than the laryngoscopist forcing a way to the cords. Finesse, not force, wins here.

8. Often with the proper assistance, I can see the cords but cannot pass the endotracheal tube itself. Any tips?

Try some type of stylet, to finesse not force the tube into proper position. Flexible gum elastic bougies have been developed to place through the vocal cords similar to the guidewire in central line placement, and a tube is positioned in place over this stylet through the cords. If you do not have such an introducer, try using the lidocaine jet apparatus originally described for topical anesthesia of the cords and the trachea beyond them. First, place this through the Murphy's eye of the endotracheal tube, and visualize the cords using direct laryngoscopy. Pass the lidocaine jet tubing through the cords, and follow this by wiggling the endotracheal tube over this stylet into proper position.

9. What if I fail with standard intubation techniques? Any suggestions on surgical airway placement?

First, find the proper landmarks for the procedure. Make a vertical incision over the cricothyroid membrane, and digitally palpate the tissues for the cricothyroid membrane again. Pop through the membrane with your scalpel, and place your finger into the incision. This prevents you from getting sprayed with bloody secretions and helps prevent you from losing your tract to the airway itself. Advise the person bagging to hold off a second when you do place the tube. The tract is now dilated to the size of your finger and should accept the airway tube itself. If you are worried about losing the tract when you remove your finger, you can use a long nasal speculum placed into the trachea to keep the tract open while placing the airway itself. Often one uses a tracheal hook from the operating room to immobilize and isolate the airway itself. A quick trick as a substitute is to use a towel clamp, easily found in most surgical trays in the ED. Use one arm of the towel clamp to immobilize the airway, and you will not lose the hole when placing your tube.

10. Central line placement in the nonarrested patient via internal jugular route often gives me problems. Any tips?

Depending on your route (anterior, central, posterior), you can use carotid palpation to define a medial boundary structure so as not to hit with your needle. I often go back to my physical examination, using visual clues to guide my needle placement. Look carefully at the neck and visualize the internal jugular venous pulsations with indirect light, just lateral to where you palpated the carotid artery. In most patients, you can see this venous pulsation and hit it with your seeker needle. Use the anesthesia needle itself as a finder needle to access the internal jugular, then slowly remove the needle from the skin in the same plane in which it was inserted, dropping off a few drops of blood in a straight line to show where to insert the larger vascular access needle. Another tip, especially in the hypovolemic patient, is not to press too hard with your nondominant fingers while palpating the carotid. Often this pressure can obliterate the lumen of the internal jugular vessel effectively so that your needle passes completely through both walls of the vessel without any blood being aspirated. The best way to show yourself how little pressure is required for lumen obliteration is to put an ultrasound probe on a model's neck, and simply show yourself how little transducer pressure occludes the lumen. Simple finger compression by the ultrasound technician in venous vascular studies compresses normal vessels, and your fingers do the same when doing procedures.

11. After successful intubation, I often cannot place a nasogastric tube, as I instead follow the endotracheal tube into the lower airway. Any suggestions?

Often just simple airway manipulation of the larynx itself to lift the larynx off the esophageal inlet allows successful nasogastric tube passage. Difficult placement may require finger manipulation of the tube posteriorly into the esophagus. Use your fingers, much like digital intubation of the trachea, to guide the nasogastric tube posteriorly and down into the esophagus. If these maneuvers are unsuccessful, try transient deflation of the endotracheal tube cuff during the nasogastric tube insertion.

12. Feeding tube replacement in patients from nursing care facilities often ties up the clinician's time. How can I make this process easier?

Often the problem with G-tube replacement is compounded by a time delay between evaluation and event. In this time, the tract may close down, making it more difficult to replace. Gentle dilation of a stenosed tract is the key here; be it with gentle pressure from a hemostat, gentle dilation using otoscope speculum heads, or the use of percutaneous tracheostomy dilators over a guidewire placed into the gastrointestinal tract lumen. Don't get frustrated in attempts to replace it quickly because this may lead to complications such as bleeding and perforation.

Many of these patients present with a tube in place but clogged. Often forceful irrigation is attempted, creating a mess as fluids spray about. The clogging material is often thick like toothpaste. The clinician can lubricate his or her gloved fingers and milk the material out, starting at the distal end and moving proximally to the patient. This may clear enough obstruction so that irrigation is possible. You may need the assistance of a flexible guidewire to help break up the more proximal concretions. But be aware that the standard guidewire found in most central line kits is not of sufficient length to clear the tube, and the last thing you want to do is lose a guidewire in the intestinal tract. You also do not want to use a stiff guidewire that could perforate the soft lumen of the feeding tube and damage anatomic structures. Replacement with a simple Foley catheter may serve better as a temporizing measure, with preplacement of the catheter through a plastic buttress before its placement. This allows you to fix the feeding tube up against the anterior wall of the stomach and prevent its possible migration intraluminally to cause a possible bowel obstruction.

13. Any tricks to the identification, location, and removal of foreign bodies?

With any laceration, clinicians typically explore the wound and look for objects with their eyes. This ideally requires a bloodless field, so as not to obscure vision. It also requires extreme luck because objects typically align along anatomic structures and may be hiding in the wound depths. Instead of using just visual clues (and looking right through the glass fragment), gently feel with a hemostat or probe in the wound depths; grittiness may be noted. Often a cotton applicator is used to probe the wound tract and results in residual cotton or Dacron fibers, which serve as a nidus for infection. In probing a wound tract, a pearl is to use the wooden or plastic end of a cotton swab, to prevent leaving parts behind.

Another trick is to use radiography to detect glass or metal. Either conventional films or fluoroscopy can be used to assist with your search and removal mission. Set an opened paper clip over the entry site, open the clip into a triangle shape, and trace on the skin with an indelible marker. This way you get a quick three-dimensional view of where the object may lie, using the double-pronged base of the opened paper clip as a landmark. The marking helps preserve landmarks on patient return from radiography because more often than not someone will remove the taped paper clip on patient return. But be forewarned, set time limits for your mission: It's amazing the amount of time that we spend looking for some small object that we know is in the tissues but we can't find. Set a time limit beforehand, using the "needle in a haystack" analogy to the patient. That way appropriate referral in the operating room is understood by the patient if you fail to retrieve the object.

If the object is in the ear canal, you can use a metal operating otic speculum to direct light into the ear canal itself. Then it is a relatively simple task of using a hemostat or preferentially an alligator forceps to remove the object. Many clinicians attempt removal through the standard otoscope head, with minimal results.

Nasal foreign objects can be difficult to remove in the squirming child. Two procedural tips are particularly helpful. First, you can use positive-pressure ventilation through an Ambu-bag over the child's mouth or the parent's mouth to blow a puff of air into the child's mouth. Either approach effectively forces air out the nostrils and occasionally blows the child's nose with the object in the secretions. Another slick trick is to place a Ward catheter into the affected nostril with some lubrication to pass gently beyond the object in the nasal passage. Gently inflate the balloon of the Ward catheter, and pull steady traction to remove the object. The catheter's shorter length does not stimulate the hypopharynx as does a Foley or Fogarty catheter and is readily accessible in the ED.

14. On my possible meningitis or subarachnoid hemorrhage patients, I sometimes get a traumatic spinal tap. How can I prevent or limit this?

Any time you pass through a vascular structure and remove your stylet, blood will tract toward the needle hub. Typically, if no cerebrospinal fluid (CSF) returns, you should replace the stylet, and advance the needle until you pop into the subarachnoid space. CSF returns, but it is sometimes blood tinged with red blood cell contamination. Unless the blood is mixed into the CSF itself (subarachnoid hemorrhage), it comes from the needle itself. Classic teaching is to let the CSF flow until time and volume clear the CSF. Simple turning of the needle 180° often allows gravity to eliminate most of the remaining blood. You also can insert the sterile pointed end of a 2 × 2 gauze into the needle hub to remove the last remains of the blood meniscus layer, eliminating the constant contamination that adds red blood cells to the CSF. This gauze must be sterile and not coated with iodine, or you will introduce contamination to the subarachnoid space. You will be amazed at how quickly this simple technique clears the CSF.

15. Any tricks on doing a digital nerve block in a 4-year-old?

You can use an ice cube over the needle entry site for 60 seconds; children usually tolerate the sensation of cold well. Then enter the chilled skin immediately after removing the ice because often the continued perception of cold masks the pain of a needle stick.

16. How about creating a bloodless field for wound exploration of the fingers?

Many clinicians use Penrose drains or rubber bands applied at the finger base as a tourniquet to achieve hemostasis and a bloodless field. After injection of anesthetic solution, using a nonsterile latex glove is invaluable in repair. Place all digits of the patient's affected hand into the glove, then cut just a small hole at the distal end of the affected finger. By rolling the glove tip (not just pushing it down) toward the metacarpophalangeal joint, one effectively exsanguinates all blood, arterial and venous, out of the finger, and the rolled-up latex glove now acts as a tourniquet of the digital vessels at the level of the metacarpophalangeal joint. Now you can explore the laceration adequately for foreign objects and tendon injuries and treat accordingly. This works especially well on vascular nail bed repairs that usually otherwise tend to ooze and obstruct the repair.

BIBLIOGRAPHY

1. Haydel M, Preston C, Mills T, et al: Indications for computerized tomography in patients with minor head injury. N Engl J Med 343:100–105, 2000.
2. Kidd JF, Dyson A, Latto IP: Successful difficult intubation: Use of the gum elastic bougie. Anaesthesia 43:437–438, 1988.
3. Knill RL: Difficult laryngoscopy made easy with a "BURP." Can J Anaesth 40:279–282, 1993.
4. McCarroll SM, Lamont BJ, Buckland MR, et al: The gum elastic bougie: Old but still useful [letter]. Anesthesiology 68:643–644, 1988.
5. Morrison WG: Transthecal digital block. Arch Emerg Med 10:35–38, 1993.
6. Relle A: Difficult laryngoscopy-'BURP'[letter]. Can J Anaesth 40:798–799, 1993.
7. Sarhadi NS, Shaw-Dunn J: Transthecal digital block: An anatomic appraisal. J Hand Surg Br 23:490-493, 1998.
8. Stiell I, Wells G, Vandemheem K, et al: The Canadian CT head rule for patients with minor head injury. Lancet 357:1391–1396, 2001.
9. Takahata O, Kubota M, Mamiya K, et al: The efficacy of the 'BURP' maneuver during a difficult laryngoscopy. Anesth Analg 84:419–421, 1997.

INDEX

Page numbers in **boldface type** indicate complete chapters.